UNLOCK THE HEALING POWER OF NATURE

DISCOVER THE WORLD OF MEDICINAL PLANTS

VOL.1

DR. WATHEK ZAIR
DR. INDRE HOWARD

Table of Contents

Introduction

Traditional and modern medicine rely on the vital presence of medicinal plants, which form the bedrock of healthcare in many cultures worldwide. The significance of these plants cannot be understated. More than half of the world's inhabitants rely primarily on plants for their healthcare, and medicinal plants are the mainstay of traditional medicine across Asia and Africa and in many cultures in the Americas and Pacific Islands. Numerous studies have demonstrated the efficacy of medicinal plants. The World Health Organization has reported that an estimated 80% of the populations in developing countries use traditional medicine for their primary healthcare needs. The medicinal plant trade is valued at several billion dollars annually and is growing apace.

For instance, tropical rainforests are home to many medicinal species like Andrographis paniculata (noted for its anti-inflammatory properties). Even botanists marvel at the marvels and manifold miracles of rainforests. Who wouldn't? Deserts—temperate rainforests, too, for that matter—are right up there with the tropical rainforest concerning the dizzying array of life forms they hold. And in all of this proverbial sea of plants, some are what herbalists call "the good stuff."

Medicinal plants have been employed since ancient times and are still used extensively around the world. They formed the basis of medical treatments for millennia, until the discovery of synthetic drugs. The compositions and effects of herbs and spices have been known for thousands of years and have been documented by ancient civilizations. Until today, the knowledge passed down through oral and written traditions has made natural medicine an important part of the healthcare system in many countries. In plants, "the key to the Drug problem" – which is what the great British chemist William Henry Perkin called medicinal plants – is something that most people and even health professionals have probably forgotten.

About a quarter of modern medicines come from plants, and a good many originate from the compounds of those plants. Take aspirin, for instance. The compound at the heart of the analgesic and anti-inflammatory properties of aspirin derives from willow bark (Salix spp.) that has been used for millennia to "make one's tongue feel strange" as the ancient Roman Pliny the Elder put it, or in other words, for its numbing effect, which is offered by both aspirin and its close relative, salicylic acid. Another example: the poppy plant from which morphine is derived has been cultivated for millennia, yet only in the past 200 years have we really harnessed its power in a way that allows us to better understand it as a potent pain reliever. And the work goes on.

Medically significant plants are important to the survival of biodiversity, and yet they are threatened by unsustainable collection practices, habitat loss, and population growth that exert too much pressure on the ecosystem. The collection of medicinal plants often is not governed by guidelines that ensure the viability of populations living in their natural habitats. In a century when the potential for catastrophic climate change threatens the survival of ecological niches and the plant populations that inhabit them, it is madness not to have in place a network of plants that can offer viable, inexpensive, and nonsynthetic alternatives to pharmacological approaches that already have proven harmful in many cases.

What lies ahead for medicinal plants is the combination of time-honored knowledge with contemporary scientific investigation. That marriage could produce something quite extraordinary: a treasure trove of new drugs. It could help us grasp the intricacies of therapies long since touted as beneficial. And it might even serve as a dependable blueprint for understanding how to mind the sustainable resource that is medicinal plants. ... Yet, plants are more than pretty vessels for holding tea. They are the future of a class of natural products that may save our lives.

Moreover, encouraging cooperation between researchers, conservationists, and indigenous communities can help promote the sustainable use of the wealth of plants long revered for their medicinal properties. These collaborations are conservation in action—and essential to Usher & Medical's mission of ensuring that knowledge continues to serve all of humanity. "It's all about making sure that the next generation has access to the wealth of knowledge that is passed down through medicinal plants," explains Shannon Wei, an anthropologist at Usher & Medical who is studying the habitats of medicinal plants.

Chapter One: Plant Families and Species

Acanthus mollis L.

Acanthus hispanicus hort. ex Loudon., *Acanthus latifolius* hort. ex Goeze. , *Acanthus longifolius* Poir., *Acanthus lusitanicus* auct., *Acanthus niger* Mill., *Acanthus platyphyllus* Murb., *Acanthus spinosissimus* Host.

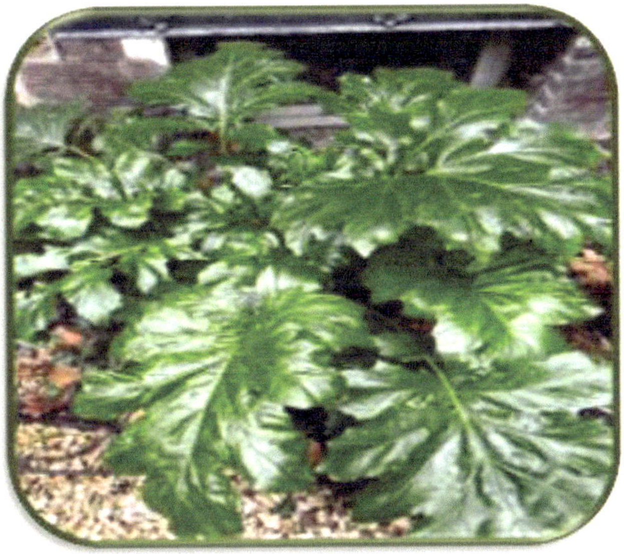

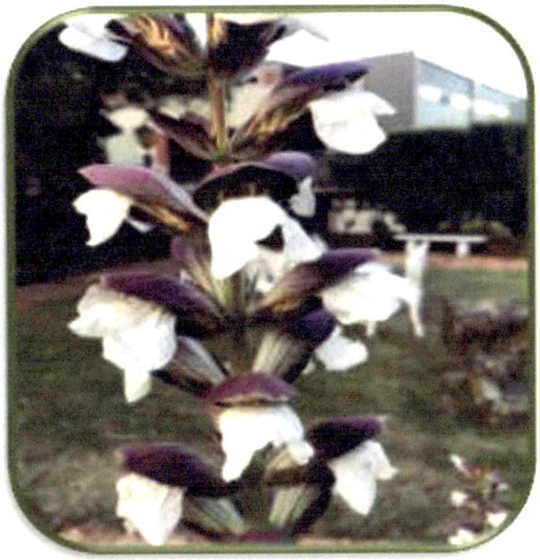

Family: Acanthaceae.

Common names: Frog, Acanthus slack, Bear's foot, Jew's thorn.

Foreign names: Eng. Acanthus, Bear's Breeches, Fr. Acanthe molle

Occurrences : 23,477occurrences

Distribution in the world

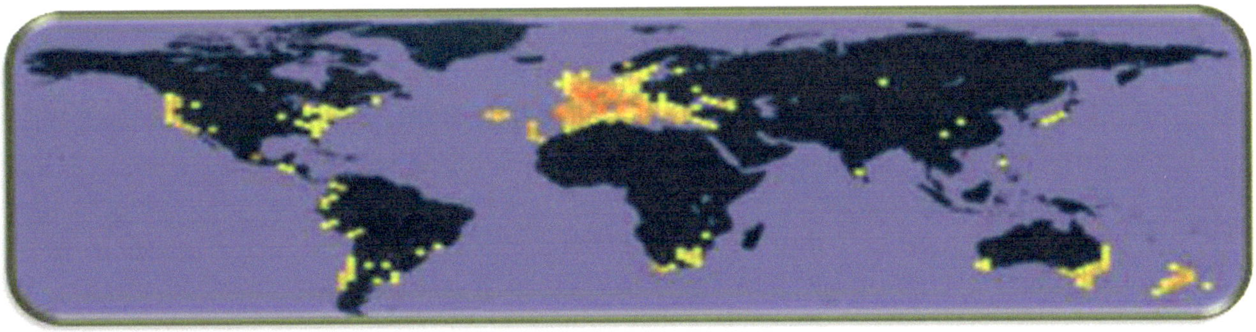

Botanical description:

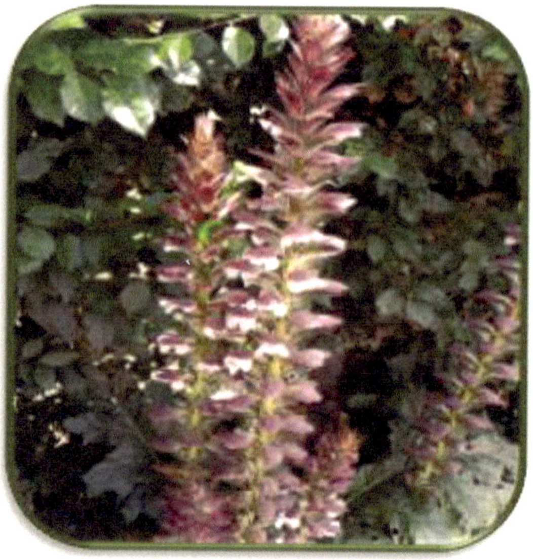

A perennial herb, 30-80 cm tall (can reach 150 cm including the length of the inflorescence.) The leaves are basal, long-stalked, very large, their length with the stalk can approach 1 m, dark green and shiny, soft to the touch, not thorny, and divided into oblong-sinusoidal lobes - serrated on the edge. The inflorescence is a terminal spike, 30-60 cm long. Each flower is surrounded by a large, thorny, serrated bract, slightly shorter than the calyx, and two smaller bracts, linear to lanceolate. Flowers are white, tinged with purple, sessile, 5-6 cm long. The calyx is composed of 4 unequal sepals, the upper and lower sepals are broad and oblong, protecting nerves, the first ending in three teeth, the second in two teeth tinged with purple, the upper sepal forming a helmet-like shape above the corolla; The lateral sepals are short, rounded or inverted oval. The corolla segments are united in a short tube that soon splits to form a single wide lip, ending in three lobes. Male: 4 unequal stamens (two long stamens and two short stamens), anther covered with dense hairs, shaped like a toothbrush. Female: bicarpel, ovary superior bichambered, each chamber containing two ovules. The fruit is a capsule, oval in shape, smooth, leathery in texture, opens stolonically, contains 2-4 large seeds, black when ripe.

Flowering: from late spring to early summer.

Habitat and geographical distribution:

It is widespread in the Mediterranean basin, especially in the northern part of it, rare in its natural state. Among its species is also the Syrian Acanthus syriacus A., and it is distinguished between them through the texture and shape of the leaf, its homeland is the eastern Mediterranean, and it has ornamental value.

History and Heritage:

The scientific name of the genus is the ancient Greek name for this species, which is derived from the Greek word "akanthos" which is derived from "akantha" meaning "thorn" in reference to the thorny bracts, while the species name "mollis" means "soft or tender." The harmonious shape with elegant division of the plant's leaves was a source of inspiration for artistic ideas embodied in the manufacture of metals and the art of architecture by the Greeks, and this shape inspired the Greek sculptor Callimachus to decorate the capital of the Corinthian column known in the art of architecture. The plant has been known since ancient times, and the leaves of this plant have been seen throughout history in sculptures, columns and furniture, and it is believed that the acanthus is the plant mentioned in the Holy Book.

Part used: Flowers, leaves, and roots.

Chemical components:

Mucilage or salivary substances, tannins, pectins, sugars, the most important of which is glucose.

Medical properties and uses:

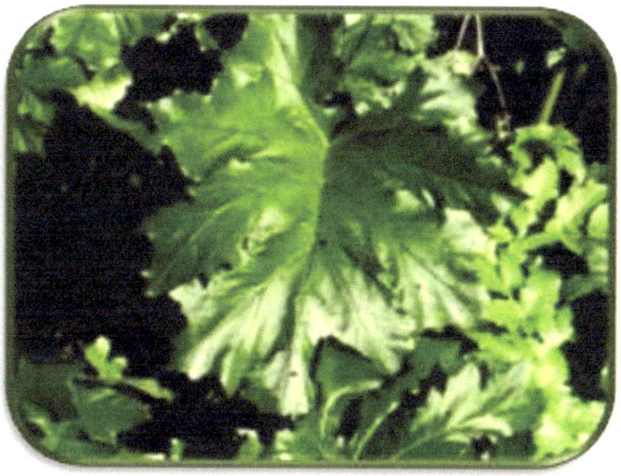

Diuretic, laxative, decoction of its leaves and flowers is useful in treating bronchitis and cystitis. Studies have proven the benefits of the mucilage and tannins found in the leaves and roots of the plant in treating wounds, burns, skin infections and arthritis (compresses). Decoction of the flowers is used as an appetite stimulant and a stimulant for bile secretion. It is similar in its components and uses to the species syriaca A.

The Greek physician Dioscorides, in the first century AD, recommended using the roots to prepare medical plasters to treat burns, and compresses to treat joint pain. Its infusion was used as a diuretic, carminative, antispasmodic, and to calm the nerves. The gum and tannin present in the plant allow it to be used externally to relieve skin irritation and redness. A decoction of the leaves is useful in calming the abdomen and improving blood flow.

The decoction of the leaves was used to heal broken bones and strengthen joints. The properties of the rain plant are useful in treating irritation of the mucous membranes of the digestive system and urinary tract. It is used in folk medicine in Africa for urinary and reproductive system infections.

Environment:

It grows in forests, rocky hillsides and sunny garden edges. The plant prefers to grow in deep loamy soils in wind-protected and sunny places, and can tolerate partial shade. The plant grows well in heavy clay soils if they are well drained, but it does not like heavy, waterlogged soils. The mature plant tolerates drought and temperatures down to -15°C, but young plants are sensitive to frost. The leaves may wilt on hot summer days when the plant is in direct sunlight. The plant may become invasive and difficult to get rid of due to its deep roots.

Cultivation and productivity:

The plant is propagated by seeds in spring in a cold greenhouse or directly in permanent soil as soon as it is ripe. The seeds germinate within 3-4 weeks at 10°C. The seedlings are transferred to permanent soil after the appearance of true leaves, and the plant is about 7-8 cm long, planting is done at a distance of 90 cm. The plant can also be easily propagated by dividing it in the fall, in which case the plants are planted directly in permanent soil. The plant can also be propagated by root cuttings. The plant is collected in the fall.

Blepharis ciliaris (L.) B.L. Burtt.

Ruellia ciliaris L.*, B. edulis* (Forssk.) Pers.*, B. persica* (Burm. fil.) O. Kuntze., *Acanthus pecti- natus* Willd. ex Nees.*, Ruellia persica* Burm.f., *Acanthus tetragonus* R.Br., *Acanthus edulis* Forssk.

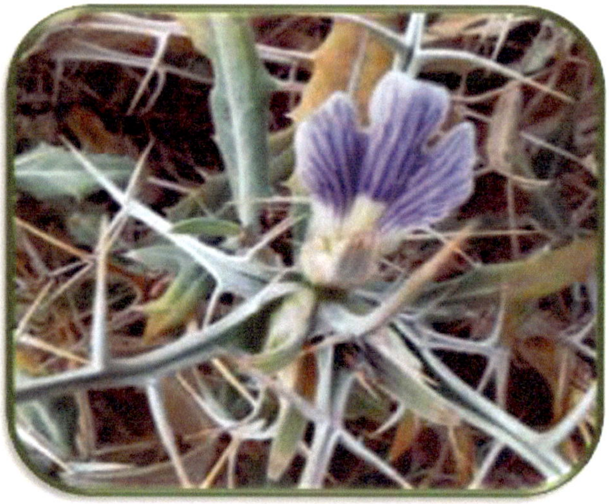

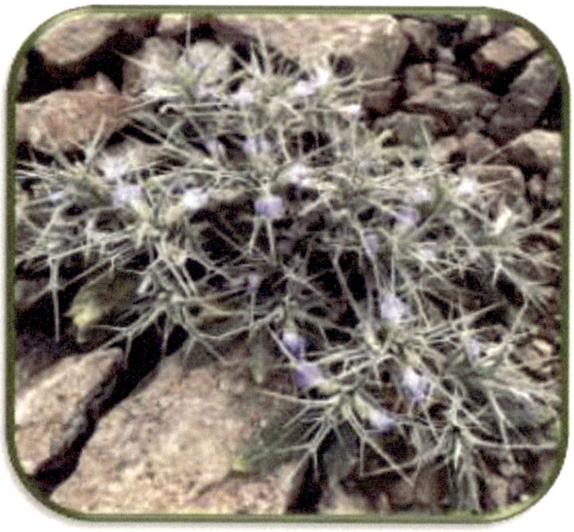

Family: Acanthaceae

Common names: Kanab, Wolf's thorn, Za'af al-Naqi', Lizard's thorn, Old Woman's kohl, Nagi

Foreign names: Ruellia Fr. Tree, Rohida .Eng

Occurrences : 1,720 occurrences

Distribution in the world

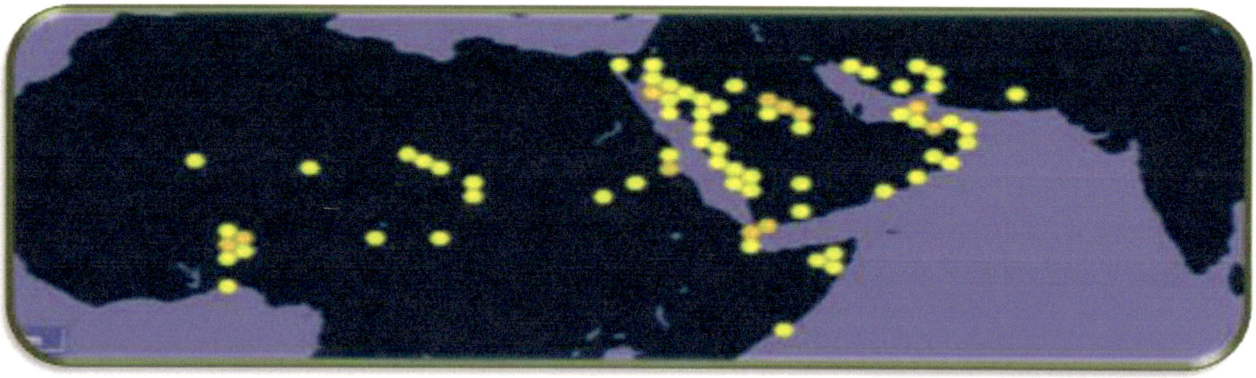

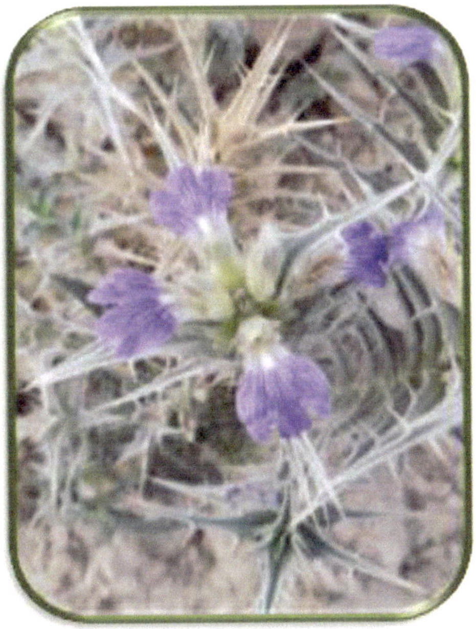

Botanical description:

Perennial herb, 20-40 cm tall, covered with short gray hairs, or almost hairless, branched abundantly from the base. Stem is solid. Stem leaves are oblong to lanceolate, gradually tapering to form a spike, about 1 cm long, entire margin or bearing small spines, dimensions 2-8.0 x 6-2 cm, appearing arranged in whorls of 4 leaves, falling quickly. Flowers are gathered in dense spikes. The flower is supported by a bract and several bracts. Bract 3-5 cm, flat, bearing 5 nerves, ovate and pointed at the apex, its apex terminates in a spine, with 3-5 pairs of lateral spines whose length does not exceed the width of the bract. Bracts 1-1.5 cm. Calyx membranous, dry, hairy, persistent, composed of 4 unequal lobes. Corolla united in a very short tube, which soon splits to form a single lip, 20-28 mm long, divided into three lobes, blue to purple, bearing dark veins, turning white when withered. Male 4 stamens, thick filaments. Fruit capsule, ellipsoid, compressed, 6-7 mm long, bare, containing two seeds. The seeds are covered with a bundle of twisted hairs, which later spread out and become sticky when wet.

Flowering: May to December.

Habitat and geographical distribution:

An Arabian and Sudanese desert plant, spread in the eastern part of tropical Africa, the Arabian Peninsula, Egypt, and southern Iran, and extends to India and Pakistan in the east.

History and heritage:

It is believed that the scientific name of the plant is of Greek origin, and means "eyelashes" or "cilia."

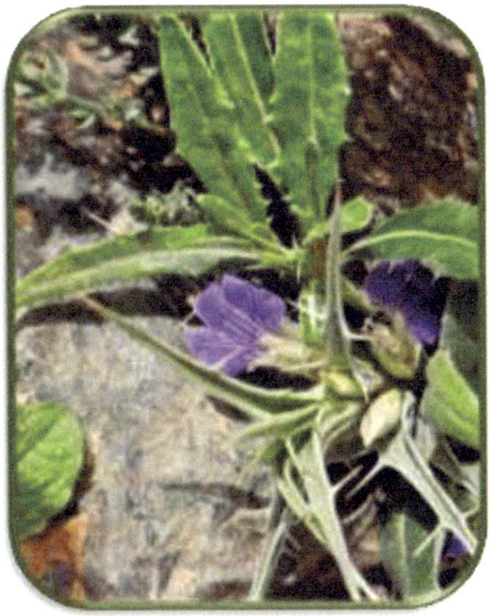

Part used: Fruits, leaves, and roots.

Chemical components: The plant contains alkaloids, phenols (naringenin, apigenin), sterols, and tannins.

Properties and medical uses:

The plant, especially the leaves, is popularly used as an aphrodisiac. The roasted seed powder paste is used for its antiseptic properties to stop bleeding, heal wounds, and treat eye infections. A decoction of the roots is used as a diuretic and to treat chronic coughs. The dried and roasted roots are ground and used as an eye ointment that is beneficial for strengthening eyesight.

Environment:

It grows in deserts, on stony and rocky soils. It is widely spread in the deserts of the Arab world, such as the Arabian Peninsula and Sinai.

Cultivation and productivity:

The plant is propagated by seeds that are collected in summer and autumn, and planted in spring.

***Sambucus ebulus* L.**

Ebulum humile)Mill.(Garcke., *Sambucus herbacea* Gilib., *Sambucus humilis* Mill., *Sambucus ebulus* subsp. *ebulus*., *Viburnum ebulus*)L.(Martinovský.

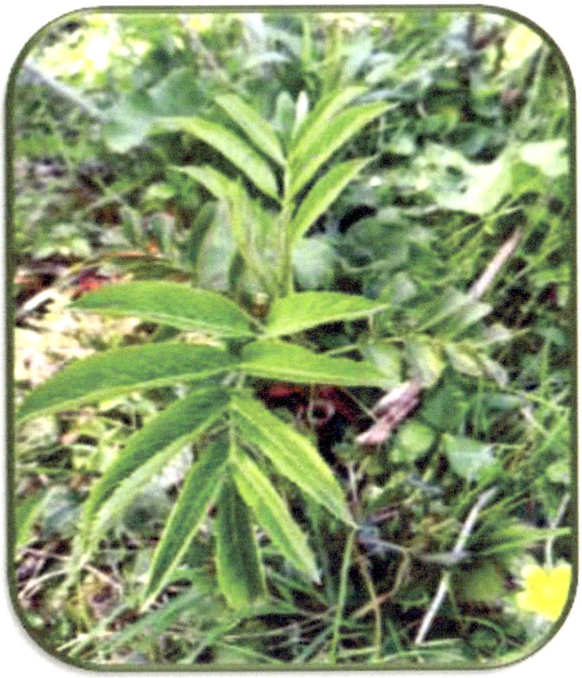
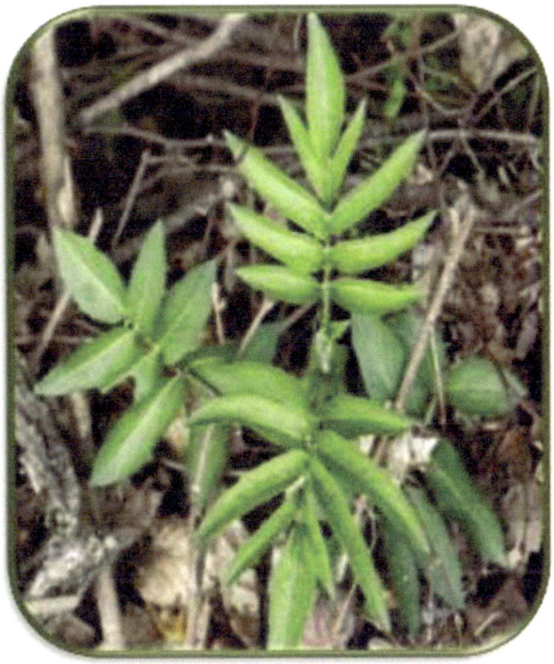

Family: Adoxaceae (formerly Caprifoliaceae)

Common names: Elder, small or dwarf elder.

Foreign names: Eng. Dwarf elder, Dwarf elderberry, Fr. Hieble

Occurrences : 141,605 occurrences

Distribution in the world

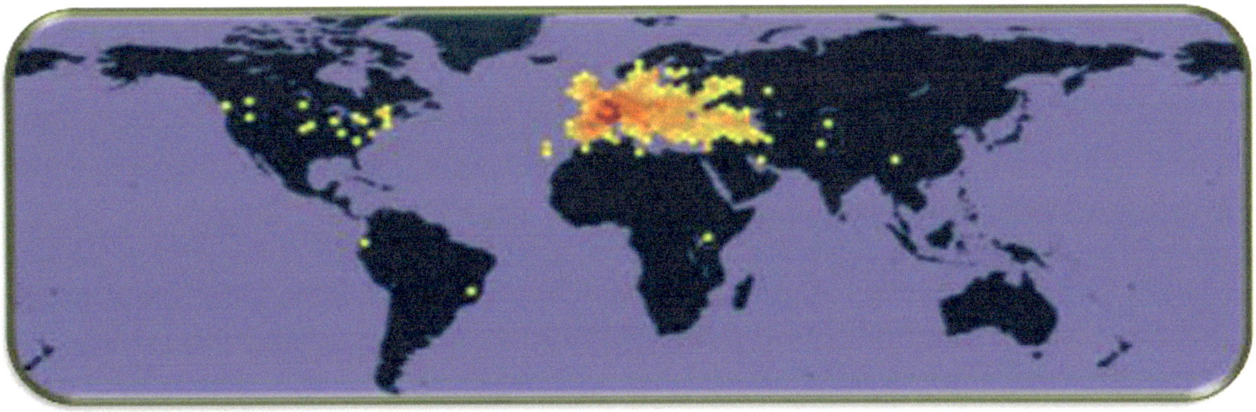

Botanical description:

A perennial plant, reaching a height of one meter or more, the branches are woody, branched, and bare, bearing compound leaves composed of 5-9 serrated leaflets, the flowers are aromatic and have a scent similar to that of bitter almonds, gathered in a large hump, the corollas are white and reddish in color, the fruit is black and reddish, filled with red juice.

Flowering: July to August

Home and geographical distribution:

Europe, southwest Asia, north Africa, the Mediterranean Basin, Iran, and is cultivated in large areas in Spain.

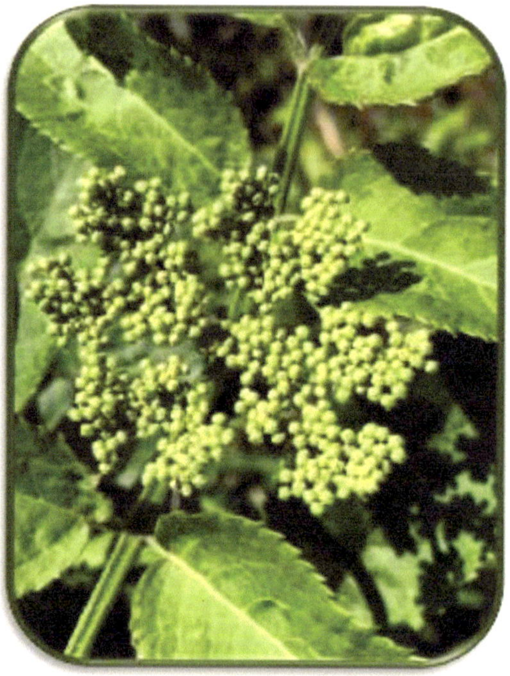

History and heritage:

The scientific name of the genus is the old Latin name of this plant. A group of traditions, customs, stories and popular sayings are associated with this plant, and it is often described as "the complete medicine cabinet", due to its many ivory and preventive properties. Known to the ancient Egyptians, it was a common medicine for removing phlegm in the seventeenth century. Nicholas Kleber wrote in 1653 that a decoction of the roots cures snake bites.

Part used: Leaves, fruits, flowers, and roots.

Chemical components:

The plant contains various phytochemicals, including flavonoids and lectins. The leaves contain volatile oil (balsam oil), bitter compounds, cyanogenic compounds, emulsin yeast, and sugars. The fruits contain volatile oil, cyanidins, sterols, cyanogenet-glycosides, some aliphatic alcohols, and unsaturated fatty acids. The green fruits also contain the free and polymerized forms of epolein. The flowers contain traces of volatile oil, cyanogenic glycosides, and sugars. The seeds contain α-linolenic, linoleic, oleic, and palmitic acids, which are essential polyunsaturated fatty acids (PUFAs). The roots contain iridoidglycoside such as ebulosid and isoswerosid, traces of volatile oil, sucrose, inositol, catechin tannins, and cyanogenic glycosides.

Properties and medical uses:

It is used in folk medicine to treat many diseases including joint pain, colds, wounds, and infections. All parts of the plant are poisonous, especially the seeds, and the fruits of this species may cause stomach disorders. The toxic substance contained in the fruits is broken down by cooking. The leaves are widely used in Turkish folk medicine in cases of inflammation, where the prepared compresses are applied externally directly to treat burns, edema, eczema and abscesses. The leaves are anti-inflammatory, diuretic, diaphoretic, expectorant and laxative. The fruits are also sometimes used, but they are less effective than the leaves. This herb is widely used to treat liver and kidney diseases, and can be used as compresses to treat edema and bruises.

The root is diaphoretic, moderately diuretic and laxative. It is dried, then crushed and taken as a tea. The leaves, flowers and bark are used for their diuretic, laxative and diaphoretic properties. All parts of the plant except the fruits are considered laxatives. The leaf extract has antibacterial properties. It is popularly used in cases of dropsy, rheumatism, chronic joint pain, colds, constipation, and as an emetic. Other uses: The fruits of the young elderberry are used in the manufacture of beverages, and a blue dye and ink are obtained from the fruits. The root liquid is also used to dye hair black.

Pharmaceutical forms: Medicinal tea.

Side effects and warnings for use:

Because it can cause nausea and dizziness. It should be used under medical supervision. It is necessary to pay attention to the toxicity of the plant because it contains epolein. Elderberry fruits should be avoided, as they may cause special toxicity (cyanide poisoning). High doses cause a drop in blood pressure, nausea and vomiting, bloody diarrhea, tinnitus, blue face, headache, loss of consciousness, and may cause death. Environment: Elderberry is widespread in temperate and cold regions of the world, and grows wild in bushy areas. It is an invasive plant, tolerates most types of soil, including calcareous, and prefers moist clay soil, and grows well in heavy clay soil. It grows in neglected lands and forests, and grows in light, medium and heavy soils, grows in moderately acidic, moderate and basic soils. It can grow in shady forests, and can tolerate strong winds but cannot tolerate sea winds, and can tolerate air pollution.

Cultivation and productivity:

The plant is propagated by seeds, by scattering them directly in the soil or by planting in the nursery, and then the seedlings are transferred to the permanent ground. It can also be propagated by root cuttings in winter, and needs irrigation in summer.

Sambucus nigra L.

Sambucus graveolens Willd., *Sambucus nigra* subsp. *nigra*., *Sambucus nigra* f. *pendula* Dippel., *Sambucus nigra* f. *luteomarmorata* Geerinck., *Sambucus laciniata* Mill.

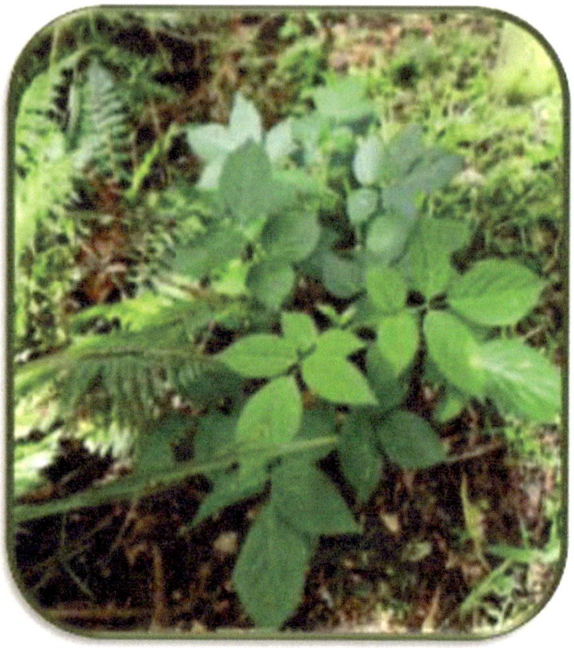

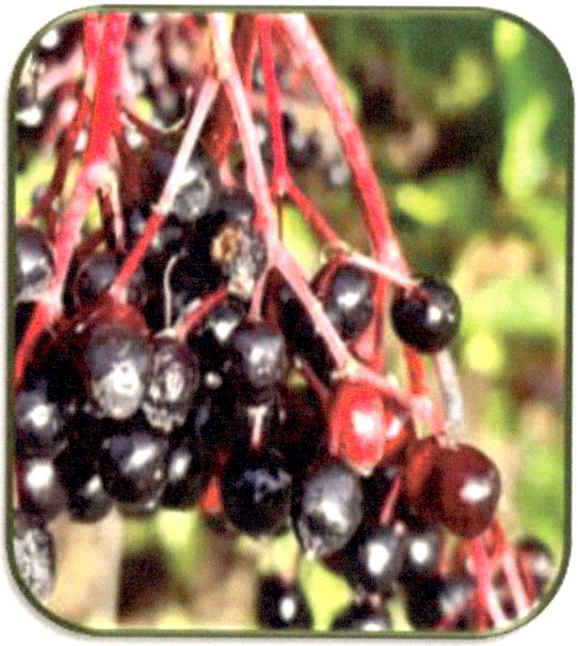

Family: Adoxaceae (formerly Caprifoliaceae)

Common names: Black elderberry, elderberry

Foreign names: Eng. Black Elder, elderberry, Fr. Sureau noir

Occurrences : 829,394 occurrences

Distribution in the world

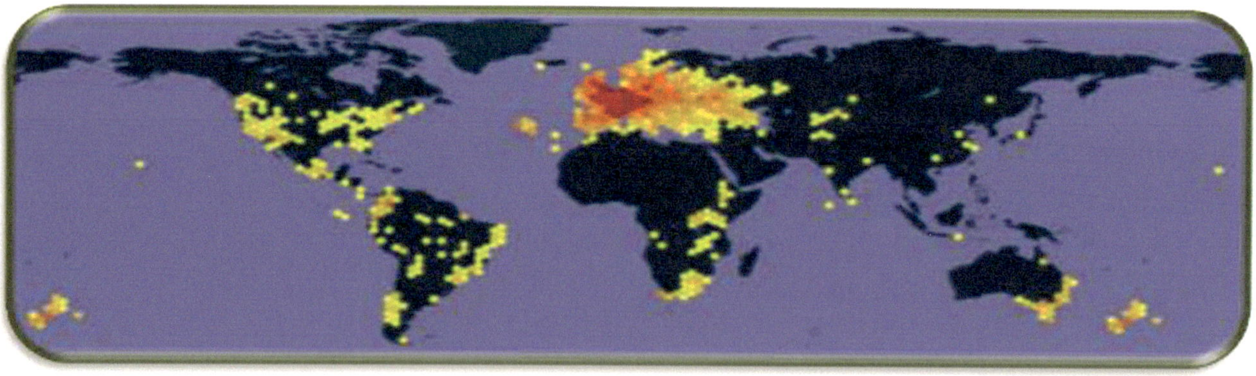

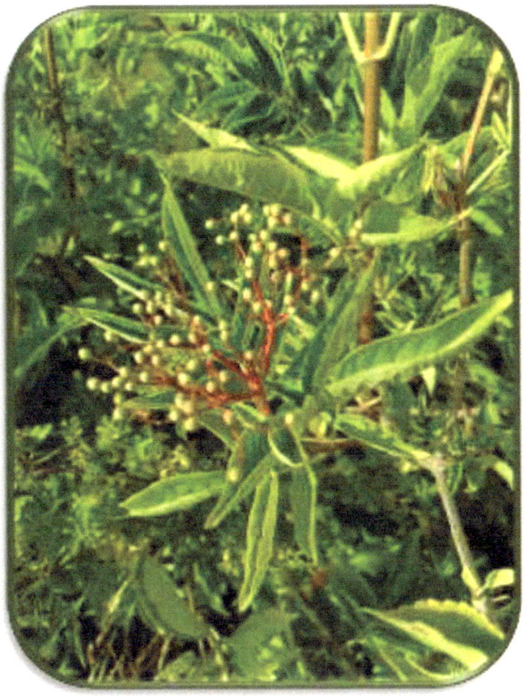

Botanical description:

Shrubs (or trees), 1-6 m high. The roots are shallow and not deep. The bark of the young branches is green, covered with a hyoid, consisting of gray lenticels, the old branches are light brown to gray, and fissured. The leaves are compound pinnate from 3 to 7 leaflets, dull green on the upper surface, and bluish-green on the lower surface. The leaflet is ovate or oblong, pointed at the apex, serrated at the margin, glabrous, and auricular. Flowers fragrant, yellowish to white, gathered in terminal racemes, erect, flat and wide, can reach 20 cm or more in width, densely flowered, has 5 main branches. The calyx is very short, fused sepals, 5-lobed. The corolla is cyclopsic, 5-lobed. The male has 5 stamens. The female has 3-carpels, the ovary is inferior, the pistils are three in number.

Fruit: Grape, black to purple, containing red to blood-red juice. Seeds: 3-5, brown, oval.

Flowering: April to May

Habitat and geographical distribution: The plant is widespread in Europe and western Asia, and is cultivated in many parts of the world.

History and heritage:

The scientific name of the genus is the old Latin name for this plant, and the name of the species nigra means "black" in reference to the black color of its fruits. It is often described for its many ivory and protective properties, and the ancient Egyptians knew it, and it was a common treatment for removing phlegm in the seventeenth century. In 1653, Nicholas Kléber wrote that a decoction of the roots heals snakebites.

Part used: Dried flowers (aromatic), fresh or dried leaves, fresh or dried ripe fruits, branch bark (removed in spring without cork.)

Chemical components:

Flowers: Flowers contain volatile oil -0.1-0.3%, sterols, triterpene compounds (alpha and beta amyrin), fatty acids and their esters. Flavonoids such as astragalin, nicotiflorin, in addition to hydroxycinnamic acid and cinnamic acid derivatives.

Leaves: contain flavonoids, triterpenes, sterols, cyanogenetic compounds, the enzyme prunasin, and some alkanes. Fruits: flavonoids, anthocyanids, volatile oil, and cyanogenic glycosides in the seeds especially (possibly toxic), with the enzyme pronazin, organic acids, and minerals (potassium, phosphorus, and calcium.)

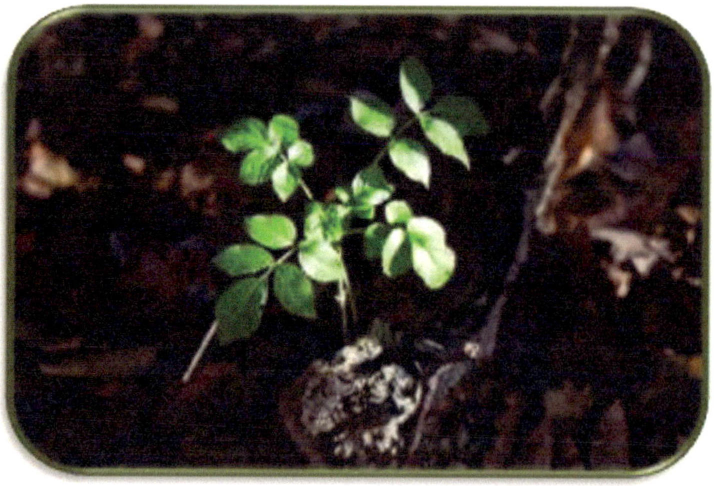

Seeds: fatty oils and lectins.

Barks: triterpene compounds such as alpha-amyrin and betuline, ursolic acid, seryl alcohol, sterols, tannins, traces of volatile oil, and lectins. Phenols known for their effectiveness in scavenging free radicals are antioxidants, and natural phenols extracted from Bellis are beneficial for diabetics who suffer from insulin deficiency, and reduce the inflammatory condition and pancreatitis.

Note:

Parts of the plant except for flowers, fruits and mature seeds are toxic to mammals, and contain cyanogenic glycoside, and the bark contains calcium oxalate crystals.

Properties and medical uses:

Bellis plant has been used in folk medicine as a diaphoretic, antipyretic and diuretic. The plant has anti-inflammatory, antibacterial, antiviral, antidiabetic, antidepressant, and antitumor properties. Elderberry flowers are laxatives that increase bronchial secretions and are used in cases of cough, asthma, bronchitis, fever, colds, and rheumatism.

The decoction of the dried fruits is used as a laxative, and the fresh fruit syrup is used as a sedative for nervous tension and sciatica pain.

The bark and leaves are used to treat rheumatism and increase urination. The flower decoction is used topically as a mouthwash to treat sore throat and toothache, or as ointments and compresses to treat scratches, skin infections, wounds, burns, and psoriasis.

bark:

Elderberry is available in the form of an ointment, an aqueous solution of the bark and leaves, an oil, and alcoholic solutions, sold under trade names such as power Elderberry, flowers Elder

Other uses:

Elderberry juice is used to dye hair, and is included in the composition of scented ointments. Children make flutes and other blowing toys from the hollow stems of elderberry, and elderberry sometimes causes cyanide toxicity in these children.

Side effects, interactions and warnings:

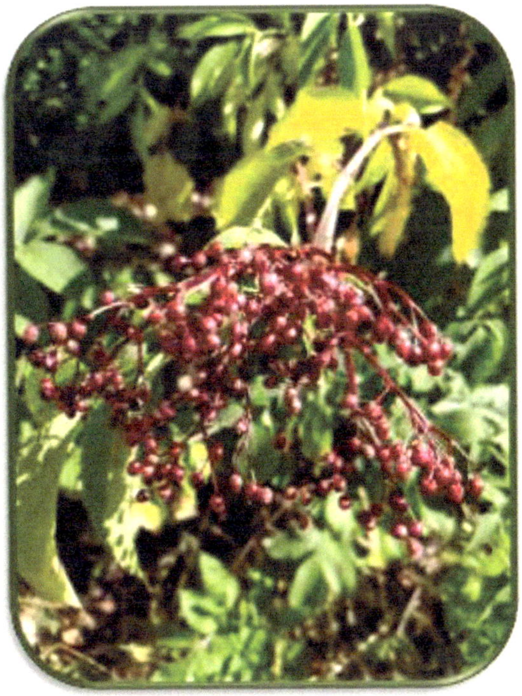

The dark blue or purple fruits are slightly toxic in their fresh state, but are edible after cooking. People with allergies or digestive system diseases should not consume the components of the plant or its products. Eating the fruits or leaves of elderberry can cause diarrhea and vomiting. Products containing elderberry should be used with caution, due to the possibility of cyanide toxicity. Pregnant and breastfeeding women should also avoid using this plant.

Environment:

Black elderberry is found in temperate and cold regions of the world, and grows wild in moist forest lands on river banks, on plateaus and mountains, among forest trees, on fertile, moist and dry soils and in sunny places.

Cultivation and productivity:

The plant is propagated by seeds and root cuttings. The seeds are scattered directly in the soil or planted in the nursery, and then the seedlings are transferred to the permanent land. Root cuttings can also be planted in winter, and need irrigation in summer.

Allium cepa L.

Cepa vulgaris Garsault., *Cepa esculenta* Gray., *Porrum cepa*)L.(Rchb., *Kepa esculenta* Raf.

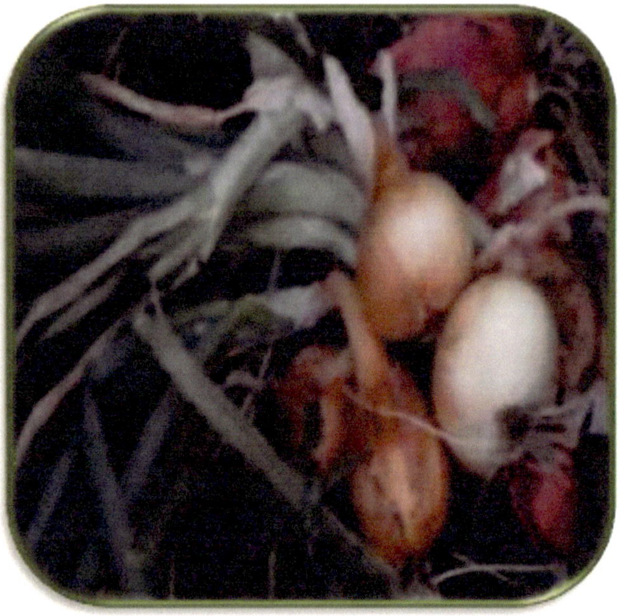

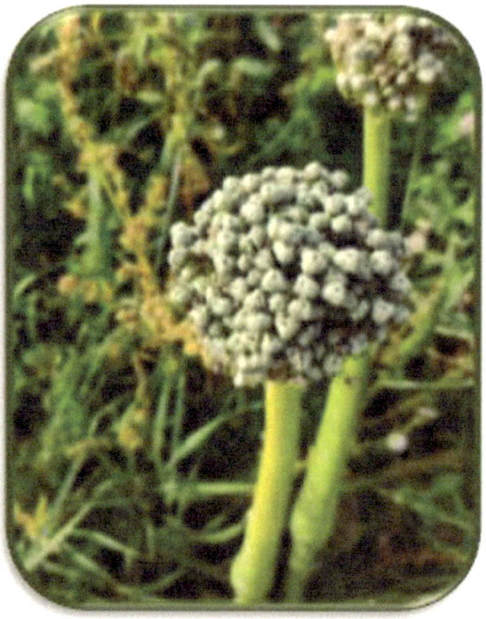

Family: Alliaceae (formerly Liliaceae)

Common names: Onion

Foreign names: Oignon Fr. Onion, Eng

Occurrences : 19,864 occurrences

Distribution in the world

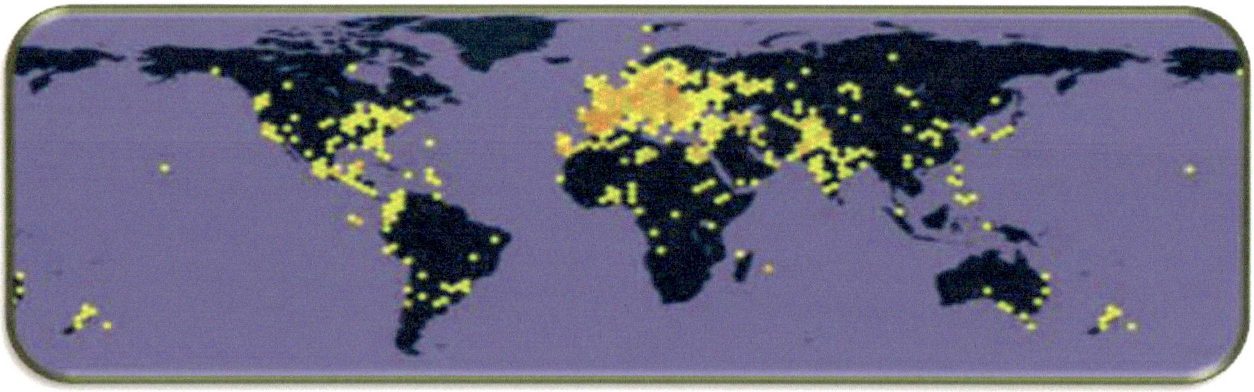

Botanical description:

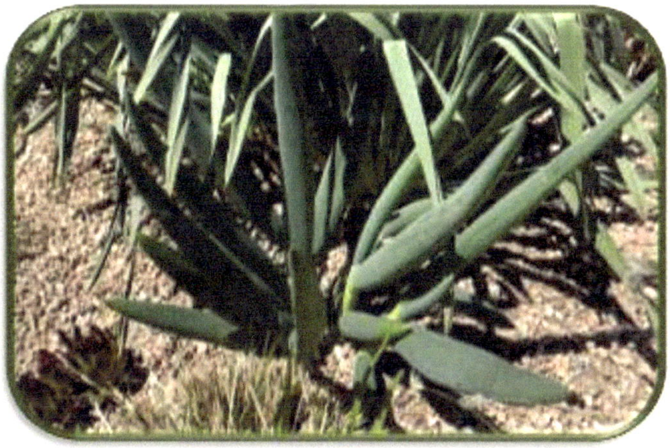

A perennial plant with a bulb that takes multiple shapes (spherical, oval or oblong), depending on the variety. The stem is erect and hollow, and can reach a height of up to 1 m. The leaves are shorter than the inflorescence, tubular or slightly flattened and hollow. The stem ends with a leafless scape, hollow, gray to blue in color, carrying the inflorescence at its end. Flowers are white, greenish to purple, long-stemmed (about 3 cm), composed of 6 sepals and 6 stamens, arranged in two whorls, and longer than the sepals, and three fused carpels, forming a three-chambered ovary. The flowers are gathered in a spherical, umbel-shaped inflorescence, surrounded before opening by a large bract. The fruit is a three-chambered capsule, containing black, angular seeds.

Bulb: A terrestrial plant part consisting of a flat, dwarf disc stem, surrounded by fleshy leaf bases filled with storages, which are in turn surrounded by dry, scaly leaves. The disc stem produces a terminal bud (and sometimes two buds) that later gives an aerial branch, and fibrous lateral roots are formed on its lower part.

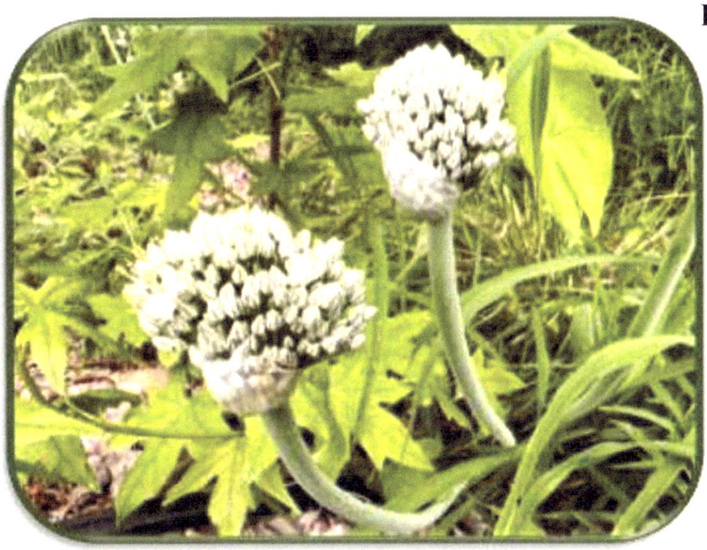

Homeland and geographical distribution:

Syria is the original homeland of the onion plant, it is spread in the eastern Mediterranean and southern Europe, and is widely cultivated in many countries of the world, and Syria and Egypt are the most productive Arab countries. History and heritage: The scientific name of the genus Allium is the old Latin name for these species, and most likely its source is the word all, meaning "stinging", while the name of the species cepa is derived from the Latin cep or cepa meaning "head", in reference to the shape of the onion. Onions are a food and ivory plant known for a long time, and were known to the oldest human civilizations, and the history of its murals dates back to three thousand years BC. The Pharaohs used it, and it is said that it occupied a position close to sanctification among them to the point that they used to swear by it, and they carried it on their chests as a talisman against diseases of envy, and it was one of the main foods for the builders of the pyramids, and they used it to treat rheumatism and stimulate the heart, and it was included in the composition of embalming materials. Onions also had a high status among the Greeks, and their doctors talked about onions and prescribed them to treat many diseases, and Dioscorides used them to purify the blood. The Chinese used them as food and medicine, and the Arabs also knew many of the benefits of Laxative for the stomach, and if cooked, it becomes more diuretic,Thirsty, Softener, Onions, Ibn al-Baytar mentioned: "Onions stimulate the appetite,

For urine, and the smell of onions is covered by roasted walnuts and fried cheese." Al-Antaki mentioned about onions that they: “open obstructions, eliminate jaundice, increase urination and menstruation, and break up stones.” Ibn Sina also advised using them to stimulate the appetite and treat weakness and emaciation of the body. The current onion does not exist wild, and it is believed that it was cultivated in Iran or Afghanistan 4-6 thousand years ago.

Part used: Onion

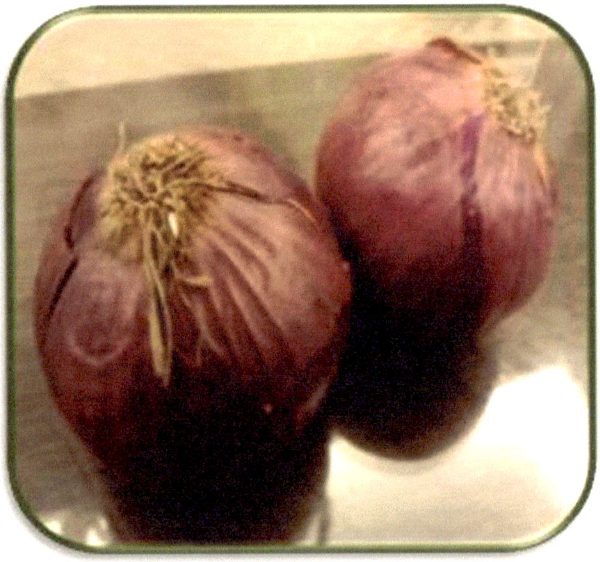

Chemical components:

Onions contain volatile oil that includes many sulfur compounds similar to alliins, especially allyl alliin, as well as thiosulphinate (decomposes to give antibacterial compounds), and thiopropionic aldehyde (responsible for eye tearing.)

Favoneoids: quercetine, prostaglandins, steroidal saponins, fructosaccharides (10-40%), sucrose, protein and vitamin A and C, along with mineral salts such as sodium, potassium, calcium, magnesium, cobalt and phosphorus.

Properties and medical uses:

Thiosulphinate has antibacterial properties, and various onion compounds reduce blood lipids, reduce atherosclerosis and high blood pressure. Studies have shown a reduced risk of stomach cancer, cholesterol and triglycerides with increased onion consumption. The sulfur compounds in onion volatile oil reduce platelet aggregation. Onions are used to treat laryngitis, bronchitis, sinusitis, and respiratory mucous membrane infections, and to eliminate harmful bacteria in the digestive system, especially Bacillus subtilis, Salmonella typhi, Pseudomonas aeroginosa, and Escherichia coli. Onions or their juice are popularly used to treat coughs, asthma, croup, tonsillitis, stimulate the secretory functions of the gallbladder in cases of digestive disorders, and reduce blood sugar levels. They also help get rid of intestinal worms. Onion juice or its alcoholic tincture is used topically as an antiseptic for minor wounds and burns, and is useful in treating warts, boils, and abscesses, in addition to being used to strengthen hair.

Environment:

Onions are cold-tolerant vegetables. The ideal temperature for plant growth is 18-26. A sufficient amount of moisture in the soil, especially during the period of seed germination, the formation of the green mass and the formation of bulbs. Onions tolerate drought during the ripening stage, and increasing humidity delays their ripening. Onions need fertile, loose and good moisture-retaining soil, due to the weakness of their root system. The appropriate pH is 6-7.

It is recommended to store the bulbs at a temperature below 26°C or more so that the flower spikes do not appear.

Cultivation and productivity:

The plant is propagated by seeds and small bulbs (Qazah, Qannar). The seeds are planted in 2X3 m basins or in rows in the fall. Onion seeds germinate within 10-16 days when the humidity and temperature are suitable, and onion seeds are characterized by a low germination rate. Onion growth in its early stages is very slow, the first true leaf appears within 10-15 days of germination, and the leaves continue to grow slowly until the plant forms 4-5 true leaves, which occurs within a month of the appearance of the seedlings. The rapid growth of the leaves begins, and their number increases in the vegetative growth stage, and the growth and formation of the onion begins with the swelling and enlargement of the leaf bases. The small onions are taken out to be planted in the field in the fall or spring in rows with a distance of 25 cm between them. The required services are provided to them, such as irrigation, fertilization, and weeding, until the onions swell, dry up in the soil, and their leaves wither above the soil. The onions are then taken out and dried. The production of a dunum of regular onions ranges between 2-3 tons.

Allium sativum L.

Porrum sativum)L.(Rchb., *Allium sativum* var. *vulgare* Döll.

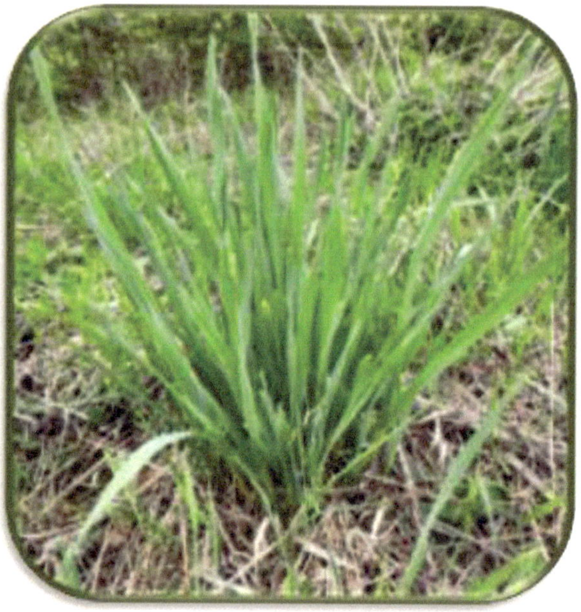

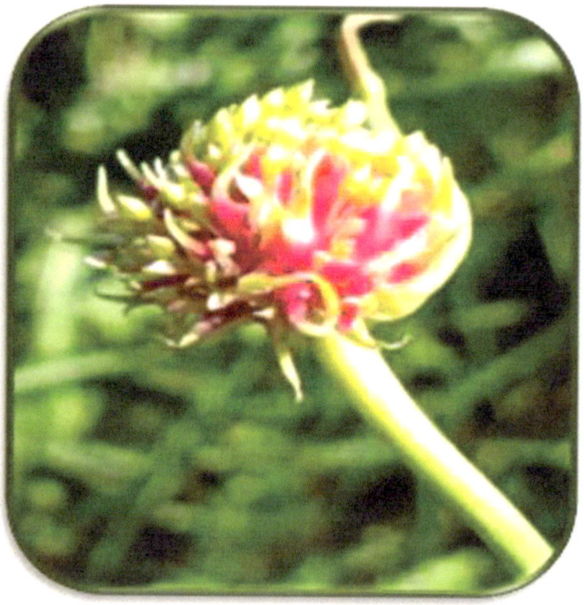

Family: Alliaceae (formerly Liliaceae)

Common names: Garlic

Foreign names: Ail Fr. Garlic, Eng.

Occurrences : 11,846 occurrences

Distribution in the world

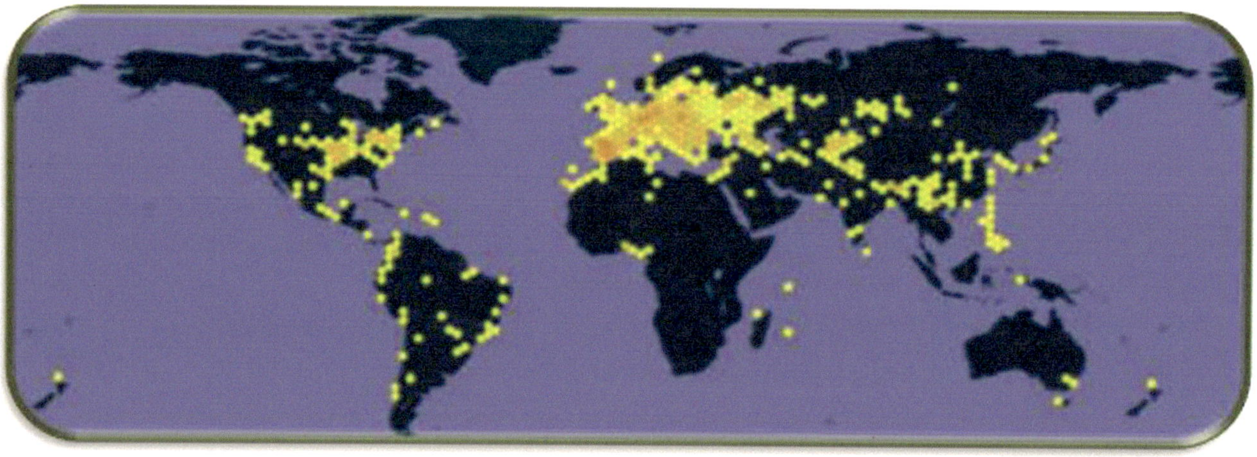

Botanical description:

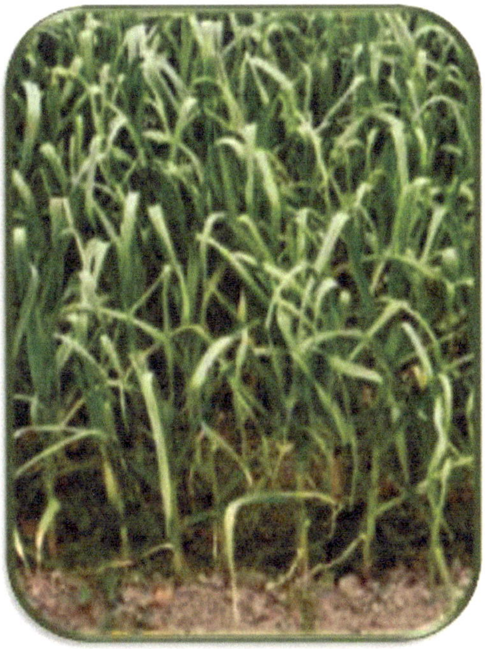

Perennial herb with bulbs, 25-70 cm high. The aerial stem is erect, solid, full, bearing leaves up to about halfway. The leaves consist of a sheath surrounding the stem, and a ribbon-like blade, 4-25 mm wide, with a smooth or rough edge. The flower stalk ends with an umbel-shaped inflorescence, consisting of a single flower, surrounded by violet florets or buds, called aerial bulbs, fixed by a weak spike, which facilitates its separation from the inflorescence, and is able to grow directly after falling without going through a state of dormancy. The inflorescence is surrounded by a pointed bract at the top. The stamen is simple, consisting of 6 reddish or greenish white petals, located in two whorls. The male has 6 stamens in two whorls.

The fruit is a three-chambered capsule. The seeds are triangular in shape. At the end of summer, a large number of secondary, arched bulbs are formed next to the main bulb, which the public calls "garlic teeth or cloves." The compound bulb and bulbs are covered with dry, scaly leaves, forming a continuous clod, white or white-purple in color. The bulb consists of an oval, arched disc stem, masked by a thick saving leaf, surrounded by a number of dry, scaly leaf bases that form a continuous thicket around the disc. The disc stem produces a terminal bud, which later gives an aerial branch, and fibrous adventitious roots are formed on its lower part.

Homeland and geographical distribution:

Central Asia and the countries of the Eastern Mediterranean, and its cultivation is widespread throughout the world.

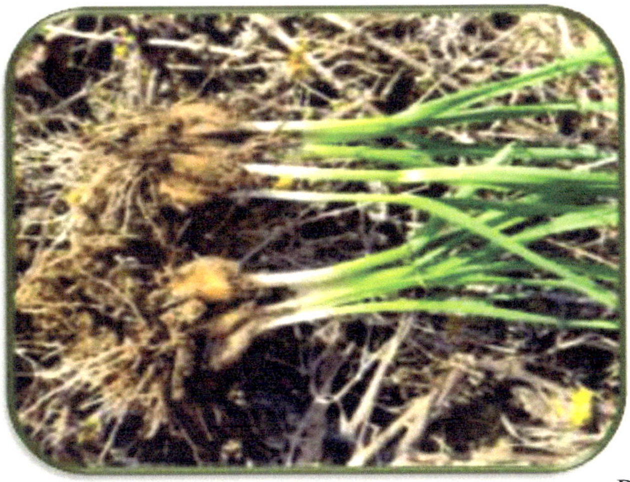

History and Heritage:

The scientific name of the genus is the old Latin name for this plant, sativum meaning "cultivated." Garlic is one of the most important and oldest plant species used as food and urn at the same time. The importance of garlic has been known for more than 5000 years. The pharaohs used to offer it as offerings to their gods. They also used to eat a large amount of garlic before doing any hard work. The first labor strike in the world was because of garlic. During the construction of the Pyramid of Khufu, the provision of garlic to the workers was stopped, which led to the workers refusing to work because of their belief that garlic It provides them with activity, vitality and strength, and prevents them from diseases and infections.

The Greeks also knew garlic, and gave it great importance in their food and medicine. A mixture of garlic and vinegar helped save the lives of thousands from the plague epidemic in France in 1720.

Part used: Garlic cloves, fresh or dried, volatile oil of the cloves.

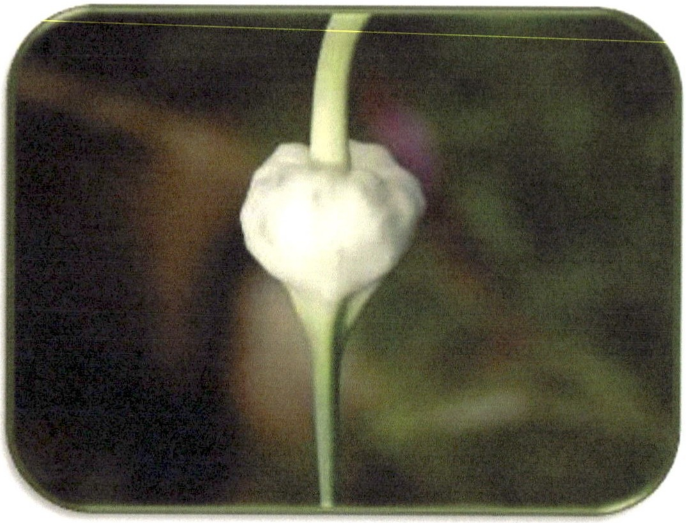

Chemical components:

Fresh garlic cloves contain a volatile oil, which consists mainly of a mixture of mono-, di- or poly-sulfur derivatives, called alliins (alkylcysteine sulphoxides), which are odorless compounds, including alliin allyl, alliin propenyl and alliin methyl. These compounds are transformed when the fresh cloves are cut or crushed in the presence of the enzyme alliinase into a compound unstable, distinctive-smelling compound called allicin (a sulfur compound responsible for bad breath), which in turn turns into allyl disulfide in the presence of water and air. The cloves also contain fructosans (polysaccharides), saponins, yeasts, and anti-fungal compounds, including allicin, garlicine, vitamins A, B1, B2, D, minerals, and compounds that resemble sex hormones in their effectiveness.

Properties and medical uses:

Garlic has many properties and medical uses, the most important of which are:

1. Antimicrobial and antiseptic for the respiratory tract, protects against colds and flu, and alleviates their symptoms.

2. Treats vascular diseases, stimulates blood circulation, and lowers blood pressure.

3. Reduces hardening of the coronary arteries, high cholesterol, and lowers blood fats. It also reduces the risk of heart disease and protects against blood clots. Scientists confirm that the best types of medicines for heart diseases are those that contain garlic, as the breakdown of allicin produces sulfur compounds that interact with red blood cells to produce hydrogen disulfide, which helps the cells communicate with each other better, and activates the cells lining the blood vessels, working to relax and expand them, allowing blood to flow easily in them, which leads to lowering blood pressure and allowing the load to be carried. More oxygen to the vital organs in the body, and reduces the burden on the heart, and garlic also increases the level of glutathione, which is a compound that resists premature cell aging.

4. Antioxidant, reduces the risk of cancer (Allicin compound.)

5. Garlic (Allicin compound) is a broad-spectrum antibiotic, eliminating many microbes (bacteria, fungi, viruses) and parasitic worms.

6. It improves the performance of natural killer cells (NK), which are important in improving and protecting the body's immunity, and which attack cancer cells, viruses, and some types of bacteria that cause infections.

7. It has properties that lower blood sugar.

8. Garlic, with its sulfur compounds, has been proven effective in protecting the liver, treating indigestion, cleansing the intestines, and removing their infection. Dried garlic powder is used to treat food poisoning caused by several types of bacteria. Such as Escherichia coli, Staphylococcus aureus, Pseudomonas aeruginosa, Bacillus subtilis. Experiments have proven the ability of garlic po.wder to kill Bacillus anthracis, which causes anthrax.

9. Garlic has anticoagulant properties or platelet aggregation. Garlic is used topically to treat and disinfect wounds, and to treat many skin diseases (boils, alopecia), and is useful in treating hair loss.

Note: To get the desired benefit from garlic, it should be used without Cooking or processing, because it loses many of its bactericidal properties when exposed to high temperatures, so it is dried in the shade, then crushed and dried at a temperature of 60°C. Garlic retains its antioxidant properties after cooking and high-temperature treatment, but it loses its antibacterial and anti-blood-clotting properties after high-temperature treatment.

Pharmaceutical forms:

Garlic is available in several forms, including garlic oil infusion, dry form, water form, and volatile oil extracted by distillation with water vapor.

Drug interactions and warnings for use:

Garlic may pose a risk to the health and lives of AIDS patients, due to its disruption of treatments designated for this disease, as it has been noted that it reduces the levels of performance of the drug "Saquinavir" in the blood to half. Caution should be exercised when consuming concentrated garlic before surgery, before labor and delivery, especially in diabetics. It should also not be used with blood-thinning medications (anticoagulants) such as heparin and aspirin. Garlic may cause indigestion, intestinal irritation accompanied by heartburn, or irritation of the urinary tract, so it should be avoided in large quantities or avoided by those suffering from intestinal disorders or kidney failure. Eating too much garlic may cause itching and hemorrhoids.

Environment:

Garlic is a long-day plant that tolerates cold. Storing garlic at low temperatures (-13°C) shortens the growing season compared to storing it at high temperatures (20-25°C). Garlic needs soil and air humidity during its growth period, especially during the period of clove germination, the period of rapid leaf growth, and the period of clove and flower spike formation. Garlic requires loose, fertile soil, and is best grown in light soils, but does not grow well in sandy soils because they do not retain enough moisture for growth.

Cultivation and productivity:

The plant is propagated by cloves, which are planted in rows 40-50 cm apart, with a distance of 10-12 cm between cloves, or in basins or basins, the dimensions of which vary according to the level of soil and the amount of water available. The required service operations are provided, including fertilization, weeding, and irrigation, with gradual reduction of irrigation, and stopping it when signs of maturity begin to appear, represented by yellowing of the leaves, drying of their tops, and bending to the ground, in addition to drying of the outer covering of the heads. Productivity varies according to the variety and service operations provided to the plant, and ranges between 1.2 and 3 tons per acre.

Pistacia atlantica Desf.

Pistacia mutica Fisch. & C.A.Mey., *Pistacia atlantica* var. *mutica* Rech. f., *Terebinthus at- lanticus*) Desf.(Dum.Cours., *Pistacia atlantica* subsp. *kurdica* Rech.f

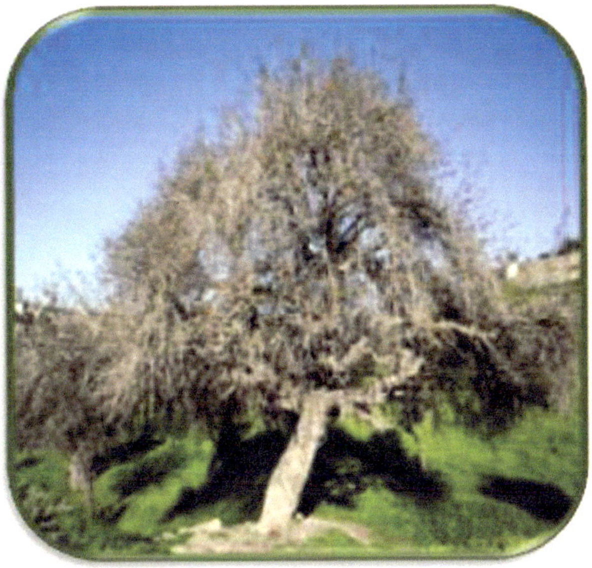

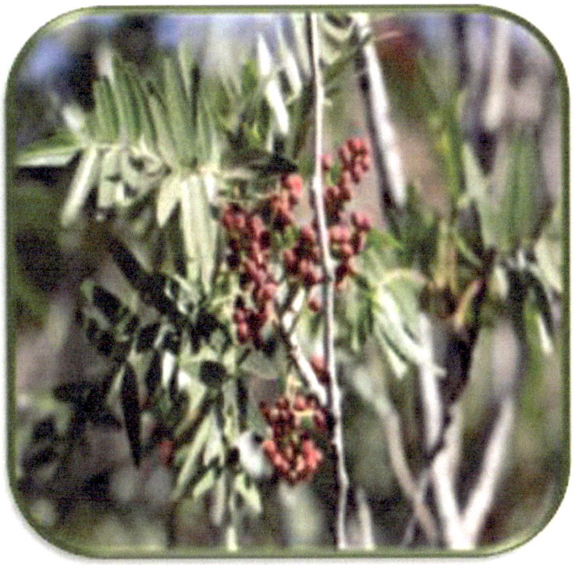

Family: Anacardiaceae

Common names: Atlantic pistachio

Foreign names:

Occurrences : 5,123 occurrences

Distribution in the world.

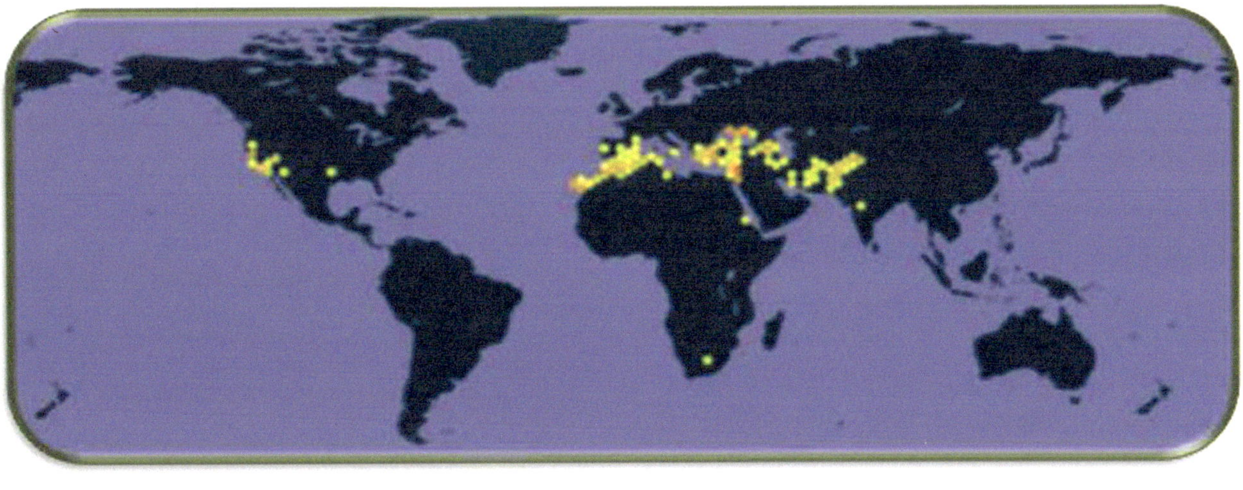

Botanical description:

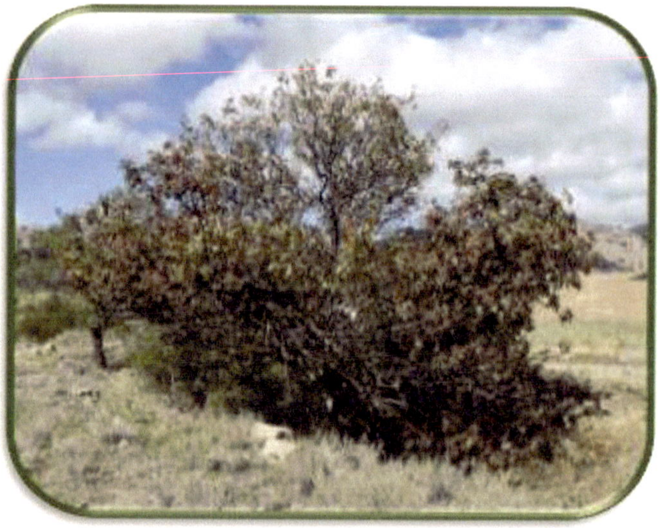

A perennial deciduous tree, 4-20 m tall. Branches are brown to grey. Leaves are alternate, compound and serrate. Leaflets are ovate to oblong in outer shape, leaf stalk is flat. Leaflet 25-70 pinnate 6-20× mm, lanceolate or oblong, blunt at the apex. Flowers are unisexual. Plants are dioecious. Male flowers are gathered in paniculate inflorescences, 3-10 cm long, compact, later becoming slack. Female inflorescences Compound racemes, 8-15 cm long. Semi-subdural flowers. Male flowers are surrounded by bracts and bracts, which together form a five-lobed false bract. Male has 5 stamens, very short filaments, and long anthers. Female flowers Include a bract composed of several overlapping dry membranous segments, female 2-3 mm, ovary monochambered, and ovule monochambered. Fruit is nuclear, 6-5×7-5 mm, inverted ovate to spherical. The outer pericarp becomes wrinkled when dry, the inner pericarp is bony. Seeds are compressed, cotyledons are large and oily.

Flowering: From March to April.

Habitat and geographical distribution:

Iranian-Turanian. Its original habitat is the Arab Maghreb, the Arab Levant, and Western Asia, reaching Iran. The Atlantic Pistachio is naturally distributed in North Africa, the Middle East, and the Canary Islands in the Atlantic Ocean. It is also found in the Batam Valley in the Sinai Desert, which is the driest location for its natural distribution, and it is also found in Syria and Jordan.

History and Heritage:

The name Batum is derived from the Akkadian language, and has been used since the second millennium BC in Mesopotamia, where the Babylonians used it to name these trees, and called it "Batmu", and other civilizations that succeeded one another in the region in the eastern Mediterranean have used it until the present time. The Atlantic Pistachio tree was strongly present in the history of the peoples who inhabited the deserts of the Levant and the Arab Maghreb. The scientific name of the genus Pistacia, comes from the Greek word Pistake, which is probably derived from the Persian word "Fustaq", which refers to the species P. vera (meaning true pistachio), which is the famous pistachio, which is widely cultivated for its fruits in Aleppo. As for the species name Atlantica, it means "Atlantic", in reference to the Atlas Mountains in North Africa, where it is

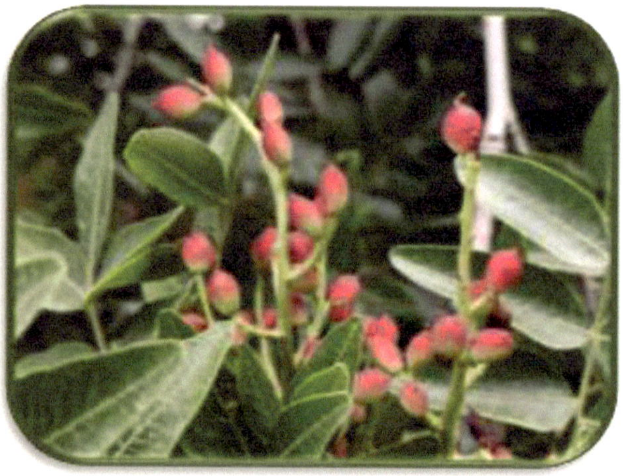

found in its natural state, and was first described. A tree that used to form vast forests in North Africa and the Middle East, and is now in severe decline due to excessive cutting (Nahal, 2009).

Part used: Leaves, fruits, and the oil resin secreted by the plant.

Chemical components:

The leaves, fruits, and resin contain volatile oil, at a rate of 0.2%, 0.8%, and 32.6%, respectively. The volatile oil compounds differ according to their source. The volatile oil produced from the oleoresin is rich in monoterpene hydrocarbon compounds, including α-pinen 43%, and β-pinen 13%. The volatile oil produced from the fruits contains α-pinen 8.3% and monoterpene oxygenated compounds, including bornyl acetate 21% bornylacetate. The volatile oil produced from the leaves is rich in monoterpene and tetraterpene oxygenated compounds: odesmol 20%, elemol 4.8%, eudesmol 4.8%. The seeds contain fixed oil, which constitutes 52% of their dry weight, and is characterized by its richness in unsaturated fatty acids 73% (oleic acid, linoleic acid), and it also contains nitrogenous compounds 27%, and fibers and minerals Na(Mg, Mn, P, .) Fe, The leaves contain tannins (tannins) 22%, and the bark of the trees (the tissues swollen by some insects) contains tannins.

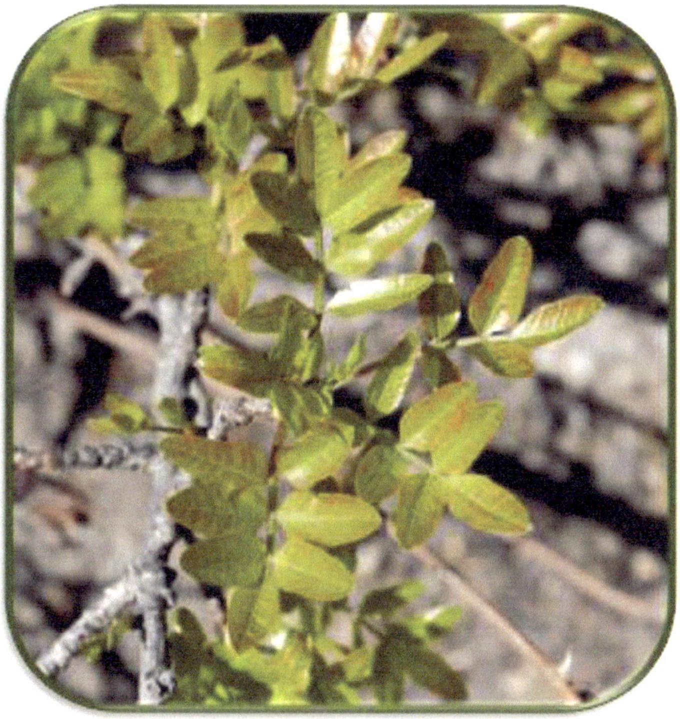

Properties and medical uses:

The fruits and leaves are used in folk medicine as an anti-diarrheal and antiseptic. Some research has shown the benefits of the aqueous extract of the plant in reducing blood sugar levels. Atlantic terebinth has been widely used in the Middle East and Mediterranean regions since ancient times for various purposes, such as stomach diseases, kidney disorders, wounds and cough. Modern studies have shown that it has many medical properties, such as antioxidants, diabetes, hyperlipidemia and others, and it can also be effective in diseases of the digestive system.

The pistachio, its oil and gum have a prestigious medical status, as mentioned by Ibn Sina and Ibn al-Nafis al-Dimashqi, in treating tumors, liver diseases, and the disease of the eyelid, in addition to its great benefit for the joints. It is also a strong antiseptic, and useful in treating insect bites and repelling them. The large tannin swellings (nuts) caused by some insects on tree buds are antibacterial and antifungal.

Other uses:

The fruits are sold in the markets as a food item that is roasted, salted and consumed as nuts. The fatty oil extracted from the seeds has many nutritional uses. The resin that oozes from the tree is used in the manufacture of wax and soap, and is also included in the composition of cosmetic ointments, pastes and compounds used in the film industry. Tannic compounds extracted from the bark and leaves are used in the manufacture of ink, dycs and leather tanning.

Environment:

The Atlantic Pistachio is naturally distributed in dry and semi-dry areas in valleys and on sunny slopes. Up to an altitude of 1500 m, it resists cold and drought. The tree is characterized by its slow growth and its tolerance of poor, calcareous and stony soils, while preferring light, deep soils (silty, sandy) with good drainage, moderate acidity, and tending to dryness. It is a light-loving plant, and leaves abundantly after cutting. The roots and stem of the pistachio are sometimes infected by some insects (wasps), which generates swollen tissues in the form of galls. It contributes to enriching wildlife, as it is a refuge for various animals, especially in the hot times of the summer.

Cultivation and productivity:

An excellent type for afforestation, and suitable for dry environments. It is propagated by seeds, which are preferably treated with scratching or acid, then soaked in water for 24 hours. The seedlings are produced in the nursery, then transferred to the ground Perennial with adequate irrigation when planted.

Pollination in the Atlas Pistachio tree is mixed and wind-borne, which justifies its presence close to the pistachio trees (P. vera), and it can also be a rootstock on which these trees are grafted. The Atlas Pistachio enters the economic production phase at the age of 5-7 years, and its fruits are harvested during the fall season (September-October).

Pistacia lentiscus L.

Lentiscus vulgaris Fourr., *Terebinthus lentiscus*)L.(Moench., *Pistacia lentiscus* subsp. *Lentiscus.*, *Pistacia brevifolia* Gand., *Pistacia gummifera* Salisb.

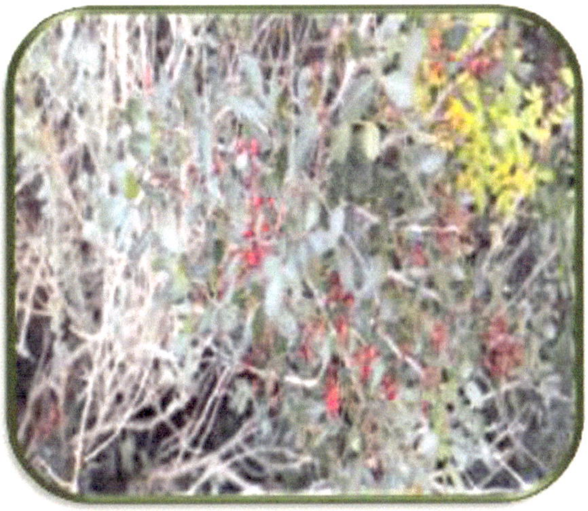 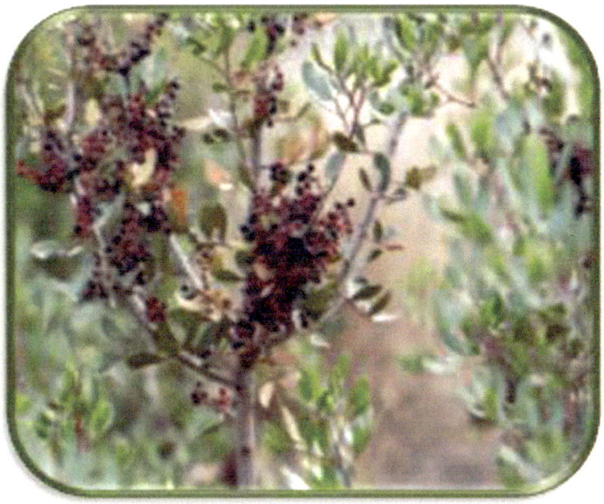

Family: Anacardiaceae

Common names: Pistachio ligaceae, Pistacia lentisca, Pistacia lentisca, Mastic, Gum lentisca, Gum lentisca

Foreign names: Eng. Lentisk, Fr. pistachier lentisque

Occurrences : 271,457 occurrences

Distribution in the world.

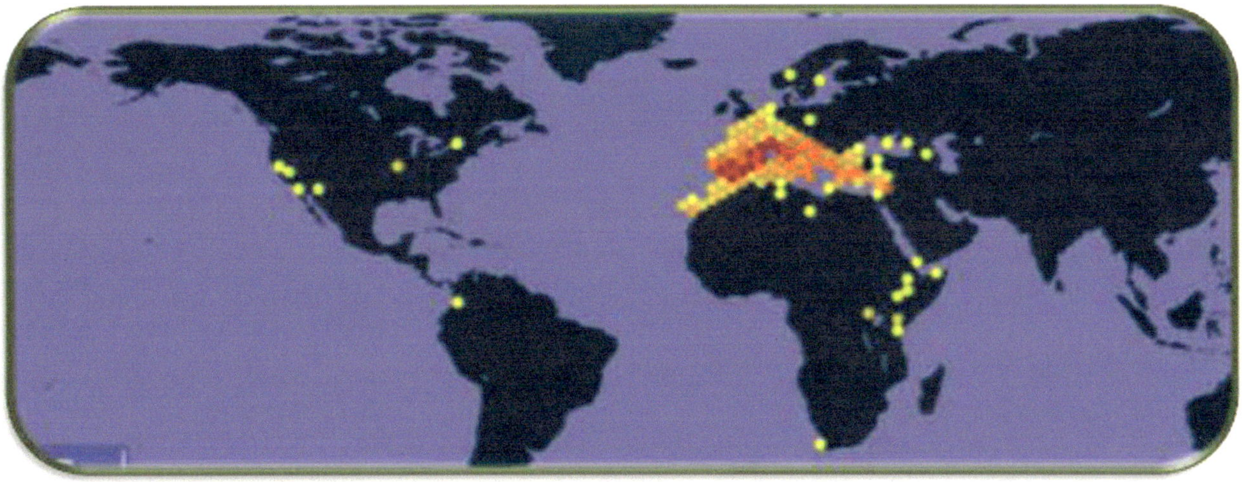

Botanical description:

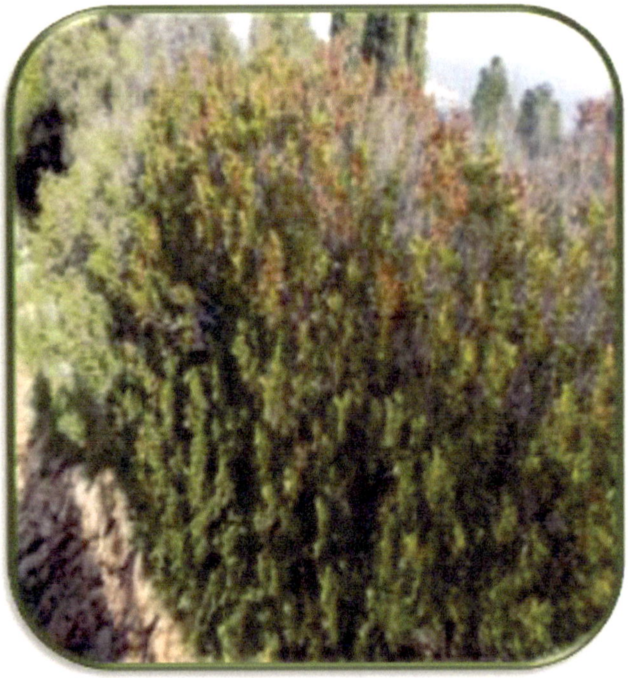

Evergreen shrubs (rarely trees), 1-3 m tall. Leaves 5-10 cm, perennial, compound pinnate, with 2-4 leaflets, winged axis. Leaflet 0.5-1×1.5-3 cm, leathery, ovate to oblong or elliptic, rounded at the apex, stalked, glabrous. Flowers unisexual. Male inflorescences spike-like and compact. Female inflorescences are axillary, gathered in bunches, each consisting of 1-4 semi-spike inflorescences. Male flowers are short-stalked, containing 4-5 stamens and a vestigial pistil. Female flowers are tall, the length of the sleeve is about 1.5 mm, the style is short. The fruit is nuclear, semi-spherical, 3-4 mm in diameter, reddish in color, tending to black when ripe, its surface is reticulate, topped with 3 stigmas.

Flowering: From March to April.

Habitat and geographical distribution:

Mediterranean countries from the Canary Islands and Portugal to the Middle East to western China. It is distributed at altitudes not exceeding 300 m in the forests of the temperate coastal areas of Syria, Cyprus, Greece and Sicily.

History and Heritage:

The word "Pistacia" comes from the Akkadian language from the second millennium BC, and was used by the Babylonians to name these trees. The descriptive name for the species, lentiscus, is the ancient Greek name for this species. The Ligasian Pistacia is considered one of the species representing an ancient flora, as it is one of the elements whose roots extend to the Tertiary period. In the past, a resinous substance called mastic was extracted from it to make a chewing gum known as "Shiu" chewing gum. The Pharaohs used it to whiten teeth. Ibn Sina mentioned it as Al-Daru, and it is a perfume used in women's perfumes in Aleppo. Its watery properties are used to increase saliva and treat mouth ulcers. Ibn al-Baytar described it: (The toothpicks of the neem are good, and its gum is also useful in perfume. The oil of its seeds expels phlegmatic winds.)

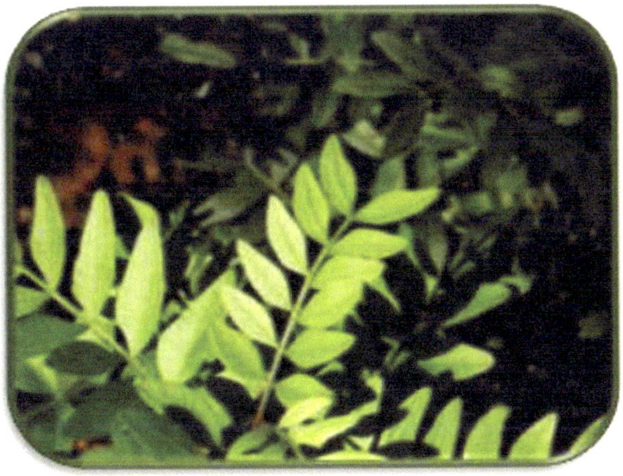

Part used:

The resinous gum or mastic (resin), the leaves, and the fruits. Mastic: spontaneous resinous secretions, or artificial secretion by removing strips of bark, or by making long slits in the tree trunk and large branches, from which a liquid, yellow resinous juice flows, part of which remains attached to the tree in the form of fragile tears Oval or elongated, and the rest falls to the ground. Mastic is extracted three times a year, the first crop is whitish in color, and is the best type of mastic, the second crop is bright yellow, and the last crop is gray.

Chemical components:

Mastic consists of a mixture of resin, volatile oil, and bitter substances. Resin constitutes 90% of the mixture, its most important compounds are mastic acid triterpenes,isomastic acid a., and oleanolic acid a. Tirucallol. Volatile oil 1-3%, its most important compounds are alpha and beta pinene - beta alpha-, myrcene, beta-caryophyllene, terpinene, cardinene, linalool. The leaves contain phenolic compounds, tannins, and volatile oil, and the fruits contain fatty oil.

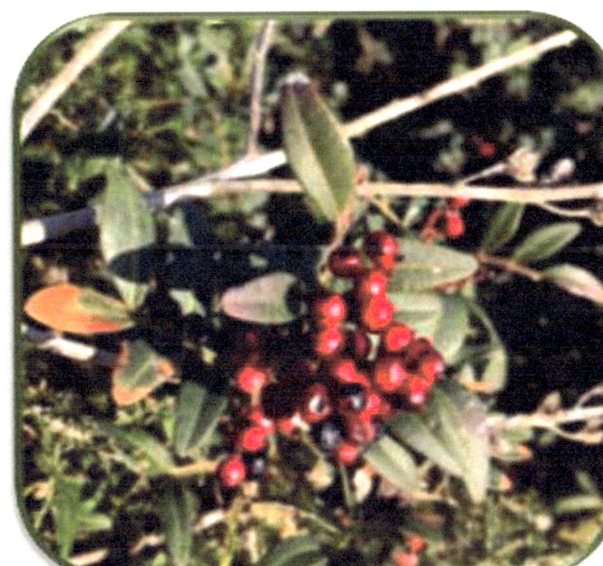

Properties and medical uses:

Mastic has been used since ancient times in folk medicine, and the people of the Levant used it as a chewing gum to give the mouth a pleasant smell,to treat indigestion, intestinal cramps, liver diseases, strengthen and tighten the gums, keep teeth white, to stop bleeding, and treat rheumatic pain, gout, and nerve pain. Mastic preparations are used internally to treat sinusitis, bronchitis, and urinary tract infections. Mastic, which contains bitter substances and volatile oil, has digestive properties, protects against stomach and intestinal ulcers caused by Helicobacter pylori bacteria, and is an astringent that helps reduce diarrhea and vaginal discharge locally in the form of a lotion. Mastic preparations are used locally in the form of gum to clean and perfume the mouth, treat gingivitis, wounds, hemorrhoids, congestion and stagnation of blood, varicose veins, and relieve rheumatic and joint pain. The decoction of the leaves is popularly used to treat stomach ulcers, and the fruit oil is used to treat digestive system disorders and constipation.

Other uses:

Mastic is considered one of the finest and most expensive types of resins. It is currently used to flavor many types of sweets and drinks, and is also used in the manufacture of incense, perfumes, cosmetics, and dental adhesives. A fatty oil is extracted from the fruits and is used in the manufacture of high-quality soaps and the preparation of some cosmetics.

Environment:

The pistachio is found in semi-arid, semi-humid, humid, hot, moderate, and somewhat fresh bioclimatic layers, in the Mediterranean thermal plant layer up to an altitude of 300 m above sea level, as it does not tolerate frost. It grows on different types of soils (clay, marsh, sandy, calcareous), and prefers clay soils, and resists salty sea winds and sea spray.

Cultivation and productivity:

The plant is propagated by seeds and cuttings. The seedlings are produced in the nursery and then transferred to the permanent land and planted in holes about 35 cm deep and 2 m apart. The seedlings are irrigated in the summer in the first year of planting.

Pistacia vera L.

Pistacia nigricans Crantz., *Pistacia variifolia* Salisb., *Pistacia macrophylla* Pers., *Len- tiscus vera*) L.(Kuntze.

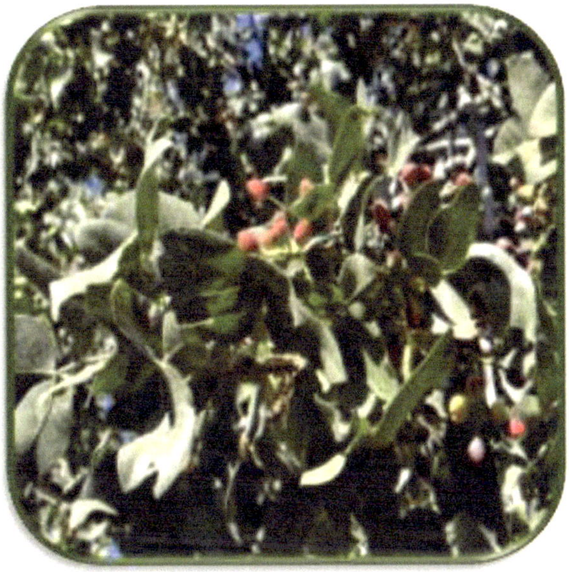

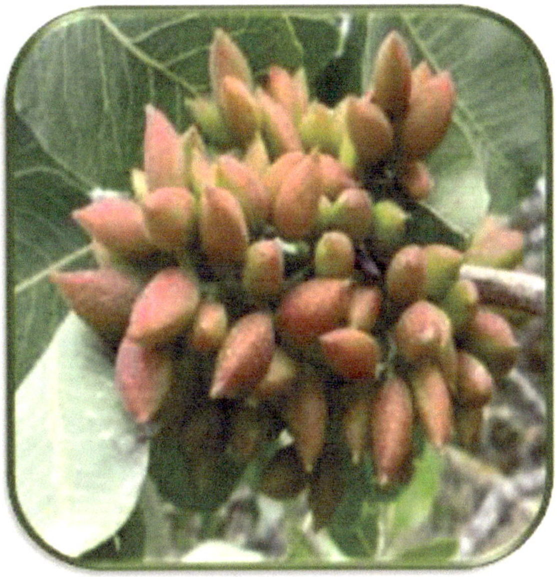

Family: Anacardiaceae

Common names: Aleppo pistachio

Foreign names:

Occurrences :4,154 occurrences

Distribution in the world

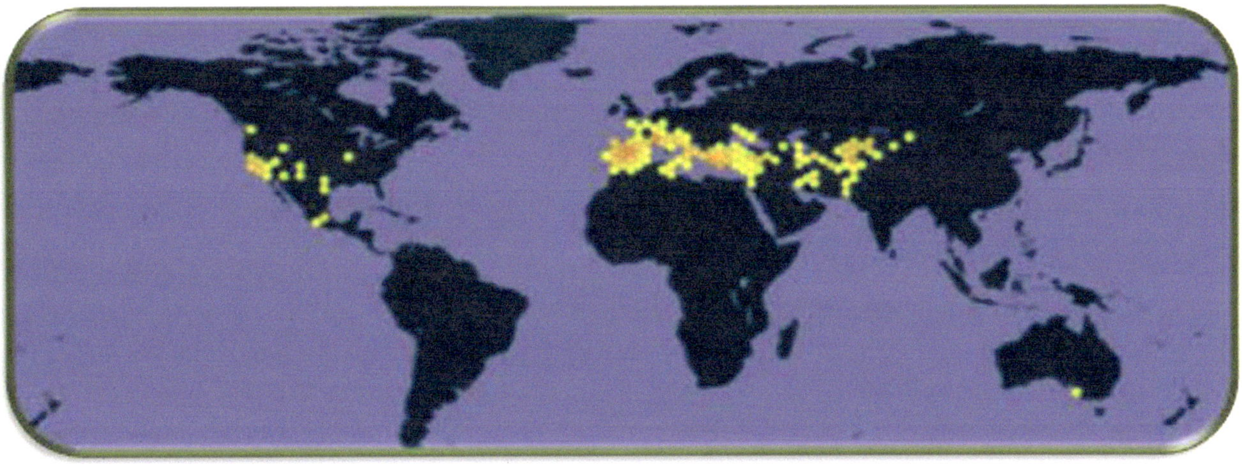

Botanical description:

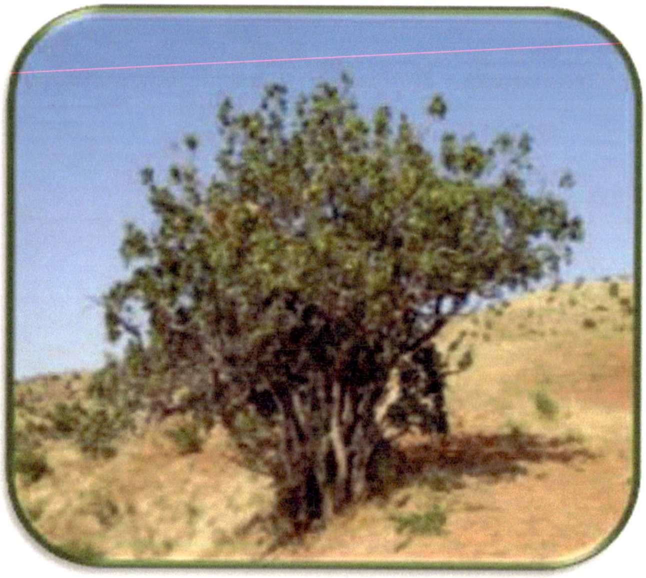

A small, deciduous, dioecious shrub, usually 3-6 m high. The stem is grey, resinous, covered with small, hard lenticels. The leaves are compound pinnate, consisting of one or two pairs of leaflets in female trees. The leaflet is oval, rounded at the top, initially hairy, then becomes bare, leathery in texture. The leaves of male shrubs are smaller in size, and fewer in number of leaflets. Flowers unisexual, male usually appears about a week before female and are gathered in conical inflorescences. Calyx 5 sepals. Corolla absent. Male 5 stamens, filaments short, free at the top and fused at their bases. Female flowers are gathered in clusters, larger than male flowers, calyx consists of 3-5 sepals. Style short, ending in three pistils; ovary inferior. The fruit is nuclear, about 2 cm long, oblong to rounded in shape.

The species includes a group of agricultural varieties that differ from each other mainly in fruit specifications (size,cracks, color, winter cold and accumulated heat requirements for fruit ripening.)

Flowering: In March.

Habitat and geographical distribution:

The original homeland of pistachios is Central Asia, and its distribution extends from the Mediterranean Basin to Central Asia. It grows wild in Iran, Afghanistan, Uzbekistan and Iraq. The cultivation of commercial varieties of the species has spread to many areas of southern Europe, the Levant and the Caspian Sea. It is currently also cultivated in California and in some Mediterranean countries, such as Greece and Italy. The most important countries producing pistachios are Iran, the United States and Turkey.

History and heritage:

The scientific name of the genus is mentioned previously (from the Greek word pistake, which is most likely derived from a corruption of the Persian word "pistachio"), while the species name vera means "true." The species p. vera is the only species cultivated commercially, and the rest of the species are mostly used as rootstocks.

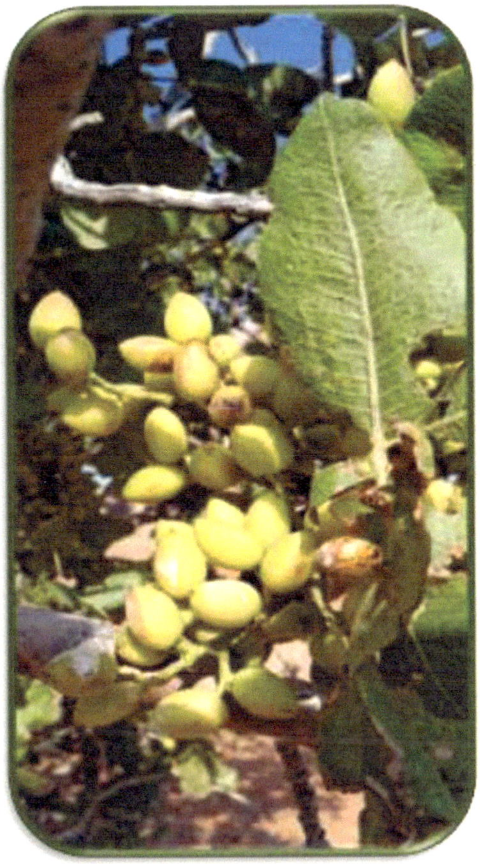

Chemical components:

Pistachios contain antioxidant compounds, proteins, starch, oils, cellulose fibers, and minerals . Phosphorus, potassium, and sodium. They are also rich in vitamins A and B.

The leaves and fruits contain monoterpene hydrocarbon compounds, alpha-pinene, limonene, alpha-terpinolene, and osimene.

The resin oil contains monoterpene compounds that are antibacterial, the most important of which are: camphene, limonene, and carvacrol.

It also contains diterpene compounds Abietadiene and abietatriene. The seeds contain (Edible part) Phenolic compounds, the most important of which are: gallic acid, catechin, epicatechin, gallic acid methyl ester and phenolic fats, the most important of which are cardanol compounds and flavonoid compounds (quercetin and rutinose). It should be noted that the flavonoid content decreases during fruit ripening.

The seeds contain fixed oil, 50-60% of their dry weight, which is rich in unsaturated fatty acids 73% (the most important of which are oleic acid, linoleic acid), and also contain other fatty acids, the most important of which are: linolenic, palmitic, palmitoleic, myristic, eicosanoic, behenic, lignoceric, arachidonic, and margaric acid. The most abundant sterols in the fruits are beta-sitosterol, cafesterol, avenasterol, stigmasterol, brassicasterol, and cholesterol. Monoterpenes, diterpenes and triterpenes present in oleoresin are the most abundant compounds in the essential oil of various parts, and these compounds are associated with anti-inflammatory and antimicrobial effects. Naringenin, eriodyctyol, daizein, genistein, quercetin, kaempferol, apigenin, and luteolin were isolated from the fruit. The fruit also contains anthocyanin pigments, the most important of which are: quercetin-3-O-rutinoside, cyanidin-3-galactoside, Cyanidin-3-O-glucoside,

Properties and medical uses:

Pistachios help reduce the level of bad cholesterol (LDL) in the blood and prevent heart and blood vessel diseases. They also significantly reduce inflammation. Its fresh or roasted seeds have been used as food for a long time.

Different parts of pistachios have been used in traditional medicine as antihypertensives, digestive system, liver, urinary tract, and respiratory system disorders. Scientific results have also revealed its antioxidant, antimicrobial, antiviral, anticholinesterase, anti-inflammatory, antidiabetic, antitumor, hyperlipidemia, sclerosis, and liver activity effects, as well as its beneficial effects on digestive system disorders. The essential oil and gum extracted from pistachios showed antibacterial activity against various types of gram-positive and gram-negative bacteria. It was noted that alpha-pinene, verbenone, terpineol, linalool, carvacrol, and favone are the main antibacterial compounds, especially Helicobacter pylori. The seeds showed beneficial effects on the levels of HDL and LDL, which affect atherosclerosis. Pistachios can be considered a functional food, as it has been proven that pistachios contain different groups of valuable phytochemicals that have biological activities, the most important of which are anthocyanins, flavones and phenolic acids. Its fresh or roasted seeds have been used as food and in the food industry for a long time, in addition to being a delicious nut.

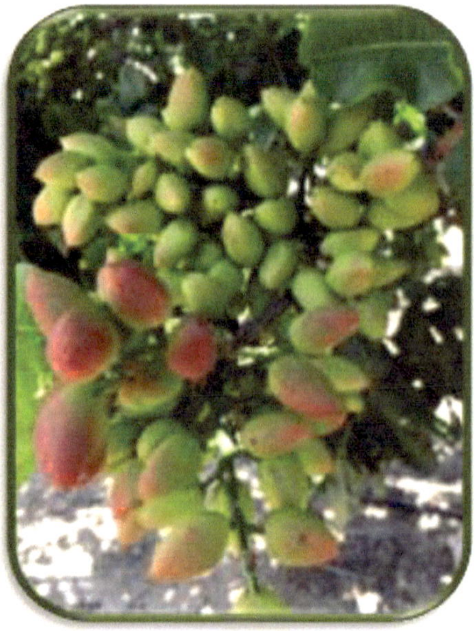

Environment:

Pistachio is a drought-tolerant, light-loving shrub that prefers areas with cold winters and long, hot, dry summers. Pistachio trees tolerate frost periods during winter and spring. It grows in different types of soils, and is found in low-salinity, highly fertile and porous soils with good drainage. It is successfully cultivated in areas with an annual rainfall of 200-400 mm, on rocky and limestone hills and plateaus. Pistachios tolerate high levels of alkalinity (pH=7.7-8.5).

Cultivation and productivity:

Pistachios are propagated by seeds in order to obtain rootstocks for grafting or afforestation, while they are propagated vegetatively by grafting for fruit production. They can also be propagated by layering. Good seeds are taken from the new crop and are laid out for a short period if their shells are not cracked. As for those whose shells are cracked, it is sufficient to soak them in water for two days before planting. Cultivation. Seeds are planted in the nursery in lines 120 cm wide and at 20 cm distances inside the line. The seedlings are transferred to the permanent land after a year or two, and grafting is done before or after the transfer, by grafting with a pen, and the seedlings can be grafted with a ring or shield bud.

The method of cultivation in the permanent land depends on the variety, soil fertility and the purpose of cultivation, as the cultivation distances are less in case of desire to obtain resinous oil Including in case of desire to obtain fruits or fruits and oil together, as these distances differ according to the varieties and fertility of the soil. Pistachios do not need irrigation except in the first years, as they are irrigated once a month until the third year. Pistachios respond to moderate fertilization with basic elements, especially nitrogen. Production begins after 8 years of planting, and increases gradually until the age of 25 years, and it is generally a perennial species. One tree produces 15-30 kg of fruits annually, and one ton of leaves and stems produces 15-18 kg of raw resinous oil.

Rhus coriaria L.

Rhus heterophylla C.C.Gmel., *Rhus sumac* O.Targ.Tozz., *Rhus variifolia* DC. *Toxicodendron coriaria* (L.) Kuntze., *Rhus amoena* Salisb.

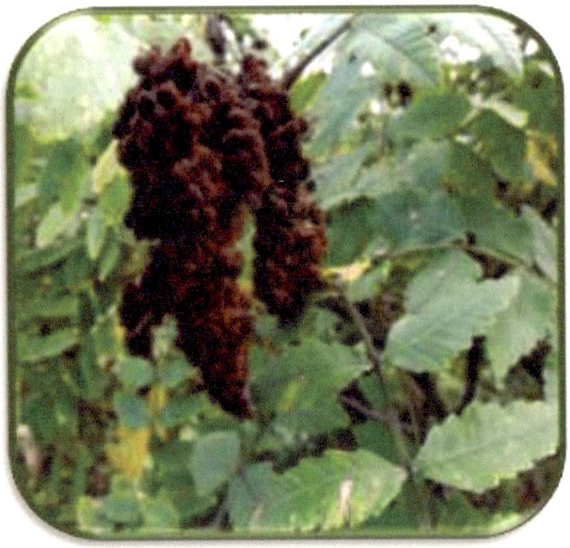

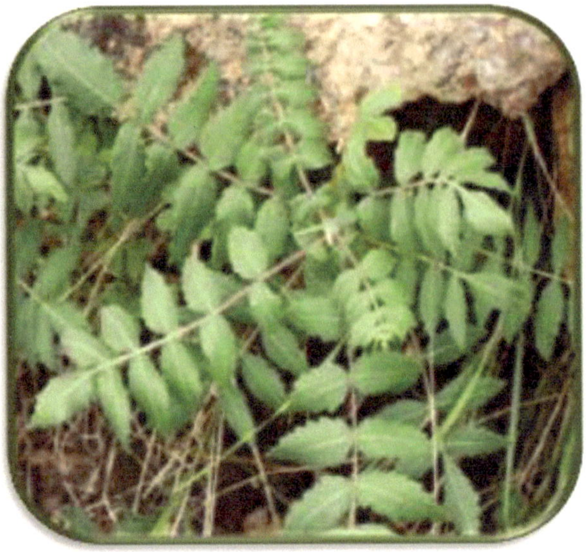

Family: Anacardiaceae

Common names: Sumac, vinegar sumac, tanners' sumac, damkh, tamtam,

Foreign names: corroyeurs de Sumac Fr. Sumach, Eng.

Occurrences :13,265 occurrences

Distribution in the world

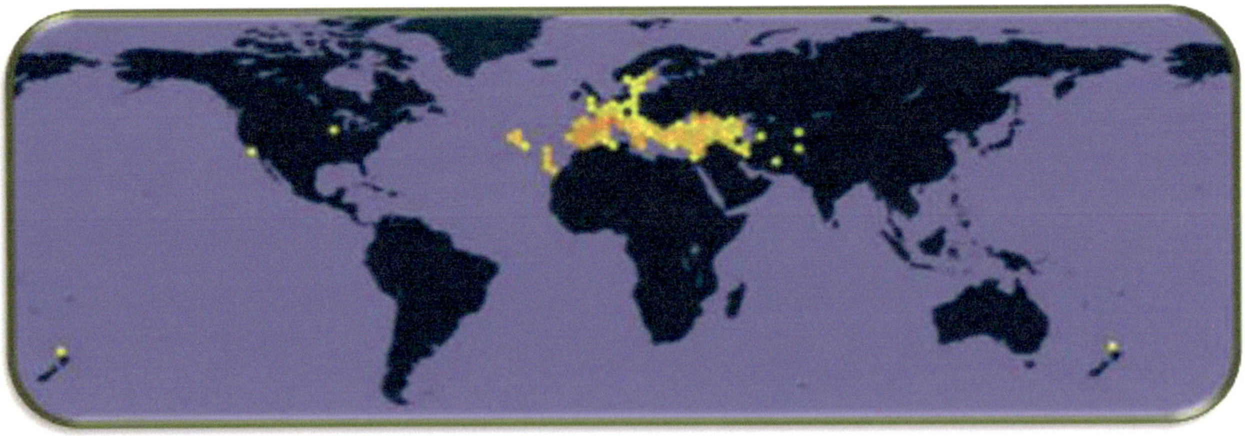

Botanical description:

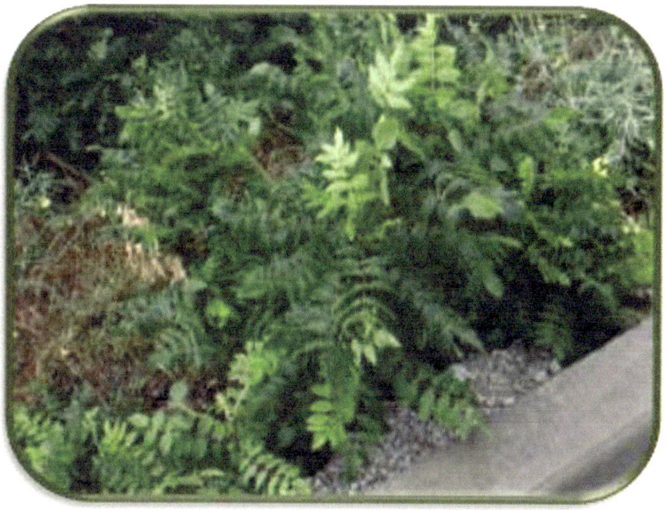

Shrubs or trees, Hybrid. Leaves 5-7 pairs, 2-4 cm long, 0.7-2 cm wide, petiole, oblong to general, pinnately compound Fluffy on both sides. Inflorescence paniculate, terminal or axillary Oval, acute or blunt-topped, serrated margin, Position, densely flowered. Flower 3-4 mm, unisexual or hermaphrodite, greenish to white. Calyx 5-lobed, hairy. 5. The stamens are twice as long as the calyx, white, ovate. 5. The fruit is 4-6 mm, spherical Villi bearing glandular hairs. To kidney-shaped, brown in color,

Flowering: April to May.

Habitat and geographical distribution:

Iranian-Turanian, Mediterranean, widely distributed in Syria, Lebanon, Jordan, Palestine and Turkey. The most important types of sumac spread in the Mediterranean basin: Rhus coriaria L., Rhus cotinus L., Rhus tripartita

History and heritage:

The scientific name of the genus Rhus is derived from the ancient Greek "rhous", which is the ancient name for sumac, while the descriptive name for the species coriaria goes back to its use in tanning, as the Latin word corium means "skin." The ripe fruits were well known to Europeans since the time of the ancient Romans, who liked their acidity and used them in vinegar like lemons today.

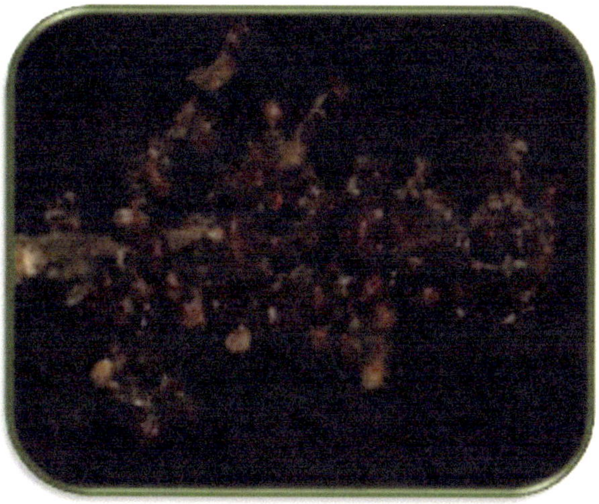

Part used: Fruits and leaves.

Chemical components:

The leaves contain phenolic compounds, the most important of which are: tannins, which constitute 25-33% of the dry weight, and consist of tannins of gallic acid at a rate of 15% and tannins of gallic acid, in addition to flavonoid compounds: myricuitrine, kaempferol, quercetin, myricetin.

The fruits contain phenolic compounds, the most important of which are: - flavonoid compounds, including: kaenpferol, quercetien, myricetin, and tannines, the most important of which is tannic acid or gallic acid and flavonoid compounds Anthocyanidin, including: delphinidin, petunidin, peonidin, cyanidin.Organic acids, including malic and citric acids, etc.

Properties and medical uses:

Sumac fruits have antioxidant properties due to the phenolic compounds (tannins) they contain, which contribute to protecting the liver from toxins, and are antibacterial and antiviral.

Tanins generally have astringent, antiseptic and anti-inflammatory properties, and are used to treat inflammation of the digestive system.

Experiments on laboratory rats have shown the properties of the fruits that reduce sugar, and help stop urinary incontinence, The extract of the leaves protects the heart and arteries. It is used popularly as a soak Experiments on rabbits have shown the effect of sumac fruits topically in the form of gargles to treat inflammation of the membranes of the mouth and throat and laryngitis, and is used in the form of solutions or ointments to treat burns and skin ulcers, and is also used to treat acute diarrhea. The decoction of sumac barks is used topically to treat skin fungi, and as a gargle to get rid of laryngitis. Sumac is used in homeopathy to treat weak bladder problems. Sumac solutions (tannin) are given in cases of poisoning by alkaloids and heavy metal salts.

Food uses:

The fruits are used as a popular appetizing spice, and sumac is added to some Arab dishes.Different parts of the plant are used.Dyes can be made in different colors: red, yellow, black and brown. The oil extracted from the seeds can be used to make candles.

Other uses: The tannins separated from the leaves are used in tanning leather.

Environment:

It grows in different types of soils, especially in the red Mediterranean soil (terra rossa), yellow, and clayey sandy, and it tolerates lime and soil salinity. Sumac is a shrub with strong roots that penetrate the soil and spread quickly, so it can be used to stabilize the soil in sloping and rocky lands and valleys, but it can compete with fruit trees if planted next to it, and it becomes difficult to get rid of it when it spreads in a certain area.

Cultivation and productivity:

Sumac plants are propagated by seeds or root or vegetative cuttings. The seeds retain their vitality for a year or more, and are generally difficult to germinate due to the infection of their sap and the dormancy of their embryos, so it is necessary to mechanically or chemically scarify the seed coat, and then stratify it in moist sand for 24 hours. The treated and stratified seeds are planted directly in plastic bags at a rate of 3 seeds per bag in late winter and early spring, and they germinate within one to two weeks. The germination rate is sometimes weak, due to the presence of empty seeds. The seedlings are transferred to the permanent ground at the age of 6-12 months at the end of winter and the beginning of spring, and they can be transferred throughout the year if irrigation water is available, while preserving their long roots. The seedlings need light and weeding. The plant blooms at the beginning of summer and its fruits ripen in August and September. Seeds are collected when they turn brown in autumn from trees 4-5 years old. This is done by cutting the fruit clusters, spreading them out and drying them under the sun. Then the fruit covering (the bark) is removed by pounding the dry fruits or rubbing them on a sieve.

Ammi majus L.

Ammi majus var. genuinum Gren. & Godr., *Apium ammi* Crantz., *Carum majus*) L.(Ko- so-Pol., *Visnaga major*)L.(J.Vick

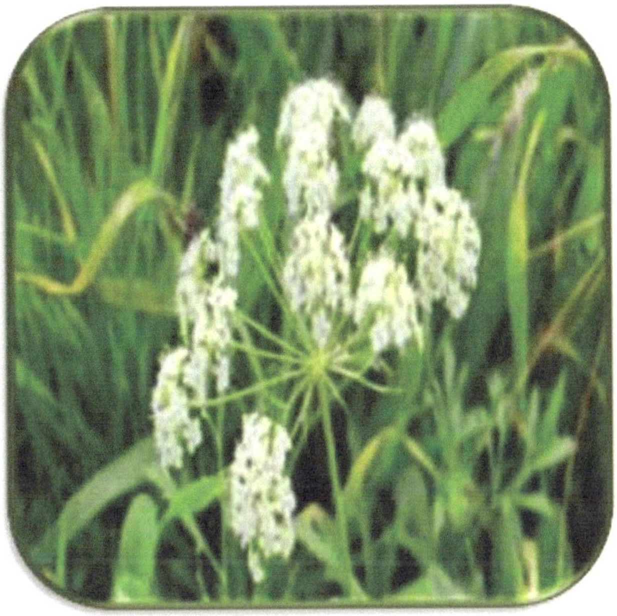 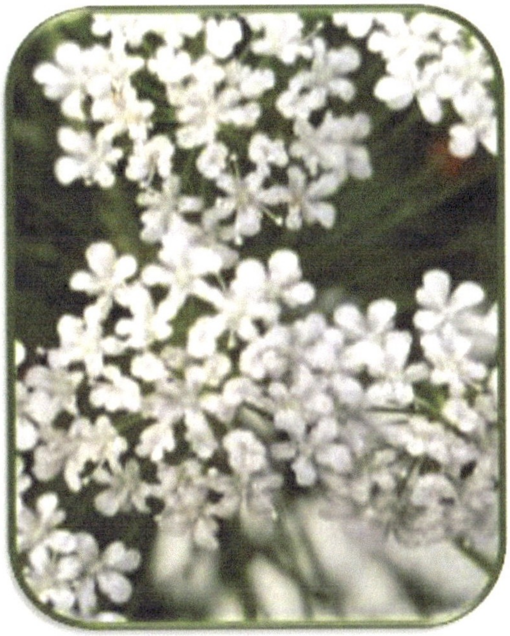

Family: Apiaceae

Common names: Devil's pickle.

Foreign names:Eng. Common Bishop, Fr. Ammi des boutiques

Occurrences :20,939 occurrences

Distribution in the world

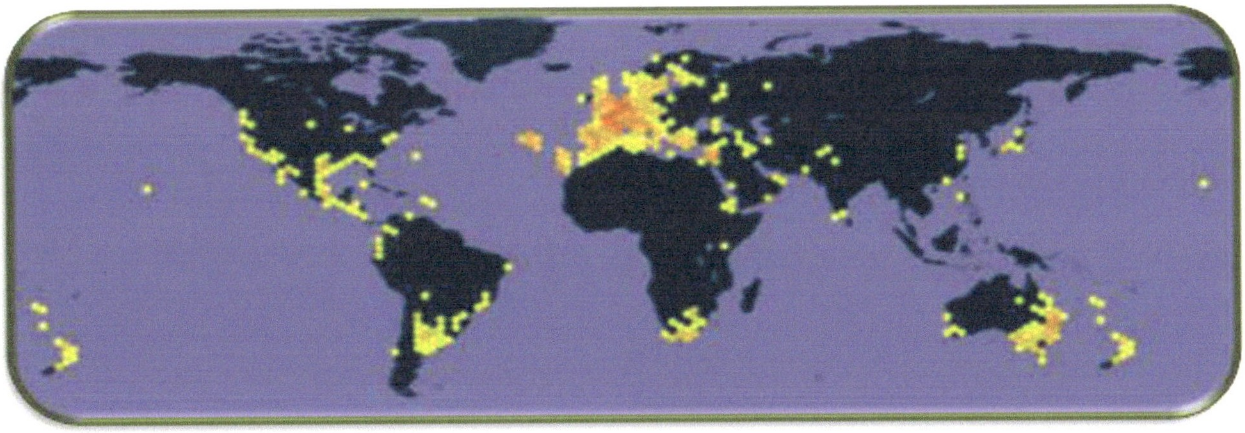

Botanical description:

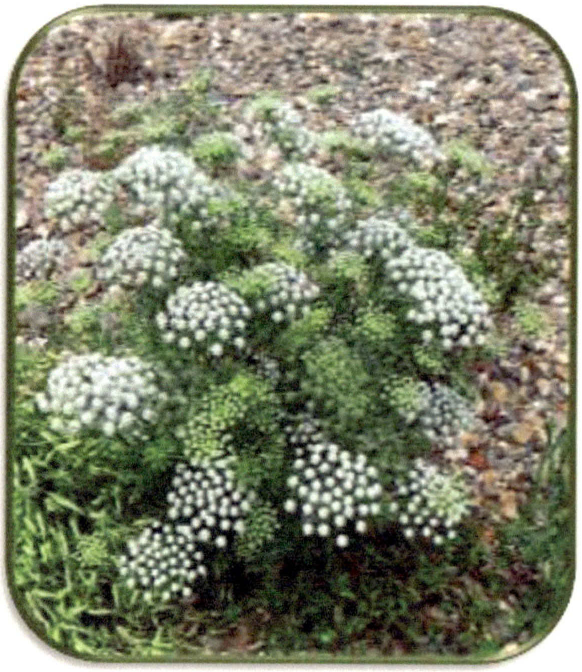

An annual herb, glabrous, 30-70 cm tall. Stems erect, highly branched, especially at the top, tough, notched. Leaves up to 10 cm long or more, ovate in general shape, green to bluish green in color. Lower leaves long-pinnate, tripartite, deeply divided into oblong to linear lobes, serrated margin. Upper leaves less divided. The compound tent is tall and pubescent, reaching a diameter of about 10 cm.

Flowering: March to August.

Habitat and geographical distribution: Nile basin (Egypt and Sudan), Mediterranean basin (Syria, Morocco, Algeria, Libya.)

History and heritage: The scientific name comes from the Greek for an unidentified oriental plant, a genus of the Apiaceae family. Ibn al-Baytar used the plant of Khalla in the treatment of vitiligo in the thirteenth century, and mentioned it in his book "Mufradat al-Adwiyya" under the name of Astral, which is the raven's foot, the devil's root, and the devil's Khalla. A Berber word meaning "bird's foot", and is known in Egypt as As for Galen, he called it Amir. One of the tribes in the Maghreb knew its benefits for vitiligo, and its members used to sell the medicine to vitiligo patients, but they kept it secret. It is worth noting that the ancient Egyptians were the first to talk about vitiligo in the Ebers Papyrus.

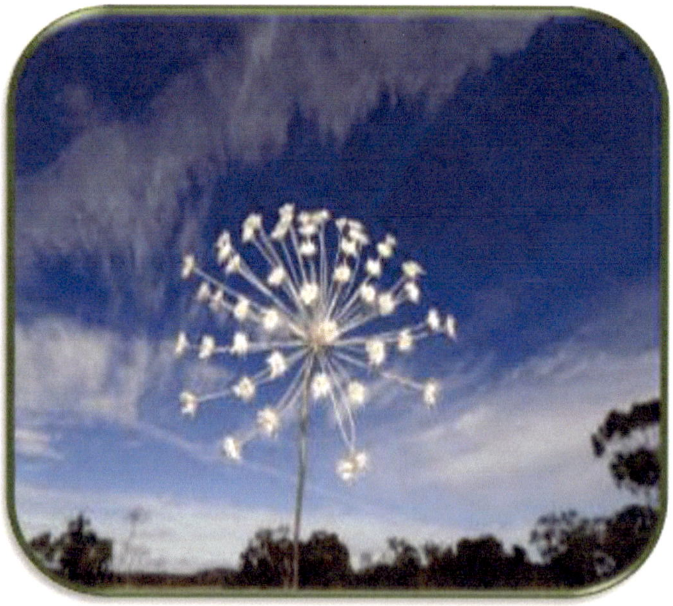

Part used: Ripped fruits, collected in late summer.

Chemical components:

The fruits contain coumarins and coumarin glycosides 1%, ammoidin 5% (xanthotoxin), ammidin 0.3%, majudin 0.01% (bergapten). It also contains biologically active compounds such as furanocoumarin and flavonoids. The devil's thorn does not contain the khellin compound.Three new types of coumarin have been isolated from the aerial parts of the thorn, including pyranocumarin.

Properties and medical uses:

Devil's trumpet seed preparations are used topically in the form of creams with caution in cases of skin spots, leprosy, vitiligo, and psoriasis. After using the drug, one should be exposed to the sun for an hour or two daily.

A decoction or soak of the seeds is popularly used to relieve asthma attacks, lower blood sugar, digestive disorders, and expel gases.

The ethanolic extract of A. majus seeds showed hypolipidemic, anti-inflammatory, analgesic, and antipyretic activities.

Pharmaceutical forms:

Different pharmaceutical forms containing: meladinine, neo-meladinine, and can be in the form of tablets and ointments.

Use warnings:

Side effects were observed during use, the most important of which is kidney inflammation.

Environment:

The khella plant is a light-loving species, belonging to areas with a moderate winter. Grows on neutral to slightly alkaline soils.

Cultivation and productivity:

It is planted by seeds, at a rate of 4-5 kg/hectare, and the productivity of the khella ranges from 0.6 to 1.2 tons/hectare. During the growing season, it needs sufficient moisture, except during the flowering and fruit ripening period, because excess moisture reduces production.

Ammi visnaga (L.) Lam.

Visnaga daucoides Gaertn.

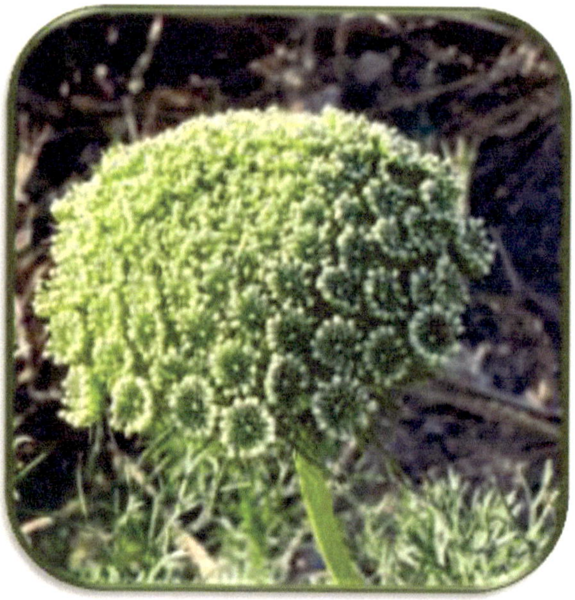

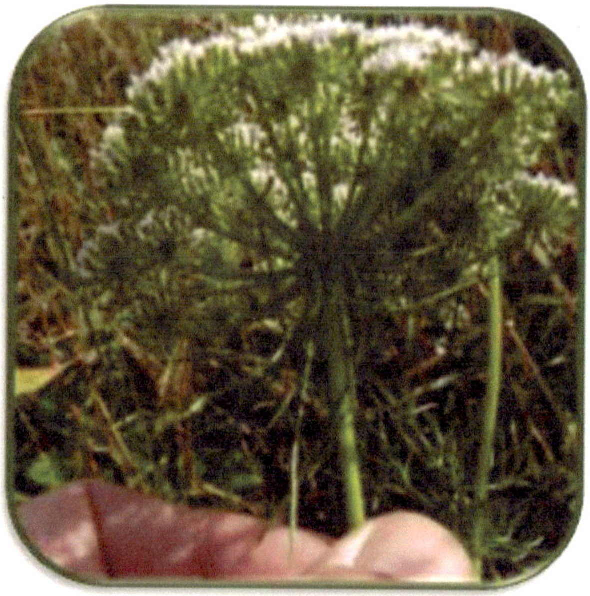

Family: Celery, Apiaceae

Common names: Khella, Khella local, Khella medicinal, Ethiopian cumin, Miswak herb.

Foreign names: Khella Fr. pick, Tooth Visnaga, Eng

Occurrences : 4,235 occurrences

Distribution in the world

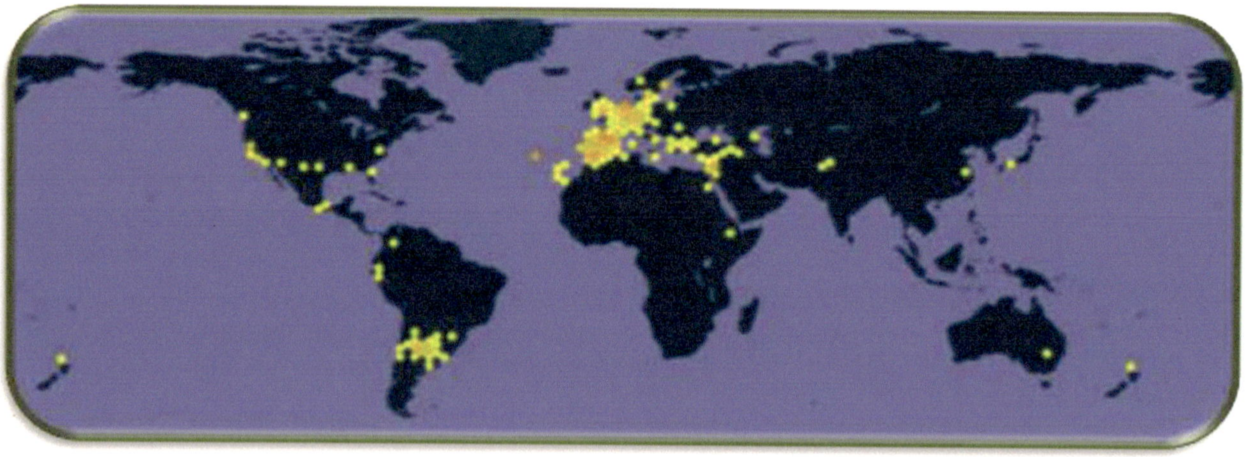

Botanical description:

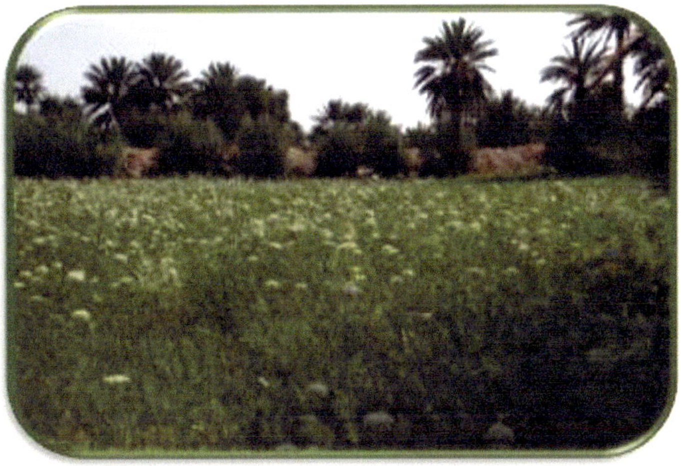

Annual herb, glabrous, 50-100 cm tall. Stems erect, branched, notched. Leaves are oval in general shape, basal compound pinnate, stem bi- or triply pinnately divided, leaf blade parts linear to filiform, entire (not serrated), branched dichotomously, length 1-3 cm × 0.5-1 mm. Flowers are white, gathered in terminal, long-stalked, flattened, umbels when flowers open, 3-13 cm in diameter, then shrink when fruiting and their stalks harden. The length of the outer inflorescence stalks is 3-7 cm. The bracts of the compound inflorescence are as long as the stalks or longer, deeply divided into threadlike lobes, which later hang down. The bracts of the simple umbels are complete. The flower stalks are longer than the flowers and the fruits. The petals are equal in size. The stalks are long, set back. The fruit inflorescence is compact,semi-spherical, nest-like, opens in the presence of moisture after rain. The fruit is double acorn, about 2 mm long,ovate to oblong, glabrous, with thick ribs.

Flowering: April to August.

Homeland and geographical distribution:

Mediterranean basin, Middle East and North Africa (Nile Basin, Egypt and Sudan), extending to the western Iranian-Turanian region, grown in Mediterranean countries, especially in Egypt and Morocco, and also grown in some areas of North America.

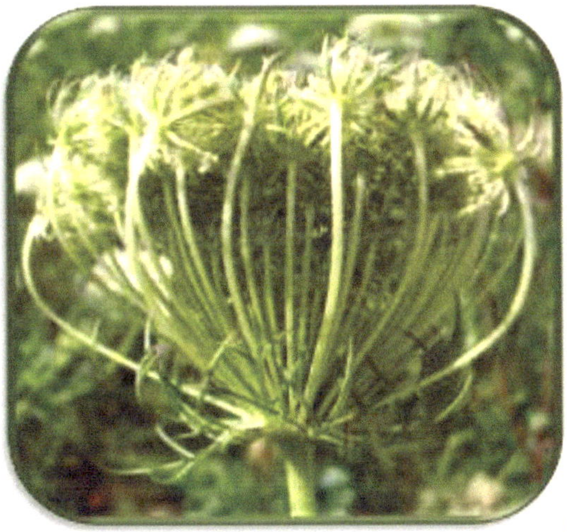

History and heritage:

Ammi is the Greek scientific name for an unidentified oriental plant, belonging to the Apiaceae family. The plant was mentioned in the books of Ibn al-Baytar and Ibn Sina as containing very bitter substances, which are useful in treating kidney colic. The khella was mentioned in the Egyptian Ebers Papyrus 1500 years before Christ for its benefits in treating diseases of the heart, respiratory and urinary systems (kidney stones). Tea prepared from the fruits of the local khella was traditionally used by kidney stone patients in Egypt. The local khella plant has been used in folk medicine by the inhabitants of the eastern Mediterranean since ancient times. The decoction of the fruits was used to treat renal colic among the ancient Egyptians, and to treat kidney inflammation in Iraq and Palestine, and to treat urinary retention and prostate pain in Algeria, and its use became widespread to the point that it was the most recommended species to treat urinary tract infections.

Part used: The fruits, collected before full ripeness in late summer, the volatile oil of the fruits.

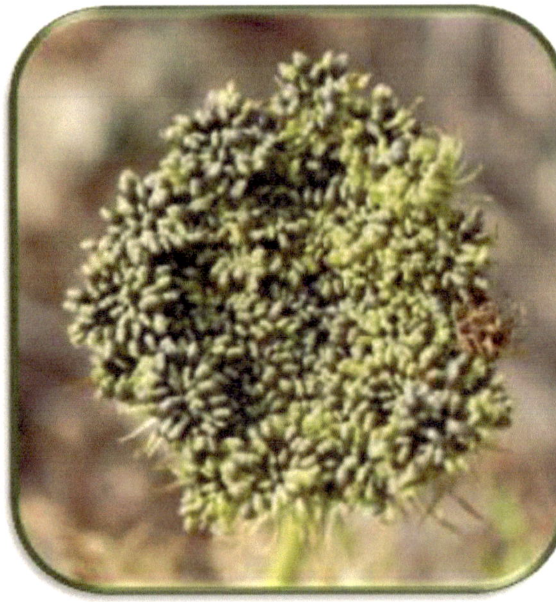

Chemical components:

The fruits contain: - Furanochromones compounds 2-4%, including khellin (visammin = 1%), visnagin 0.3 - 0.05%, khellol and its glycosides (khellinol, khellenin, ammiol). - Pyranocoumarins compounds (visnaganes) 0.2 - 0.5%, including visnadin, samidin and others. - Furanocoumarins, including traces of xanthotoxin. - Favonoids 0.02 - 0.03%, including quercetin, kaempferol and sorhamnetin. - Fixed fatty oil 12-18%, proteins 14%. Volatile oil 0.02 - 0.03% rich in 2-methylbutyle methyl butanoate. -

Medical properties and uses:

The compounds of khellin, visnadine and visnagen stimulate the work of the heart muscle and strengthen its perfusion by expanding the coronary vessels (coronary vasodilator). It has been used The drug was until recently used to treat angina pectoris, heart failure and tachycardia. The compounds in the fruits of the local khella, especially khellain, are known for their antispasmodic effect that works to relax the muscles. Smooth throughout the body, the fruits of the khella are used to relieve whooping cough attacks, bronchial asthma, bronchitis, and calm stomach and intestinal disorders.

Khellan, visnagen, and khella glycoside help increase the volume of urine output and treat urinary tract spasms resulting from the presence of kidney stones, as they work to relax the muscles of the ureter and expand it, facilitating the passage of small kidney and ureter stones, and reducing the pain of their irritation of the ureter. The plant's properties show an antibacterial effect against gram-positive bacteria. The volatile oil of the khella is popularly used as an antispasmodic, and is used in cases of asthma and renal colic, and is also used externally to treat many skin diseases. The fruits and their main components (khellan and physnagin) have shown beneficial effects on kidney stones caused by hyperoxaluria in male rats by reducing the occurrence of calcium oxalate crystal deposition and increasing urine excretion. Khaleen is commercially available in the form of tablets and ointments.

Side effects, interactions and precautions:

During the use of the drug, the skin becomes sensitive to sunlight (phototoxic), so exposure to sunlight should be avoided during the period of taking the drug, and it should not be used for a long period.

Research has shown that the use of khellin for a long period is not free of side effects manifested by the toxic accumulation of khellin in the body,which has limited its current use in America, which causes insomnia, nausea and vomiting, and may lead to To an increase in liver enzymes, But it is still popularly used in Mediterranean countries.

The local khella should not be used by patients who use blood thinners or vasodilators except after consulting a specialist doctor. Stagnation of bile secretion and jaundice may occur.

Other uses: The buds of the khella plant are used in many countries to clean teeth.

Environment:

The khella grows wild on heavy alluvial soils, on roadsides and swamps, and among Rocks, On neglected soils, and is suitable for dry, semi-dry and semi-humid climates, resistant to drought. Its vegetative and fruit production is high at low temperatures in winter (15-5 C) accompanied by high atmospheric humidity, as this leads to a clear increase in the content of the active substance in the plant. It is planted in all types of soils, Preferring fertile, sandy, yellow, well-drained soils, resistant to salinity. Suitable soil acidity 8.6-8.3 (pH)

Cultivation and productivity:

The plant is propagated by seeds that are planted during the fall, and it is also possible to plant in the spring, where the land prepared for cultivation is divided into basins or basins, and one hectare needs 4-7 kg of seeds.

Plants need to be separated when their length reaches 10-15 cm, and they need moisture (irrigation) at the beginning of the flowering season, noting that increased moisture during the flowering period affects Negatively in production. The plant responds to fertilization. The plant blooms at the beginning of summer, and the fruits and seeds ripen at the end of it. The plants are harvested in the early morning, dried under the sun for a week, then the fruits are separated, sieved and stored. The inflorescences of the khella are collected before the stage of full maturity, because its mature inflorescences are scattered, which causes loss of the crop. The productivity of the local khella from seeds reaches up to 1 ton/ha.

Anethum graveolens L.

Anethum arvense Salisb., *Angelica graveolens*)L.(Steud., *Ferula graveolens*)L.(Spreng., *Pastinaca graveolens*)L.(Bernh., *Peucedanum graveolens*)L.(Benth. & Hook.f. ex Hiern., *Selinum graveolens*)L.(Vest.

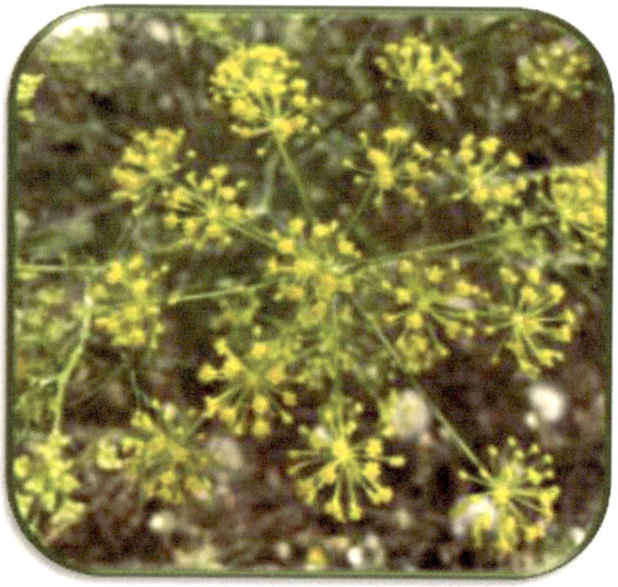

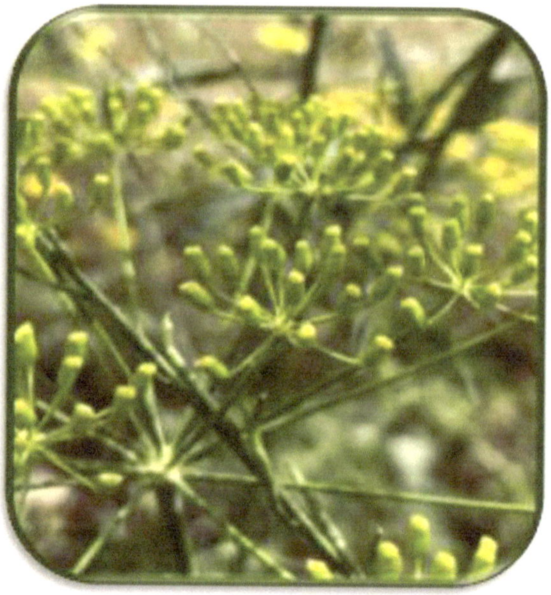

Anethum graveolens L. Anethum arvense Salisb., Angelica graveolens (L.) Steud., Ferula graveolens (L.) Spreng., Pastinaca graveolens (L.) Bernh., Peucedanum graveolens (L.) Benth. & Hook.f. ex Hiern., Selinum graveolens (L.) Vest.

Occurrences :13,710 occurrences

Distribution in the world

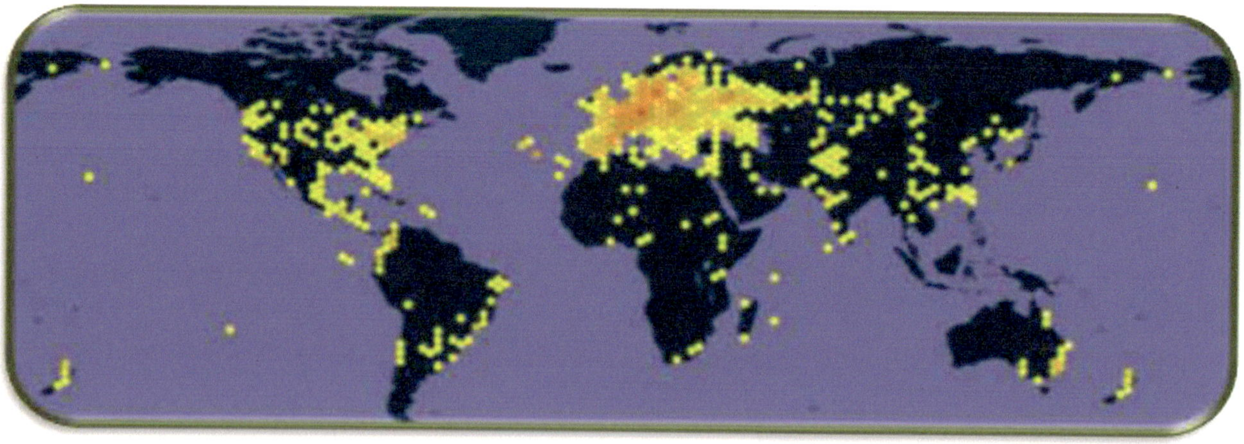

Botanical description:

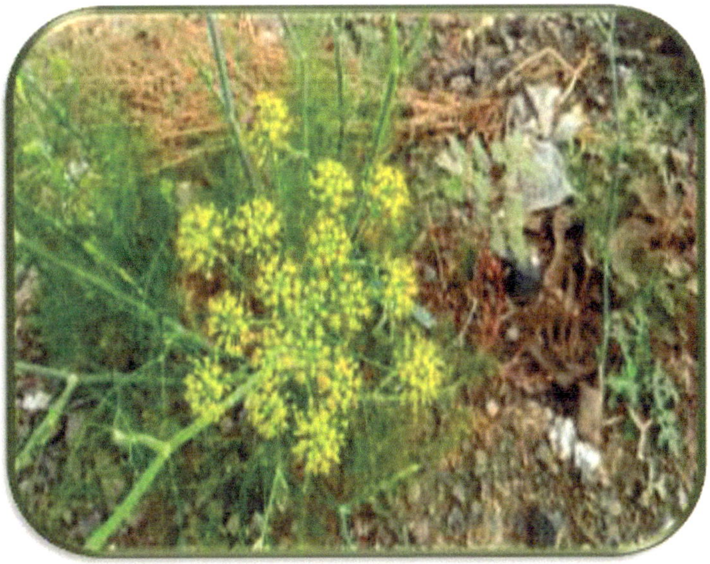

An annual herb, with a strong aromatic smell, tending to bluish-green in color, glabrous, 30-60 cm long. Stems are erect, branched from above. Leaves are oval to oblong in general shape, 10-30 cm long, pinnately divided into 3-4, lower leaves are oblique, upper leaves have a broad sheath, membranous margin, and fine thread-like lobes, ending in a hard hair. The compound umbel inflorescence contains 15-30 rays, almost equal, each 3-7 cm long. Bracts absent, either at the level of the compound or simple umbel. The calyx is absent. Corolla 5-petaled, yellow, almost rounded, notched at the apex. Stamens 5. The stylopedes are conical-compressed, the stigmas are short, erect at flowering time, bending downwards later. The fruit is biconical, compressed, 3-6 mm long, elliptical, the ribs are prominent, and the edge of the rib is winged.

Flowering: From April to June.

Habitat and geographical distribution:

Its original habitat is believed to be the countries of southwest Asia. It is widespread in southern Europe and the countries of the Mediterranean basin. It is cultivated in the countries of eastern Europe, central Asia and Egypt.

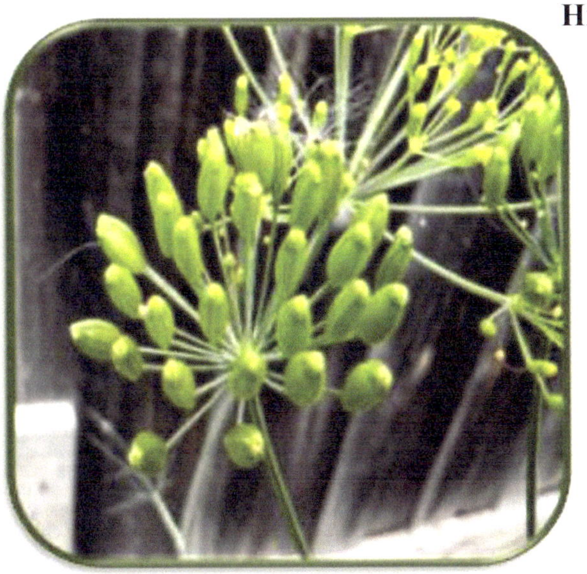

History and heritage:

Anethum from Anisum, which is dill, false anise, false anise, and the origin of the scientific name is from Greek. The name of the species graveolens means its taste, which is similar to the taste of spices. It has been used for centuries in traditional Asian medicine. Al-Antaki mentioned it in his Tadhkirat: "Dill with honey is useful for crippling diseases such as hemorrhoids, and it is specifically used to treat the reproductive organs. Sitting in its decoction cleanses the womb of all diseases, and its juice dissolves ear diseases in drops, and its oil cooked in it dissolves fatigue and all cold pain such as numbness and paralysis."

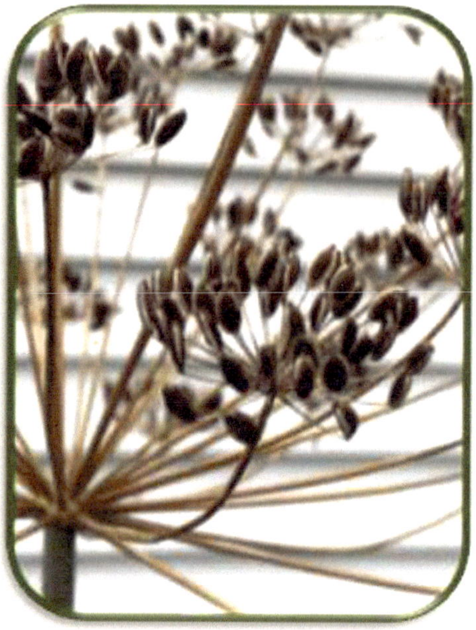

Part used:

The fruits and the green group, and are characterized by their aromatic smell. For its taste that resembles the taste of caraway.

Chemical components:

The fruits contain volatile oil, the percentage of which reaches 4%, containing about 63% carvone, in addition to apiol and myrsticine, and the seeds contain an essential oil rich in carvone, limonene, and trans-anitole, In addition to phenols and flavonoids.

Properties and medical uses:

Dill is used to treat digestive disorders, expel gases, and as a flavoring in grip's water. Boiled fruits are popularly used to treat respiratory disorders, insomnia, muscle spasms, digestive problems (improving digestion), stimulating milk production, hiccups, intestinal gas, stomach pain, improving appetite, and strengthening nails. Dill extract is also effective in thyroid function, and has beneficial effects on diabetes, cardiovascular disorders, hypolipidemia, and hypoglycemia. Recent studies have shown that dill is effective in treating hepatocellular carcinoma.

Pharmaceutical forms:

Dill is available in the form of dried fruits, distilled or concentrated dill water, or dill oil. It is sold under the trade names Mixture Barker's, Water Dill Concentrated, and others.

Warnings for use:

Dill should be avoided when following a low-salt (low-sodium) diet, because dill contains a large amount of sodium. Also, caution should be exercised when using dill if there is an allergy to other spices, because it can cause allergies.

Environment:

Prefers light, sandy or medium clay soils with good drainage, pH 7.8-5.3, loves moist soils, does not tolerate shade.

Cultivation and productivity:

The plant is propagated by seeds, which are scattered in lines 45-70 cm apart, on well-drained, light soil rich in organic matter. One hectare needs 25-30 kg of seeds. The plant is cultivated for its green leaves and seeds for food use.

Apium graveolens L.

Apium lusitanicum Mill., *Carum graveolens*)L.(Koso-Pol., *Celeri graveolens*) L.(Britton., *Helosciadium graveolens*)L.(Rojas Acosta., *Selinum graveolens*)L.(E.H.L.Krause., *Seseli graveolens*)L.(Scop., *Sium graveolens*)L.(Vest.

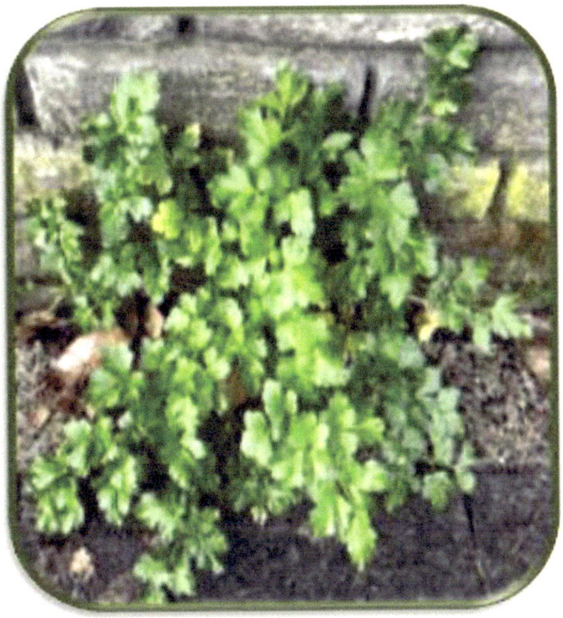
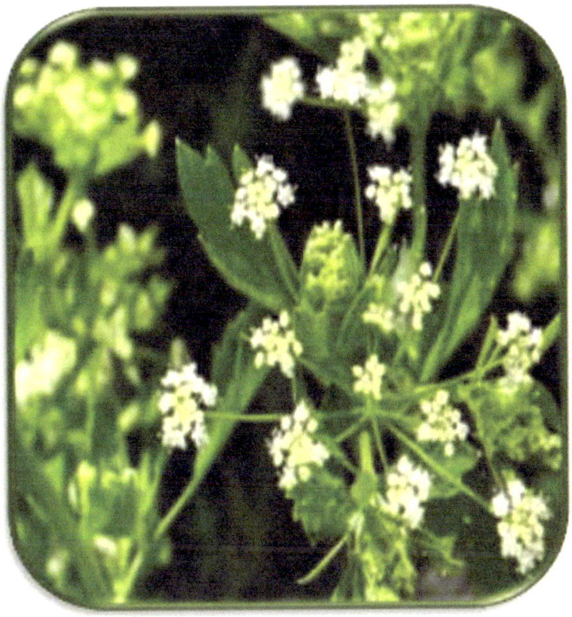

Family: Apiaceae

Common names: Wild celery. Fr. Celery, Ache odorante

Foreign names:

Occurrences :25,281 occurrences

Distribution in the world

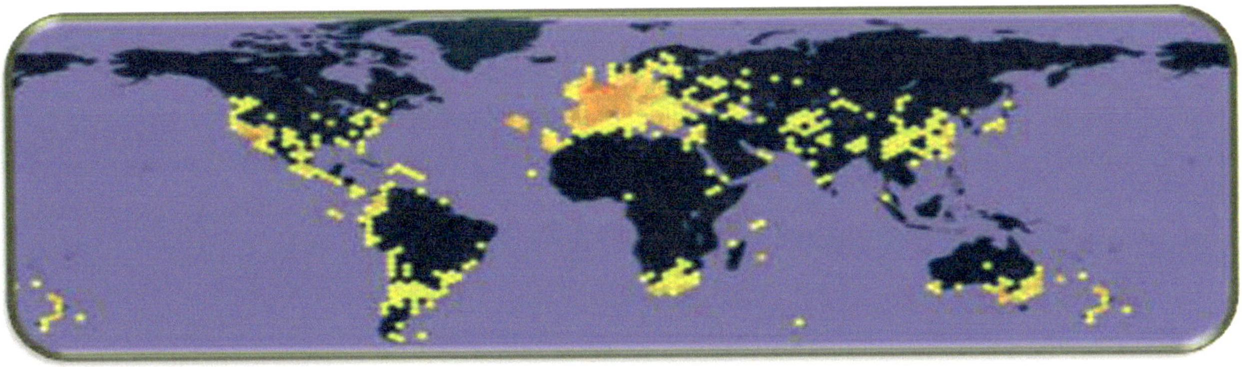

Botanical description:

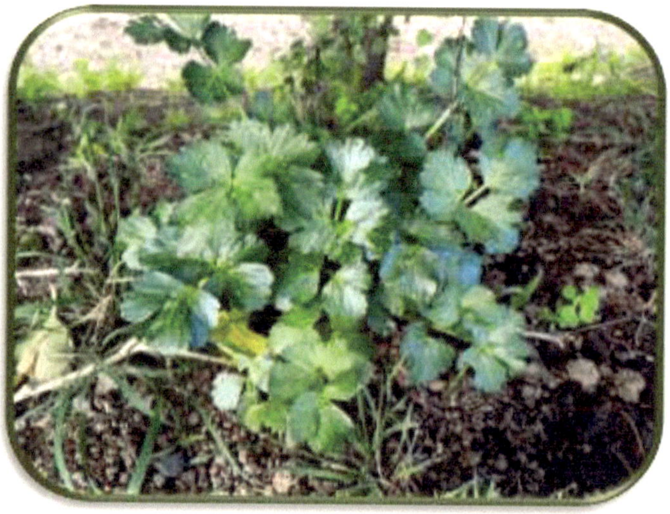

Annual or biennial herbaceous plant, glabrous, with a strong aromatic scent, 30-100 cm high, highly branched. Roots are spindle-shaped. Stems are erect or ascending, angularly notched, hollow, branched dichotomously. Leaves are somewhat fleshy, glossy, pinnately compound; The lower ones are obtuse, pentagonal, the leaflets are rhombic to triangular, the margin is serrated, the stalk is semi-palatine or palatine, its blade is three-parted, each part is rhombic to lanceolate. The flowers are small (5 mm), white, gathered in axillary, compound, umbelless, bractless, short-stalked or palatine inflorescences. The calyx is absent. The petioles are white or green to whitish, elliptic. The stems are longer than the pen foot. Fruits are double cylindrical, 2-×1.5 1.5 mm, fruiting bodies are spherical, fragrant, appear on old stems, have 5 prominent lobes.

Flowering: May to September.

Habitat and geographical distribution:

It is believed that the original homeland of celery is central and southern Europe, although it is found wild in Asia Minor band northern Africa. Several varieties are cultivated for food consumption in many regions of the world.

History and Heritage:

Celery A. graveolense, also known as the wild celery, is a long-standing name for other species of the Apiaceae family, such as Smyrnium olusatum (wild celery) and Sium latifolium (water celery).

Celery has been known as an important winter vegetable and medicinal plant for a long time, and historical documents indicate that the plant was used in Egyptian tombs. The Italians used it

The braids of the wild origin of celery were found dating back to 850 BC, and it was in the seventeenth century, and Nicholas Kleber mentioned in 1653 AD that it is "one of the herbs that are eaten in the spring to sweeten and purify the blood", and the Russians used it in the eighteenth century to increase the body's vitality and raise the ability to work. The plant was also used in folk medicine for kidney diseases and treating wounds.

Part used: Fruits (specific smell and slightly bitter taste), aerial herbaceous part (sweet aromatic taste, specific aromatic smell.)

Chemical components:

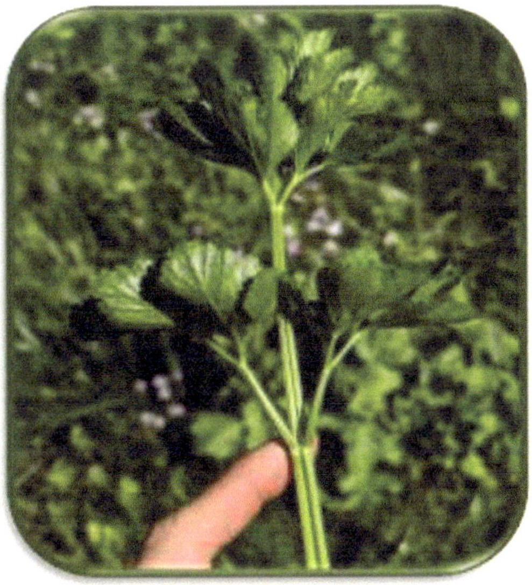

The fruits contain: 3% volatile oil, golden yellow to greenish yellow in color, and flavonoids, including apigenin, grvaebiosid B A, apinin, and isoquercetin. Coumarins, such as ber-gaptene, dihydrofurocoumarin, apoetin, sesquiolene, and silyroside, and a 29% yellow-green, slightly astringent, fatty oil containing petroselinic acid, in addition to linoleic and oleic acids, caffeic acid, coumaric acid, ferulic acid, luteolin, tannin, saponins, and campherol. Other phytochemicals of celery include carbohydrates and phenols, such as flavonoids, and alkaloids. The presence of compounds such as limonene, selenin, furanocoumarin glycosides, flavonoids, and vitamins A and C is the reason why celery is one of the most widely used plants in traditional medicine. The aerial part of the herb contains: volatile oil 0.8%, flavonoids, including apinengraffitopiside. In addition to coumarins, phenolic compounds, and steroids. It also contains vitamin C. Celery seeds contain 2% volatile oil, which is used in food seasonings, as well as in the perfume industry, and limonene and selenine constitute about 60% and 20% of the oil, respectively.

Properties and medical uses:

The fruits have diuretic, sedative and anticonvulsant properties, and the volatile oil has antibacterial and antifungal effects. The fruits are popularly used for their diuretic properties, and in treating kidney and bladder pain, gout and rheumatism. It is also used to treat nervous conditions, as an stomach tonic, a carminative, and a cough suppressant. The green parts are popularly used to reduce high blood pressure, treat arthritis, bronchitis, cough, asthma, fever, expel intestinal gases, aid digestion, treat liver and spleen disorders, soothe headaches, muscle and nervous spasms, allergies, amenorrhea, toothache, cleanse the urinary tract, urinary retention, and vomiting. Celery extracts have antioxidant properties and lower blood sugar and fats. Celery can also be used to treat some bacterial skin infections (MRSA) and psoriasis. Celery can protect against cardiovascular diseases, jaundice, liver diseases, and urinary tract obstruction. Gout and rheumatic disorders. Research conducted on rats shows that ethanol extracts from celery leaves increase sperm formation and improve their fertility.

Pharmaceutical forms:

Celery is available in the form of anti-rheumatic capsules, under the names of pain rheumatic lesurd, Cashets and others.

Side effects and warnings for use:

Allergic reactions such as laryngeal constriction, facial edema, skin rash, dermatitis, often increased by exposure to sunlight. Large doses may cause a slowdown in the activity of the nervous system, resulting in side effects such as dizziness. The plant should be avoided by pregnant or breastfeeding women. It is not given in case of kidney inflammation.

Other uses:

The green parts are used in cooking to flavor food, and in the manufacture of soap and chewing gum. The plant is included in diets because it is rich in fiber. Celery fruits are used in the manufacture of cosmetics as a hair fixative and in perfumes.

Environment:

Celery grows well in cold and moderately hot areas. It tolerates low temperatures ranging between 10 and 15°C during the vegetative growth period, and can withstand frost for short periods, while high temperatures lead to a decrease in the amount of leaves and oil. The plant grows in soils rich in organic matter, and does not tolerate acidity (pH), but tolerates relative soil salinity, and is a moisture lover.

Cultivation and productivity:

The plant is planted by seeds directly or by seedlings, at all times in warm areas, while in cold areas, planting is done after the end of winter. It is recommended before planting the seeds to soak them in warm water for 4 days in the presence of light if possible. The plant is watered at close intervals During green growth, and at intervals during flowering and fruiting, and basic fertilizers are added. The leaves are cut from the beginning of autumn until the end of winter.

A hectare needs 1.2 kg of seeds in the case of winter cultivation, and 2.4 kg when planting seeds directly. A hectare yields about 10 tons of fresh green grass before the flowering stage, and 25 tons of green fruiting in the milky ripening stage, and one ton of dry fruits. A ton of grass yields The fruit yields about 1.5-2 kg of oil, while one ton of dry fruits yields 13-15 kg of oil.

Carum carvi L.

Carum gracile Lindl.

Carum carvi var. *gracile*)Lindl.(H. Wolff., *Carum carvi* f. *carvi.*

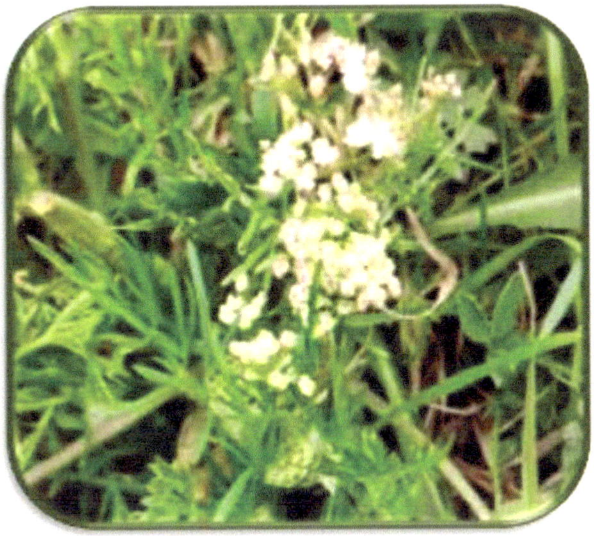

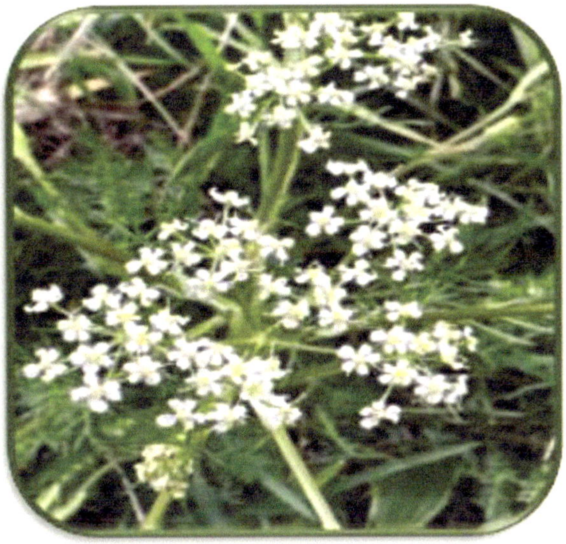

Family: Apiaceae

Common names: Caraway

Foreign names: Carvi Fr. Caraway, Eng.

Occurrences : 120,887 occurrences

Distribution in the world

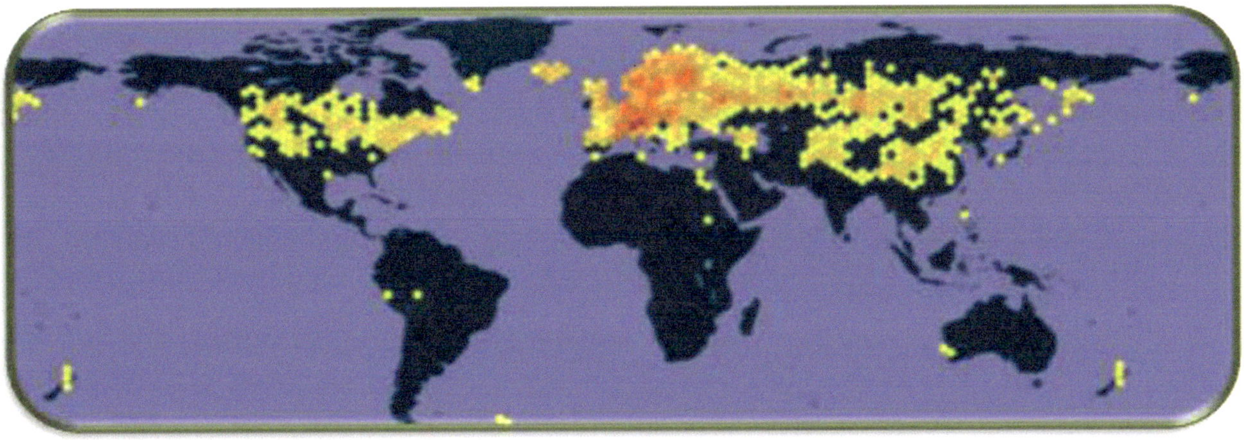

Botanical description:

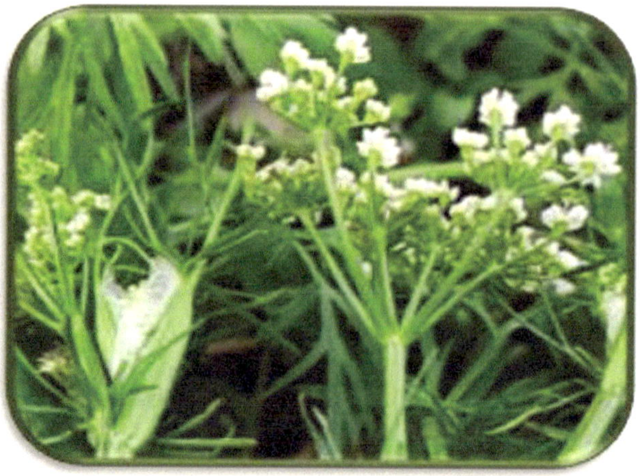

Annual or biennial plant, up to 1 m tall, glabrous. Stem is mostly simple, branching from above. Leaves are light green, compound, double pinnate, deeply divided, terminal lobes finely threadlike, 3-5 mm long, 1-2 mm wide, lower ones are obtuse, upper ones are flat, with a wide sheath with a white edge, forming the largest part of the blade. Compound umbel 3-6 cm wide, composed of 5-9 unequal rays (axes), bract 1-5 linear bracts, may be absent altogether. Bracts at simple umbel level minute or absent. Flowers small, white to pale pink. Calyx teeth indistinct. Corolla slightly blunt. The fruit is biconical, ovate to oblong, pointed at both ends, glabrous, yellowish to brown in color, 3-5 mm long, 1-2 mm wide, prominent tips.

Flowering: From May to July.

Habitat and geographical distribution:

It is widespread in central and northern Europe and some areas of the Mediterranean basin, and is also found in Asia in the Himalayas and Mongolia. The most important Arab countries that produce it are Morocco and Egypt.

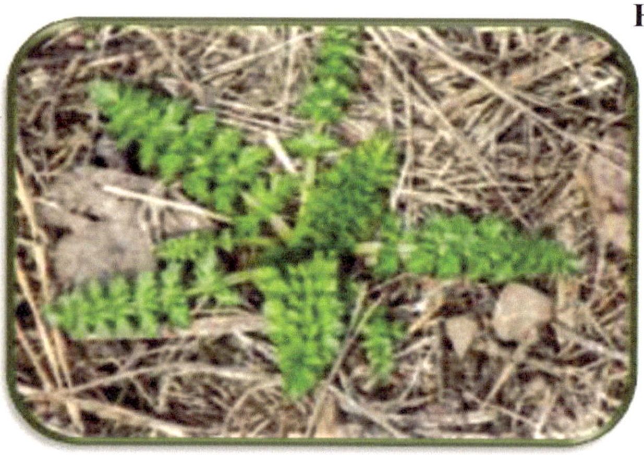

History and Heritage:

The scientific name is of Greek and Latin origin, and was formerly given to an unspecified aromatic plant from the Apiaceae family. This name applies to C. carvi. The word carvi is from the Greek karon, which is taken from the Arabic "caraway." References mention that the origin of the name for this genus is from the Arabic word "Qura'an" or "Ra's", which refers to the shape of the seed. It was cultivated in Asia Minor before the birth of Christ, and its medical benefits were known since the time of the ancient Egyptians.

Ancient manuscripts speak of Emperor Julius Caesar's use of caraway, and of his soldiers' food rich in it. The famous physician Dioscorides advised girls with pale faces to take caraway oil. Caraway was cultivated in Europe in the century 9th AD, and it was very popular and widespread. The Arabs used it to expel gases, and to treat colds and flu.

In Germany, it is used to flavor cheese, cabbage, soup, and bread, and in Norway and Sweden, black bread mixed with caraway is eaten in rural areas.

Part used: The ripe, dry fruit, and the volatile oil extracted from the fruit.

Chemical components:

Caraway fruits contain furocoumarins (antiviral compounds), and volatile oil 4-7%, the most important of which is carvone 40-60%, limonene, and α, β-Pinene. The remaining pulp after extracting the volatile oil contains 20% fatty oil, proteins, and polysaccharides. γ-Terpinene (37.2%) was identified as a major component of the oil, in addition to polyphenols and flavonoids.

Properties and medical uses:

Caraway fruits have volatile oil that has digestive properties, anti-gas and antispasmodic properties, anti-depressant, anti-anxiety effect, in addition to its antioxidant properties. Volatile oil and coumarin compounds also have properties that kill microbes such as pseudomonas bacteria, Bacillus, and some types of Candida fungi. The volatile oil is used topically to treat skin fungi. It is used in the composition of mouthwash and sterilization preparations. The aqueous extract and essential oil of caraway have anticonvulsant and diuretic properties. Caraway fruits are used as a flavoring in foods and drinks, and have various traditional uses in folk medicine. A decoction of the fruits is used in cases of flatulence, colic and stomach cramps in children. It strengthens the body and increases milk production in nursing mothers, and is also an emmenagogue. Caraway extracts are sometimes mixed with other medicines to add a pleasant flavor, as in the case of mixing them with laxatives.

Warnings for use:

Excessive consumption of caraway or use of its oil in large quantities and for a long period may lead to disturbances in the functions of the kidney and liver. Pregnant women should not use its volatile oil.

Food uses:

Caraway is used as an appetite stimulant, its fruits are used to prepare a nutritious hot drink, and its powder is used in the manufacture of sweets. It can be used frequently as preservatives in the food, cosmetics and pharmaceutical industries.

Environment:

The plant grows in dry meadows, on the sides of roads, and in mountainous areas. The optimum temperature for vegetative growth is between 10 and 20°C, while the suitable temperature for flowering and fruit formation is around -20-22°C. Sunny and dry weather leads to a decrease in the amount of volatile oil, while cool and humid weather increases the amount of oil. The plant grows well in calcareous, highly alkaline soils, and prefers well-drained silty soils. Heavy, fertile soils encourage vegetative growth at the expense of fruit growth. It tolerates high levels of alkalinity, and caraway cultivation succeeds in saline soils provided they are well-drained.

Cultivation and productivity:

The plant is propagated by seeds that are planted in the fall in temperate regions, and after the frost in cold regions. Cultivation is done in lines or in 5X4 m holes, at distances of 75X30 cm, with several seeds placed in one hole if the goal of cultivation is to obtain fruits. One hectare needs 10-15 kg of fresh and healthy seeds. It is necessary to irrigate the plants moderately and stop when the fruits are ripe. Fertilization with essential elements increases fruit production and the percentage of aromatic oil. One hectare yields about 1.5-2 tons of dried fruits.

Conium maculatum L.

Cicuta maculata)L.(Lam., *Cicuta major* Lam., *Cicuta oficinalis* Crantz., *Conium macu- latum* var. *barceloi* O. Bolòs & Vigo.

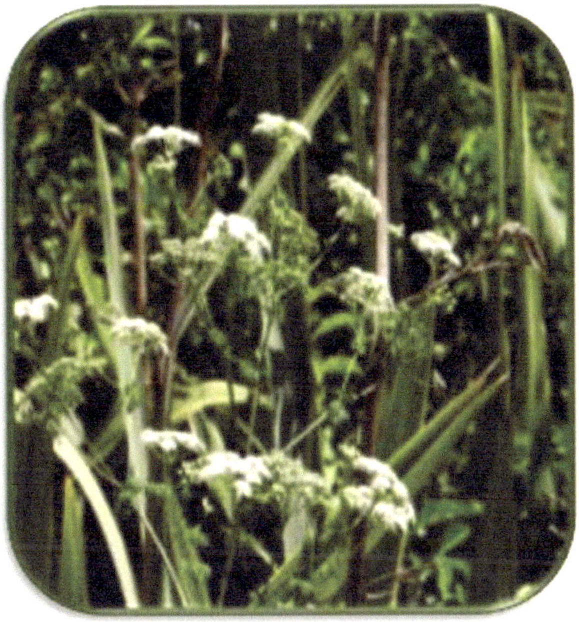

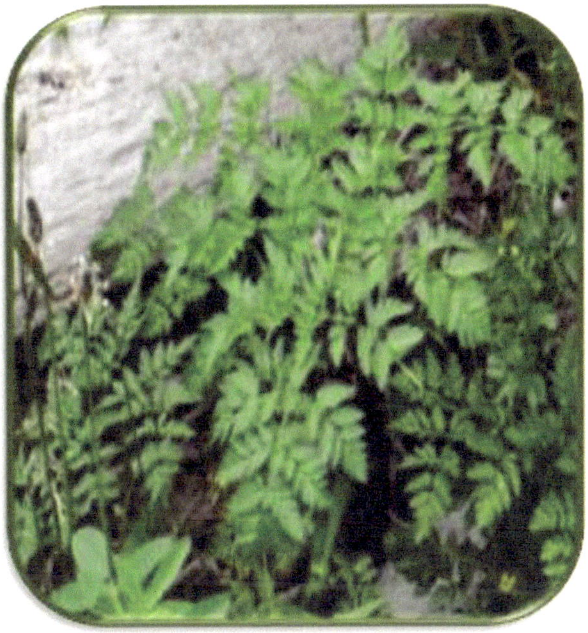

Family: Apiaceae

Common names: Hemlock, poison parsley

Foreign names: Cigue d'Athenes Fr. Hemlock, . Eng

Occurrences :111,170 occurrences

Distribution in the world

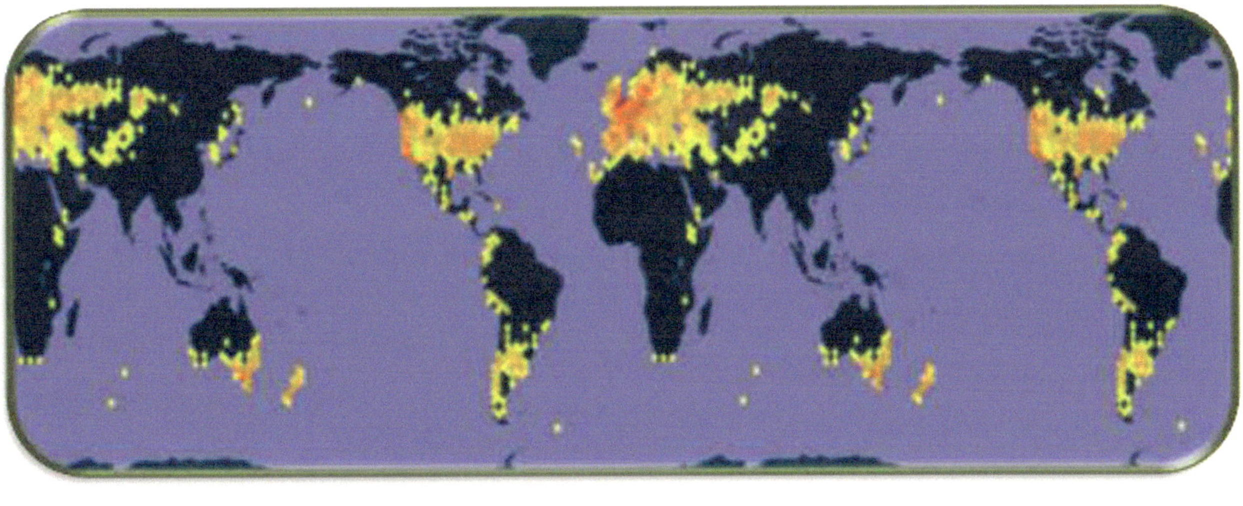

Botanical description:

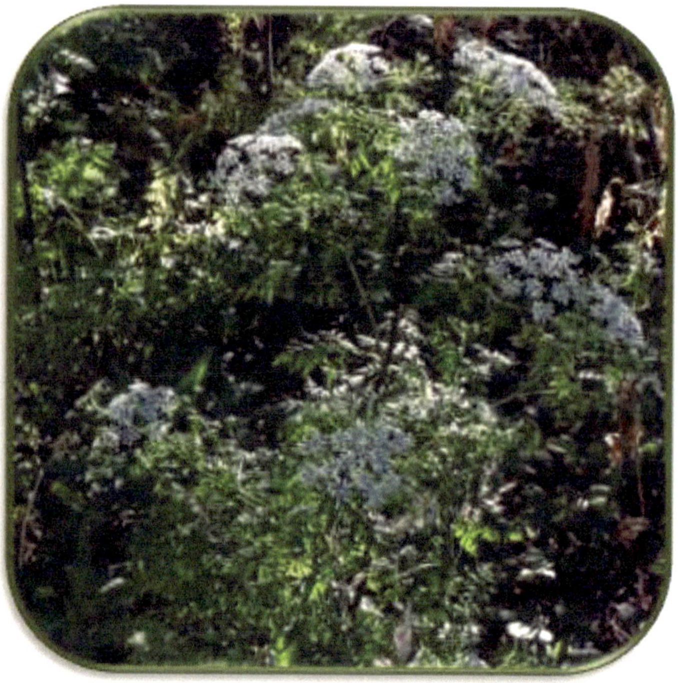

Biennial or perennial herb, 60-150 cm tall and sometimes more, glabrous. Roots are spindle- shaped. Stem erect, branched, especially at the top, hollow, notched, spotted. Branches are often opposite or sessile. Lower leaves arc 20-40 cm long, 5-10 cm wide, long-stalked, triangular in general shape, divided more than once (2-4 times) into oblong or oval-shaped lobes. Upper leaves semi-pinnate, compound, double pinnate, lobes linear. Inflorescence compound, opposite leaves, terminal, long-branched, consisting of 8-20 rays. Bracts 4-5, falling, lanceolate, pinnate. Simple bract bearing 12-20 rays. Bracts 3-6, 2-3 mm long, shorter than fruit bracts, unilateral. The fruit is a double nut, 2.5-2×4-3 mm, broadly oval, the fruit pods become arched when ripe, the ribs are very prominent and wavy.

Flowering: April to June. - Siberian and Mediterranean, extending to the Iranian-Turanian region.

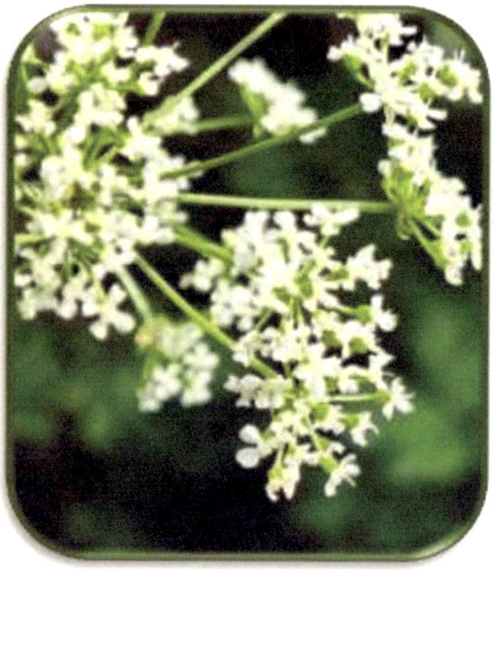

Habitat and geographical distribution: Europe

History and heritage:

The scientific name of the genus Conium is the ancient Greek and Latin name for the poisonous hemlock, while the species name maculatum means "stained with red." The toxicity of the plant has been known since ancient times, and the Greeks used it to execute criminals. It is said that the philosopher Socrates died by drinking hemlock juice in 399 BC.

Part used:

The herbaceous plant, flowering tops, and fruits.

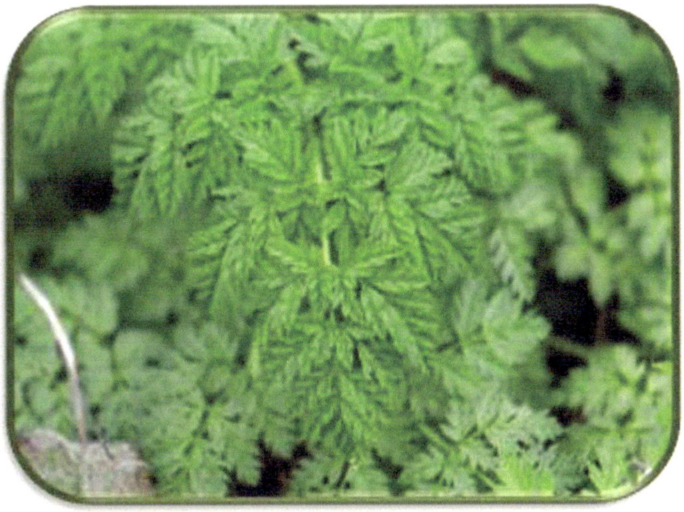

Chemical components:

The entire plant contains alkaloids belonging to the Piperidine group, reaching 2%, the most important of which are coniine = (cicutine), coniine methyl, coniceine, and conhydrine (toxic alkaloids). It also contains polynes, the most important of which are falcarinol, furanocoumarins, including bergaptene, and flavonoids, including diosmin. The fresh leaves and inflorescences contain a transparent, yellow aromatic oil with an unpleasant odor. The main component in the oils of flowers and leaves was germacrene D (27.2) and 41.0% respectively. In the oil of leaves, the compound β-ocimene was found, while in the oil of flowers, the compounds β-ocimene Z (14.3%) and β-myrcene (9.3%) were found. The oils of green leaves and flowers were characterized by the presence of volatile substances composed of unsaturated fatty acids, and those found in the oil of flowers. It may be an attractive factor for pollinators. Insecticides, and volatile alkaloids similar to the compound coniine in its chemical structure, for which hemlock is known for its toxicity.

Properties and medical uses:

A very toxic plant, not currently used, small doses of it cause a decrease in blood pressure and rapid breathing. It was previously used in folk medicine as a sedative, antispasmodic, and to treat coughs. It was also used topically to treat back pain, bruises, and lack of perfusion.

It is traditionally used to treat pain Weak rheumatism, stomach pain, peptic ulcer pain, nervousness, and insomnia. It has been used topically to treat back pain, bruises, and chronic peripheral ischemia. Conium maculatum extract is used as a traditional medicine for cervical cancer.

The alkaloid part of the plant has shown analgesic activity at a dose of 200 mg/kg, and also showed anti-inflammatory activity at a dose of 200 mg/kg. Hemlock essential oil can be used as a general antimicrobial.

Side effects and warnings:

It is not used during pregnancy. Taking high doses of it causes respiratory depression, back pain, tension, and then paralysis, and toxic doses cause burning of the mouth, drooling, visual disturbances, muscle weakness and other symptoms that end in death.

Environment:

It grows wild in meadows, wet places, near river banks, canals and irrigation channels, roadsides, agricultural fields and heavy lands in general.

Cultivation and productivity:

It is propagated by seeds, where planting is done by scattering in basins after mixing them with soil or sand at a rate of 1:4, to regulate their distribution or in lines at a rate of 60 cm between each line and 20-15 cm between holes. The seedlings are thinned when they reach a height of 5 cm. The plant requires regular irrigation during its growth period, and it responds well to fertilization

Coriandrum sativum L.

Coriandrum majus Gouan., *Coriandrum sativum* subsp. *indicum* Stolet., *Bifora loureiroi* Kostel., *Coriandropsis syriaca* H. Wolff.

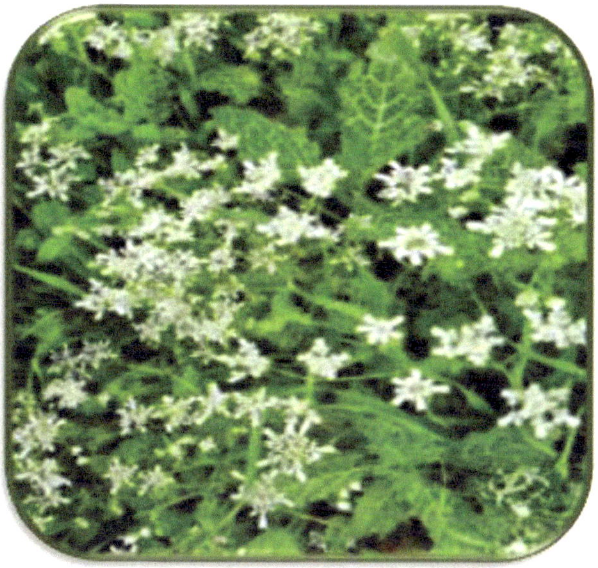

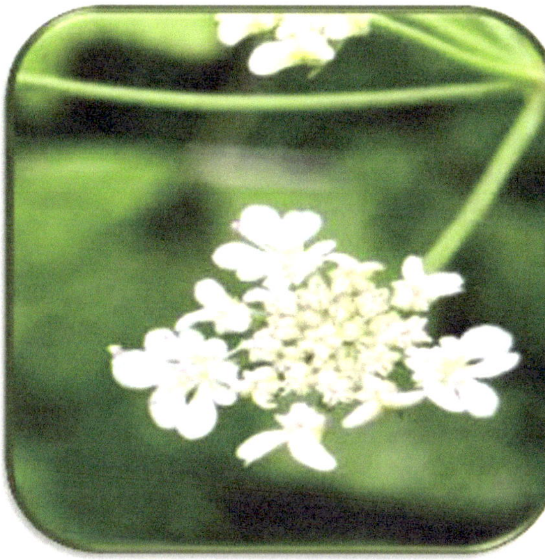

Family: Apiaceae

Common names: Coriander, Chinese parsley, Coriander, Coriander, Coriander

Foreign names: English Coriander, Fr. Coriander cultivé

Occurrences :16,847 occurrences

Distribution in the world

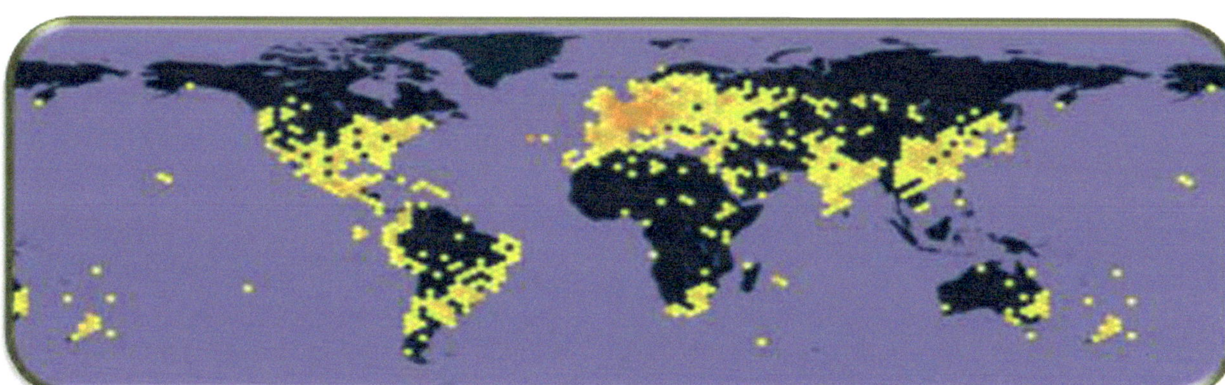

Botanical description:

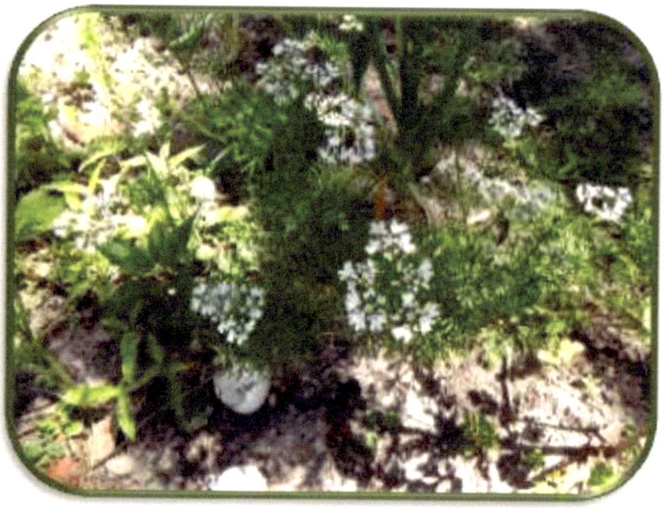

An annual herb, 10-50 cm tall, stems erect, slender, grooved, branching dichotomously starting from the base. Glossy leaves, three types: basal, long-stalked, app earing withered, undivided or three-lobed, and the lower stem leaves, deeply divided more than once into ovate to pedicel-shaped lobes, with serrated edges, and the upper leaves, petiole, deeply divided more than once into thread-like lobes. Flowers small, white, in compound racemes, 3-5 rays. Bracts 1 or absent. Simple umbel 3-5 rays. Bracts 3 or more, linear-conical. Calyx reduced to small teeth. Receptacles 5, notched, not quite equal in size. The fruit is composed of two fruiting parts, spherical in shape, 1.5-5 mm in diameter, showing 10 flat, slightly convex primary ribs on the surface of the fruit, and 8 thin, straight, more convex secondary ribs, which only become flat when they dry.

Flowering: From March to June.

Original habitat and geographical distribution:

Eastern Mediterranean and western Iran Turan, from where its cultivation spread to most temperate and semi-hot regions of the Old World.

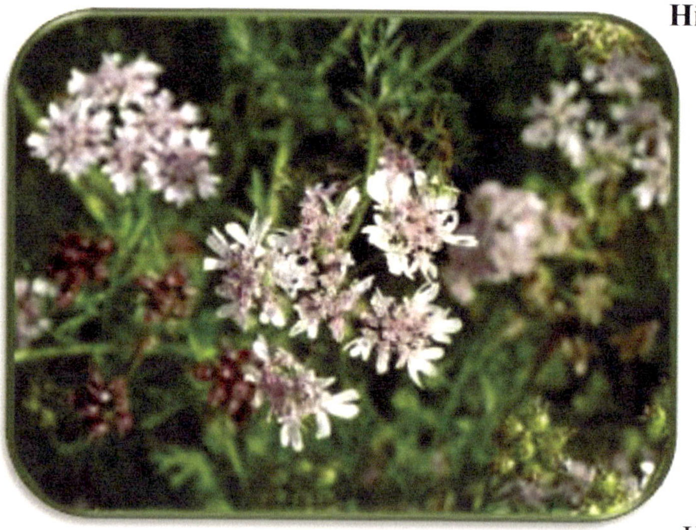

History and Heritage:

The Arabic name "Kazbra" is derived from Syriac, the scientific name of the genus is derived from the Greek koris meaning "fosphos" or "fos" referring to the smell of the fresh plant, the descriptive name of the species sativum means "cultivated." Its medicinal value has been recognized since ancient times. The fruits have been used for more than two thousand years, and the species was mentioned in the Ebres Papyrus, which dates back to the Pharaonic civilization, as well as in the Hanging Gardens of Babylon, and in ancient Indian texts written in Sanskrit, as it was known to the Greeks, Romans, and Chinese.

Part used: Ripe, dry fruits, volatile oil extracted from the fruits. oil. coriander

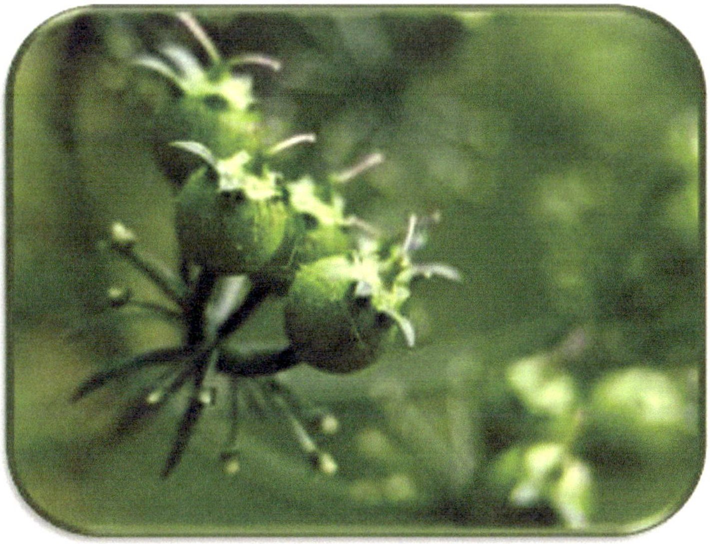

Chemical components:

Coriander fruits contain biologically active phytochemicals such as essential oils, fatty acids, tocols, sterols, and carotenoids. The fruits contain volatile oil -0.4%1.4, the most important components of which are: linalool, coriandrol 70%, geraniol, borneol, p-cymene, camphor, and limonene. And fixed oil 21-13%, the most important components of which are: oleic acid, linolenic acid a., and parsley acid a. .petroselinic and hydroxy coumarins compounds, the most important of which are: umbelliferone, scopoletine. .Favonoids, including: campherol, quercetin and their glycosides, Favonoid compounds, terpenoids and phenolic acids.

Properties and medical uses:

Coriander is used as an antibacterial, anti-inflammatory, anticancer, anticonvulsant, neuroprotective, analgesic, to relieve migraines, lower blood fats, lower blood sugar, and lower blood pressure. Coriander seeds are a famous appetizer and digestive spice, and are antioxidants due to the presence of many flavonoids. Coriander seed oil shows antimicrobial activity against gram-positive and gram-negative bacteria, some yeasts, dermatophytes, and filamentous fungi. The volatile oil stimulates the secretion of digestive juices, expels gases, and relieves colic and cramps. Studies have proven the benefits of the fruit for diabetics, as it stimulates the pancreas to secrete insulin. Coriander is included in diets, due to the effect of its fixed oil in lowering blood fats and cholesterol. Its oil is used as a fragrance in some pharmaceutical preparations. The ground fruit is popularly used to freshen bad breath, especially eating garlic, and is used in cases of indigestion, cough, fever, and cystitis. Coriander oil is also used topically to treat epistaxis (nosebleeds), and as an ointment to treat hemorrhoids and rheumatism.

Environment:

The plant tolerates cold and high temperatures, but its green and fruit production is high in temperate and semi-hot areas compared to hot or cold areas. It grows in the form of scattered colonies in the mountainous and stony areas in the Damascus countryside (Syria). The plant grows in yellow or heavy and stony lands, provided that they are well drained and ventilated. It also grows well in fertile black lands, and does not tolerate high levels of alkalinity or acidity of the soil.

Cultivation and productivity:

The plant is planted in the fall as a winter crop in warm areas, and in the spring as a summer crop in cold areas. It is propagated by fresh seeds that are no more than a year old, in lines or in holes within pits. 3-4 seeds are placed in the hole, and the hectare needs 15-25 kg of fruits.

Seeds start germinating at temperatures of -6-8°C, and the germination stage under these conditions takes 20-25d ays. Seedlings are thinned when they reach 6-8 days. Seedlings tolerate low temperatures up to -7-8°C below zero. They are thinned, and two seedlings are left in each hole.

Cuminum cyminum L.

Cuminum aegyptiacum Mérat ex DC., *Cuminum sativum* J.Sm., *Cuminum odorum* Salisb.

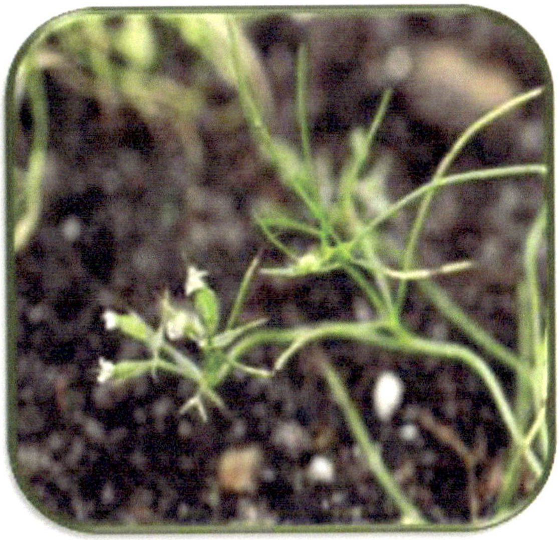 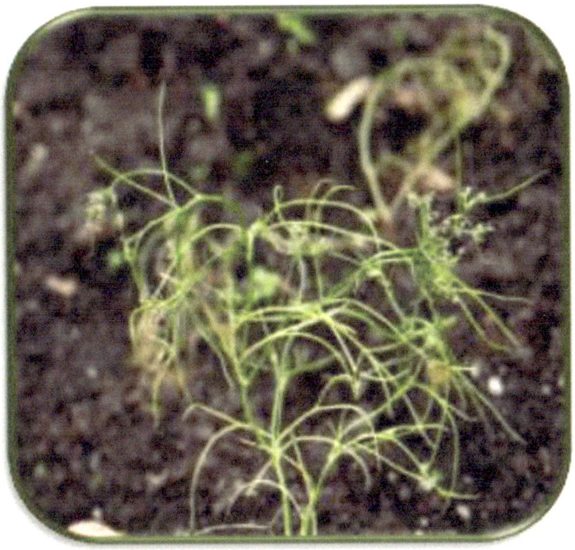

Family: Apiaceae

Common names: Cumin, Snoot, Zeera, Whale cumin

Foreign names: Cumin Fr. Cumin, Eng.

Occurrences :629 occurrences

Distribution in the world

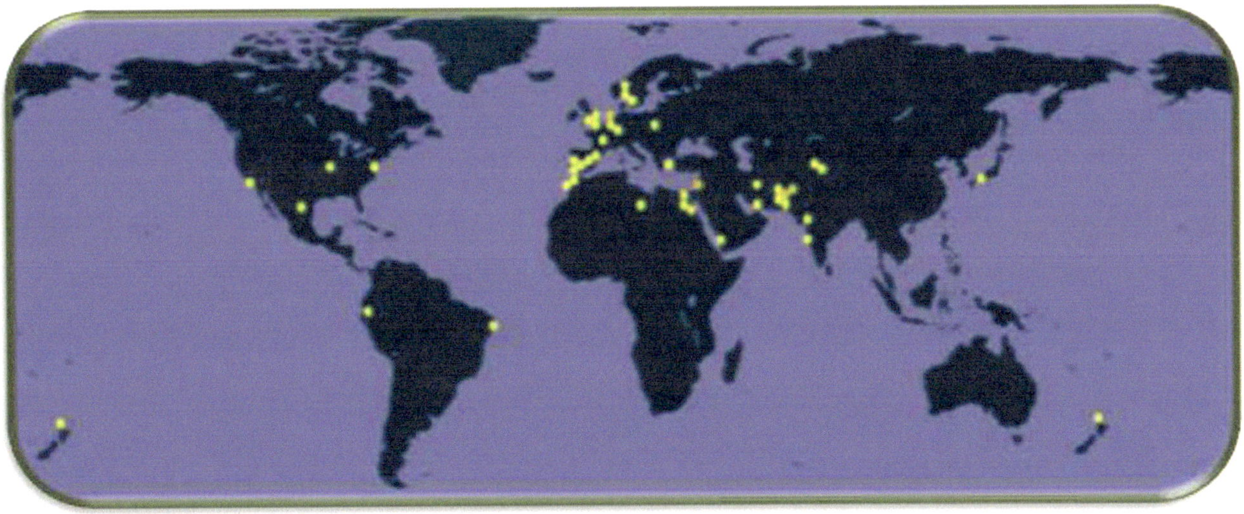

Botanical description:

Annual herb, glabrous, 10-50 cm tall. Stem dichotomous at the base, cylindrical. Leaves glabrous, small, deeply divided into oblong to linear lobes. Flowers white or pink, gathered in compound tents. Calyx reduced. Sepals 5, oblong, serrated at the apex. Male 5 stamens. Female bicarpal, ovary inferior. The fruits are double, spindle-shaped, 3-6 mm long, and about 1.5 mm wide, yellowish-brown in color, and have an aromatic smell and a pungent taste.

Flowering: From April to June.

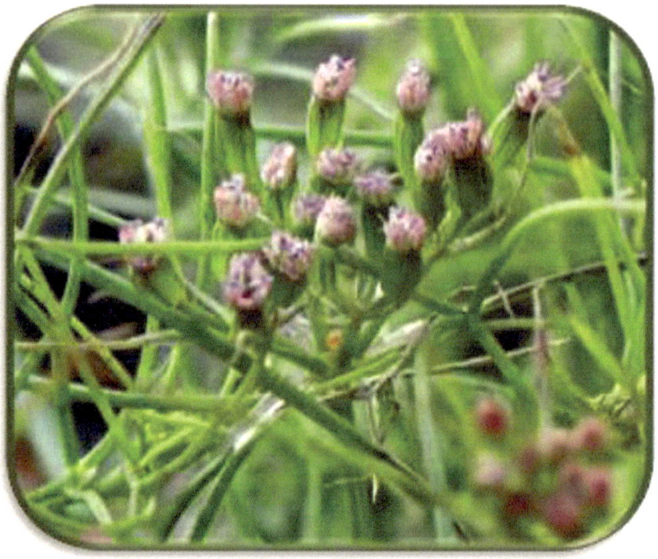

Habitat and geographical distribution:

It is believed that the original home of the plant is the Nile Valley, especially Egypt and Sudan, although it is widespread in Asia, especially India and Pakistan. It is cultivated in most hot and dry regions of Asia and Africa, and in the southern United States of America.

History and heritage:

Cumin is an ancient Arabic word, most likely from Babylonian. The scientific name is the Greek and Latin name of this plant, which is derived from Babylonian. The Pharaohs knew the properties of cumin and planted it abundantly on the banks of the Nile, and they called it "Qamni." It was mentioned in ancient papyri in more than 60 ivory descriptions. The Greek physician Dioscorides wrote about it: "Cumin has a warming power, expels wind, has astringent and drying properties, and is used when crushed with vinegar and smelled to stop nosebleeds." Galen wrote about it: "Cumin with oil or honey to heal wounds, and if it is mixed with oil or honey, it breaks up stones, removes colic, flatulence, and bloody urine. Cumin is used with oil as an ointment for swollen testicles." The Arabs introduced it to the western Mediterranean in the twelfth century. Ibn Sina mentioned it, and distinguished between Its various types.

Used part: Ripe and dry fruits, volatile oil extracted from the fruits.

Chemical components:

It contains volatile oil 2-5%, the most important components of which are aldehyde cumin, gamma terpinene, β-pinene, ρ-cymene, and ρ-menthandial, and fixed oil 10-15%, the most important fatty acids are petroselic acid, palmitic acid, oleic acid, proteins 15-20%, and flavonoids.

Main components of cumin fruit oil cyminum C. are: 4-dien-7-al,p-mentha-1, cumin aldehyde, gammaterpene, and betapene. The research results indicate the possibility of using the above-mentioned essential oils in compounds to control bacterial and fungal plant diseases.

Properties and medical uses:

Cumin fruits and their volatile oil have antioxidant properties, and some types of bacteria Baccilus subtilis and Staphylococcus epidermis, and Candida albicans fungi. Candida, especially as an appetite stimulant and digestive stimulant, increases digestive secretions, helps expel gases, and relieves intestinal spasms. Studies have shown that cumin fruits contain compounds with estrogenic effect (isoflavonoids), which affect the body's lipid reception, and thus contribute to the prevention of menopausal diseases in women, and cardiovascular diseases. Cumin extract also has an antiplatelet effect. Blood-clotting The essential oil of the fruit was found to have strong toxicity against the two grain storage insects Sitophilus zeamais (corn weevil) and Tribolium castaneum (red flour beetle) adults, and showed strong fumigation toxicity against them. The compounds Carvone R and D-limonene showed strong contact and fumigation toxicity against them as well.

Cumin fruits are popularly used as an abortifacient and emmenagogue. A decoction of the powdered fruits is used for its soothing and appetite stimulating properties, and for treating stomach acidity, flatulence, colic, digestive disorders, and cramps resulting from intestinal worms. It is also used to increase urine and milk production in nursing mothers, and to relieve rheumatic pain. A decoction of cumin fruits is used topically to wash the face to remove facial spots and obtain clear skin, and to wash inflamed eyes. The fruit powder is also used to make oils, which are used to treat wounds, ulcers, scabies and itching. The fruit powder is often used mixed with oil to stop nosebleeds. Cumin is sold in the market in the form of fruits, pharmaceutical preparations and nutritional supplements. Drug interactions and warnings: Cumin interacts with some sleeping medications. Using volatile oil for long periods causes skin irritation. It should not be taken by kidney patients.

Food uses:

Cumin powder is one of the basic spices that are added to many foods to stimulate the appetite and give them a distinctive taste and smell. Cumin oil is added to sweets, bread, cakes and pies to perfume them, and it is also included in the composition of some types of perfumes.

Environment:

Cumin grows in hot and semi-hot, dry and semi-dry areas, and does not tolerate low temperatures even for a short period, nor does it tolerate very high temperatures. The ideal temperature for its growth is 25°C. Yellow and light clay soils with good drainage and ventilation are the most suitable soils for the growth of cumin. Heavy clay and sandy soils are not suitable for its cultivation, because the former leads to infection with diseases that cause wilting and suffocation, and the latter causes the fruits to ripen quickly and reduce their weight. Cumin tolerates degrees of salinity and slight alkalinity, but it prefers moderate soils.

Cultivation and productivity:

Cumin is propagated by seeds, and it is recommended not to plant seeds stored for a period exceeding two years. The seeds are scattered in the fall before the temperature drops after mixing them with sand (3:1). Planting is done in holes in rows. The plants are thinned when they reach a height of 5-8 cm.

Eryngium campestre L.

Eryngium vulgare Lam., *Eryngium campestre* var. *genuinum* Rouy & E.G.Camus., *Eryngium campestre* var. *latifolium* Mariz., *Eryngium campestre* var. *parvifolium* Merino.

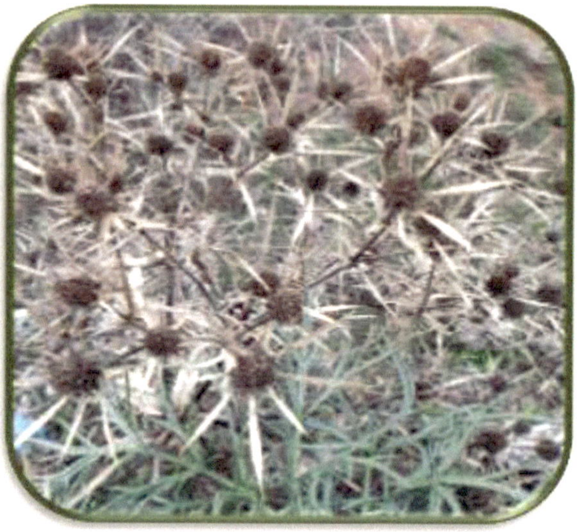

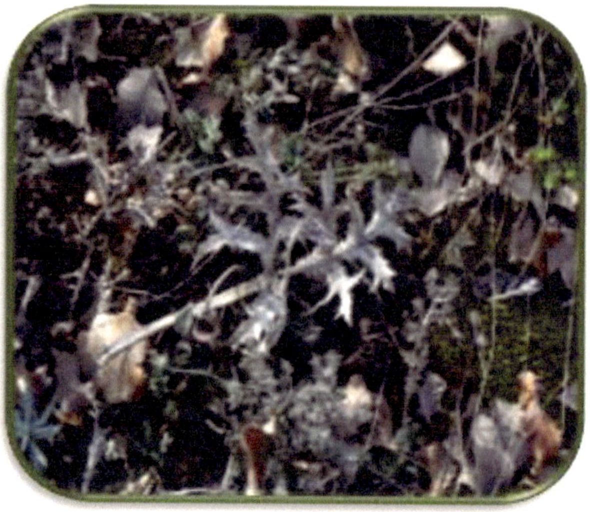

Family: Apiaceae

Common names: Pirate's thorn, Egyptian thorn, Fentaje', Goat's beard,

Foreign names: Rolland Chardon Fr., Eryngo Eng

Occurrences :270,287 occurrences

Distribution in the world

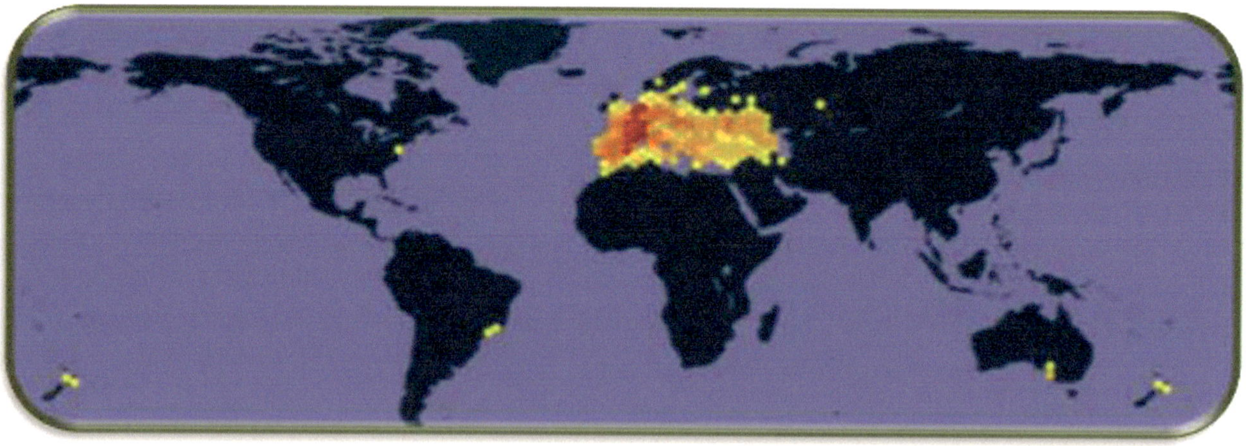

Botanical description:

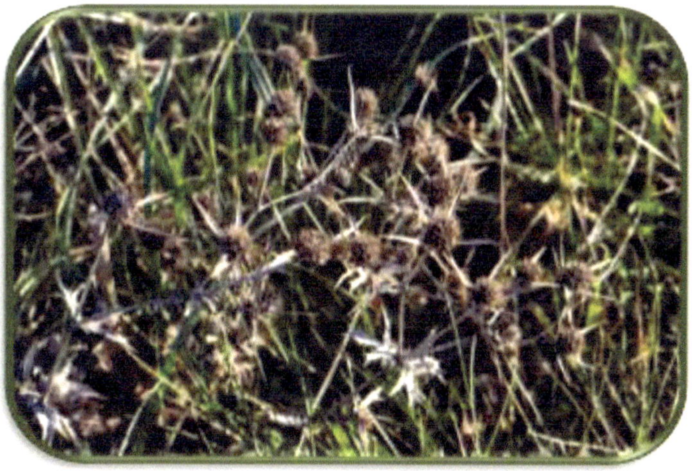

Perennial, thorny, bluish-green herb, 20-60 cm tall, numerous branches, in the form of a co mb-like inflorescence. The basal leaves are broadly oval in shape, trifoliate, pinnately divided, lobed, serrated and thorny. The inflorescence is simple, semi-capital, surrounded by a bract composed of 6-7 lanceolate bracts, bearing one or two thorns at its base, twice as long as the bract. Flowers hermaphrodite, bluish-green, sessile, surrounded by simple, spiny bracts, longer than the calyx, but much shorter than the bracts surrounding the head. Teeth of calyx conspicuous, hard, sharp. Petals erect, convergent, striated, with a long, downward-recurving apex. Stylus broad, with a high margin surrounding the filamentous bracts. The fruit is inverted oval or cylindrical, covered with scales or tubercles, the fruiting parts are not distinct.

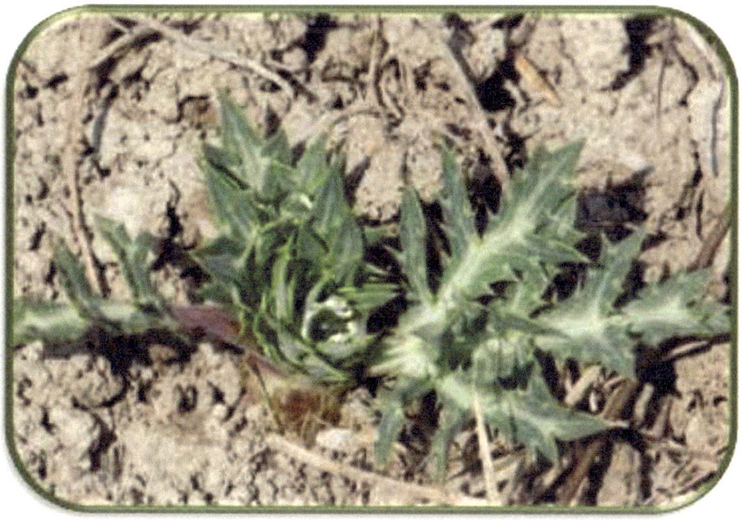

Flowering: From May to August.

Habitat and geographical distribution:

The plant is widespread in the wild in central and southern Europe, northern Africa, and the countries of the Mediterranean basin, and its distribution extends eastward to Afghanistan.

History and heritage:

The scientific name of the genus is derived from the Greek: êryggos or êryggion, while the species name campestre means "field." The plant has been used since ancient times in preparing some foods, and as a medicine for many conditions such as cough, bladder stones, and snake bites. It was mentioned by Ibn al-Baytar, al-Antaki, and Ibn Sina.

Part used: Dry leaves and flowers, and roots collected in the spring and fall.

Chemical components:

The plant roots contain: triterpene saponins, such as the glycoside barrigenol and pyranocoumarins, the most important of which are: egelinol, egelinol benzoate, agasyllin benzyl-esters, and grandivetin. They also contain monoterpene glycosides and caffeic acid esters, including rosmarinic acid and chlorogenic acid, and they contain alkaloid sugars. The leaves and flowers also contain flavonoids, potassium, calcium, manganese, magnesium, vitamins such as vitamins A, B, and C, in addition to pectins. The most important main compounds of the essential oils extracted from the aerial parts are

Germacrene D, Campestrolide, Germacrene B, Myrcene, α-Cadinol, Spathulenol, Eudesma-4-7-dien-1-β-ol (15) and Cadinol.

Properties and medical uses:

Research on experimental mice has shown that the extract of the aerial parts and roots (saponins) has analgesic and anti-inflammatory properties. It is used The decoction of the plant's roots is popular for its expectorant, antispasmodic, respiratory tract infection, and cough-fighting properties, in addition to its use in cases of urinary retention, urinary tract infection, and the treatment of kidney and bladder stones and renal colic. The methanolic extract of the plant showed antitumor activity (tumor inhibition by 86%). The roots are used as topical tinctures to treat wounds and skin diseases. The leaves and flowers are used to treat urinary tract infections, prostatitis and bronchitis. There is another species called Eryngium maritimum, which is widespread on the shores of the Baltic, Black and Mediterranean Seas, and is popularly used like this species.

Environment:

The plant grows in dry grassy areas and edges of fields. It requires well-drained soil and sunny locations. It prefers medium-light soils, and tolerates most types of soils, including poor, stony and calcareous soils.

Cultivation and productivity:

It is propagated by seeds that are scattered in the nursery in beds after they mature in early autumn or spring. Seeds usually germinate after 5-90 days at a temperature of 20°C. The seedlings are transferred to plastic bags or pots to spend the first year in the nursery, and then transferred to the permanent ground at the end of the following spring. The plant can be propagated by division in early spring or in the fall, and it can also be propagated by root cuttings in the fall or winter. The plant has deep and widespread roots, which help it spread quickly, making it difficult to get rid of it once it spreads.

Ferula hermonis Boiss.

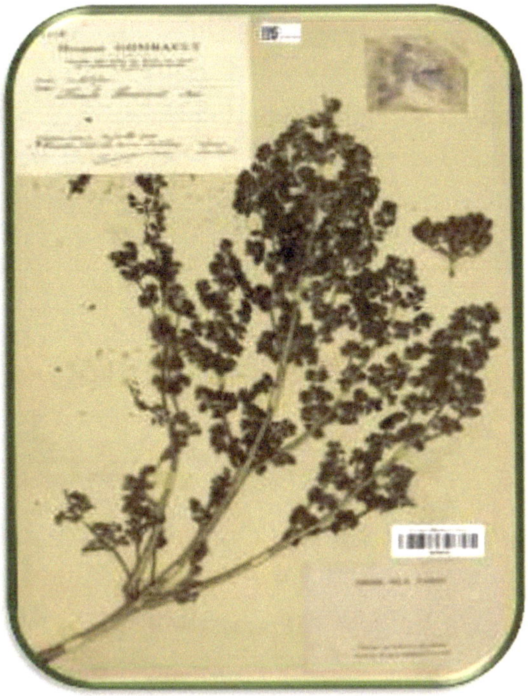

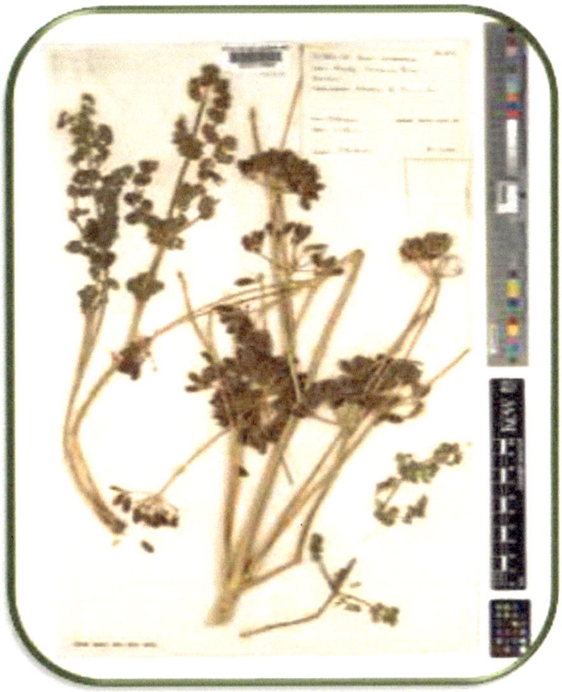

Family: Apiaceae

Common names: Zallouh, Shars al-Zallua, Shamr Abi Tayeb

Foreign names: Zallouh Fr. Sallua, Eng

Occurrences : 40 occurrences

Distribution in the world

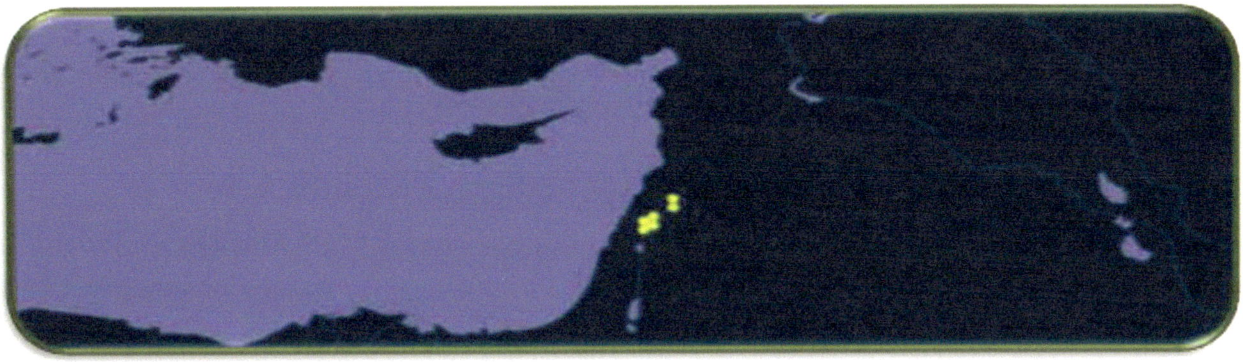

Botanical description:

Perennial herb, 1.5-1 m tall, branched, and the branching in the upper part of the plant is in the form of whorls. Leaves: Gracious, the lower ones are bluish-green, oval in general shape, the base of the petiole is broad, partially surrounding the stem, compound pinnate, the first-degree lobes have a thick petiole, the others are semi-threaded, threadlike and numerous, branching at the apex, the upper leaf blade is greatly reduced, and is almost limited to the sheath which becomes broad (its width exceeds its length), shiny, and embraces the stem.

The flowers are gathered in inflorescences composed of 6-8 short rays, the central one is semi-squamous, without a stalk, and the stalk is represented by small oblong-shaped stalks. The fruit is oval, about 10 mm long, about 5 mm wide, brown to purple in color, compressed dorsally, flattened, not thick at the edge, its dorsal stalks are equal in size, threadlike, prominent, and the lateral stalks are close to the edge. The plant has a strong scent, sometimes secreting small orange resin clusters.

Flower: May to August.

Habitat and geographical distribution:

Endemic to the mountain slopes of the eastern Lebanon mountain range in Syria and Lebanon, at an altitude of more than 2000 meters above sea level.

History and Heritage:

The scientific name of the genus is the old Latin name for this plant, and it is descended from Fero, meaning "carry", alluding to the ancient use of the stem in preserving, carrying and transporting fire. The scientific name of the species "hermonis" refers to its natural distribution in Mount Hermon in Syria.

Part used:

Roots and rhizomes (collected in the fall), the resinous gummy substance found in the rhizomes.

Chemical components:

The roots contain resinous substance, volatile oil, and gum. The most important compounds are ferulic acid, monoterpene compounds (ferutinin, teferdin, alpha-bisabolol, alpha-pinene 38%, azarecine, sulfur, in addition to triterpene and steroid saponins.

Properties and medical uses:

Zallouh is a sexual stimulant and tonic. Its properties include stimulating the heart and nervous system, and helping to renew cells. Experiments conducted on male mice showed that the compounds ferutinin and teferdin increase the level of testosterone. It was also noted that the compound teferdin increases the sexual abilities of male mice, and that the compound ferutinin negatively affects the sex hormone in female mice, and reduces their sexual desire. The Lebanese Urological Association conducted several clinical trials on the plant root, and the study concluded that the root of the plant contains elements that stimulate blood circulation, including ferulic acid, which dilates and activates blood vessels. The volatile oil found in the roots, including monoterpene compounds and semi-sesquiutespene, shows high effectiveness against Gram-positive bacteria Staphylococcus aureus and S. fecalis. The resin in the rhizomes also shows high effectiveness against bacteria, especially Gram-negative Escherichia coli and Salmonella typhi and Pseudomonas aeruginosa. The root of the saffron is popularly used in cases of general weakness, as a tonic and physical and sexual stimulant, tonic for the nerves, in the treatment of asthma and whooping cough, as an expeller of gases that cause colic, and in the treatment of diseases of the urinary system. It is also attributed to the benefits of zalu'a in delaying aging, strengthening hair, and regrowing hair that has fallen out. Zalu'a is available in the markets mixed with honey and royal jelly, in the form of capsules of zalu'a root powder.

Side effects and warnings:

Irritations of the colon have been observed when used for long periods. Some people who have used the plant have also felt flushing and headaches resulting from the effects of the plant in stimulating blood circulation. Doctors advise against using the plant root for people who suffer from high blood pressure, heart disease and diabetes except after the approval of a specialist doctor.

Environment:

Zalou grows in high mountainous areas, on cold hills, slopes and plateaus. It is spread in humid and semi-humid to semi-arid environments, where cold or moderate heat is available, and is considered one of the light-loving species. It grows in agricultural lands and even rocky mountainous lands. It prefers medium-fertility, loose, well-drained soils.

Cultivation and productivity:

The plant is propagated by seeds, and cultivation is done in regular rows at the end of winter and the beginning of spring. The plant blooms in spring, and the roots are collected in autumn and early winter and dried in the sun.

Foeniculum vulgare Mill.

Anethum pannorium Roxb., *Ligusticum foeniculum*)L.(Crantz., *Anethum dulce*)Mill.(DC., *Anethum foeniculum* L., *Anethum rupestre* Salisb.

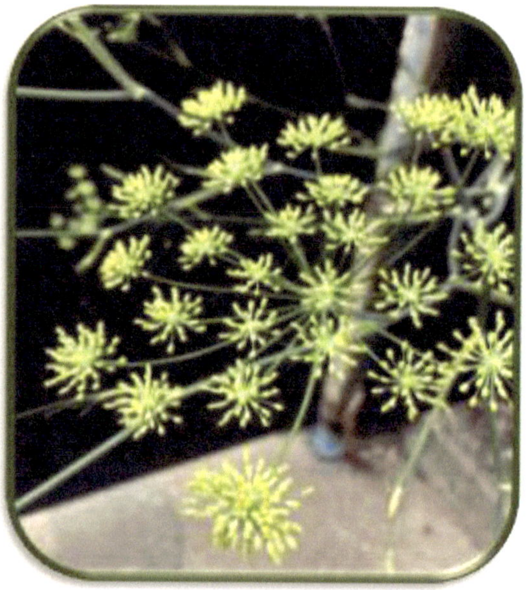

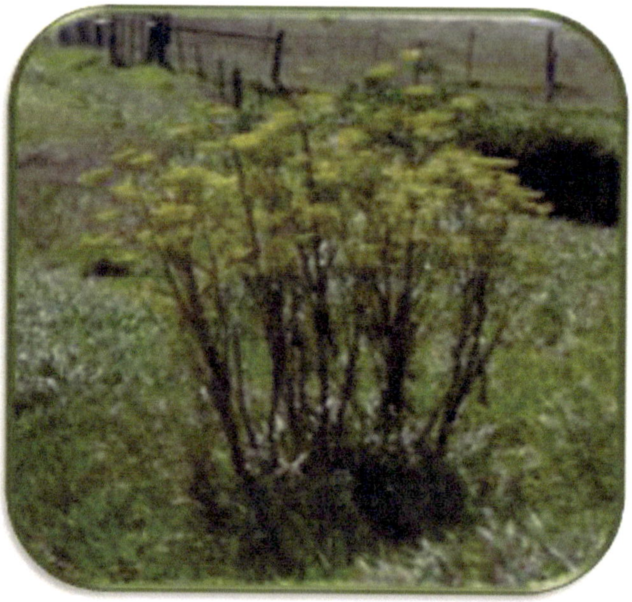

Family: Celery, Apiaceae

Common names: fennel, pepper, senut, sweet, sweet seed, sweet fennel, bitter fennel.

Foreign names: fenouil Fr. Fennel, Eng

Occurrences : 124,097 occurrences

Distribution in the world

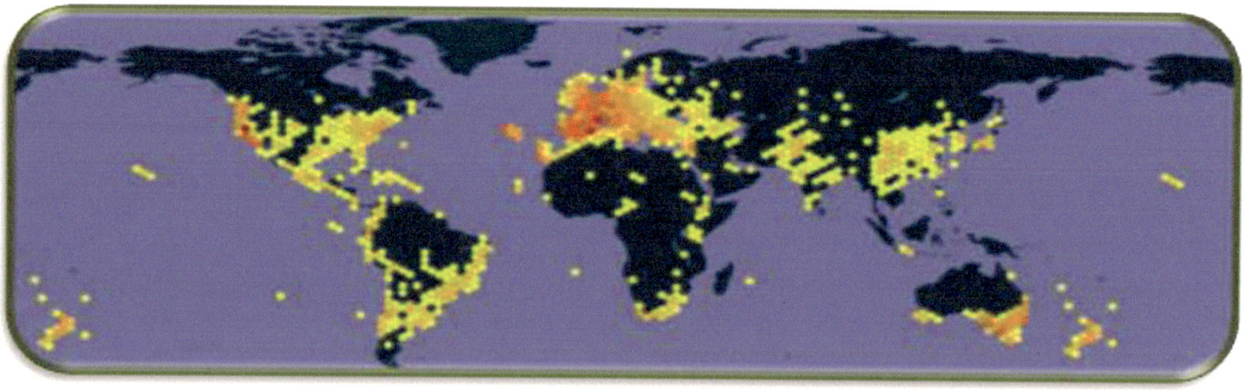

Botanical description:

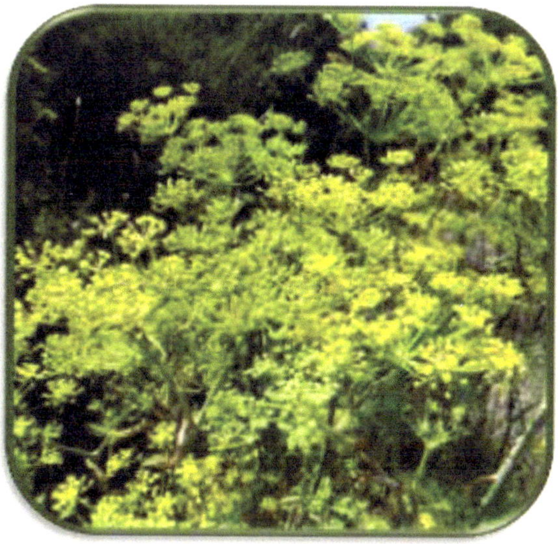

A fragrant herbaceous plant, biennial to perennial, 0.8-1.5 m tall. Stem erect, branched, solid, smooth, glabrous. Lower leaves are obtuse, divided into very thin, thread-like lobes, and upper leaves have a long, broad sheath. Inflorescence is compound, umbel, consisting of 5-10 unequal rays, about 15 cm in diameter, bract absent. Flowers are yellow, small, hermaphrodite. Calyx reduced to a circular ring. The petals are externally coiled. Male 5 stamens. Female bicarpal, ovary inferior.

Fruit is double acorn, greenish-yellow, ellipsoid to cylindrical in shape, with 10 prominent lobes on its surface, 6-8 mm long, 2-3 mm wide, with a strong aromatic smell when ripe. There are several varieties of fennel that were bred from the wild type, the most important of which are: (Bitter fennel) Foeniculum vulgare subsp. vulgare var. amara: Bitter fennel, (Sweet fennel) Foeniculum vulgare subsp. vulgare var. dulce: Sweet fennel

Habitat and geographical distribution:

The Mediterranean Basin and southern Europe are the original homeland of the plant. It is grown in France, Britain, Germany, America, and southern Argentina, and in Asia in India, China, and Iran. Egypt and Syria are among the most producing countries of good quality sweet fennel.

History and heritage:

Name The scientific name of the genus is derived from the Greek and means "short hair." Fennel and fennel are common names, and have similar names in Aramaic, Hebrew, and Assyrian. The scientific name of the genus Foeniculum is derived from the Latin "Fenum" meaning "fodder" for the softness of the leaves. Fennel is a common and well-known word in the Levant. The descriptive name for the species vulgure means "common." Fennel has been used for thousands of years to treat many diseases. The Pharaohs used it under the name Shammari, and its fruits were found in their tombs. It was mentioned in the Harris Medical Papyrus under the name "Shamarn", and its name in ancient Coptic is known as "Shamarhot". It was also mentioned in another papyrus under the name "Basbas", which the Arabs kept and later changed to Basbasa. The ancient Chinese, Hindus and Romans cultivated it, and ate its fragrant, sweet-smelling roots and leaves. The senna was one of the best medicinal materials used in the Middle Ages, and its fresh leaves were added to fish and vegetable dishes by the rich, and the poor used to eat its leaves as an appetizer during fasting days. It was mentioned in ancient medicine that the senna plant has two types; wild and garden, and two types; Nabataean and Roman, and Arab and other doctors praised its benefits. Ibn al-Baytar, al-Antaki, and Abu al-Qasim al-

Ghasani mentioned it as an antispasmodic, digestive, appetite stimulant, stomach tonic, milk stimulant, worm repellent, and wound healing aid.

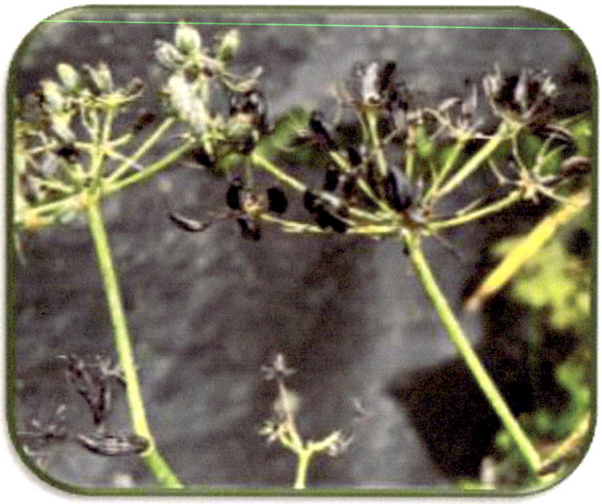

Part used: Fruits, seeds, and the essential oil extracted from them.

Chemical components:

Fennel fruits contain volatile oil, the proportions and components of which vary according to the variety, geographical origin, and extraction method (water vapor, hexane). The most important components of the volatile oil in bitter fennel are trans-anethole 50%-75%, fenchone 33-12%, estragole 5-2%, limonene 2%, alphapinine, alpha and beta phellandrene beta alpha-, myrcene, and paracymene p-. While fennel oil contains Sweet fennel: Anethole increases to 80-90%, astragol to 3-10%, and fenchone decreases to 1-10%.

Both sweet and bitter fennel seeds contain volatile oil, which has the same composition as the fruit oil in both varieties, in addition to traces of hydroxycoumarins: scopoletin, umbelliferone, osthenol, scoparin, and traces of furocoumarins and pyranocoumarins, xanthotoxin, columbianetin, psoralen, bergapten and flavonoids. It also contains fixed oil 12-18%, consisting of 60% petroselinic acid, 22% oleic acid, 14% linoleic acid, and 4% palmitic acid, in addition to vitamins C, B, A, and minerals phosphorus, calcium, sulfur, iron, and potassium.

Properties and medical uses:

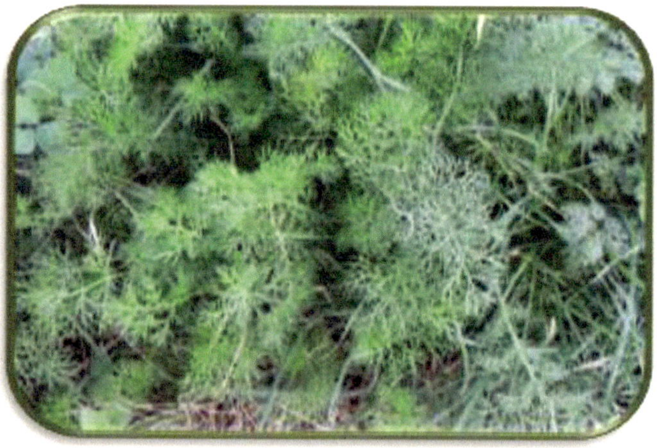

Fennel is used in traditional medicine for a wide range of diseases related to the digestive system, endocrine glands, reproductive system, and respiratory system. It is also used as a galactagogue in lactating mothers. Results based on traditional uses and scientific evaluation indicate that fennel is still the most widely used herbal plant, and has been used for more than forty types of disorders. Fennel essential oil has stimulating properties for the stomach and intestines, antispasmodic in cases of indigestion, anethole has a carminative effect, and anethole and fenchone have an expectorant effect and a condition for mucous secretions of the respiratory tract. Studies have proven that fennel essential oil has an antibacterial effect against some types of bacteria, and it is used to stop diarrhea caused by bacteria.

The effect of estragole has been proven to be similar to that of female hormones in stimulating increased milk production in lactating mothers, and as an emmenagogue, in addition to stimulating the sexual aspect in women. Sweet fennel oil is added to some laxatives to improve their effectiveness and taste. A decoction of fennel seeds is popularly used as an appetite stimulant, diuretic, and stomach pain reliever. It is given to children to help them get rid of gas and indigestion, and as an expectorant that is beneficial in cases of colds, coughs, and flu. The volatile oil sweetened with honey is used in cases of laryngitis, bronchitis, and asthma. The decoction of the plant powder, including the roots, is used topically as a gargle in cases of mouth and gum inflammation and as an eye wash for conjunctivitis (conjunctivitis). Fresh fennel leaves are used to treat breast and genital abrasions by placing them over the affected area and securing them with a bandage. The boiled leaves are used by placing them hot over the abdomen to expel gases and relieve intestinal colic pain in children.

Precautions for use:

Pregnant women should not use concentrated fennel oil, both bitter and sweet, and should be used with caution by people with peptic ulcers and diabetics. Using a high dose of the oil causes congestion and heart failure, as well as cramps, dizziness, nausea, and vomiting, in addition to the appearance of a skin rash, and may cause a seizure similar to an epileptic seizure.

Environment:

Fennel prefers light, fertile, well-ventilated soils with moderate acidity (pH), and is sensitive to salinity. The plant grows abundantly vegetatively at low temperatures ranging between 15 and 20°C, and flowering and fruiting growth require temperatures ranging between 20 and 25°C accompanied by rain and moderate atmospheric humidity during growth and development periods.

High fruit production requires frost-free weather during the period Green growth, moderate temperature, and long day to encourage floral growth, fruiting and setting. Dry and hot weather leads to the formation of under-full fruits, low weight, and low oil content.

Cultivation and productivity:

Fennel is propagated by seeds that are planted in the fall in temperate areas, and after the frost in cold areas. Planting is done at distances of 75X15 cm, with several seeds placed in one hole if the goal of planting is to obtain fruits. However, if the goal of planting is to obtain Green leaves, so the seeds are first planted in pits, then transferred to the permanent land after about 6 weeks, seedlings are done at 70X20 cm distances. Irrigation and fertilization with essential and rare elements improve the production of fruits and aromatic oil. Irrigation is prohibited when the seeds are fully formed and before the fruits are ripe. It is preferable to harvest the plants and fruits while they are green and tender; that is, before they are fully ripe and dry; because the amount of oil is greater. The plants are cut before sunrise, then dried, threshed and sieved.

One hectare yields about 80-95 tons of fresh grass in the milky stage, and 5-7 tons of fruits. One hectare yields 120-140 kg of aromatic oil resulting from distillation of the green mass, and one ton of dry fruits yields 10-15 kg of aromatic oil.

Petroselinum sativum Hoffm.

Petroselinum crispum)Mill.(Fuss.,*Petroselinum crispum subsp. Crispum.*

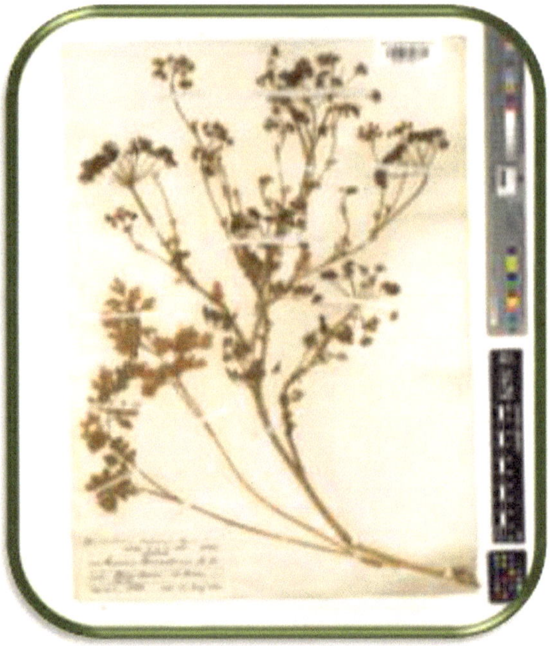

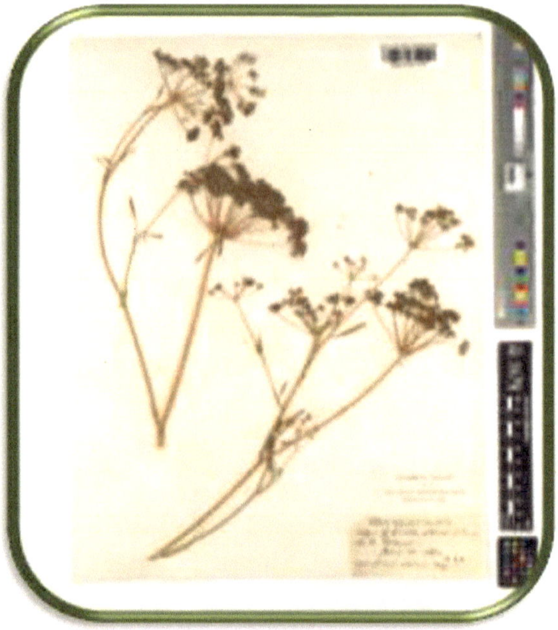

Family: Apiaceae

Common names: Parsley, Parsley, Celery, Parsley

Foreign names: Persil Fr. Parsly. Eng.

Occurrences : 876 occurrences

Distribution in the world

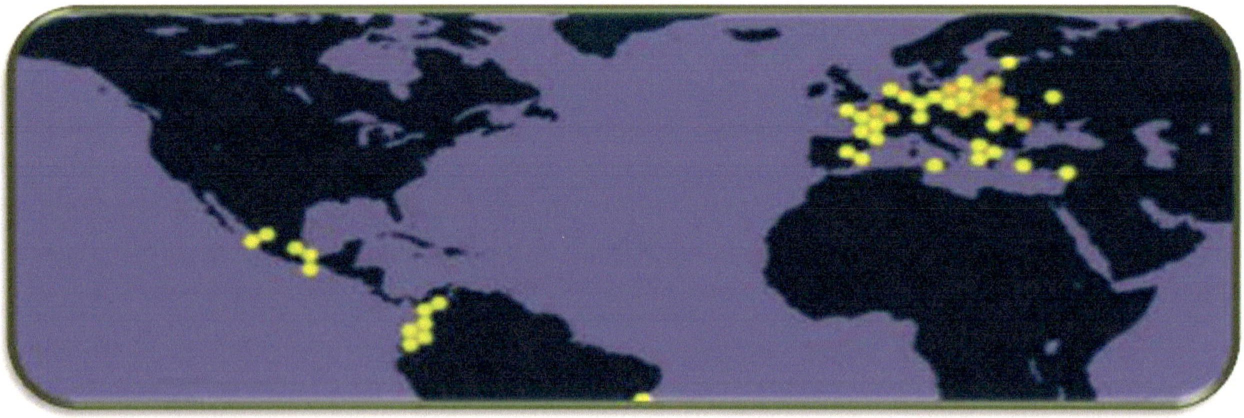

Botanical description:

An annual herbaceous plant, 30-100 cm tall. The lower leaves have a long petiole (3-7 cm), its base forms a narrow sheath; the blade is 5-8 cm long, 4-7 cm wide, divided 2-3 times, its terminal lobes are serrated, elliptic or ovate, shiny green in color, 4-12 mm long, the leaves are reduced towards the top to become three-lobed. Inflorescence umbel-complex, 3-6 cm wide, bracts 1-2 or absent, linear,

2-5 mm long, rays 10-25, almost equal, bracts 6-8, linear, shorter than flowers. Simple umbel contains about 20 flowers, bracts 1.5-4.5 mm. Petals greenish. Fruit double ovate, ovoid, 2-4 mm long, 1.5-3 mm wide, grey to brown.

Flowering: June to July.

Homeland and geographical distribution:

It is believed that the original home of parsley is the Mediterranean region. From there, its cultivation spread to all parts of the world.

History and heritage:

The scientific name of the genus "Petroselinum" is the ancient Greek name for this plant, while sativum means "cultivated." The Greeks, Romans, and medieval doctors used parsley in food as a spice and medicine to treat epilepsy and cough. The roots were also used as a diuretic and to treat kidney diseases.

Part used:

The fruits, the volatile oil extracted from the fruits, the fresh herb (leaves and stems at the beginning of the flowering period), and the dried root.

Chemical components:

The fruits contain 2-5% volatile oil, the most important components of which are: apiole 20%, myristisin 43%, alpha-beta-pinene alpha 20%, beta-phellandrene 4%, and furanocoumarins, including: bergapten, psoralen, isopimpinellin, psoralen, xanthotoxin, imperatorin. Fixed oil 20-22%, the most important acids are parsley acid 60-75%. The herb contains Green contains less volatile oil than the fruit, 0.02-0.3%, in addition to other compounds found in fruit oil. Flavonoids constitute 1.9-5.6%, the most important of which is apiin and vitamins, especially vitamin C. Ascorbic acid also contains large amounts of iron, calcium, phosphorus, manganese, sulfur, potassium, sodium, iodine and copper. The roots contain 0.12-0.5% volatile oil, the most important components of which are apiol, myristicin, terpineol, pinene, limonene, beta-bisabolene, and phtalides, including ligustilide. 0.2-1.3% flavonoids, the most important of which is apiin. Furanocoumarin compounds similar to those found in the young herb. And Polyynes (long-chain organic compounds), the most important of which are: falcarinol, falcarindiol (fatty alcohols).

Properties and medical uses:

Parsley is often used in Morocco to treat high blood pressure, diabetes, heart and kidney diseases. Parsley's antioxidant and antibacterial activities make it useful in diets. Parsley leaves and roots (flavonoids) have antioxidant and anti-inflammatory properties, which are useful in treating urinary tract infections, and help get rid of kidney and bladder sand and stones. Furanocoumarins and phthalides found in the leaves and roots of the plant have a hypotensive effect by relaxing and dilating the muscles surrounding the blood vessels. The plant, with its volatile oils (myristicin and apiol), is a diuretic and can help reduce high blood pressure. The oil extracted from parsley fruits helps increase digestive secretions, get rid of gases and intestinal colic, in addition to its activity in inhibiting the growth of some types of bacteria.

Apiol has astringent properties for smooth muscles in the digestive system, bladder and uterus, so the seeds or its volatile oil are used to treat menstrual problems. Parsley (leaves, seeds and roots) is popularly used due to its many benefits; It is an appetite stimulant, expectorant, and its decoction is used internally as a digestive and intestinal stimulant and bile secretion stimulant. It is also useful in reducing rheumatism pain, arthritis, and anemia. It is considered a diuretic that helps in getting rid of urinary sand. Parsley juice is used topically in the form of drops to treat eye inflammation, skin spots, pimples, and boils, and to clear the skin. The juice of its fresh leaves is used as a disinfectant for wounds and ulcers.

Drug interactions and warnings:

It is not recommended to use it when using blood pressure lowering medications, as it may lead to a sharp drop in blood pressure. It is not used by people who are allergic to the apiol compound. It is not prescribed for pregnant women, people with kidney inflammation, or children.

Nutritional uses:

Parsley is one of the main ingredients in salads. The young leaves are high in nutritional value because they contain vitamins and minerals that the body needs. Parsley fruits and young leaves are included in some foods, giving them a distinctive taste and smell. Parsley leaves have a high ability to remove bad breath, especially the odors emanating from eating garlic and onions.

Environment:

The plant grows mainly in sunny, humid environments. It tolerates both high and low temperatures during different growth periods, but it gives better vegetative and fruit production in areas with moderate temperature conditions, and frost and snow have a harmful effect on vegetative production if they continue for a long period. Parsley cultivation is good in most lands, provided that they are well drained and ventilated, but it does not tolerate high salinity. The appropriate soil acidity for it is pH=6-5.5.

Cultivation and productivity:

The plant is propagated by seeds throughout the year in temperate and hot areas. Cultivation is done by spreading in basins measuring 3X5 m after mixing them with soil or sand at a rate of 1:4. It can also be planted in lines at a rate of 60 cm between one line and the other, and 15 cm between holes. Seedlings appear above the soil surface 16-25 days after planting, and may be delayed until after 35 days under unfavorable conditions.

Pimpinella anisum L.

Anisum odoratum Raf., *Anisum oficinale* DC., *Anisum vulgare* Gaertn., *Apium anisum*) L.(Crantz., *Carum anisum*)L.(Baill., *Pimpinele anisa* St.-Lag., *Selinum anisum*) L. (E.H.L. Krause., *Sison anisum*)L.(Spreng., *Tragium anisum*)L.(Link

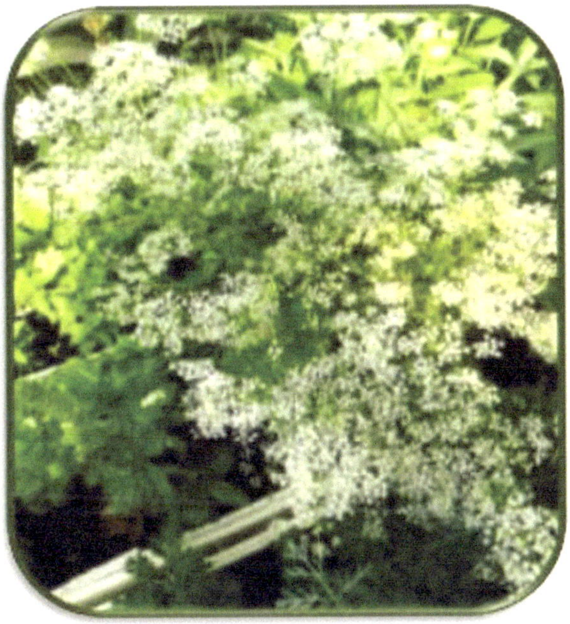

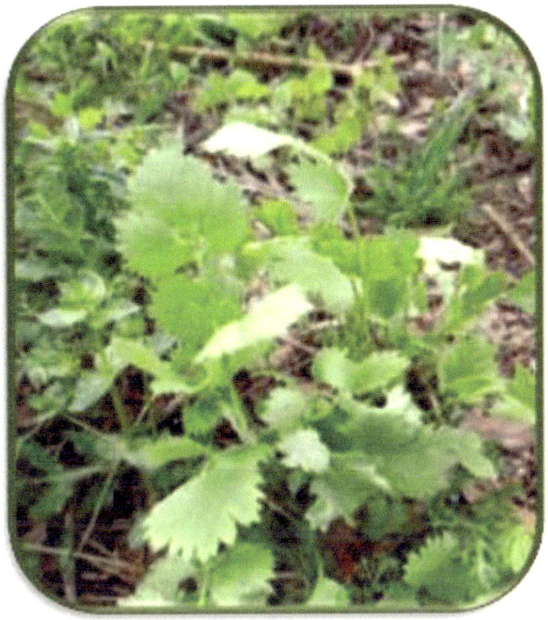

Family: Apiaceae

Common names: Anise, Anise, Sweet Cumin, Sweet Cumin

Foreign names: Anise Fr., Anise Eng.

Occurrences : 1,140 occurrences

Distribution in the world

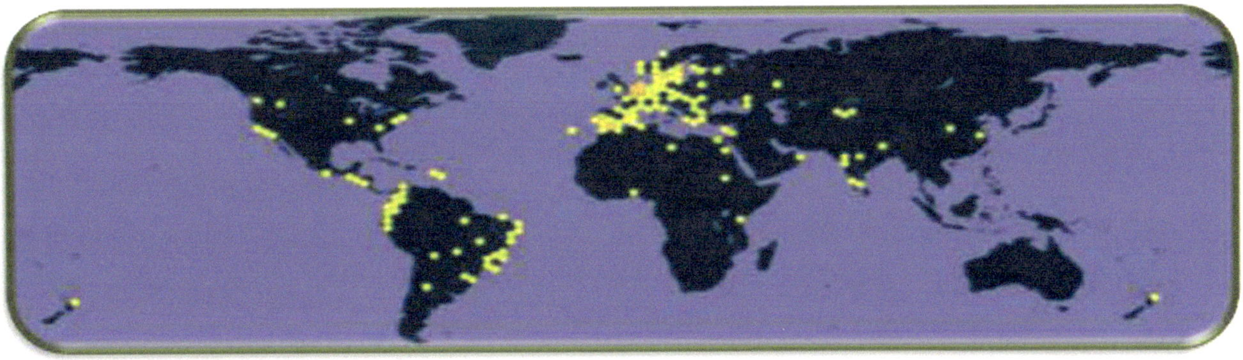

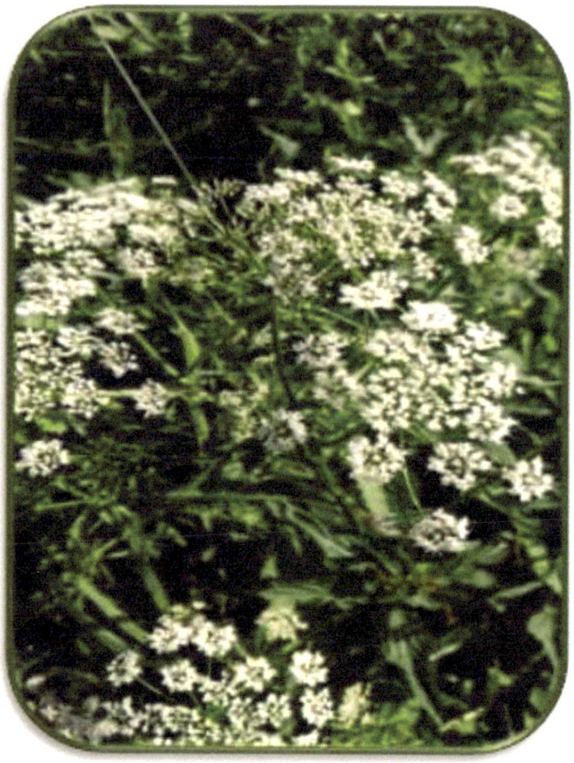

Botanical description:

An annual herbaceous plant, aromatic, The basal is obtuse, round-kidney-shaped, serrated to lobed at the margin, not divided, the lower stem leaves are ovate-rounded in general shape, three-lobed or three-leafed, the leaflets are ovate or obtuse-ovate and serrated in shape, the upper leaves are short-obtuse or obtuse, with a narrow sheath, deeply divided into linear-lanceolate lobes. Inflorescence is umbel-complex, composed of 7-15 rays, lacking bracts, either at the level of the umbel-complex or simple. The calyx is reduced. Corolla 5-petaled, white, fringed at the edge, hairy at the bottom. Male 5 stamens. Female Acacia, bicarpelic, inferior ovary. Fruit acorn, 3-5 mm long, ovate-oblong, prominent ribs and distinctive scent.

Flowering: April to June.

Homeland and geographical distribution:

Unknown, but it is likely to be native to the Middle East. It grows spontaneously in Egypt, and is cultivated in the countries of southern Europe, Turkey, Syria, Tunisia, Central Asia, India, China, Central and South America. Egypt and Morocco are among the Arab countries that produce the most of it. History and Heritage: The scientific name of the genus Pimpinella is the ancient Roman name given to the species, meaning "with two wings" in reference to its feathery leaves, while the species name anisum is the ancient Arabic name for anise. The aromatic properties of anise have been known since the earliest ages of Egyptian civilization.

Part used:

Dried fruits (with a sweet taste and distinctive flavor), and the volatile oil extracted from the fruits.

Chemical components:

The plant contains volatile oil, the percentage of which varies according to the variety and climate, and generally ranges between 2-6%. Its most important components are: anethole (phenolic ether) 80-90%, estragole 2%, anis aldehyde 1%, linalol, and alpha-terpineol. It also contains organic acids from caffeic acid derivatives: chlorogenic acid and caffeoylquinic acid. Favonoids: apigenin glycosides, and isovitexin. Isovitexin, luteolin, isoorientin, quercetin, rutin, fixed oil 20%, proteins 20%, sugars, gums and fibres.

Properties and medical uses:

The fruits have the properties of anethole, which has the properties of a general stimulant, appetite stimulant, expectorant, antifungal, antibacterial and antiviral. Volatile oil is used to treat respiratory diseases (runny nose, laryngitis, pharyngitis and bronchitis, dry cough), as a carminative and antispasmodic, and is useful in cases of indigestion, colic and intestinal laziness. Flavonoid compounds enhance the effect of anise oil in addition to its antioxidant properties. Anise fruit alcoholic tincture and oil are used in the composition of many pharmaceutical forms such as cough medicines and expectorants, giving them an acceptable taste. The oil is also used in the composition of ointments used to treat acne and pimples. Anise is used in traditional medicine for its medicinal properties that include cardiovascular function. Anise fruit is used in the form of a boil, or an alcoholic tincture is prepared from it. The aqueous extract (AE) reduces blood pressure.

Other uses:

Anise fruits are used to add flavor and taste to some types of sweets, and scent to perfumes and soaps.

Precautions for use:

It should not be used by pregnant women, and it should not be used by people who are sensitive to the anethole compound.

The oil is considered a sedative in high doses and has a slowing effect on blood circulation.

It is warned against giving it to children, and anise fruit decoction is considered a sedative.

Environment:

The plant is found in cold and moderate areas, as cold the vegetative and floral growth is coordinated during the winter and spring seasons, while the moderation in temperatures is suitable for fruit set, fruit formation and seed maturation. High temperature and low humidity lead to rapid flowering, early ripening, and low fruit size and aromatic oil content. The critical period for temperature extends from the beginning of flowering until maturity. It is planted in different types of soils, and prefers light and heavy yellow soils (provided that they are fertile and good drainage) and moderate in terms of acidity and alkalinity (pH=7.4-6.8), and does not tolerate soil salinity.

Cultivation and productivity:

The plant is propagated directly by seeds, which are planted in autumn in temperate areas, and in spring in cold areas, in lines 40-50 cm apart, or in rows 3-4X10-20 m apart, and 3-4 seeds are placed in the hole. The seedlings are thinned when they reach a length of 6-8 cm, and two seedlings are left in each hole. A hectare needs 15-20 kg of fresh and healthy seeds. The plant needs 3-4 irrigations, and various service operations (weeding and fertilization) are important to obtain high productivity. The green mass or fruits are collected from the plant. The green mass is harvested or mowed during the flowering stage and the beginning of fruit formation, and the fruits are collected when they are ripe and before they are completely dry. One hectare yields about 25 tons of green grass and 1-1.5 tons of ripe fruits.

Atriplex halimus L.

Atriplex halimoides Tineo, *Atriplex capensis* Moq., *Obione halimus*)L.(G.L.Chu , *Schizotheca halimus*)L.(Fourr.)

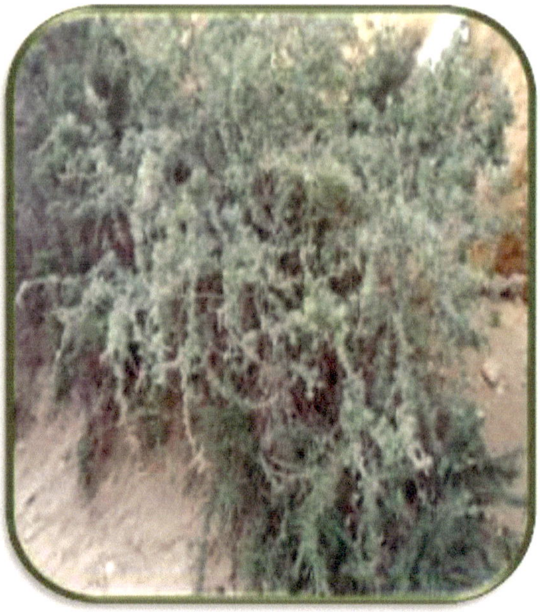

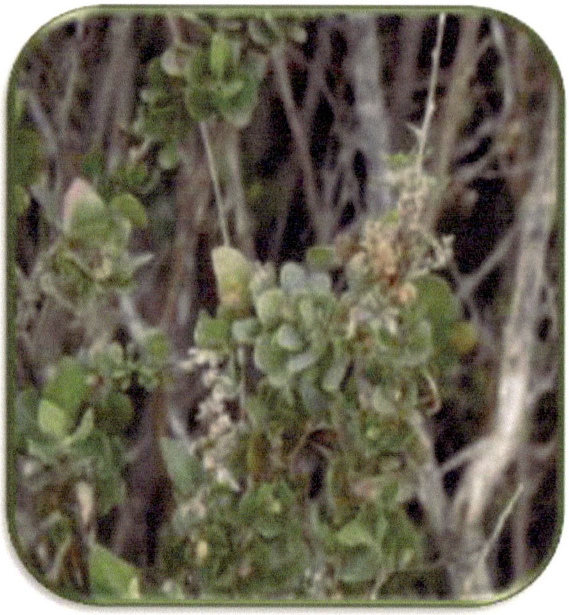

Family: Cockscomb (formerly Amaranthaceae, Chenopodiaceae). Saltwortal

Common names: Saltwortal, Arroche mari time.

Foreign names.Eng. Saltwortal, Fr. Arroche mari time.:

Occurrences : 21,159 occurrences

Distribution in the world

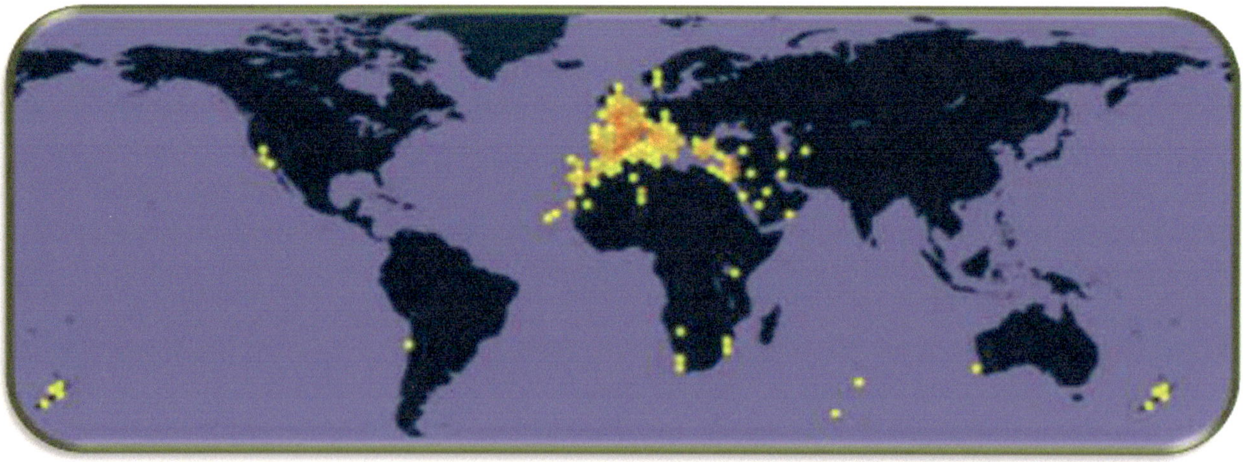

Botanical description:

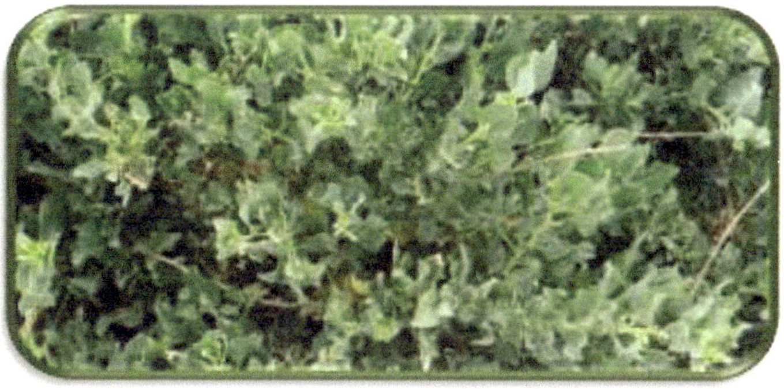

A shrub 1-2 m tall, covered with vesicular hairs. Stems erect, much branched, woody, cylindrical or angular, whitish. Leaves Simple, obtuse, 40-4 × 60-10 mm, alternate (semi-opposite below), ovate to ovate-rhomboid to triangular, petiolate or arrow-shaped, with entire, wavy or serrated margin, silvery-white, no prominent nerves, upper leaves narrow, lanceolate. Flowers are unisexual, gathered in dense groups, forming terminal spikes, without leaves. Male flowers are indistinct, their 5-parted, membranous, located at the apex of the inflorescence. Female flowers are at the bottom of the inflorescence axis, without a sac, but they have two leathery bracts, called "valves." The fruit is a sacculus (acine) completely surrounded by two valves, its fruit periphery is free membranous. The peduncle is round or semi-round or kidney-shaped, its base is short, scalloped, its margin is entire or serrated, its surface is smooth or reticulate, its length and width are about 4-5 mm. The stems are free-linear. The seeds are 1-2 mm, vertical, lenticular, dark brown in color, the embryo is round.

Flowering: from April to October.

Habitat and geographical distribution:

Mediterranean and desert-Arab. It grows naturally in the Mediterranean basin, and in central Africa, and the Atlantic part of Europe. It is widespread in the Levant, the Arabian Peninsula, Kuwait, Egypt, Libya, Tunisia, Morocco, Mauritania, Cyprus, and South Africa.

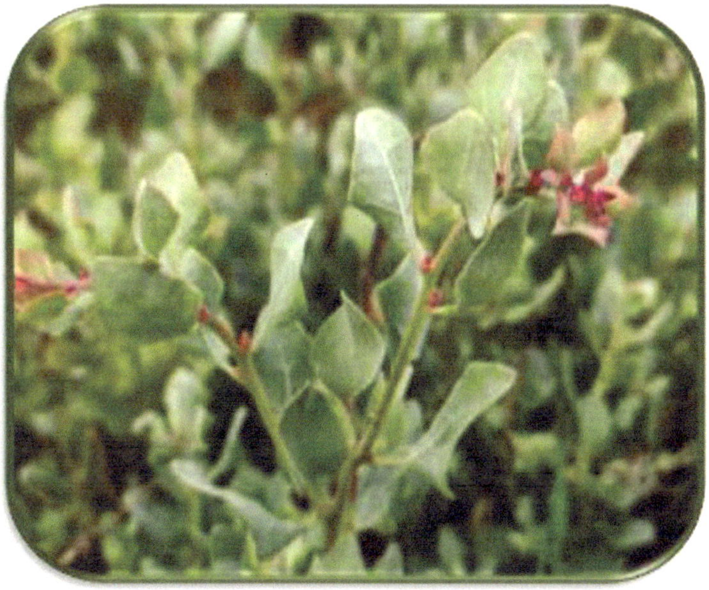

History and Heritage:

The Arabs knew the pastoral value of the salty harvest since ancient times and considered it the best pastoral species for camels, goats, and sheep.

However, increased drought reduces the palatability of sheep due to salts and oxalates. Ibn al-Baytar mentioned that its seeds are useful for treating jaundice and tumors.

Part used: The entire plant.

Chemical components:

The plant contains many nutritional compounds (proteins, vitamins A-C-D, and minerals, the most important of which is chromium.)

The plant does not contain toxic compounds. The aerial parts extract contains: myristin, quercetin, isoramentin glycosides, phenolic acids and simple esters.

The aqueous extract of the salt pick contains tannins, flavonoids, saponins and alkaloids. The total phenolic content is 12.47 mg/g of expensive phenols.

Properties and medical and nutritional uses:

The plant is popularly used to treat diabetes (possibly because it contains chromium), and it has carminative and antacid properties. It is used in traditional Algerian medicine to treat thyroid disorders. The aqueous extract of the leaves of the ragal has beneficial effects in reducing high blood sugar levels. It may be a good candidate for anti-cancer agents.

Other uses:

The buds and young leaves are used raw in the form of a salad due to their salty taste, or cooked like spinach leaves, and they retain their distinctive salty taste if cooked over low heat. The seeds can be roasted, mixed with honey, and used to prepare some types of soup, or mixed with grains to make bread.

A red dye is extracted from the decoction of the plant's leaves, similar to the henna dye, and is used to dye hands and feet.

The ashes of the plant are used alkaline in the soap industry.

Precautions for use:

It should not be consumed by children, nursing mothers, and patients with kidney and liver diseases.

Environment:

It is a dry plant, tolerant to salt (Halophyte), although it grows well in non-salty environments. It prefers areas with winters ranging from cold to hot, and tolerates temperatures down to -10°C. It is suitable for well-drained sandy and loamy soils, and can grow in poor lands. It is found in open, sunny, unshaded places on coastal sandy hills. It resists winds and moving sand, and is used to stabilize moving sand. It is considered one of the important shrubs that can be used in reclamation and rehabilitation programs for saline lands in dry and semi-dry areas. The leaves retain their salty taste in low-salinity soils as well.

Cultivation and productivity:

An easy-to-germinate plant, propagated by seeds. It is best to remove the fruit covers or soak them in water for 36 hours. Seeds germinate in 1-3 weeks at 13°C. It can be easily propagated by cuttings, and it is recommended that the cuttings used have leaves.

Chenopodium ambrosioides L.

Dysphania ambrosioides (L.) Mosyakin & Clemants

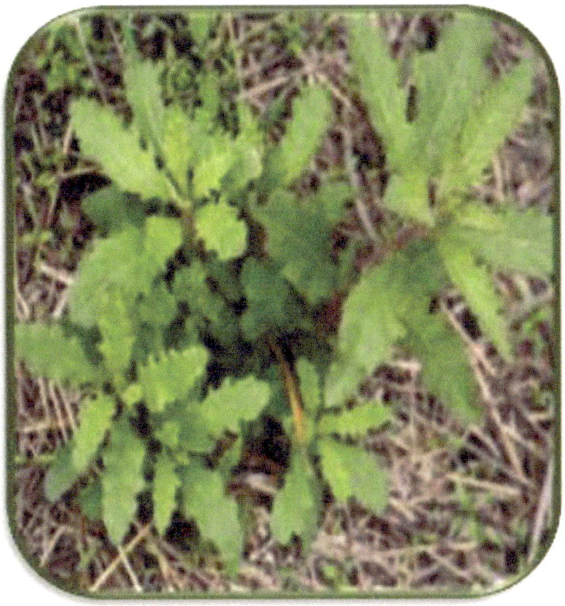 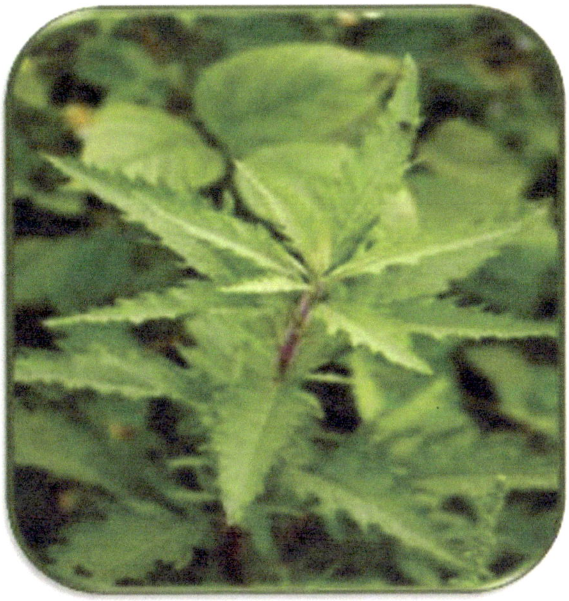

Family: Amaranthaceae (formerly Amaranthaceae, Chenopodiaceae).

Common names: Mexican tea, Zarbikh, Worm-repellent wormwood, Gunpowder (in the Damascus countryside)

Foreign names: Anserine, Fr. oil Wormseed Eng.

Occurrences : 24,872 occurrences

Distribution in the world

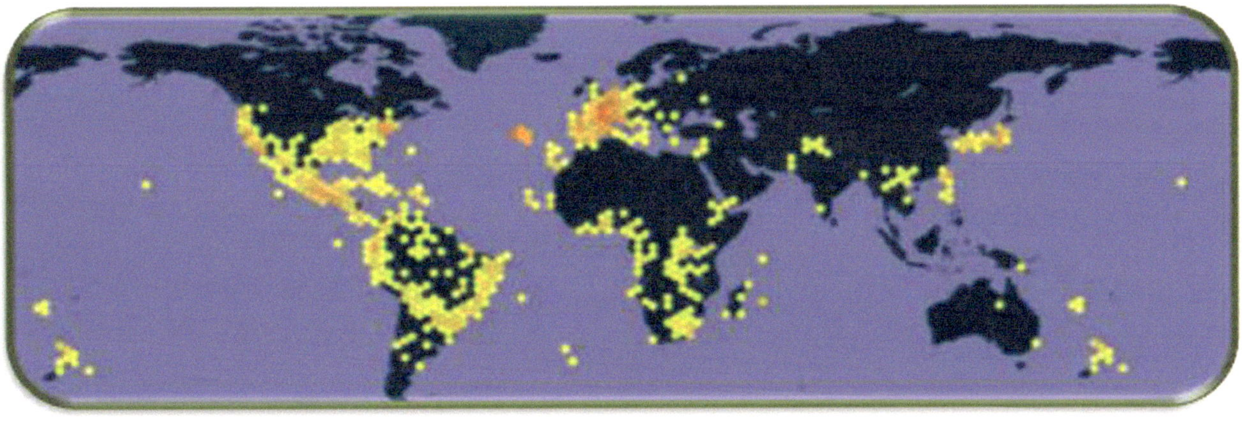

Botanical description:

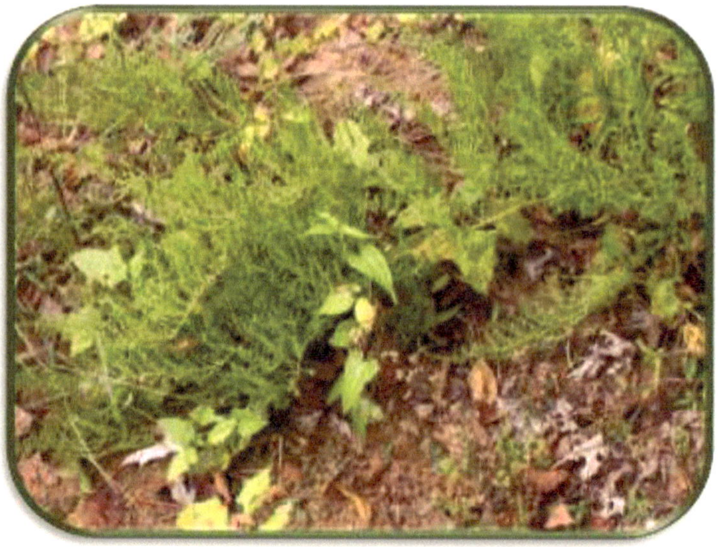

Annual or biennial herb, velvety. Leaves short-pinnate, oblong to lanceolate, sinusoidal-toothed, upper leaves entire, all bearing yellow glands on the lower surface. Flowers hermaphrodite, green, gathered in dense groups, forming elongated spikes, arranged in a long leafy cluster. The bract is simple, about 1.5 mm long, includes the fruit, its segments 4-5, free or fused to their bases, velvety-glandular. Male 5-4 stamens. Female carpels, ovary superior, single-chambered. Fruit is ovate. Seeds horizontal, shiny.

Flowering: March to October.

Habitat and geographical distribution:

Central and South America are the original homeland of the plant, and it has spread to most parts of the world. The United States of America occupies an important position in the production of the plant and its oil, followed by India.

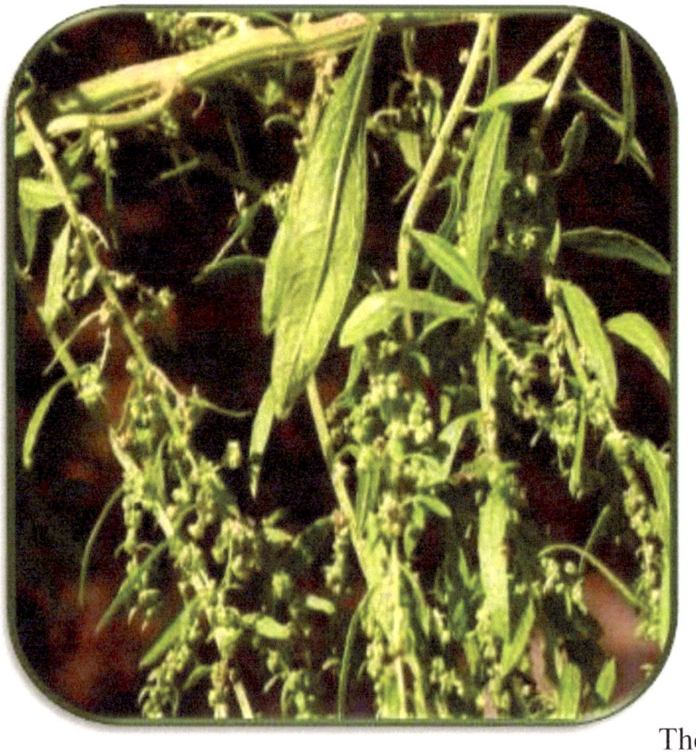

Man, History and Heritage:

The name of the genus is derived from the Greek, meaning "goose foot", the word: chêne means "goose", and podion means alluding to the shape of the plant leaf, which resembles a goose foot.

The Red Indians used the plant extract for diseases of the digestive system in particular. The plant was introduced to Europe in 1900 AD, and was one of the most important drugs used to expel worms. Interest in it increased during World War I, then decreased after it was replaced by industrial compounds.

Part used: Seeds and leaves.

Chemical components:

The seeds contain a yellow volatile oil, the percentage of which reaches 0.6 - 1% and is known commercially as "chinopodium oil", the most important compounds of which are ascaridole 80%, para-cymene, alpha-pinene, alpha-terpene, and limonene. In addition to a fatty oil, the most important of which is butyric acid.

The compounds of C. ambrosioides oil were discovered, and the most abundant compounds were: carvacrol, phytol, and squalene, in addition to the presence of vitamin E and sucrose.

Properties and medical uses:

The plant has toxic properties, especially the compound ascaridole. The plant was used to get rid of Ascaris worms and hookworms, but its use has declined due to the availability of many less dangerous alternatives. The seeds and leaves of the plant are used in South American folk medicine to treat asthma. The oil is used in Chinese medicine to treat joint rheumatism, eczema and uterine bleeding. Anti-inflammatory, analgesic, anthelmintic, antiparasitic, and immunomodulatory against the different stages of schistosomiasis, reducing the granulomatous inflammatory manifestation resulting from infection. The volatile oil of the plant is effective in reducing the parasite load and lesion size in c/BALB mice infected with Leishmania amazonens L. The extract of C. ambrosioides at its lowest inhibitory concentration was effective against Candida albicans. The plant extracts have an anti-larval effect against the infective nematode Haemonchus contortus also known as the hookworm, and it has anti-arthritic, anti-acidic, anti-cancer, anti-oxidant, anti-diabetic, anti-diarrheal, anti-fertility, anti-leishmaniasis, anti-malarial, anti-ulcer, antipyretic, anti-anxiety, insecticide and molluscicide, and helps in bone regeneration.

Warnings for use:

Poisonous plant, the lethal dose of the plant is estimated at 10 mg for adults, and less than that for children. Taking the plant may lead to damage to the nervous system in general, and damage to the sense of hearing in particular, this damage may last for years, so taking the plant is not recommended

Environment:

The plant grows wild in fields, neglected places, and on the edges of canals, drains, and roads. Sarmic is a summer crop from the temperate regions located between 40-70 latitudes north and south of the equator, and from the plants of the humid environment and short rivers. It lives in most types of soils, but prefers light soils rich in nitrogen. It also tolerates soil salinity, and is suitable for a pH between 5.2 and 8.3. It is a harmful weed in fields, especially with potato crops.

Cultivation and productivity:

The plant is easily propagated by seeds. The seeds are scattered in the nursery soil at the beginning of spring, and the seedlings are transferred to the permanent soil at the end of spring when they reach a height of 5-10 cm. The seedlings are planted in holes in lines at a rate of 10-15 cm between the two holes and 75 cm between the two lines in the presence of water. The plant responds to nitrogen fertilization in particular due to its great appetite for this element. The plant is harvested by cutting it above the soil surface when the seeds turn black and before the plant turns brown, as delaying harvesting leads to the fruits falling and the loss of a large part of the crop. One hectare yields about 900 kg of fruits, which produce 50-60 kg of oil.

Haloxylon salicornicum (Moq.) Bge. ex Boiss.

Hammada salicornica)Moq.(lijin ‹*Caroxylon salicornicum* Moq.,

Haloxylon schweinfurthii Asch. &Schweinf, *Hammada elegans*)Bunge(.

Occurrences : 2,035 occurrences

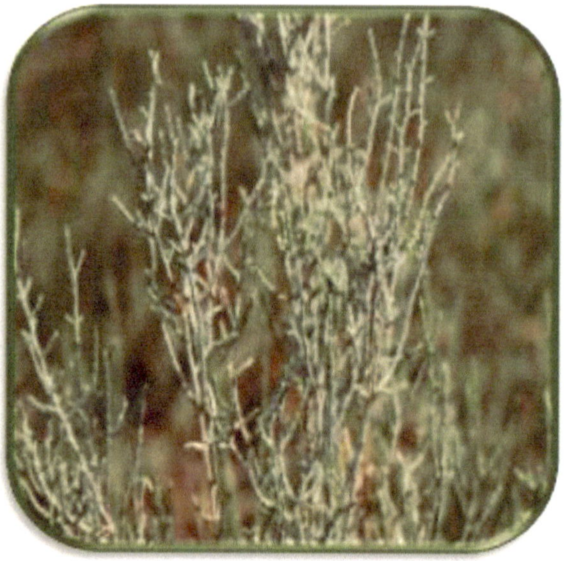

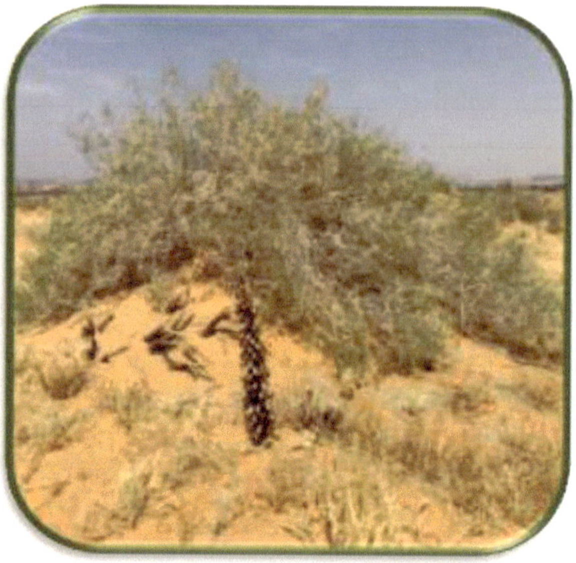

Family: Amaranthaceae (formerly Amaranthaceae, Chenopodiaceae).

Common names: Ramth, Hamd

Foreign names: Saxaoul Fr. Saxaul, Eng

Distribution in the world

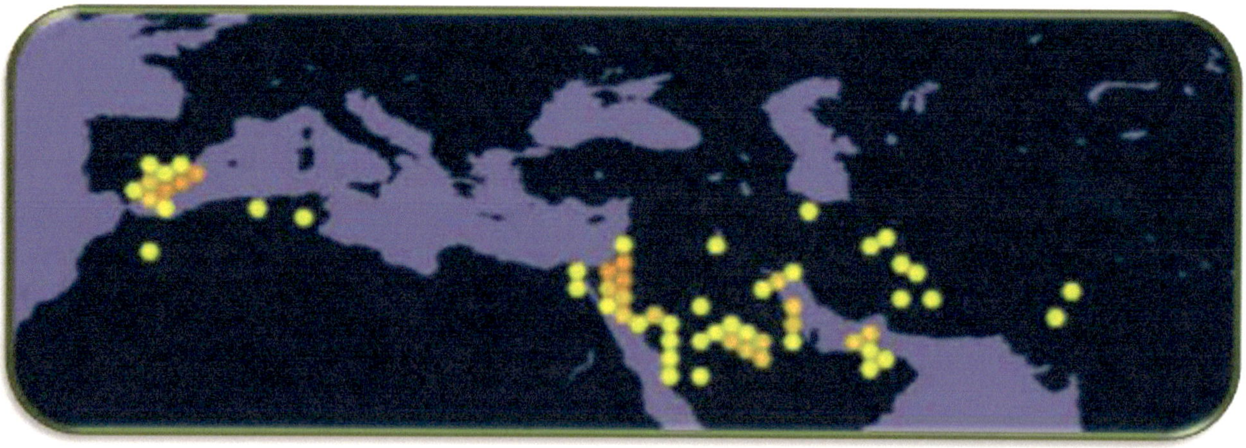

Botanical description:

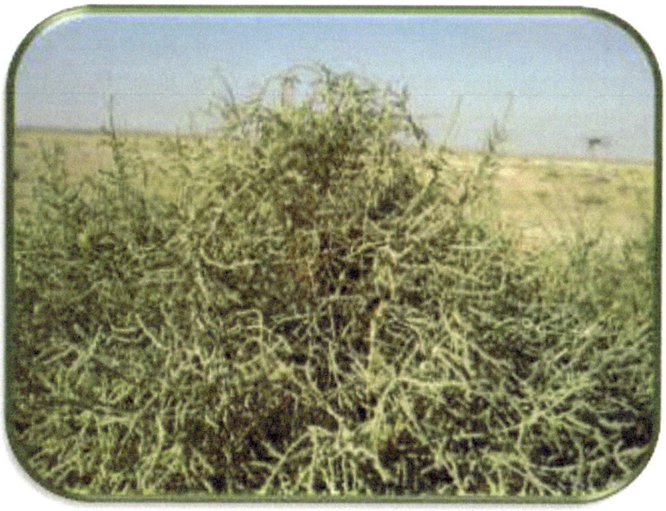

A shrub, 30-60 cm tall, the woody lower stems produce new branches every year, irregularly. The branches are articulated, ascending, solid, light to ivory in colour, turning waxy yellow when dry. The leaves are reduced to small, triangular scales, united in the form of a short, membranous funnel, with woolly hairs inside. Inflorescences are widespread, consisting of short, scattered spikes, 3-6 cm long, most of which are found at the ends of green main or lateral branches that are formed annually. The flower is hermaphrodite, surrounded by two concave bracts, woolly-haired from below. The stamen is simple, consisting of 5 sepals. The male has 5 stamens, free, alternating with five linear-ovate, papillary-apex stamens. Female bicarpal, ovary superior, stigmas short, ending in two papillary stigmas. Fruit 7-8 mm (including wings length). Wings inverted-ovate-rounded, upwards, strongly overlapping, unequal, tinged pale brown. Seeds horizontal.

Flower: September-November.

Habitat and geographical distribution:

Iranian Turanian, spread in the dry Arab regions, Kuwait, Qatar, the United Arab Emirates, the northern Arabian Peninsula, Iraq, Palestine, Syria, Algeria, Mauritania, the Sultanate of Oman, Egypt, Libya, and Tunisia, and is also found in southern Iran and Afghanistan.

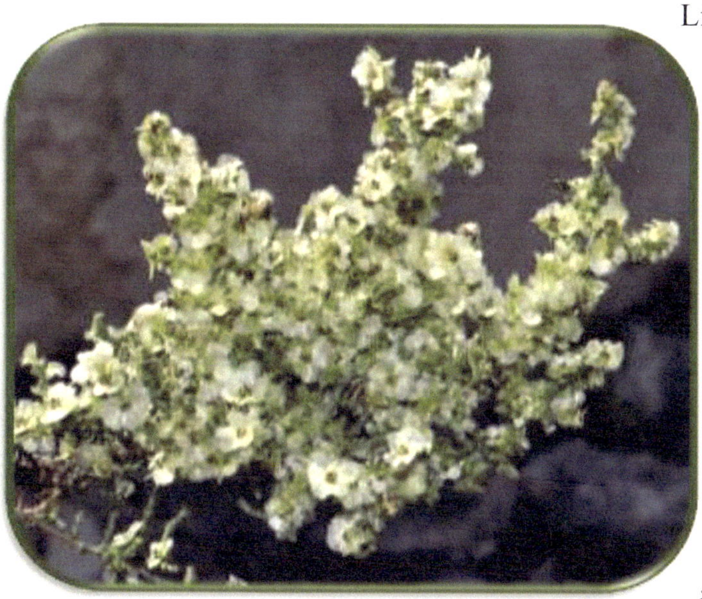

History and Heritage:

The genus comes from the Greek, where halio means "salty" and xylon means "wood", while salicornicum means "similar to lilac".

Part used: Aerial parts (tasting sour and salty).

Chemical components:

The aerial parts contain several alkaloids from the piperidine group, the most important of which are: haloxynine, anabasine, halosaline, and haloxine. It also contains coumarins, saponins, sterols, cardiac glycosides, and flavonoids. Volatile oil, tannins, and anthraquinone. The tips of the plant branches begin, just before the flowering period, to secrete a sticky, sugary-tasting, white substance called "manna, honeydew honey, or honeydew." Chemical analysis of H. salicornicum plant showed that it contains alkaloids:

methyli- sosalsoline, salsolidine, sosalsolidine, dehydros- alsolidine, N-methyltyramine, oxedrine, tyramine, carnegine, tryptoxine, scordenripine, and diterpene and coumarin compounds such as: scopolitin, umbelliferone, xanthotoxol, isoxyimperatorin, and esculitin.

Properties and medical uses:

The plant has anti-inflammatory properties due to its piperidine alkaloids. Research has shown the positive effect of the plant in treating diabetes. It has also shown the positive effect of boiled ramth plant in experimental animals suffering from diabetes, which explains its popular use in treating diabetes patients. The ash of the tamarisk tree is used popularly to treat wounds, burns, and suppurating ulcers. The powder of the plant is also used to treat colds, weakness, fever, and bone pain in the body. The steam of the tamarisk water is used to treat rheumatism. It has antiseptic effect and is used to treat peptic ulcers. The stem and leaves can be used as respiratory stimulants, vasoconstrictors, muscle relaxants, laxatives, analgesics, antioxidants, antipyretics, antimicrobials, antihypertensives, anti-inflammatory, anticancer, and reduces high blood cholesterol.

Other uses:

It is a pastoral plant, and a source of firewood. It was used as a substitute for soap.

Environment:

The tamarisk grows in hot, dry and very dry areas, on plateaus and valleys on medium-depth sandy, gypsum-sandy or sandy-loamy soils, with a limestone layer underneath, as well as on silty soils. It tolerates difficult conditions, especially high salinity. It collects sand around it to form mounds that reach a height of more than half a meter.

Cultivation and productivity:

It is propagated by seeds. Its fruits are characterized by a short life span (9 months to a year) when stored in laboratory conditions. The period can be doubled when stored in a dry atmosphere and at low temperatures (-2 °C). Storage at prolongs the life of the fruits. The optimum temperature for germination ranges between 15 and 18 °C, and stops at 1 °C. Low temperatures of less than 3 °C do not prevent the germination of the tamarisk. It was noted that removing the fruiting covers accelerates and increases the germination rate. Most of the growth of the ramth occurs between April and September, and it is preferable to avoid grazing the plant in late summer and early autumn, because this is the critical period for it.

Salsola kali L.

S. acicularis Salisb., *S. decumbens* Lam., *S. turgida* Dumort, *Kali soda* Moench, *Salsola kali* var. *hirta* Ten., *Salsola kali* var. *vulgaris* W.D.J.Koch.

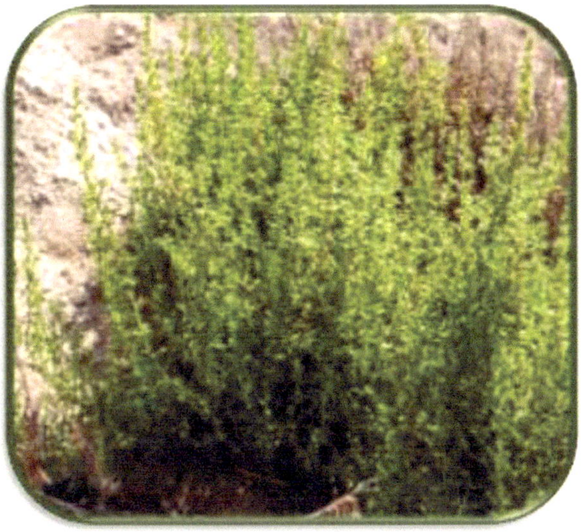

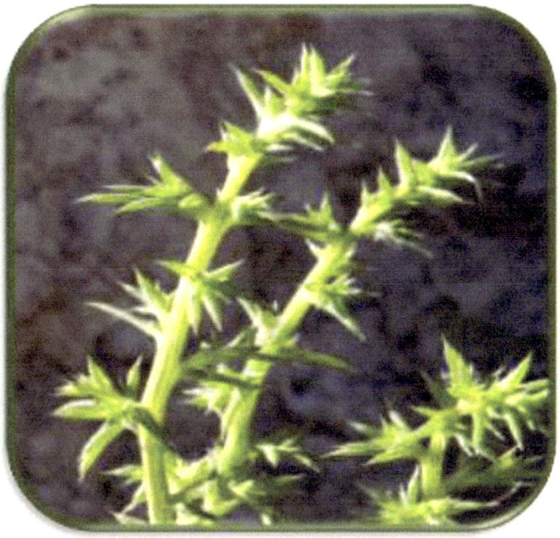

Family: Amaranthaceae (formerly Amaranthaceae, Chenopodiaceae).

Common names: Prickly saltwort, Prickly thistle, Prickly saltwort, Prickly brulee.

Foreign names: Eng. Prickly saltwort, Russian thistle, Fr. Soude brulee

Occurrences : 44,396 occurrences

Distribution in the world

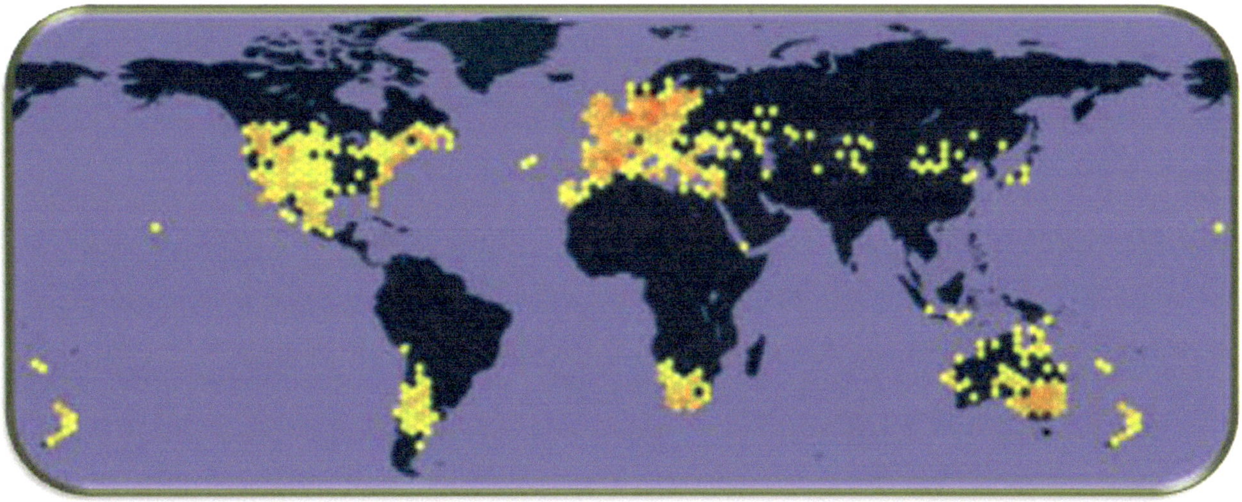

Botanical description:

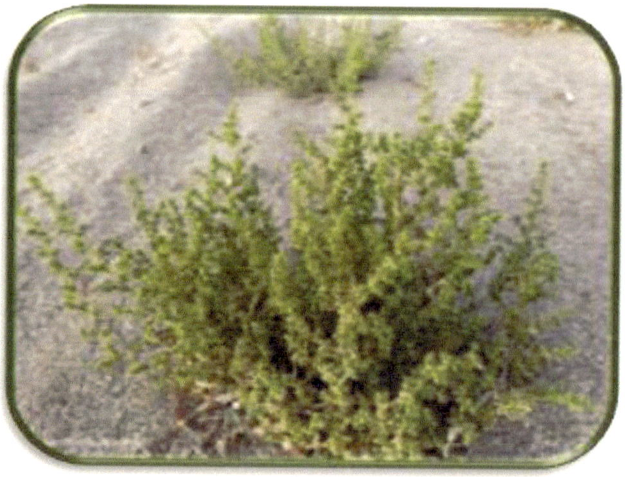

An annual herbaceous plant, fleshy in stature, especially in the early stages of growth, covered with down and hairs, to almost hairless, 20-70 cm long. Stems are simple or multiple, spreading or ascending, angular, branching dichotomously, especially from the base. Leaves are simple, 3-2×30-6 mm in size, the lower ones are opposite, the upper ones are alternate, fleshy, linear, tapering at both ends, and their ends are thorny. The bracts are oblong-ovate to triangular, slightly longer than the sleeve segments, ending in a stinging spine. Flowers hermaphrodite, solitary or in 2-3 clusters, axillary, forming a loose, leafy spike. The bract is simple, its segments 3-4 mm long, free, membranous, oblong, blunt-apexed. Male stamens 5, free. Female bicarpelic. Ovary superior, unicameral. Stigmas 2-3, long, filiform. Fruit is a drupe, 4-10 mm in diameter (including wings), wings are ovate, inverted to renal, striated, sometimes reduced. Seeds are horizontal.

Flower: July to October.

Habitat and geographical distribution:

The plant is of Eurasian origin. It has spread widely throughout the world, and has become an invasive plant in some countries such as the United States of America and Australia.

History and Heritage:

The scientific name of the genus is derived from the Latin word salsus, meaning "salty", and the descriptive name of the species kali is from the Arabic "alkali or alkali." Ibn Sina mentioned the benefits of its seeds as a stone crusher and diuretic. Al-Antaki mentioned the benefits of its ashes in stopping the bleeding of hemorrhoids and drying ulcers.

Part used: Plant

Chemical components:

Alkaloids 0.2 - 0.3%, the most important of which are: salsoline, and salsolidin. Oxalic acid 5%. Fatty oils, the most important fatty acids of which are linolenic acid (linseed oil), oleic acid a. oleic, arachidic (pistachio a.), and palmitic (palm) a. palmitic, and salts of sodium, potassium, calcium, magnesium, aluminum, iron, and sugars (glucose, fructose, arabinose, rhamnose.) flavonoids - tannin.

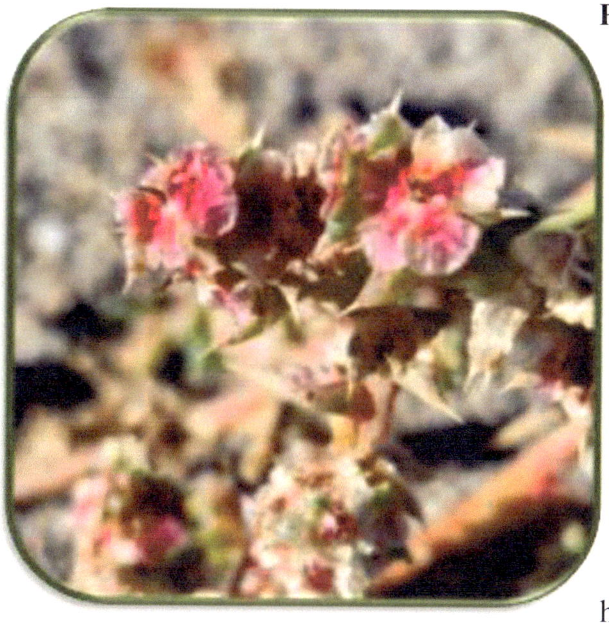

Properties and medical uses:

Salsulin alkaloid is used to reduce blood pressure as it is an arteriolar dilator. The juice of the fresh plant is popularly used for its diuretic properties, and in treating liver and bile diseases, urinary tract infections and expelling worms. The ash of the plant is used topically to treat skin diseases such as scabies, vitiligo and warts. Anti-cancer, laxative, emollient, anti-ulcer, anti-inflammatory, anti-bacterial and anti-oxidant.

Other uses:

The plant was used in the glass industry, and the ash was used in the past as a type of soap that is highly flammable. When dry, it is suitable for cooking and heating. Warnings for use: A poisonous plant, it should be used with extreme caution. Using large quantities (oxalic acid) leads to the fixation of many nutrients in the body, so that they become useless, which causes a deficiency in these elements. It should not be used by people who are prone to kidney stones or have excessive acidity or patients with rheumatism, arthritis, and gout, because it may worsen their health condition. Pollen dust can cause some respiratory allergies in some people. The thorns of the plant cause allergies in humans and animals. Oxalic acid or potassium nitrate KNo3 may be behind the poisoning cases of animals that graze it (nitrate NO3 is converted in the stomach of animals to nitrite NO2, which reacts with blood hemoglobin and converts it to methemoglobin, which prevents the transfer of oxygen to the body's organs and tissues, and leads to respiratory and cardiac disorders.

Environment:

An invasive plant, spreads in well-drained loamy and sandy soils, and can grow in saline and alkaline soils. pH (7.9-7) Prefers sunny places and does not tolerate shade, moderate temperature (9-24) suits it. Drought. It can be found in coastal sandy lands. The wind uproots it in winter and rolls to collect in valleys and low-lying areas.

Cultivation and productivity:

It is propagated by seeds that are scattered in the permanent soil in the spring. The seeds do not retain their vitality for a long period, so they must be stored in cold winter conditions.

Calotropis procera (Aiton) W.T.Aiton.

Asclepias procera Ait.,Calotropis procera subsp. hamiltonii)Wight(Ali., Asclepias pro- cera Aiton, Hort., Madorius procerus)Aiton.(Kuntze., Calotropis gigantea var. Procera)Aiton(P.T.Li.)

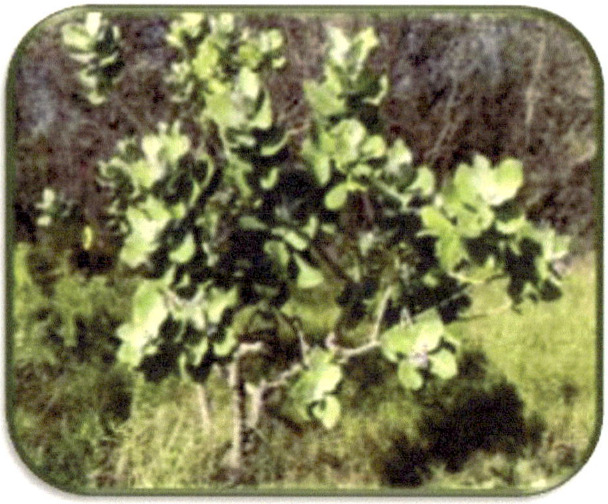

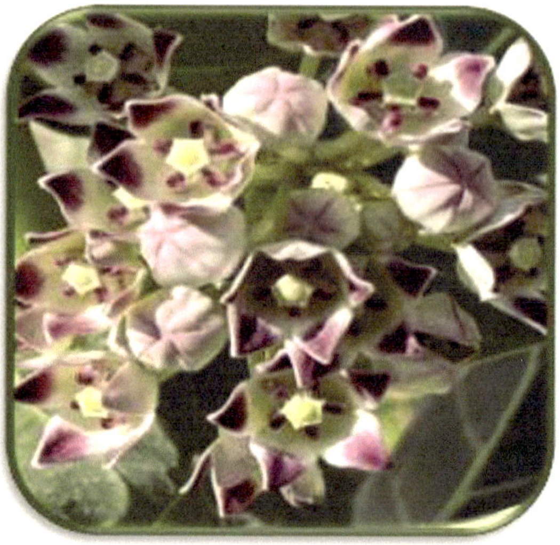

Family: Apocynaceae (formerly Asclepidiaceae).

Common names: Sakab, Shakhar, Ashkhar, Ashar, Ashar, Ashur, Ashur, Ashar, Eggs of the Ashar, Camel's Eggs.

Eng. Calotropis, Apple of Sodom giant milkweed Foreign names: Fr. calotropis , poome de sodome

Occurrences : 23,371 occurrences

Distribution in the world

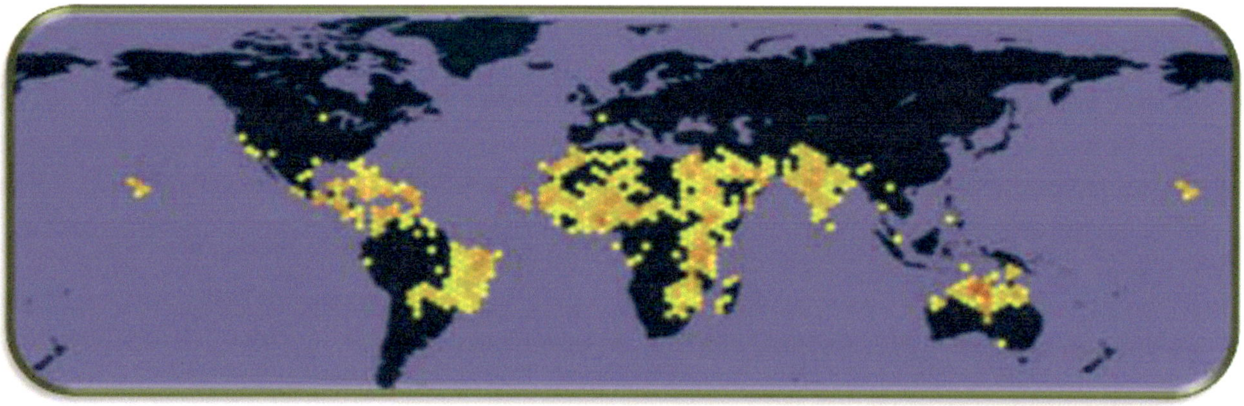

Botanical description:

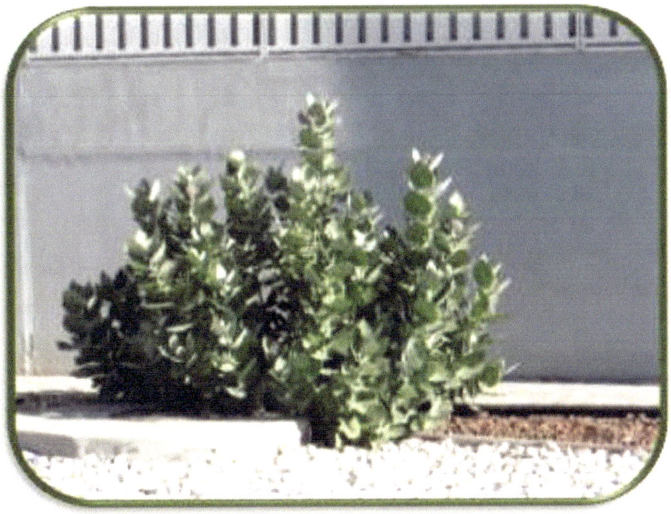

A white, 6-2 m tall, grey-green shrub. Young branches are white, woolly, hairy to almost glabrous . Stem covered with a white, corky, deeply fissured bark. Leaves 15-5×30-10 cm, simple, opposite, entire, semi-lobed, broadly ovate or elliptic or inverted ovate, with two auricles at the base, somewhat fleshy, hairy when young, especially the lower side. Inflorescence semi-semitic, axillary. Flowers radiate symmetrical, pentagonal, and hermaphrodite. Calyx perennial, segments fused at bases. Corolla cycloid-bell-shaped, about 20 mm in diameter, 5-lobed, broad, ovate, flattened, dark purple at apex, whitish in the middle, and greenish on the outside. Corolla bears a coronet composed of 5 laterally compressed segments, fused to the special structure formed by the fusion of the anthers with the apex of the style. The male has 5 stamens, the anthers of which are fused with the tip of the style to form a special structure. The female is composed of two free carpels, the ovary is superior, the styles are fused in their upper part, and they widen to form a five-fold stamen head, and the five stamen surfaces are exposed on the lower surface between the anthers. The fruit is composed of two marsupial fruits (or one marsupial fruit resulting from the abortion of one of them), semi-spherical or obliquely ellipsoidal or semi-oval in shape, green in colour, 8-12 cm long, smooth to the touch. The seeds are numerous, compressed, flat, with white hairs.

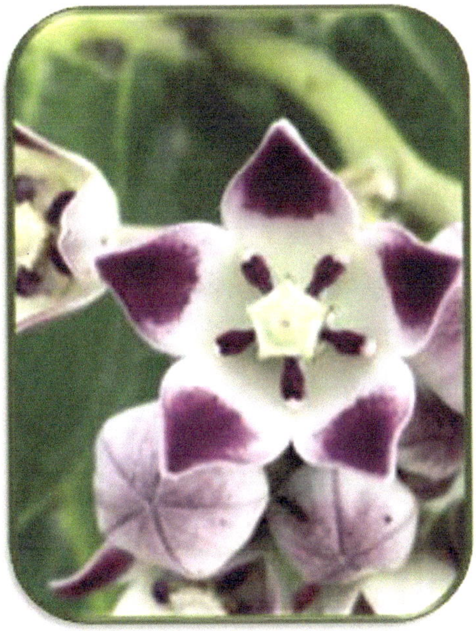

Flowering: From May to November.

Habitat and geographical distribution:

Sudanese, extending to the Arabian desert region In the Kingdom of Saudi Arabia, Egypt, Libya, Palestine, the Sultanate of Oman, Sudan, all desert countries, India, Afghanistan, and Pakistan.

History and heritage:

The genus name Calotropis is derived from the Greek, where kalos means "beautiful and wonderful", and Tropis means "boat", and the name may go back to the crown lobes. As for the species name procera, it means "high." The plant was used in medicine, as it was mentioned in ancient Egyptian medicine in the medical paper of Hirst as part of a recipe related to blood vessels. The Arabs knew it in ancient times, and they used to make ropes from its bark. Al-Asma'i mentioned it (the fruit has a skin that, when split from the fruit, appears from it like cotton, which is similar to the camel's udder). Abu Hanifa Al-Dinawari described it in the Book of Plants (as one of the large trees, it has sweet gum, it has broad leaves, and it has sugar that comes out of its flower site, it is called the sugar of the tenth, and it has bitterness.) The tenth was mentioned in the heritage of ancient Arab medicine, where it was used as a laxative for the intestines, and to expel For worms, and a medicine for ulcers, its ash is an expectorant, and a medicine for urinary retention. The hot leaves are placed on the stomach to heal stomach pain, the flowers are tonic, stimulate the appetite, and are used in treating asthma. The tree was known in ancient India to the level of sanctifying the plant, the Indians included it in medical prescriptions, so the juice of the root bark was used to treat some skin diseases, and the flowers were used to improve digestion and stimulate the appetite.

Part used:

Plant bark, root bark, and milky sap (when the stem is scratched or injured, a sticky milky liquid flows.)

Chemical components:

The plant bark and roots contain toxic cardiac glucosides, which are cardio-(cardenolids) steroids active, the most important of which are: calotropin, calactin, uscharidin, and others. It also contains alkaloids, including: asharin, furocharin, in addition to bitter substances.

All parts of the plant contain a milky juice, the most important components of which are resinous substances: trypsin, alpha and beta calotriol, digestive enzymes similar to papain, as well as trypsin enzyme responsible for the cell-lytic action. Several flavonoid compounds were isolated from the methanol extract of the plant leaves such as: rutin, kaempferol, isorhamnetin. The plant contains many substances such as glycosides (mostly cardenoids), flavonoids, triterpenes, alkaloids, saponins, proteins, and enzymes.

Properties and medical uses:

The plant is characterized by broad-spectrum biological activities such as: anti-inflammatory, antioxidant, anti-cancer, wound healing, and antimicrobial activities. A poisonous plant (accidental poisoning is common among cattle that eat the plant), especially the milky sap, due to the presence of toxic steroid compounds, to the extent that it was used to poison spears.

Research has shown the anti-tumor effect of calotropin, and the effect appeared especially in carcinoma epidermoid cells in the nasopharynx. The decoction of the flowers is used in Saudi folk medicine to treat asthma and indigestion. A mixture of powdered with honey is used to treat bronchial asthma and cough. The leaves are a strong emulsion or a strong laxative, and an external treatment for hemorrhoids. The Ashar is also used in the form of The milky juice is used topical tinctures in the treatment of chronic eczema, pimples, skin ulcers, rheumatism, and joint pain. The root barks are used for their diaphoretic, emetic, and expectorant properties. These compounds, in addition to the vegetable milk, have shown antibacterial and antifungal activity against some bacterial and fungal strains.

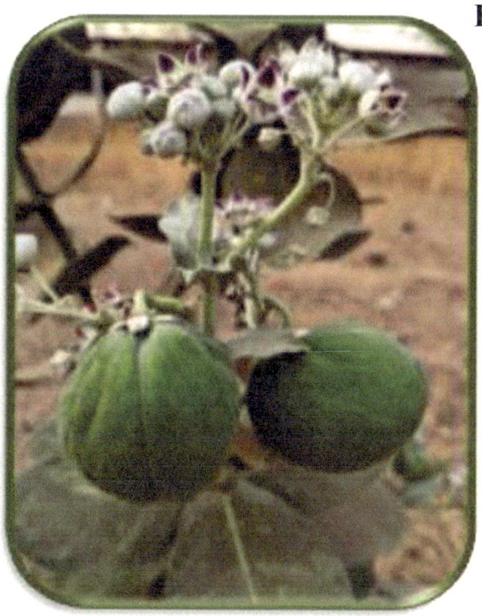

Precautions for use:

The Ashar fruit is warned against, as the sodium it contains causes eye and chest allergies.The plant is very poisonous, and should only be used under strict medical supervision. Ingestion of the juice or any part of the plant causes irritation of the digestive system, stomach pain accompanied by nausea, vomiting, severe diarrhea, slow heartbeat, and causes lung and liver damage, which may lead to death. It should be noted that small doses of the ten are diaphoretic and expectorant, while excessive doses cause severe vomiting and diarrhea, muscle spasms, and heart failure (cardiac arrhythmia). Very large doses are toxic and may cause death. The stomach must be washed immediately and the appropriate antidote taken.

Other uses:

The plant of the ten is one of the commercially important plants, as it produces strong, white, silky fibers, similar in their properties to flax fibers that are resistant to both fresh and salt water. The fibers are used in the manufacture of sewing threads for clothing, carpet threads, fishing nets and bird traps. The rubber of the ten is 80% effective in inhibiting the activity of the tobacco mosaic virus. The bark extract can be used for hair removal and tanning leather.

Environment:

A widespread plant, growing in desert areas on sandy plains in various areas such as valleys.

Cultivation and productivity:

A plant that reproduces by seeds, and may sometimes be invasive.

Nerium oleander L.

Nerium indicum Mill., *Nerium latifolium* Mill., *Oleander vulgaris* Medik., *Nerion ole- andrum* St.-Lag., *Nerium odoratum* Lam., *Nerium odorum* Salisb., *Nerium grandiflorum* Desf.

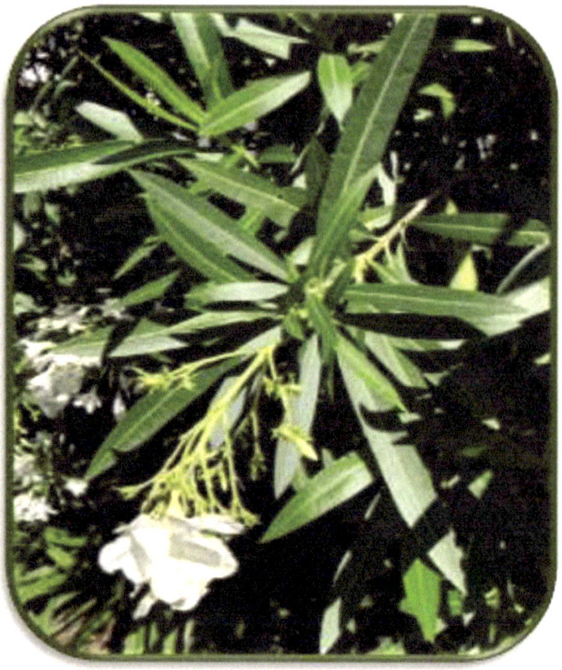

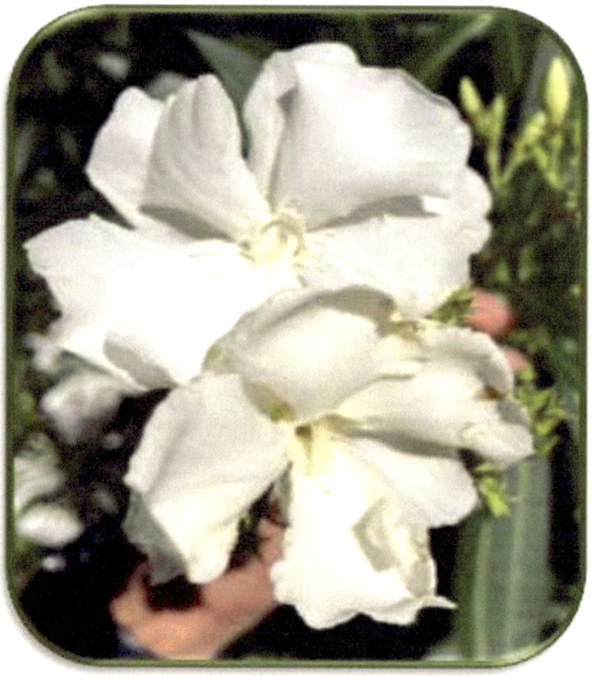

Family: Apocynaceae

Common names: Oleander, Dafla, Donkey rose, Donkey poison, Haban, Alaa, Tarish.

Foreign names: Laurier-rose Fr. Laurel, Rose Eng.

Occurrences :106,768 occurrences

Distribution in the world

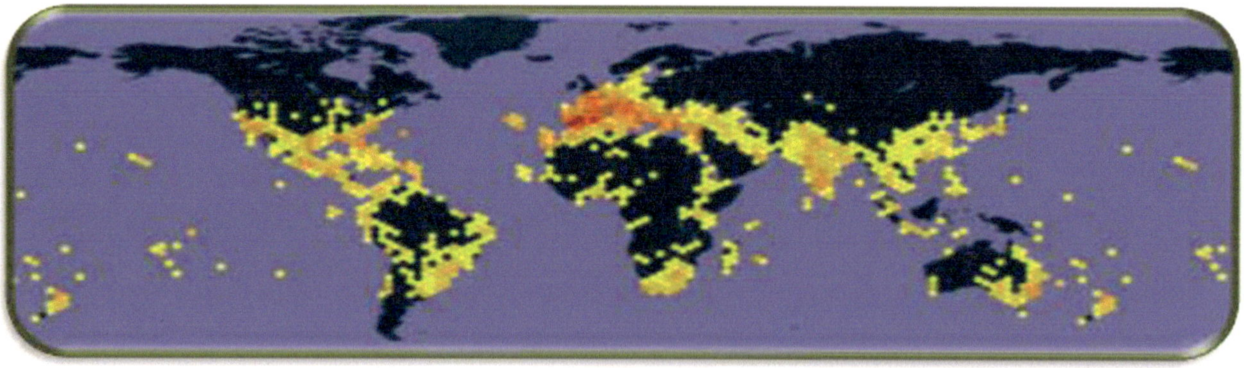

Botanical description:

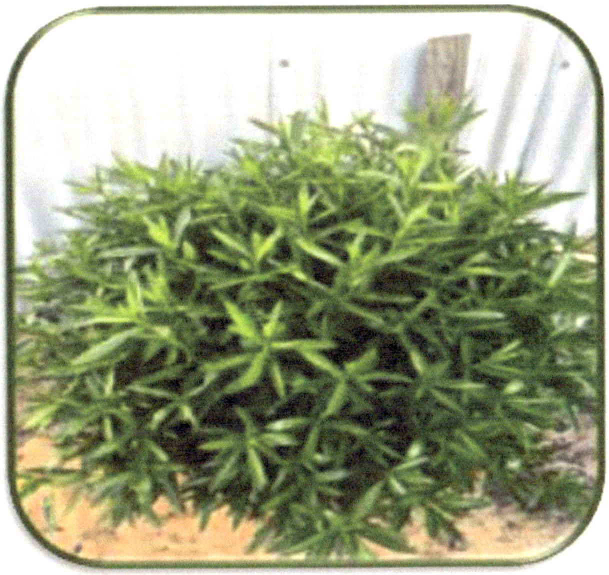

An evergreen shrub, 1-4 m tall, semi-growth, branches erect. Leaves are sessile (arranged in whorls of 3-4 leaves), about 10 cm long, leathery, linear to lanceolate, acute, short-stalked, and covered with dense hairs on the lower surface. Flowers are relatively large, gathered in terminal racemes. The calyx is divided into 5 lobes, linear to lanceolate. The corolla is white or pink, 4-5 cm in diameter, its segments are united in a tube that widens suddenly and splits into 5 lobes, around the opening of the tube there is a wreath composed of 5 serrated appendages. The male has 5 stamens, located on the corolla tube in the middle, the anthers are longer than the filaments, united in the middle with the stigma, and its apex bears appendages that are braided together. The fruit is composed of two fused marsupial fruits, which separate when ripe. The seeds are abundant, woolly, and their top ends with a bouquet of hairs.

Flowering: Oleander blooms from spring to fall.

Habitat and geographical distribution:

The Mediterranean basin is the original home of the species, where it is naturally spread in Syria, Lebanon, Palestine, Jordan, Iraq and Egypt, and grows in other parts of the world such as Japan and Korea. It is planted as an ornamental shrub in gardens and public streets.

History and heritage:

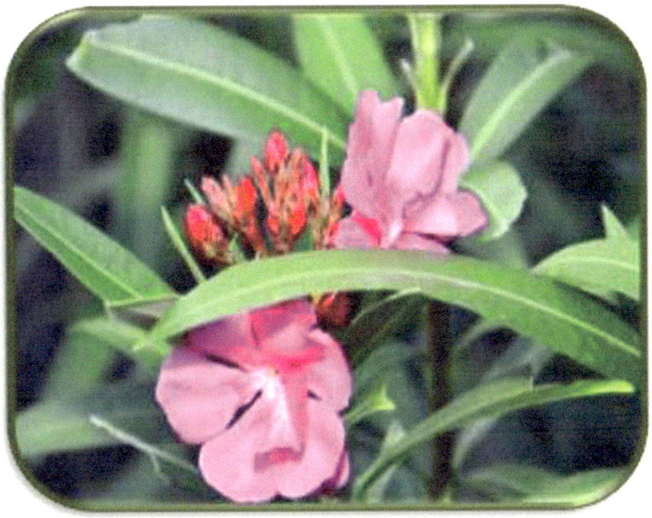

The scientific name of the genus is derived from the Greek word nêrion, which is the name of a similar plant, and then it was designated to name this genus. As for the name of the species oleander, it means "olive", due to the similarity of its leaves to the leaves of olive sp. .Olea It is used as a dressing, A plant known for its extreme toxicity. Ibn Sina and Ibn al-Baytar mentioned that oleander is good for knee and back pain if inhaling it soothes toothache. It is used as an example for bitterness, so it is said: bitter like oleander.

Part used: Leaves, picked just before flowering.

Chemical components:

The leaves contain cardiac steroid glycosides of the cardenolide type, the most important of which are: oleandrosid, nerigoside, and neriumoside. It also contains pregnane. The flowers contain cardiac glycosides (4.24%), flavonoids (4.21%), terpenes (3.76%), alkaloids (3.21%), saponins (2.41%), phenols (1.92%), and astringents (0.11%). Anthraquinones. (0.09%) In addition to the presence of chlorogenic acid, rutin, and quinic acid esters such as caffeoylquinic and decaffeoylquinic acids.

Properties and medical uses:

Oleander has a positive effect on the contraction of the heart muscle, and a negative effect on the heart clock. The glycosides cardenolide compounds found in oleander are similar in effect to digitoxin, but they are weaker than it, and this may be due to the difficulty of absorbing these compounds in the body.

It is popularly used to treat heart failure, heart disorders, and skin diseases. The juice of the leaves is used topically in Indian medicine to treat eye diseases, and is also used to treat hemorrhoids and scabies. The crude flower extract has antimicrobial, anti-inflammatory, and anticancer properties with no potential toxicity at therapeutic doses. Phenolic compounds have been extracted from oleander leaves, which have shown to inhibit the growth of colon and rectal cancer cells.

Side effects, interactions and precautions:

Oleander should not be used with quinidine, calcium salts and glucocorticoids. High doses cause toxicity manifested by nausea, vomiting, diarrhea and tachycardia.

Environment:

Oleander grows naturally on waterways, however it tolerates drought. It grows well in areas with moderate temperatures and high atmospheric humidity. It is considered a salt-tolerant species, although it leads to slow plant growth, accompanied by a high content of sodium in the leaves and a low content of potassium and calcium.

Cultivation and productivity:

The plant is propagated by stem cuttings collected during the pruning period. The cuttings are planted in basins in a slanted position in the nursery soil, or in pots or black nylon bags. The plant can also be propagated by suckers, which are long cuttings, each containing a small part of the stem of the mother plant called a heel. The cuttings or suckers are transferred to the permanent ground the following spring.

Vinca herbacea Waldst. & Kit.

V. libanotica Zucc.,*Vinca pumila* E.D.Clarke., *Vinca sessilifolia* A.DC., *Vinca mixta* Velen., *Vinca herbacea* subsp. *libanotica*)Zucc.(Bornm., *Vinca bottae* Jaub. & Spach.

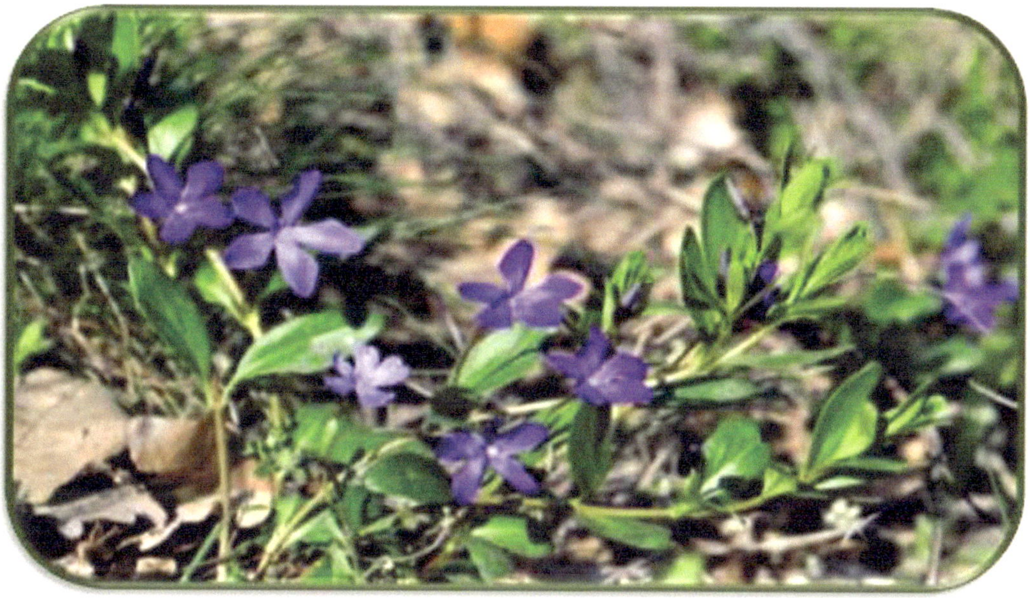

Family: Apocynaceae

Common names: Herbaceous periwinkle, Pervenche herbacee

Foreign names:

Occurrences :4,294 occurrences

Distribution in the world

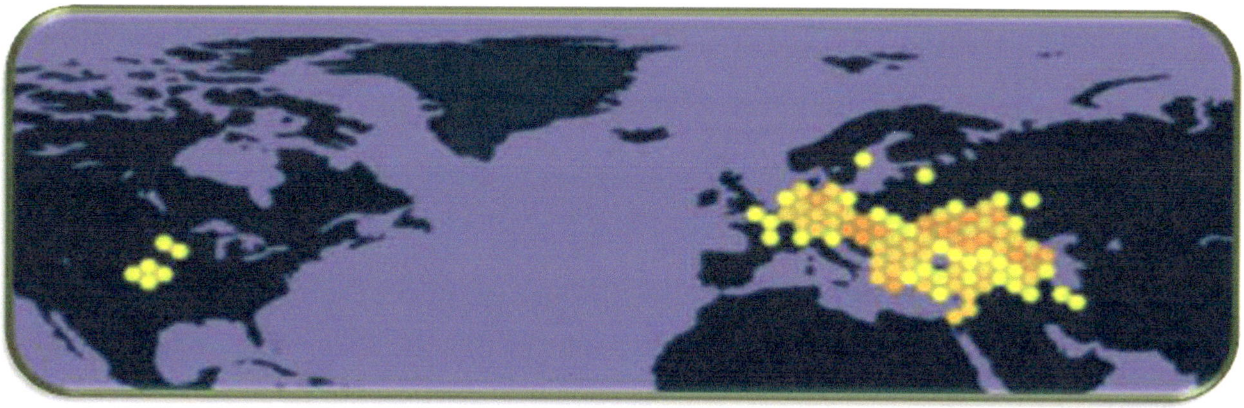

Botanical description:

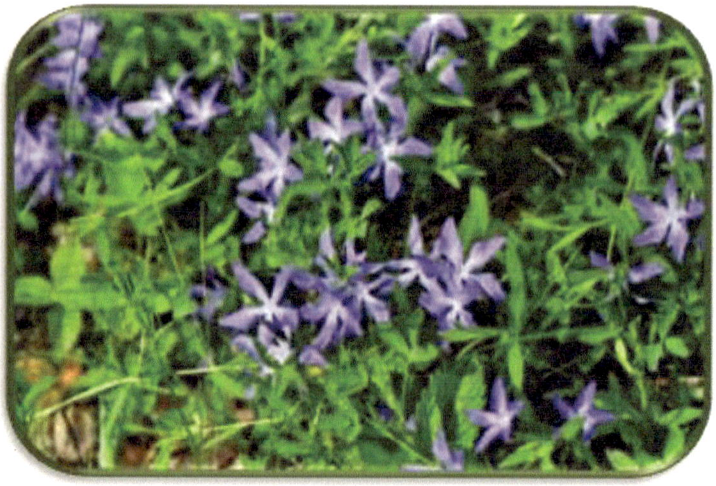

Perennial herb, 20-40 cm tall, glabrous. Stems are supine and ascending, spreading in all directions. Leaves are simple, opposite, short-petiolate, ovate to elliptic to lanceolate, semi-rough-edged or smooth. Flowers are solitary in the axils of the leaves, their panicles are equal in length to the supporting leaves or longer. The calyx has linear to lanceolate lobes, acute. Corolla funnel-shaped, blue, 20-35 mm in diameter, tube densely hairy inside. Male 5 stamens, above petal. Fruit composed of two marsupial fruits, 3-4 cm long, arched. Seeds smooth.

Flowering: March to May.

Habitat and geographical distribution:

Mediterranean and Iranian-Turanian, extending to the Euro-Siberian region.

History and Heritage:

Vinca is a modern Arabized name from the scientific name of the genus Vinca, which is the old Latin name for this species, descending from "Rabt", referring to the climbing stems in some species of the genus, while the name from the word Vincere, meaning "to embrace" or " the descriptor of the species Herbacea, meaning "herbaceous." Interest in some species of the genus has increased recently, due to the effects that have been discovered for some of the alkaloids they contain.

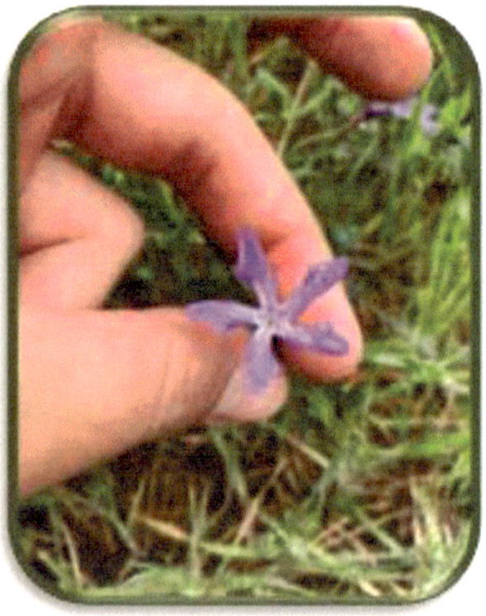

Part used: Dried leaves, and the young flowering plant.

Chemical components:

The plant contains alkaloids akuammin, ervamycin, herbain, hervin, vincarin, vincamin, and vincanin. It also contains rutin, organic acids, tannins, and simple phenols.

Medical properties and uses:

The plant has neurocardiovascular effects, effects on blood pressure, and effects on smooth muscles. It is popularly used as an anti-digestive and anti-spasmodic, and in the treatment of diabetes. It is also used topically to treat dental diseases and fungal skin diseases. The results showed that the aqueous and alcoholic extracts of the herbaceous periwinkle have antioxidant activity due to their high content of rutin. Periwinkle extracts inhibited the growth of Staphylococcus aureus by 60% in almost all concentrations. They also had an antibacterial effect against E. coli bacteria and an inhibitory effect against S. aureus bacteria.

Precautions for use: High doses cause general tremors.

Environment:

The plant tolerates high and low temperatures, and prefers a moderate climate and a long photoperiod, which stimulates the speed of vegetative growth and increases the percentage of the active substance. The plant grows well in most soils, the best of which are light, well-drained and aerated soils. Calcium in the soil improves vegetative growth and increases the percentage of the active substance.

Cultivation and productivity:

The plant is propagated by seeds and stem or root cuttings. The seeds are planted in early spring and are transferred to the permanent soil after two months. Planting is done in lines, at a rate of 80 cm between one line and the next, and 70 cm between seedlings or cuttings in one line, and they are irrigated directly after planting. Planting can also be done in basins or drains. The service operations provided to the plant are summarized in moderate irrigation during the growth period, nitrogen and phosphate fertilization in particular, as well as combating the many fungi and viruses that infect it. The green parts are cut before the flowering stage in two stages, the first in the summer and the second in the fall, and dried in the shade or in dryers with a temperature exceeding 45°C. The production per hectare reaches 2.5-3 tons of dry grass and about 2-1.5 tons of dry roots.

Vinca major L.

Pervinca major)L.(Garsault., *Vinca grandiflora* Salisb., *Vinca minor* subsp. *major*)L.(Bonnier & Layens., *Vinca ovatifolia* Stokes.

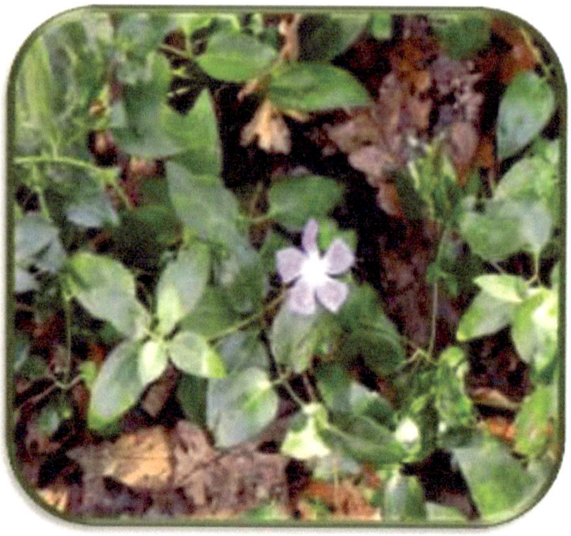

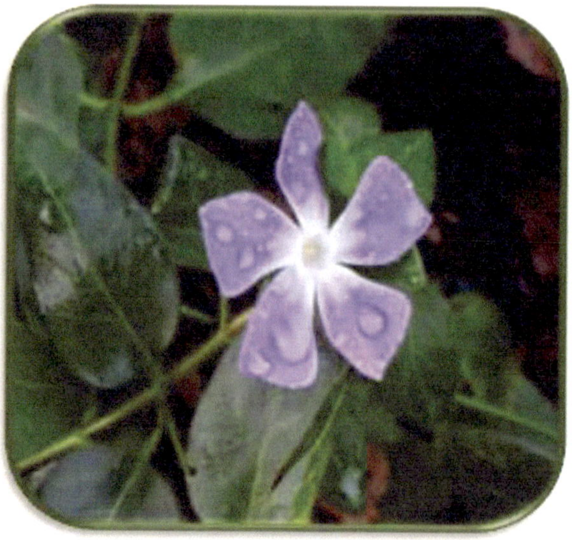

Family: Apocynaceae

Common names: Great Periwinkle

Foreign names:

Occurrences : 100,735 occurrences

Distribution in the world

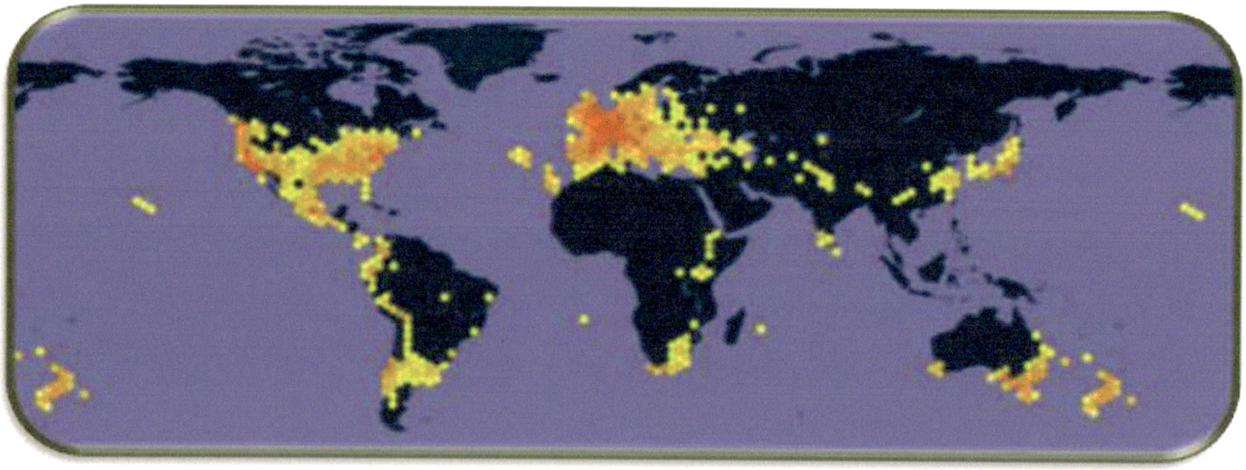

Botanical description:

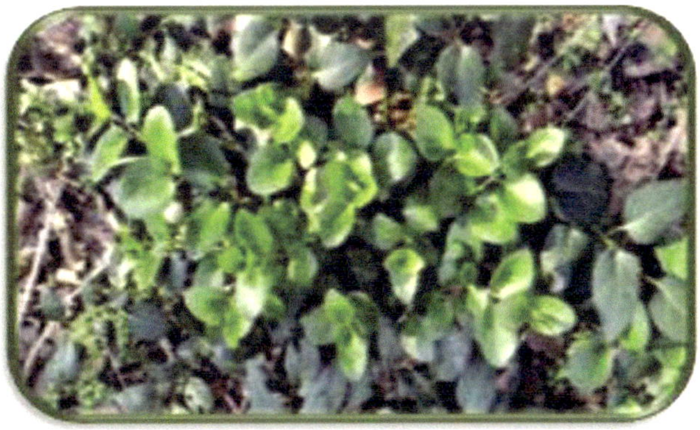

Perennial, evergreen, glabrous herb. Stem is main, forming a clump of plants, diameter 2-5 m, height 50-70 cm. Leaves are simple, opposite, ovate, 3-9 cm long, 2-6 cm wide, petiole 1-2 cm long. Flowers are solitary in the axils of the leaves, diameter 3-5 cm. Calyx 12-15 mm, lobes linear-lanceolate, acute. Corolla funnel-shaped, violet, tube slightly longer than the calyx. Male 5 stamens, above petal. Female composed of two free carpels. Fruit composed of two marsupial fruits, 3-4 cm long, arched. Seeds smooth.

Flowering: March to September.

Habitat and geographical distribution: Mediterranean.

History and heritage:

The genus name was mentioned in the previous species. As for the descriptive name of the species major, it means "large."

Part used: Herbal plant

Chemical components:

The plant contains alkaloids akuammin, ervamycin, herbain, hervin, vincarin, vincamin, vincanin, reserpinin, and jervine. Recently, 43 alkaloids have been isolated, 9 of which have been described. The herb also contains iridoid terpenoids, flavonoids, organic acids, tannins, and simple phenols.

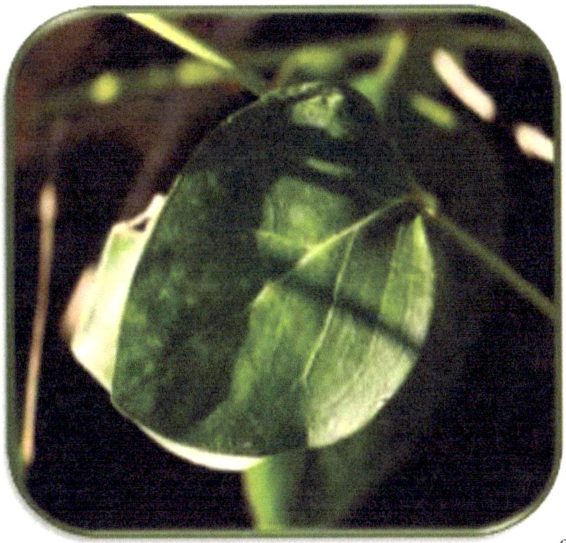

Properties and medical uses:

The plant has a blood pressure lowering effect and is an antispasmodic for smooth muscle. It is popularly used as an anti-digestive and anti-spasmodic, as well as in cases of diabetes. It is used externally to treat hemorrhoids, as a vasodilator, and as a diuretic. The plant is astringent, analgesic, brain stimulant, and vasodilator. It is used internally to treat excessive menstruation, abnormal uterine bleeding, vaginal discharge, and arteriosclerosis. It is used externally for vaginal discharge, nosebleeds (epistaxis), sore throat, and mouth ulcers. Due to the astringent effect of mature fennel, leaf extracts are used externally as a mouthwash or gargle for sore throat, gingivitis, and mouth ulcers, and as a wash, wet compress, or dressing to treat minor skin infections, eczema, vaginal discharge, and wounds. In addition, the herb has also been used to stop nosebleeds (epistaxis) by placing the leaves directly into the nostrils. It can be used to treat gastritis (inflammation or irritation of the stomach lining) and diarrhea.

Studies have shown that patients suffering from poor memory, behavioral disorders, speech disorders, irritability, insomnia, dizziness, and headaches showed significant improvement when taking vincamine.

Dosage and method of use:

Tincture: 1-2 ml three times a day.

Gargle: Two tablespoons of dried herb boiled in half a liter of water for a few minutes.

If the herb is intended for internal medicinal use, it should be done under the supervision of a specialist only.

Precautions for use:

High doses cause general tremors. Do not give to patients with constipation. Taking large amounts of the herbal substance can be harmful to the kidneys and nervous system, and cause problems in the digestive system and a severe drop in blood pressure.

Environment:

As mentioned in the previous type herbaceae.

Cultivation and productivity:

As mentioned in the previous type herbaceae.

Vinca minor L.

Pervinca minor)L.(Garsault., *Vinca humilis* Salisb., *Vinca minor* var. *alba* Weston., *Vin- ca intermedia* Tausch., *Vinca ellipticifolia* Stokes., *Pervinca heterophyla* Raf., *Pervinca repens* Raf.

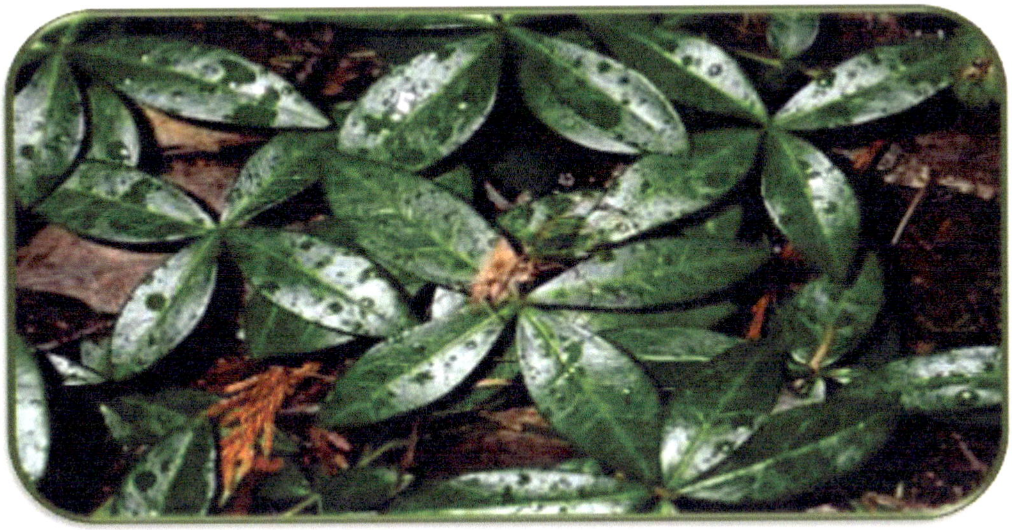

Family: Apocynaceae

Common names: Little periwinkle, Little periwinkle

Foreign names: Lesser periwinkle, Fr. Petite Pervenche

Occurrences : 245,412 occurrences

Distribution in the world

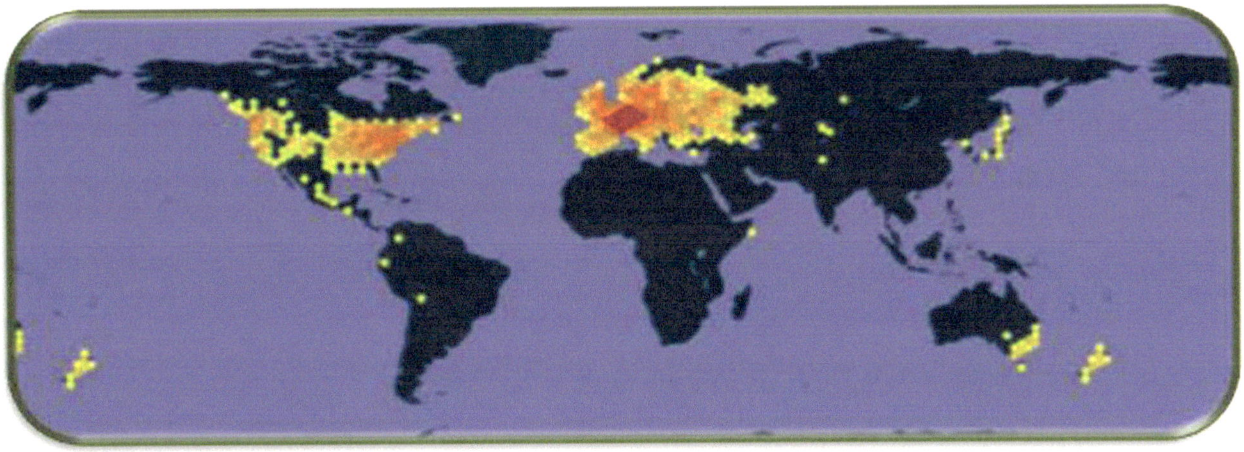

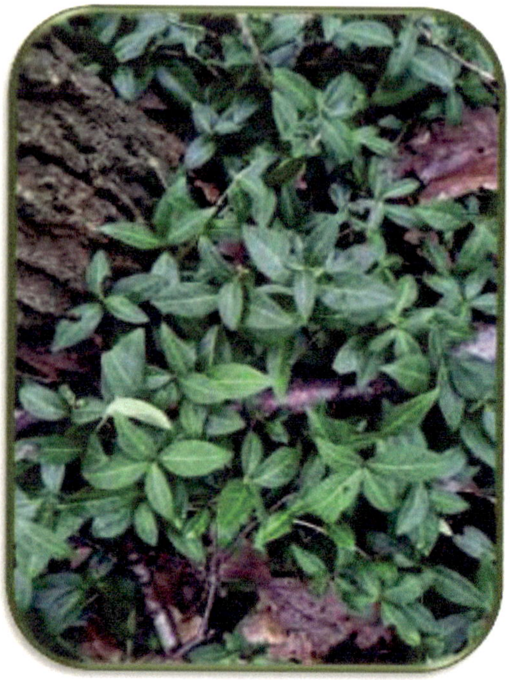

Botanical description:

A perennial herb, up to 40 cm tall, with a main stem, which contributes to its spread in the form of colonies, and secretes a colorless vegetable milk. The leaves are simple, shiny, opposite, short-petiolate, entire-edged, oblong, oval or elliptic in shape, and pedicel-shaped at the base, not fringed at the edge, their dimensions are 0.5-2.5 × 1-4.5 cm. The flowers are solitary, axillary, their panicle length is about 1 cm, five-segmented. The calyx is small, 3-5 mm long, five-lobed, apexed. The corolla is lilac to blue, funnel-shaped, the tube is cylindrical, about 1 cm long, its aperture is pentagonal, not hairy, the lobes are flattened, inverted ovate, their apex is truncated obliquely, overlapping to the left, their diameter is 2.5-3 cm. The stamens are located slightly below and in the middle of the tube. The female is dioecious. The fruit is marsupial, erect. The seeds are numerous, glabrous.

Flowering: It blooms in spring and summer.

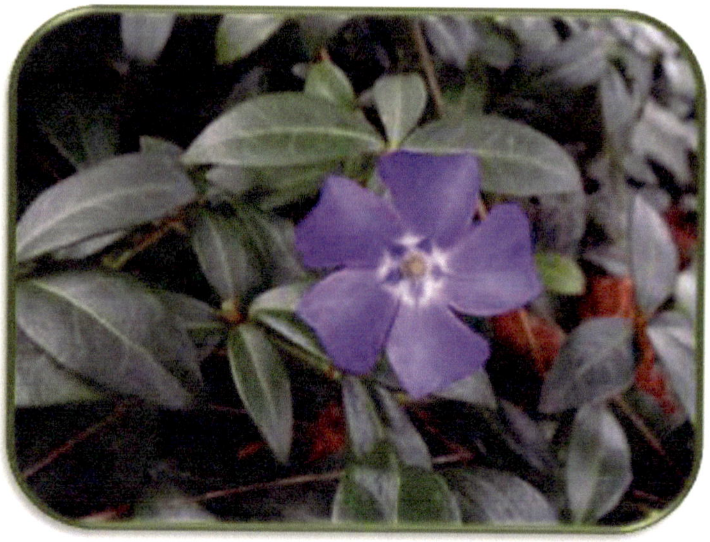

Habitat and geographical distribution:

The species of the genus are spread wild in many regions of the Mediterranean Basin countries and central Europe, and are cultivated in many countries such as the United States of America, Russia, Germany, Switzerland and France.

History and heritage:

The scientific name of the genus as mentioned in the species is herbaceae V. and the descriptive name of the species minor means "small."

Part used: Dried leaves, tender flowering plant.

Chemical components:

Indole terpene alkaloids, and Indole alkaloids 1.4-0.15%, the most important of which are vincamine, vincine, and apovincamine, in addition to flavonoids. In addition to alkaloids, there are other important natural compounds found in vinca species, which are phenolic acids, carotenoids, caffeic acid, irioid, flavonoids, amino acids, and other phenolic compounds. Chlorogenic acid (one of the phenols) is found in large quantities in all species of the genus Vinca. Other phenols have also been identified in different species of Vinca, in much lower concentrations compared to chlorogenic acid, such as coumaric acid, caffeic acid, ferulic acid, rutin, and kaempferol.

Properties and medical uses:

Vincamine alkaloid has hypotensive properties, it also has a negative effect on heart rhythm, Anticotropic, hypoglycemic, antisympathetic, antisympathomimetic, it is used in the treatment of circulatory disorders .For the action of sympathomimetic drugs (circulatory problems related to the brain in particular), memory loss, high blood pressure, and cystitis, Inflammation of the stomach and intestines.

It is used externally to treat nosebleeds, sore throat, eczema, abscesses, and bleeding. Vinbastine alkaloid is one of the chemotherapy drugs, usually derived from the alkaloid vincamine, used with other drugs to treat many types of cancer, including: Hodgkin lymphoma, non-small cell lung cancer, bladder cancer, brain cancer, skin cancer, and breast cancer. The treatment is given by injection into a vein.

All plant extracts had better inhibitory effect against S. aureus than E. coli. E. coli was inhibited by all extracts in a dose-dependent manner.

Use Precautions:

Excessive doses of the plant can cause poisoning.

Environment:

The plant is widespread in areas of the Mediterranean Basin, Latin America and North America. The United States of America is the first in the production of the lilac, followed by Germany, Russia, France and Switzerland. Some of its species are also widespread in Syria in the Jabal al-Arab, Hauran and western Damascus countryside regions, and are planted for decoration in homes and public parks. The plant tolerates high and low temperatures, and prefers a moderate climate that allows for a large percentage of vegetative growth and active substance. The length and intensity of the light period increases the size of vegetative growth and the percentage of active substance in the plant. The plant grows well in most agricultural soils, the best of which are light soils with good drainage and ventilation. Calcium in the soil improves vegetative growth and increases the percentage of active substance.

Cultivation and productivity:

It is propagated by seeds or root or stem cuttings. The seeds are planted in early spring and transferred to the permanent land after two months. Planting is done in lines at a rate of 80 cm between each line and 70 cm between seedlings or cuttings on the same line, and it is irrigated directly after planting. It is also possible to plant in basins or drains. The service operations provided to the plant are summarized in moderate irrigation during the growth period, nitrogen and phosphate fertilization in particular, as well as combating the many fungi and viruses that infect it. The green parts are cut before flowering, in two stages; the first in the summer, and the second in the fall, and are dried in the shade or in dryers with temperatures exceeding 45 ° C. The production of a hectare reaches 3-2.5 tons of dry grass, and about 2-1.5 tons of dry roots

Hedera helix L.

Hedera poetica Salisb., *Hedera helix* var. *arborescens* Lodd. ex Loudon., *Hedera helix f. poetarum*)Nicotra(. McAll. & A.Rutherf., *Hedera communis* Gray., *Hedera helix var. vulgaris* DC., *Hedera helix* f. *helix.*

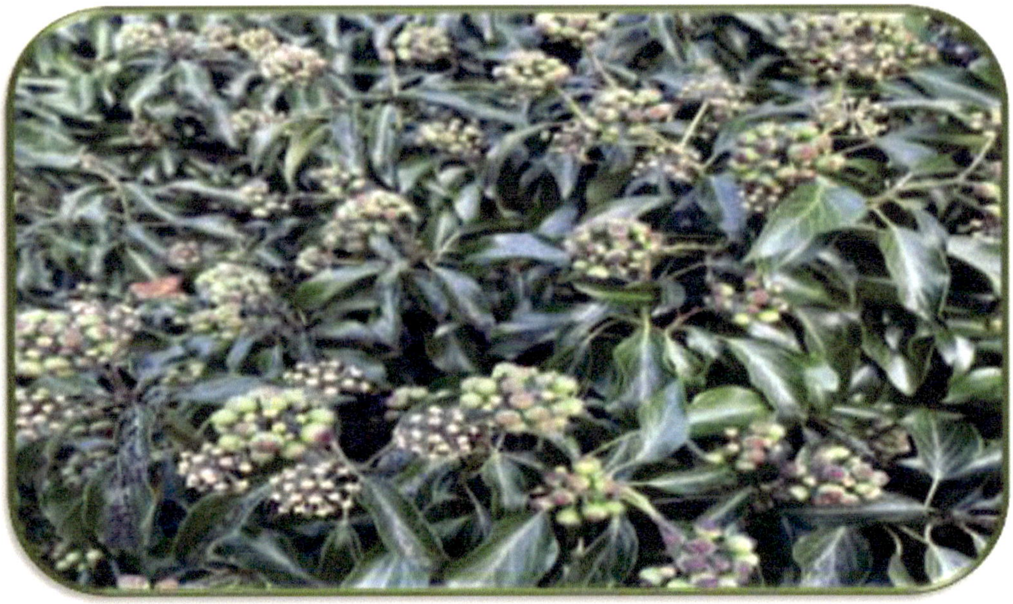

Family: Araliaceae

Common names: Liberal, climbing Liberal, poor man's rope, priest, hydra

Foreign names: grimpant Lierre Fr. ivy, English Eng

Occurrences : 990,780 occurrences

Distribution in the world

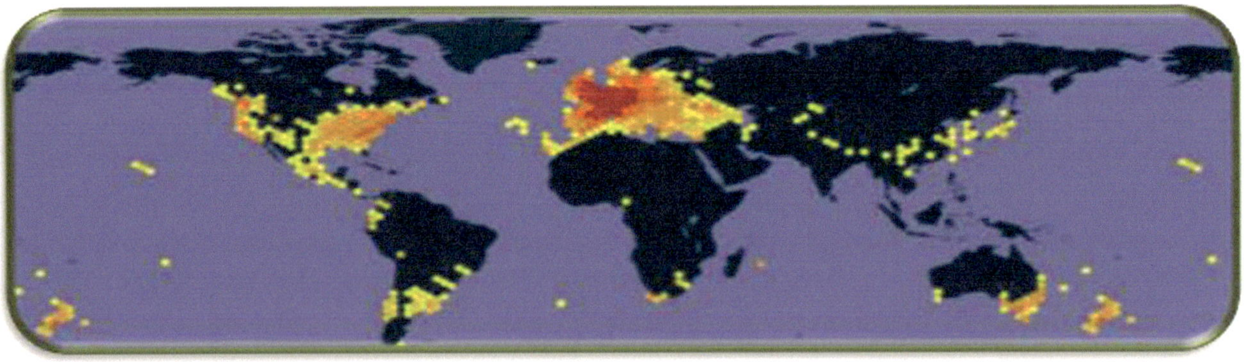

Botanical description:

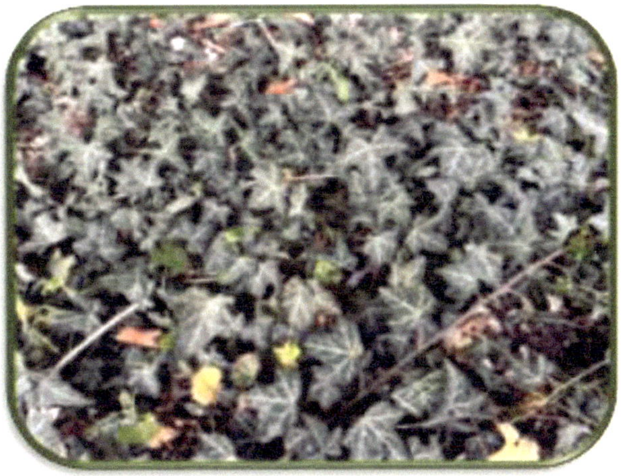

A climbing shrub, evergreen, that can excee d tens of meters in height. The stems are woody, with many branches. The branches bear brush-shaped, nail-like roots that help them cling to the supports they climb on (walls, rocks, or trees), and they do not have an absorption function. Leaves alternate, long-petioled, leathery, base wedge-shaped, cordate or rounded, dark green on the upper surface, glossy, leaf blade 6-2×12-3 cm, lower leaf blade contains 3-5 complete triangular lobes, upper leaf blade complete, ovate to rhombic, apex pointed. Flowers are paniculate, gathered in spherical umbel inflorescences. The calyx is fused to the ovary, has the shape of a cup ending in 5 triangular lobes, about 2 mm long. Corolla 5 free petals, 3-4 mm long, yellowish to green, triangular to ovate, cap-shaped. Male 5 free stamens. Female 5 carpels, ovary inferior, dome-shaped, topped by short stigma. Fruit 5-8 mm, berry-like, inverted conical to spherical, blackish in colour, composed of 5 ovatetrilobed nuclei, each containing one seed.

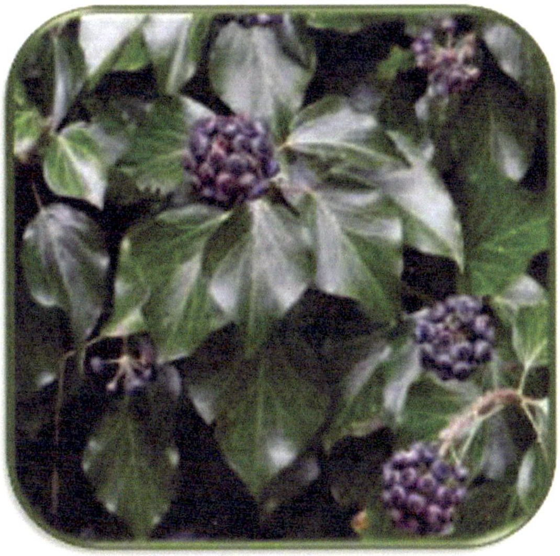

Flowering: October to February, fruiting in late winter and early spring.

Homeland and geographical distribution:

European - Siberian and Mediterranean. Its cultivation was introduced to many countries. It is naturally widespread in the forests of the eastern Mediterranean countries.

History and heritage:

The word "lablab" is of Syriac origin, and it is not the "lablab" that is given to a type of bean that grows in Egypt and is called "lablab" Dolichos. The scientific name of the genus is the old Latin name for these species, while the species name "helix" is derived from the Latin word for a plant that resembles "lablab".

Part used: Leaves

Chemical components:

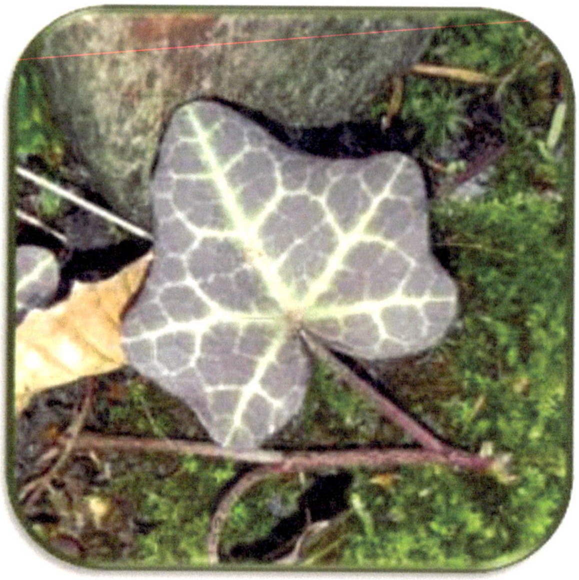

The leaves contain triterpene saponins (oleanolic acid saponins such as hydracoside), volatile oil, hydrocarbons, polyynes including falcarinol, steroids such as sterols, beta-sitosterol, campasterol, phenolic compounds (coumarin glycosides), organic acids, flavonoids, and vitamins E, A, and C. The groups included Chemicals isolated from the fruits of the plant: triterpene saponins, A helixoside, B helixoside, hederagenin, polyacetylene: falcarinone, falcarinol, panaxidol. Fatty acids, including petroselinic, oleic, sesquiquinic, palmitoleic, and β-lectins.

Properties and medical uses:

The leaves have antitussive and anti-bronchitis properties, expectorant, antiviral and antibacterial properties, worms (fasciola hepatica), and flagellates, and cytotoxic, antispasmodic, and diuretic properties. The plant extract is an astringent, digestive stimulant, and nerve sedative, especially in cases of burns. It is also used to treat respiratory tract infections (catarrh), for the symptomatic treatment of chronic infectious bronchitis, and to treat ringworm, scabies, and worms. A decoction of the leaves is used popularly to treat the liver, bile, and pancreas. Its leaves are used topically as cold compresses to treat infections, wounds, burns, parasitic diseases, rheumatic pain, gout, and phlebitis. The crushed leaves are used externally as a parasiticide and insecticide, for example against scabies and lice.

Pharmaceutical preparations:

Herbal medicines containing the leaves of the hyssop are usually available in solid or liquid pharmaceutical forms, taken orally. Medicinal tea, especially liquid, shampoo.

Precautions for use:

The young leaves may cause local allergic reactions. Do not use wormwood medicines for children under two years of age. Hydra should not be taken by people who are highly allergic to hydra leaves or other plants of the Araliaceae family.

Environment:

Hydra is a temperate plant. It grows in forests and shady, semi-shady or sunny places, climbing on trees, walls and rocks, but it does not usually flower in complete shade. It grows on different types of soils, and its presence indicates moderately acidic soils in most Sometimes. Loves soil moisture, but is tolerant to drought and pollution.

Cultivation and productivity:

The plant is propagated by seeds, the fatty pulp of the fruit is removed, as it prevents germination, and it can be stacked in the cold for four weeks, which greatly improves its germination. The seeds are scattered in the spring, when the seedlings grow a little, they are transferred to pots placed in moderately warm places during the winter, and they are transferred to the permanent ground in late spring or Early summer. It can also be propagated by semi-woody cuttings, which are planted in spring or summer in a shaded place, or in a greenhouse, in sandy, humus soil, moistened with a fine spray to stimulate them to form roots, and then transferred to planting in permanent soil, watered moderately. Wooden cuttings of 12 cm in length can be used and planted in the fall in a greenhouse as well. It can also be propagated by layering, which is what the plant usually does naturally.

Phoenix dactylifera L.

Palma dactylifera)L.(Mill., Phoenix excelsior Cav., Encephalartos pungens Lehm., Macrozamia tridentata var. pungens)Willd.(J.Schust., Palma major Garsault.

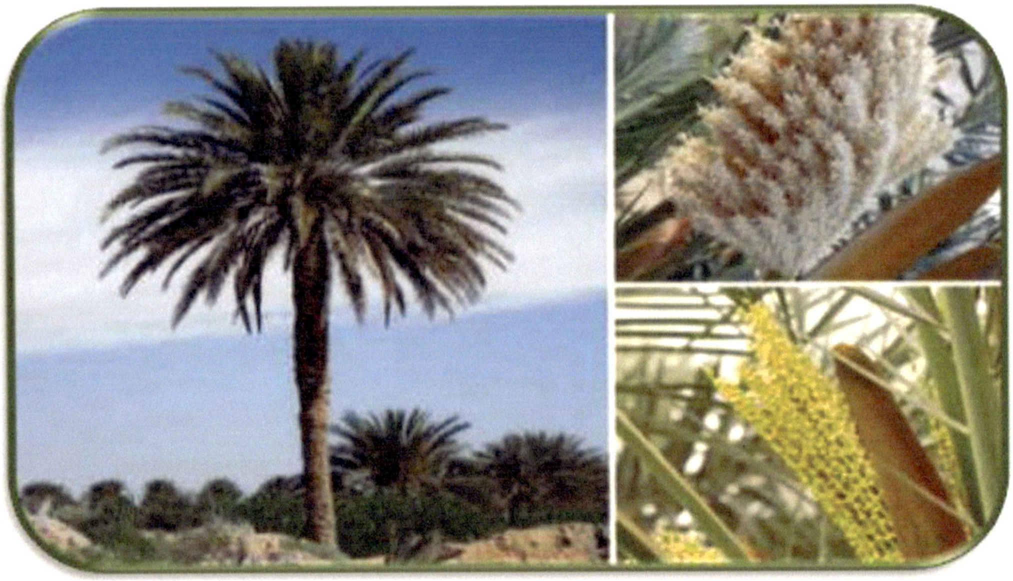

Family: Arecaceae

Common names: Palm, Date Palm

Foreign names: Dattier Fr. Palm, Date Eng

Occurrences :7,111 occurrences

Distribution in the world

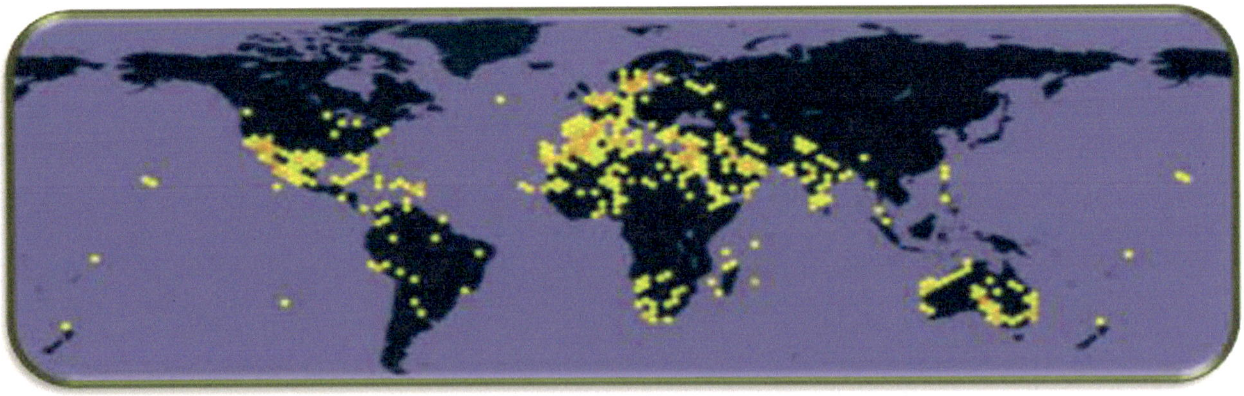

Botanical description:

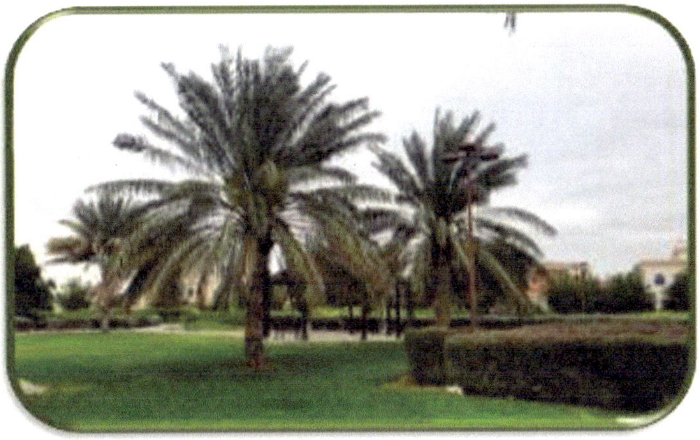

A dioecious tree, 10-20 m tall, the stem is unbranched, vertical, covered with fallen leaf bases. The leaves are large, 2-3 m long, bluish-green, oblong-lanceolate in general shape, deeply divided, the main nerve is thick, semi-cylindrical, its parts are linear-lanceolate, pointed, folded lengthwise. The inflorescence is paniculate, its branches are long, sinuous. The flowers are unisexual, sessile. Male flowers: 6-segmented in 2 whorls; outer three-toothed, cup-like, inner free. Male 6-stamens, anthers semi-segmented. Female flowers: segment similar to male flowers, female composed of three free carpels, but only one carpel matures. Fruit a single-seeded berry (date), seed ovate to ellipsoid. Seed with longitudinal slit, endosperm composed of very tough cellulose fibers.

Flowering: April to May.

Home and geographical distribution:

It is believed that the original homeland of the plant is the dry belt extending from Morocco to Pakistan, and it is believed that it has been cultivated in Iraq and Egypt since 5000 years BC.

History and heritage:

Allah Almighty has distinguished dates with many virtues, and the verses of the Qur'an have indicated the high status of dates, as He Almighty said: (And shake the trunk of the palm tree toward you, it will drop upon you fresh, ripe dates.) Surah Maryam.

The Prophet (peace and blessings of Allah be upon him) said: "Whoever eats seven dates in the morning will not be harmed that day by poison or magic." It was also reported that he said: "A house without dates will have hungry people." The ancient Greeks called the palm tree Pheonix, and the use of the name dates back to ancient times. Some believe that the name is derived from the Phoenicians who traded dates in the eastern part of the Mediterranean, or that it refers to the mythical bird Phoenix of the ancient Egyptians. The descriptive name of the species dactylifera refers to the fruits that resemble a finger (from the Greek: dactylos finger) meaning that the fruits are finger-shaped. The date palm was known as the "tree of the Arabs" The fruits of the palm were the basic food for the people of the Arab region, and they were widely spread in the Arab countries.

Part used: The fruits.

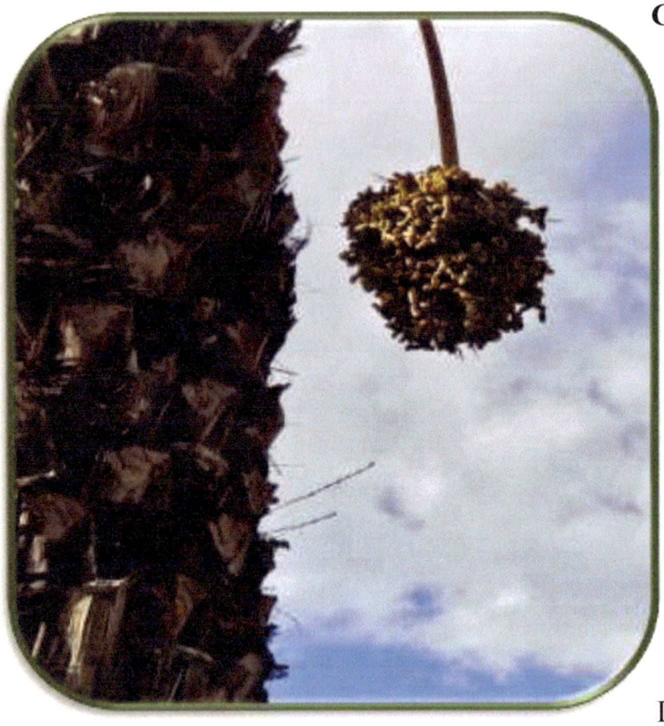

Chemical components:

Dates contain 70% sugars (grape sugar, fruit sugar, cane sugar), acids, fats, proteins, vitamins C (B2, B1, A), and mineral salts, including iron, phosphorus, potassium, boron, sulfur, manganese, copper, calcium, and magnesium. Ripened dates contain phenolic compounds.

Chemical analysis of the ethanolic extract of dates showed that it contains the following components: maltose (polysaccharide), (catechin, myricetin, quercetin, favonates), beta-sitosterol, di-galacturonic acid, chlorogenic acid, and beta-carotene.

Nutritional and medical uses:

Dates are an ideal food for humans because they contain the main nutrients, especially proteins and sugars that build the body and provide it with the necessary energy. One kilogram of it provides three thousand calories, which is equivalent to the thermal energy of an average active man in one day. Fasting people are usually advised to break their fast with dates, because the sugars are quickly absorbed and compensate the body for the lack of sugar in the blood during fasting. Dates have many health benefits, including anti-parasitic, anti-cancer, and anti-Hyperlipidemia, antiviral, liver and kidney protection, and prevention of stomach diseases. Dates cleanse and activate the liver, diuresis, and wash the kidneys (sugars, vitamin B2). The phosphorus in dates enhances mental activity, and adjusts blood acidity that causes kidney stones, gallstones, gout, hemorrhoids, and high blood pressure. Dates, with their vitamin A content, maintain eye moisture and shine, strengthen the optic nerves, and are beneficial for children's growth and weight gain. Dates activate the thyroid gland, strengthen the nerves, soften the blood vessels, moisturize the intestines, and protect them from inflammation. Dates calm the nerves, treat nervous anxiety, and increase sexual ability. They contain anti-cancer compounds (phosphorus and arginine), etc. Date cellulose fibers are a natural laxative that protects against constipation and hemorrhoids. Dates contain the hormone Pitocin, which stimulates uterine movement and increases its contractions, making it an aid to childbirth. In addition, it prevents bleeding during and after childbirth, and reduces blood pressure in pregnant women.

Environment:

The plant is widely grown in hot, dry, sunny areas, and where water is available close to the ground surface. However, it is drought-resistant.

Cultivation and productivity:

The method of propagation by cuttings, which are formed around the base of the trunk, is the common method of propagating palm trees vegetatively on a commercial scale. Recently, it has been possible to propagate it by tissues on a commercial scale, by budding, and by using floral parts. Palm trees also respond to seed propagation. The cuttings are planted after being separated from the mother tree directly in the field, whether it is an orchard or on the perimeter of fields and the sides of agricultural roads. They can be planted in all seasons of the year except winter, at a distance of 7-8 m between one tree and another, in holes 40-50 cm deep so that the root does not rot, and in a slightly tilted position opposite the direction of the wind. The top of the cutting is tied with mats or hemp to protect it from the heat of the sun and the cold until its new leaves grow. A tree that is 15 years old or more, and is in full production, can produce about 50 kg of fruits per year.

Asparagus officinalis L.

Asparagus altilis (L.)Asch., *Asparagus altilis* subsp. *oxycarpus* (Steven) K.Richt. , *Asparagus altilis* subsp. *polyphyllus* (Steven ex Ledeb.) K.Richt., *Asparagus caspius* Schult. & Schult., *Asparagus caspius* Hohen., *Asparagus collinus* Schur, *Asparagus esculentus* Salisb.

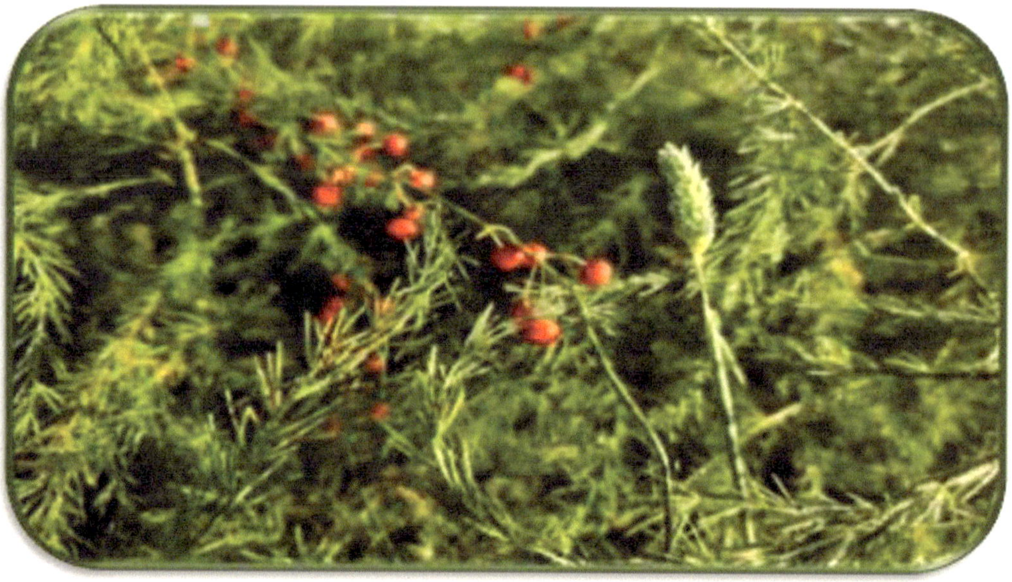

Family: Asparagaceae (Hyacinthaceae)

Common names: Rough air, asparagus, metal, hyacinth, diamond booth

Foreign names: Asperge Fr. Asparagus, Eng.

Occurrences : 105,384 occurrences

Distribution in the world

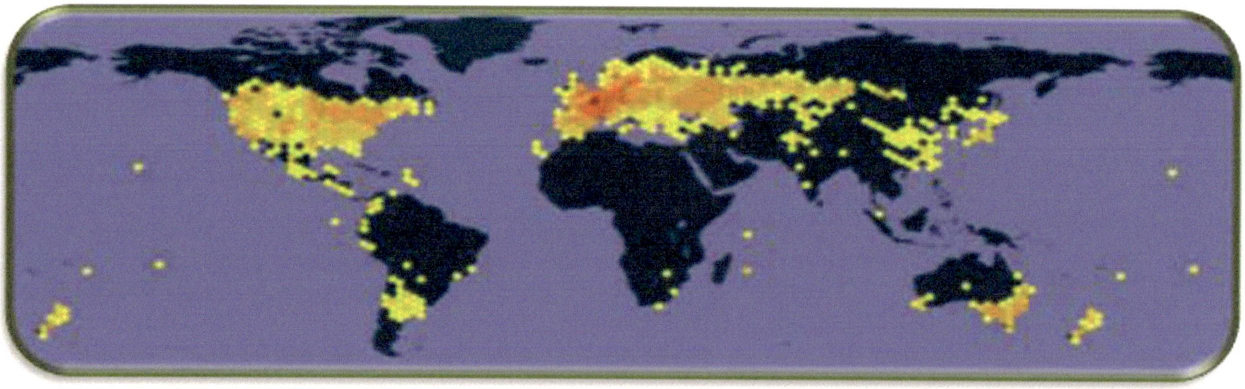

Botanical description:

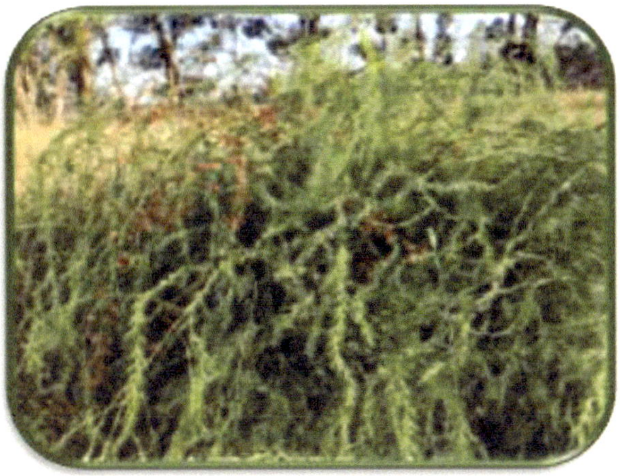

A perennial herb with rhizomes, climbing, 50-100 cm tall, highly branched, woody at the base, branches and branch ends striped, velvety hairy. True leaves are semi-scaly and are mainly in the lower part of the plant, becoming prickly with age. Leafy branches are green in color, gathered in groups of 4-12 branches, 3-9 cm long gradually forming a yellow thorn. Flowers 1-2, mm, equal or nearly equal, needle-like, solid, erect Hymenoptera. Stigma articulated to about midpoint, slightly longer than flower. Receptacle petiolate, bell-shaped, segments nearly equal, fused at base. Male in male flowers 6 stamens, free. The female in female flowers is 3 carpels, The ovary is three-chambered, in which the stamens are reduced to stamens, the pistils are 3. The fruit is a grape, spherical, about 5 mm in diameter, Green, turning black when ripe.

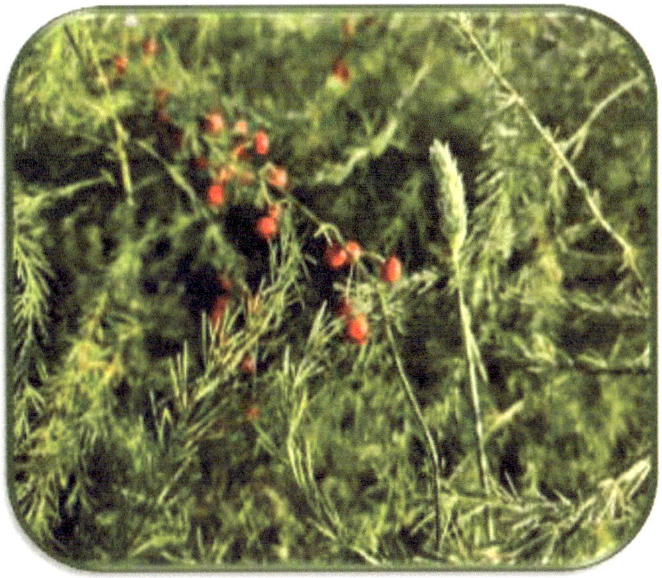

Flowering: August to September.

There are several varieties:

Sweet asparagus, grows underground (sweet in taste), pink asparagus (bitter), and green asparagus.

Habitat and geographical distribution:

Mediterranean, western Asia.

History and heritage:

The Latin name for the genus Asparagus is derived from the Greek asparagos, which is the name of the plant as it was known in ancient times, while the name describing the species "officinalis" means "medicine The genus includes several medicinal species such as A. acutifolius, meaning sharp-leaved. It was used by the Chinese, Babylonians, Persians, Greeks, It is said that Akhenaten and his wife Nefertiti declared and the ancient Egyptians, it is mentioned that asparagus is the food of the gods. It was mentioned by Ibn al-Baytar and al-Antaki, and it was mentioned in Ibn Sina's book that asparagus opens obstructions of the viscera, especially the liver and kidneys.

Part used: Roots and rhizomes.

Chemical components:

The rhizomes contain steroidal saponins, including derivatives of sarsapogenin, the most important of which is asparagoside. Various carbohydrates, such as glucose, and inulin. Fatty oils, flavonoids, amino acids and proteins, organic acids and salts, the most important of which is potassium salt. Asparagus is rich in fiber and nutrients, and is an excellent source of vitamins A, B9, C, E, K, minerals and folic acid. Studies have shown the presence of amino acids such as: L-arginine, L-asparagine and L-glutamic acid, and many soluble sugars and acidic sugars (aldonic acids) and organic acids and their derivatives, more specifically quinic acid, malic acid, and abscisic acid a. .abscisic acid.

Green asparagus contains phenolic derivatives of hydroxycinnamic acid (chlorogenic acid), and ferulic acid. The detected flavonoids belong to the flavonol group, namely: quercetin, isorhamnetin, kaempferol, and quercetin-3-O-(rutin) rutinoside constitutes 60-80% of the total phenolic content of asparagus extracts.

Properties and medical uses:

Rhizome has diuretic properties and is used in the treatment of urinary tract infections. It helps in getting rid of uric acid and urinary tract stones.

Rhizome decoction is popularly used as a medicinal tea in cases of dysuria, phlebitis, rheumatism, gout, liver and spleen diseases, bronchial asthma, and tachycardia. Asparagus protects against the formation of free radicals, which are primarily responsible for cell aging.

Other uses:

Asparagus rhizomes are included in diets designed to reduce obesity, and it is recommended to eat asparagus, which is rich in fiber and cellulose, to help cleanse the digestive system.

Side effects and warnings:

Allergic reactions may occur, especially when used topically. Asparagus has severe effects on the kidneys, so people with kidney weakness who are predisposed to forming kidney stones should not overdo it in consuming asparagus, in addition to the fact that it causes an unpleasant odor in urine and sweat due to the accumulation of the compound methyl mercaptan.

Environment:

Asparagus is widespread in dry places and on the edges of fields, especially on calcareous soils. It prefers sandy loamy soils, and can tolerate temperatures as low as -10°C.

Cultivation and productivity:

Asparagus is an easy species to propagate. It is propagated by seeds that are planted in the nursery in the spring or immediately after they ripen in the fall, after soaking them for about 12 hours in warm water. The seeds usually germinate within 3-6 weeks at a temperature of 25°C, then they are transferred to the permanent ground when they become 30 cm long, in the following spring, i.e. after about a year. Seedlings are planted in holes 20 cm deep and 35 cm apart. It can be propagated by root cuttings obtained in early spring and planted like seedlings. It is preferable not to cut any part of the plant during the first and second years, and to provide appropriate service operations during them, especially irrigation during drought.

Ruscus aculeatus L .

Ruscus dumosus E. D. Clarke, Ruscus flexuosus Mill., Ruscus laxus Sm., Ruscus aculeatus var. angustifolius Boiss., Ruscus aculeatus subsp. laxus (Sm.) k.

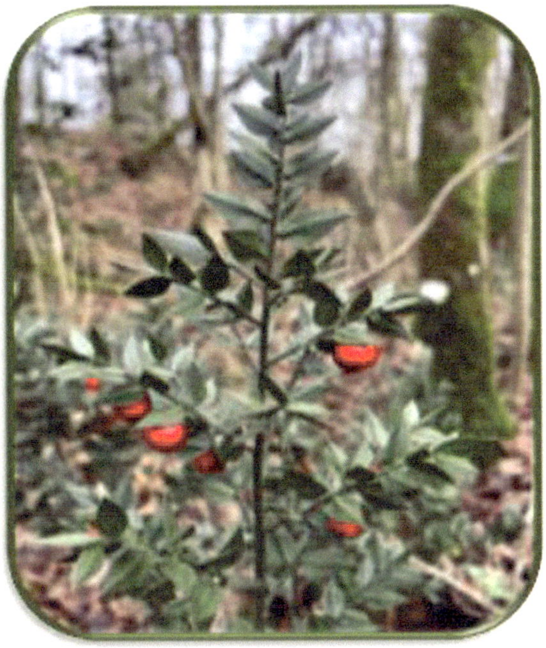

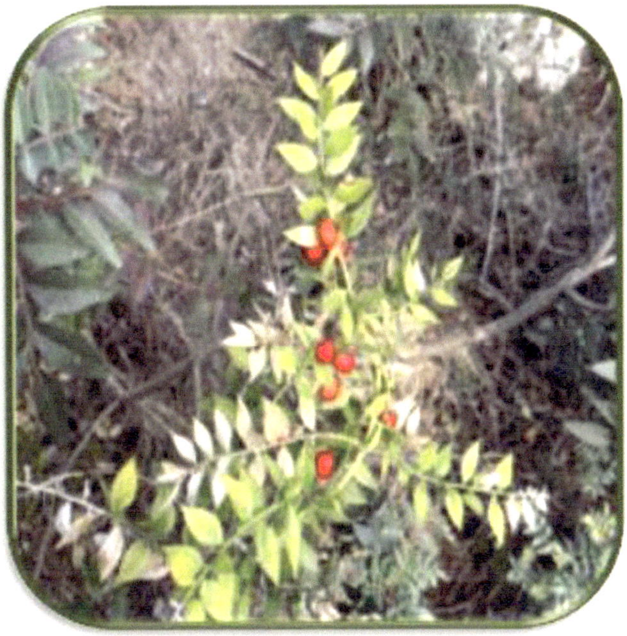

Family: Asparagaceae (formerly Ruscaceae, Liliaceae). Common names: Butcher's Broom, Savander, Wild Myrthe, Box Holly, Pettigree Foreign names: Fr. Fragon épineux

Occurrences : 195,663 occurrences

Distribution in the world

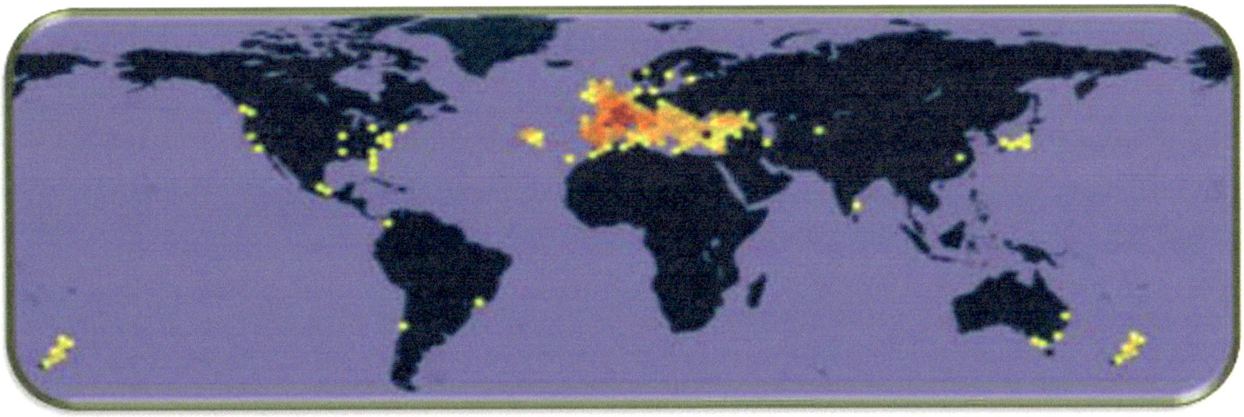

Botanical description:

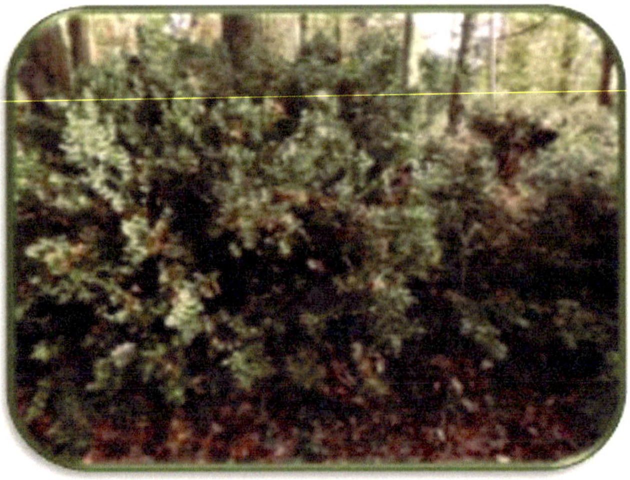

Perennial, thorny, stacked, evergreen shrub. Dioecious, dark green, 25-60 cm high. Stem stiff, branched, erect. Leaves alternate, true leaves small, membranous, semi-squamous, lanceolate or triangular, pointed at the tip. The terminal stalk that emerges from the axils of the true leaves is flat, takes a leaf-like shape and is called "leaf stalk", green, solid, ovate to lanceolate, leathery to touch, 1.5-4 cm long, gradually tapering to form a thorny tip. Flowers are greenish white. Unisexual, short-branched, born in the middle of the rib Green, composed of 6 segments, free, The average on the lower or upper surface of the leaf stalk, supported by a bract. The sleeve Flat, unequal, arranged in two whorls, the segments of the inner whorl are narrower than the outer, the sleeve length reaches 2.5 mm. The male flowers bear 3 stamens, their filaments are united in a tube. The female flowers bear 3 united filaments, but they do not end in anthers, and surround a single-chambered ovary. The fruit is a grape, about 1 cm in diameter, spherical, red in color, covered with a waxy layer, containing 1-2 semi-spherical seeds.

Flowering: March to May.

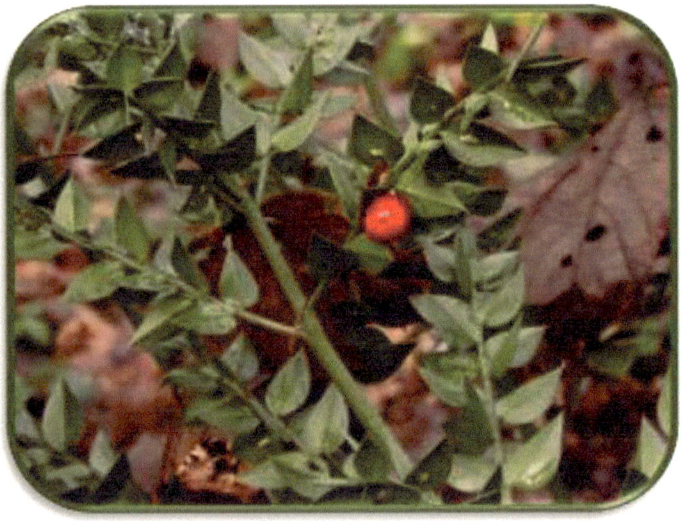

Habitat and geographical distribution:

Mediterranean region, extending to the Euro-Siberian region, and western Iran-Turania. The original homeland of the plant is the Mediterranean basin, the Caucasus, northern Africa, and western Asia.

History and heritage:

The scientific name of the genus is derived from the name of the plant in Latin, and the origin of the species name aculeatus is from Latin and means "thorny", referring to the sharp leaf stem of the plant. A medicinal plant known since ancient times, it is still sold by herbalists under the name of Dick's sarm, referring to its red berry fruits.

Part used: Rhizome (greyish in color.)

Chemical components:

4-6% steroidal soap compounds, the most important of which are: ruscine, ruscoside, and aglycones, including: ruscogenin, and neuroscogenin. It also contains alcoholic acids: glyceric clycolic acids, and potassium salts. Benzofuranes, including ruscodibenzofurane and euparone. Nine phenolic compounds were detected in all properties. Apigenin-C-hexoside-C-pentoside IIII isomer was the major compound in the aqueous properties, and in the hydroethanol extract it was quercetin-O-deoxyhexoside-hexoside followed by apigenin-C, hexoside-C, pentoside IIII isomer.

Properties and medical uses:

The rhizomes have diuretic (alcoholic acids, potassium salts), and anti-inflammatory (ruscogenin) properties.

The saponins (ruscogenin, neuroscogenin) have astringent and vascular strengthening properties. Blood, which improves blood circulation, and makes the drug preparations a supportive remedy for chronic venous insufficiency, and an urgent remedy for accompanying problems such as edema, venous stasis, lower limb spasm and slow movement, varicose veins and ulcers. The drug is available in the form of powder in capsules or liquid extracts that can be drunk, and in the form of creams (Ruscorectal), and suppositories for external use in the case of itching and burning of hemorrhoids. The roots of the plant are used in pharmaceutical and cosmetic preparations for their anti-inflammatory, anti-phlebitis, and anti-hyperthyroidism effects. It reduces edema around the lower legs and heels in adults with acquired immunodeficiency syndrome (CVII).It is mainly used as a diuretic and the rhizomes are used to treat urinary disorders and as a laxative. All properties revealed antioxidant activities. The roots did not show toxic effects on non-tumor cells. It is used as a medical product to relieve symptoms of mild venous insufficiency (heaviness in the legs).

Precautions for use:

It is preferable to use it under medical supervision, since the drug is a venous constrictor, its use may cause an increase in blood pressure in some people, digestive disorders, allergies and vomiting. It is not used by pregnant women.

Other uses:

The fruits are poisonous. The young growths do not contain any toxic substance, and are consumed raw or cooked as in the case of wild asparagus due to the soapy compounds they contain. It is grown in warm regions as a medicinal or ornamental plant.

Environment:

A forest plant that grows on dry slopes. It loves a temperate climate, and its behavior varies according to the area of spread, it can Tolerate drought and calcareous soils in Mediterranean regions. Flexible in its tolerance to light, as it grows in closed, medium or open light environments alike. The plant grows well in various types of soil except loose sandy soil, preferring heavy clay soils.

Cultivation and productivity: It is propagated by division, where the mother plants are divided into several parts, each part contains a root and a stem, then these parts are planted separately from each other at distances of 40-50 cm, and the plants are watered abundantly, since the plant loves water. After that, the roots expand and a vertical stem emerges from them that fills the spaces between the lobes with the increase in the lateral growth of the plant. The process of detailing and planting can be done at any time of the year if water is available. Safflower is not grown as a field crop. When a crop is desired, it is grown in fields between trees to provide adequate shade, or on the sides of irrigation channels, and next to walls (shaded areas). Safflower is not usually fertilized, especially in fertile soils, but when grown in poor soils, it can be fertilized with compound fertilizer. 2-2-1 To collect the crop, the plants are cut above the surface of the soil, and then dried in the open under direct sunlight. The remaining roots in the ground are watered to produce new plants.

Urginea maritima (L.) Baker.

Drimia maritima (L.) Stearn.

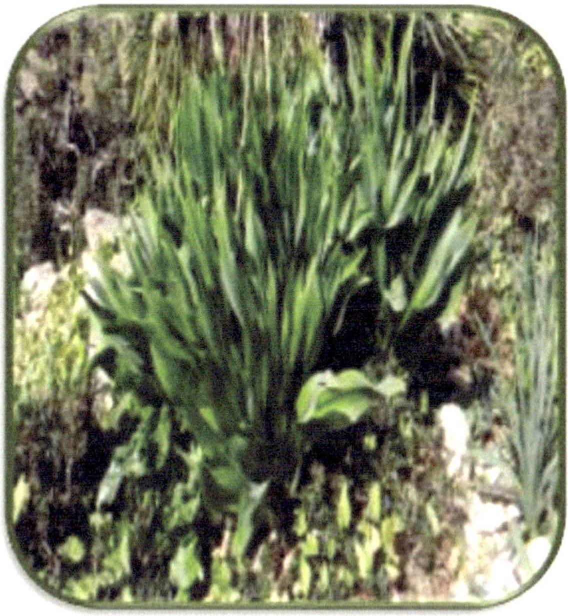

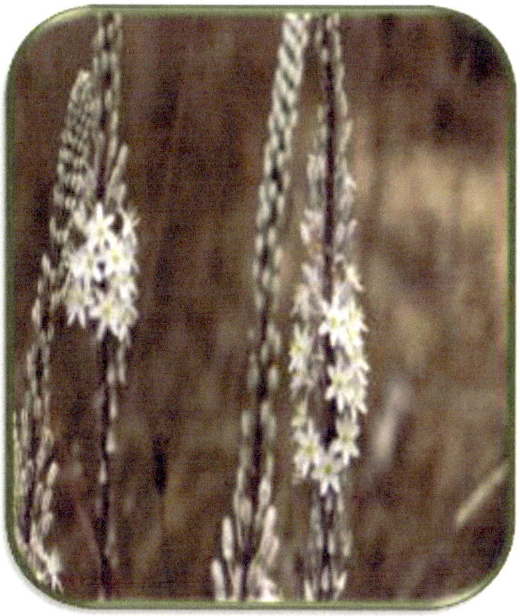

Family: Asparagaceae (Hyacinthaceae)

Common names: Sea onion, sea squill, Fr. scille maritime

Foreign names:

Occurrences : 13,584 occurrences

Distribution in the world:

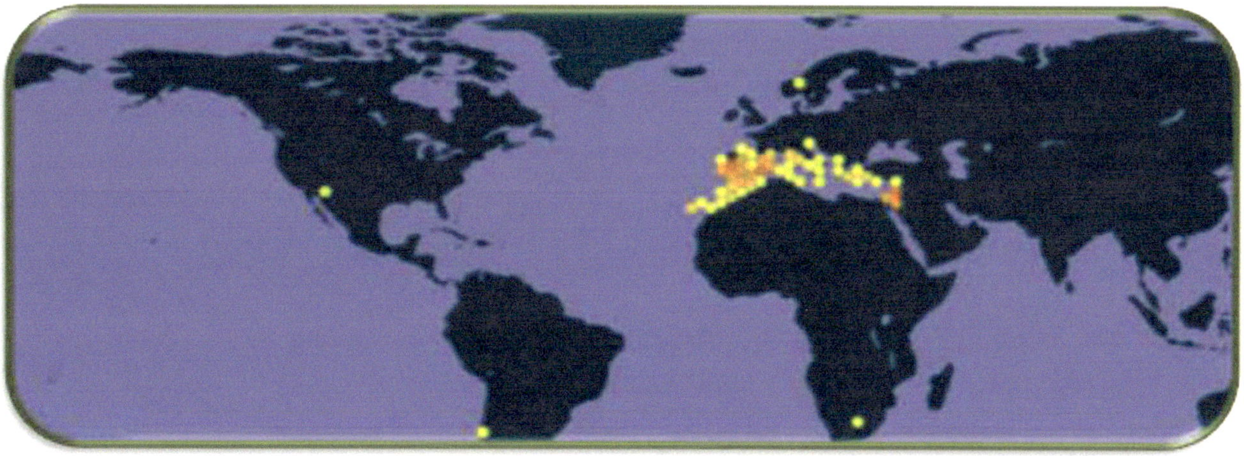

Botanical description:

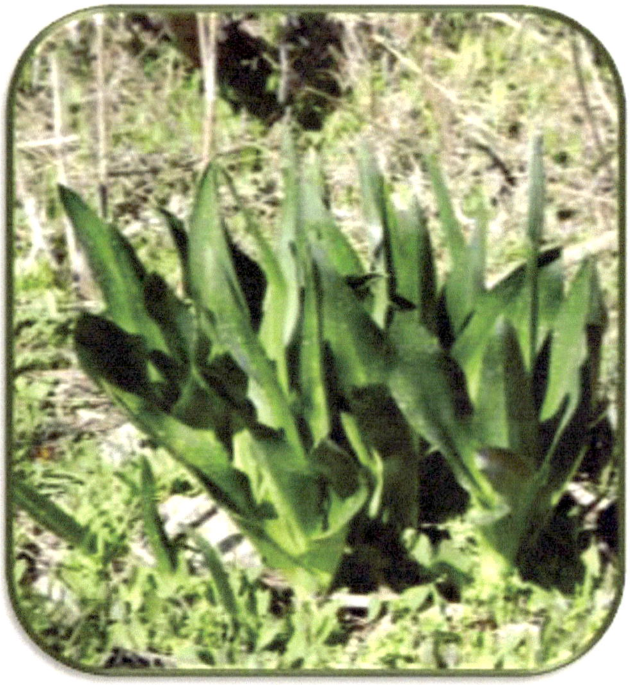

A perennial herb with bulbs, the bulb is 5-15 cm in diameter, thick and fleshy, white to reddish- brown in color. Leaves 10-20, 30-60 cm long, 3-8 cm wide, erect, broadly lanceolate, bluish-green in color, Appear early in winter (November-November) after the end of flowering, and continue until April-May.

Inflorescence axis leafless, 60-100 cm long, solid, tending to purple. Inflorescence raceme long, dense, 50 flowers or more. Bracts small, membranous, spur-shaped below the middle. Flower panicles erect, 2-3 times the length of the sleeve. Sleeve petal, star-flattened, 6-lobed, white with a medium green or purple vein, 7-9 mm long. Male 6 stamens, filaments shorter than the sleeve, widened at the base, anthers greenish. Ovary superior, tri-chambered. Fruit capsule, tri-chambered, inverted ovate in general shape. Seeds 4-1 in each chamber, black, shiny.

Flowering: July to October.

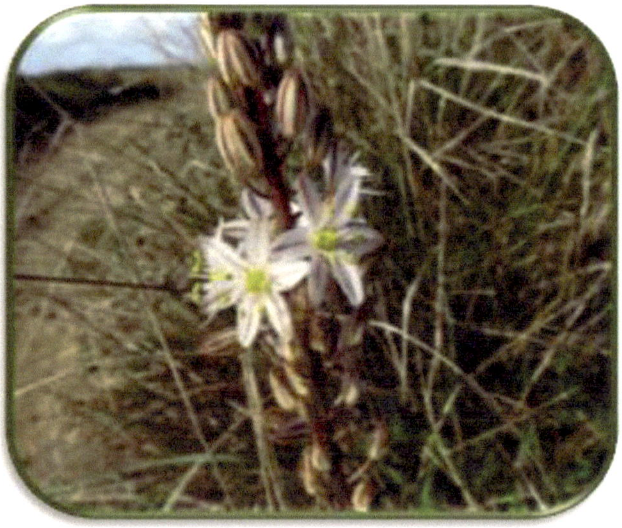

Habitat and geographical distribution: Mediterranean.

History and Heritage:

The scientific name of the genus Urginea comes from the name of the land of a tribe in Algeria known as Urgin Beni, where the plant was first collected, and the species name maritima means "sea." The squill bulb has been a medicinal plant for a long time, as it was sacred to the ancient Egyptians, who considered it a repellent of demons and evil spirits, and a medical recipe for squill was found in an Egyptian papyrus. It was also known to Greek and Arab doctors. Dioscorides described it soaked in vinegar to treat heart diseases.

Part used:

The bulb, is removed after the flowering period, in late summer and early autumn, the outer scales are removed, and the middle is kept, cut into slices 1 cm thick, then dried quickly (industrially) so that the glycosidic compounds do not have the opportunity to decompose enzymatically.

Chemical components:

There are two types of squill bulbs: the white squill, which is the medicinal type that contains cardiac glycosides, and the red-scaled squill (red squill or mouse onion), because the sap of some cells contains anthocyanin pigments, and is not used medically.

The white squill bulb contains:

Cardioactive steroid glycosides 1-3%. The main compound, glycoside Scillarene A (a crystalline compound, which constitutes two-thirds of the glycosides present in the onion), is hydrolyzed by the enzyme Scillarenase into a glucose molecule and an intermediate compound Proscillaridin A. Upon completion of the decomposition by the action of the enzyme Scillarenase, the compound Scillaridin A is released, which is responsible for the plant's heart-strengthening properties. It also contains another compound, Scillarene B, which is amorphous and constitutes the remaining third of the glycosides in the scales. It also contains mucilage, sugars (fructosan), flavones, and tannins. The red plant contains a toxic cyanogenic glycoside, which, through enzymatic hydration, gives the compound Scillirosidine, which is used as a rodent poison. Chemical examination revealed that the plant bulb contains anthraquinones, anthocyanins, steroids, and terpenes.

Properties and medical uses:

The glycosides of the white onion have properties that strengthen the heart muscle, and are used in the treatment of heart failure, venous problems, nervous heart, and arrhythmia. The glycosides of the white onion plant differ from the glycosides of the leaves of the Digitalis sp plant, in that its compounds do not accumulate in the body, unlike what happens when taking digitalis.

It is worth noting that the pharmaceutical preparations of the active ingredients are more effective than the active compound in the pure state. The onion of the sea squill has diuretic, expectorant, anti-bronchitis, anti-cough and anti-asthmatic properties. Its preparations are used topically to treat hemorrhoids, sterilize infected wounds, treat sagging gums and loose teeth. The sea squill has shown anti-inflammatory, antioxidant, antibacterial, vasodilator and antifungal effects and is suitable for wounds infected with fungal infections. It is also useful in treating digestive system disorders and rheumatic diseases.

In addition, extracts of the onion of the squill have anti-cancer effects (breast cancer cells).

Side effects and warnings for use:

A generally poisonous plant if used in large doses, and it is recommended to take its pharmaceutical preparations for fear of the inability to control the doses prepared popularly through the squill and others.

The plant or its glycosidic compounds are not used in cases of atrioventricular block, hypercalcemia, hypertrophic cardiomyopathy, hypokalemia, carotid sinus syndrome, ventricular tachycardia, aortic thoracic aneurysm, and Wolf-Parkinson-White syndrome.

Environment:

It grows in warm, sunny locations. It grows on sand and dry hills near the sea. The bulbs go through a period of summer dormancy, during which they must be kept dry. They are sometimes sensitive to humidity in winter.

Cultivation and productivity:

The plant is propagated by seeds, which are scattered immediately after ripening in pots or bags at a rate of one seed in each, and fertilized with a complete nutrient solution. It can also be propagated by dividing young bulbs as soon as the plant enters a dormant period. Every 2-3 parts of the bulb are placed in a pot and transferred to the permanent soil after a year during the dormant period. Large bulbs can be planted directly in the permanent soil. The bulbs maintain their great ability to regain growth for a long period of up to several years. The bulbs are collected after a growth period of 6 years, and their productivity is about 25,000 bulbs per hectare.

Aloe vera (L.) Burm. f.

Aloe barbadensis Mill., *A. barbadensis var. chinensis* Haworthm., *A. perfoliata var. vera* L., *Aloe elongata* Murray., *Aloe flava* Pers., *Aloe indica* Royle., *Aloe lanzae* Tod.

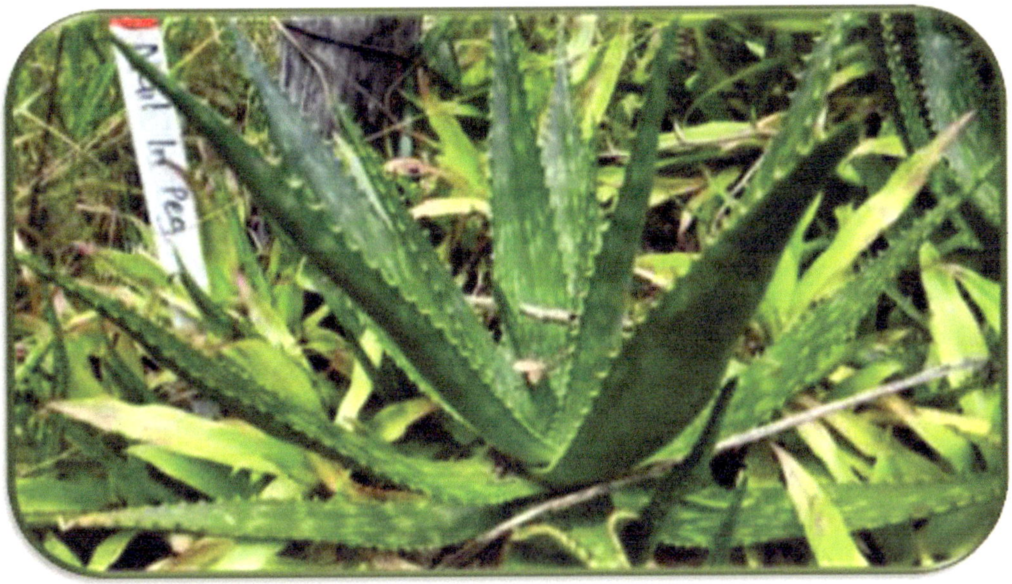

Family: Asphodelaceae (Xanthorrhoeaceae)

Common names: Barbados Aloe, Aloe vera, Polisher, Polisher

Foreign names: Bitter aloe, Barbados Aloe, Fr. Aloès

Occurrences : 3,933 occurrences

Distribution in the world

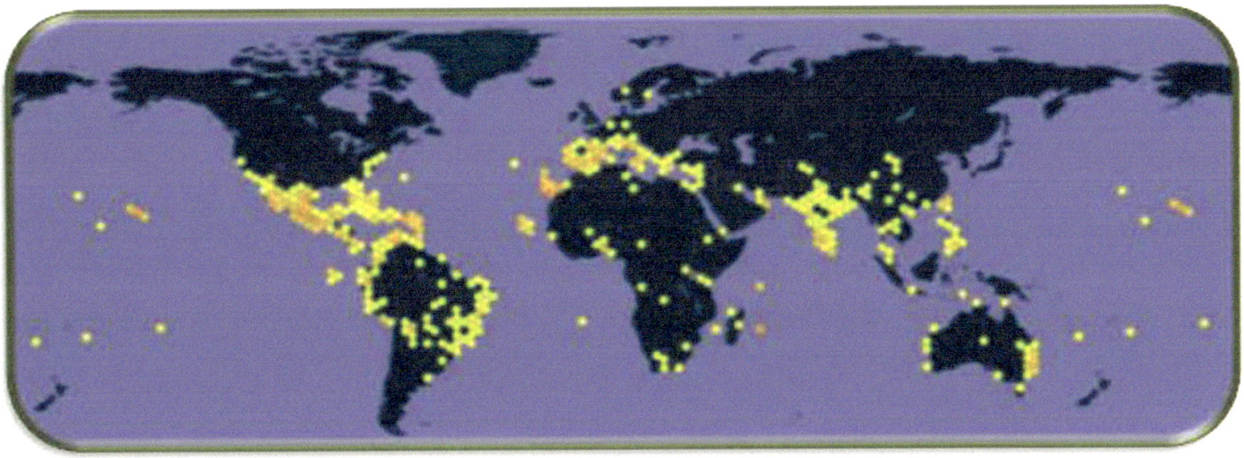

Botanical description:

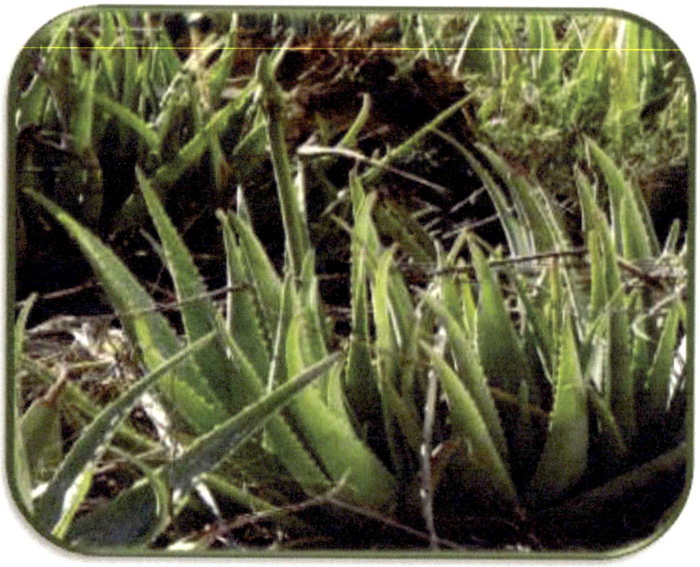

Succulent, very short stem. The leaves are fleshy Plant Thick, emerging in the form of a rosette from the base of the plant, 15-50 cm long, and 4-7 cm wide from the bottom, linear-lanceolate, serrated-spiny on the edge, the length of the tooth is about 2 mm, its upper surface is concave, green to gray in color, and its edge is a pale carnation color, pale spots can be seen on it, especially in young plants, the middle tissue is full of gum (mucus) and sticky juice Gives "Ham" patience. The inflorescence is clustered, erect, 60-90 cm long, its panicle is thick about 2 cm, one or two ascending branches can be seen on the panicle. The bracts are white, broadly lanceolate, about 1 cm long, and 5-6 mm wide, bearing 5-7 nerves. The flowers are yellow or orange-yellow, paniculate, drooping, about 3 cm long, the bract is simple, composed of 6 segments in 2 whorls. The male has 6 stamens in 2 whorls. The female is triploid, the ovary is superior, and the fruit is a slightly elongated capsule, three-chambered, about 1.5 cm long. It blooms in spring, and may extend into winter. There is another type of aloe called Cape Aloe (Miller ferox A. (capensis Aloe) after its original homeland in South Africa (Cape region), or what is known as the Cape of Good Hope, it produces the best types of drugs, and is similar to Barbados aloe in its components and uses.

Home and geographical distribution:

Barbados aloe is originally from East Africa and the coasts of the Red Sea (Asir Mountains south of Jazan) and North Africa. Its cultivation was introduced to the West Indies and the Antilles in the seventeenth century.

History Heritage:

The genus name Aloe is derived from the Greek alsos, meaning "bitter juice" contained in the leaves of the plant, and perhaps the name is of Semitic origin, or came from the Arabic Aloe, meaning "bitterness", and vera from Latin, meaning "true." The importance of the ivory plant has been known for 5000 years, and it was mentioned in the clay tablets discovered in Mesopotamia.

In 2000 BC, the ancient Egyptians knew it, and it was mentioned in the Ebers Papyrus, and they used it in preparing mummies, treating skin diseases, dressing wounds, treating inflammation, burns and ulcers, and preventing wrinkles. Cleopatra mentioned that she used to massage her face daily with aloe vera juice. Dioscorides described the medicinal properties of aloe vera, and Aristotle advised Alexander the Great to occupy the island of Sumatra, where the aloe plant grows and the islanders make juice that has medicinal benefits. He may have meant the species Aloe soetrima. The juice of the plant was included in the composition of the elixir of life among the ancient Chinese. The Arabs considered this plant a symbol of humility, moderation, patience and steadfastness in the face of heat and drought, and they called the plant's juice the name of the plant.

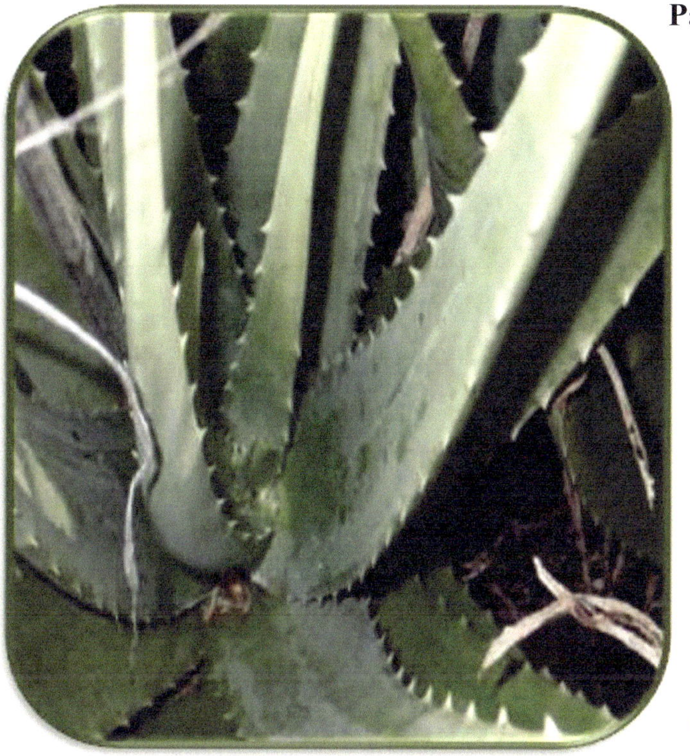

Part used:

Leaves, and ham (the bitter juice extracted from the old leaves between August and November.) Ham is obtained by cutting the leaves near their base, which allows the flow of the important substance stored in the inner cells of the leaves. The important substance (juice) is collected in a pot and boiled for several hours. The juice is left to cool and dry in the form of solid, brown, bitter-tasting masses. The drug masses are soluble in hot ethanol, and partially in b oiling water, but are insoluble in ether and chloroform. The geographical origin, method of cultivation and preparation of the juice contribute to determining the effectiveness of the drug.

Chemical components:

There is some confusion regarding the aloe vera juice, as some say that the juice contains irritating and laxative compounds, while others say that it contains soothing and calming compounds. In fact, both opinions are correct, because it depends on the part of the leaf from which the drug is taken, and the method of preparing the specific. The composition of the specific aloe vera juice depends on the method of preparing the specific. The irritating substances (anthraquinones) are found in the periphery of the leaf, while in the center of the leaf there is a light-colored sticky juice (gel) containing salivary compounds. The juice of aloe barbadensis contains two types of anthraquinone compounds:

Free anthraquinone compounds, the percentage of which does not exceed 1%, are called aloe-emodin. Anthraquinone glycosides 15-20%, the most important of which is barbaloine = (aloin A, B), and hydroxyaloin A, B, to which the laxative effect of the drug is attributed. The juice also contains resinous compounds (aloe D - C - B resins) at a rate of 10-20%. Aloe vera juice is distinguished from aloe vera juice by the presence of resinous compound B in addition to the resins found mainly in aloe vera. Favones and saponins. Amino acids: phenylalanine lysine, leucine, contribute to the renewal of skin tissues. Sugars: polysaccharides glucose phosphate, 6-mannose-acemannan, contribute to moisturizing and softening the skin and strengthening the body's immune system. It also contains enzymes, the most important of which is the enzyme bradykinase. And minerals, the most important of which are iron, potassium, sodium, phosphorus, calcium, copper, magnesium, manganese, chromium and zinc. And vitamins A (B1, B2, B3, B5, B6, B9, B12 and C) needed by the body and nervous system.

Properties and medical uses:

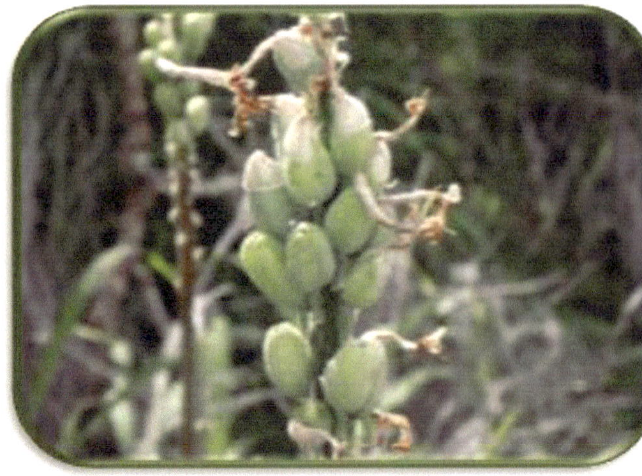

Aloe vera gum has been used in traditional medicine for a long time to treat burns, and is effective on deep second-degree burns, and promotes wound healing locally. Aloe barbadensis and aloe vera juice preparations are widely used to improve digestion and cleanse the digestive tract if taken in small doses (0.02-0.06 g). Aloe vera juice is one of the most important laxatives currently used to treat constipation in doses of 0.1 g, and it can become a strong laxative. The enzymes and vitamins present in the drug accelerate the metabolism and fat burning process (reducing the percentage of fat and cholesterol in the blood), and improve the digestion process by regulating the flow of digestive juices, and activating the work of the liver, as well as activating the production of white blood cells and strengthening the immune system. The presence of amino acids, minerals and antioxidants helps maintain the health of the body. Studies have shown that using aloe vera juice (aloe-emodin) orally reduces symptoms of inflammation in patients suffering from stomach ulcers and ulcerative colitis. Studies have shown the positive effect of the emodin compound in reducing the activity of some enzymes that help in the proliferation of some types of cancer cells (antineoplastic effects). It also indicated that the important property of aloe vera has an effective anti-inflammatory effect on infections caused by viruses, bacteria and fungi, due to the aloe-emodin compound it contains. Its benefit has been proven in treating inflammation of the throat, sinuses and conjunctiva, and also preventing the growth of Candida albicans fungi. The use of toothpaste containing aloe vera extract led to a noticeable decrease in gum inflammation and the formation of dental tartar (calculus).

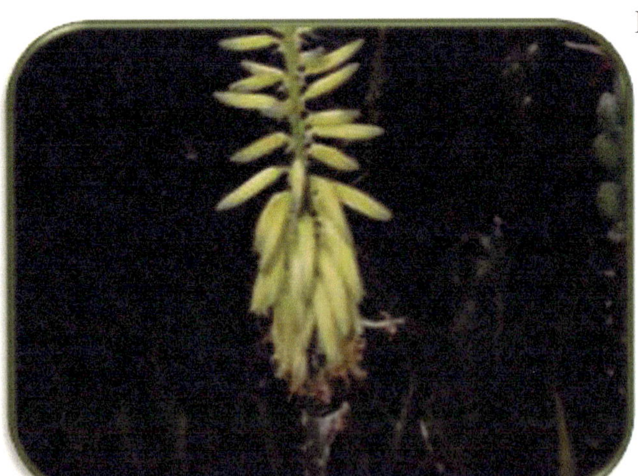

Ham is used topically to accelerate the healing of wounds, superficial burns, and purulent blisters and to protect them from infection, as the ham substance stimulates the repair of wounds and burns by accelerating the growth and renewal of skin tissue. The drug preparations are currently used to shorten the time required for wound healing in cosmetic surgery. Studies have shown the effectiveness of ointments that contain the drug in moisturizing dry skin and treating many skin diseases (ulcers, eczema, acne). Aloe vera juice components are currently a main component in many skin, complexion and lip care products, and protect them from the sun's rays. They are also used in hair loss prevention products and supplementary pastes. The drug is available in the market in several pharmaceutical forms, some of which are intended for external use in the form of ointments or ointments, or for internal use in the form of syrup. The aloe vera genus contains chemical compounds that have selective toxic effects against cancer cells. Studies indicate that Aloe vera is an antioxidant, and because of its effectiveness in scavenging free radicals, it has a protective effect against changes that occur in the testicles when using the anti-cancer chemotherapy drug Cis-platin. Aloe vera gel is an antiseptic to prevent some bacterial skin wound infections caused by E. coli, Shigella, Salmonella, and Staphylococcus aureus. Aloe vera flower and its active ingredients can also be used as a skin moisturizer to enhance skin function and improve skin-related diseases.

Side effects, drug interactions and precautions for use:

The dose should be reduced in case of gastrointestinal cramps after taking aloe vera, noting that gastrointestinal cramps are normal when taking aloe vera, due to the laxative effect of the plant. Aloe vera should not be used in cases of ulcerative colitis, Crohn's disease, appendicitis, and abdominal pain of unknown cause.

Prolonged use of aloe vera may cause pigmentation of the intestinal mucosa (pseudomelanosis), a harmless condition that can be eliminated by stopping the use of the plant. Prolonged use of the plant may cause dermatitis, eczema, or loss of potassium from the body, which affects the action of cardiac glycosides and antiarrhythmic drugs, and albuminuria (the presence of albumin in the urine). High doses also lead to From aloe vera to decreased intestinal peptide and decreased somatostatin levels, leading to tissue damage. Long-term use of anthracene found in aloe vera increases the risk of colon cancer. Aloe vera is not recommended for children, pregnant women, or patients with hemorrhoids.

Environment:

A plant that adapts to dry and hot environments. It grows in all types of soil, preferring light, well-drained, sunny, and organic-rich sandy soils. It does not tolerate excessive cold, but it tolerates heat in the summer. It is successfully cultivated in dry and semi-dry bioclimatic floors, and sometimes semi-humid in the warm variable, but in the moderate variable it does not tolerate frost, and in the sweet variable it may die completely during the winter.

Cultivation and productivity:

It is easy to propagate it by means of the offshoots that are found around the mother stem and resulting from the green buds found on the stem close to the soil surface, and it is preferable to do this during the spring. It can also be propagated by means of fleshy leaves after cutting them into suitable parts, drying the wounds resulting from the cutting process, and then planting their bases in the soil. The plant is harvested from August to October, where the leaves are cut and hung vertically or pressed to release the juice that dries in various ways. Productivity ranges between 8-25 tons/hectare depending on the cultivation method (protected or open), as well as care and services. Aloe vera is currently grown for ornamental or medicinal purposes in many countries, especially those in tropical and temperate regions, such as the Americas (southern United States, Mexico, Caribbean Islands) and Asia (Philippines and Malaysia).

Achillea falcata var. breviradiata Boiss.

Achillea falcata L.

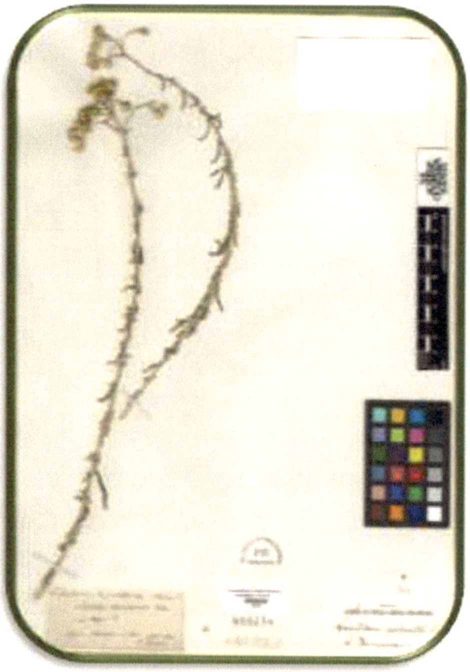

Family: Asteraceae (Compositae)

Common names: Achillea falciformis, Achillea falciformis

Foreign names:

Occurrences : 1 occurrences

Distribution in the world

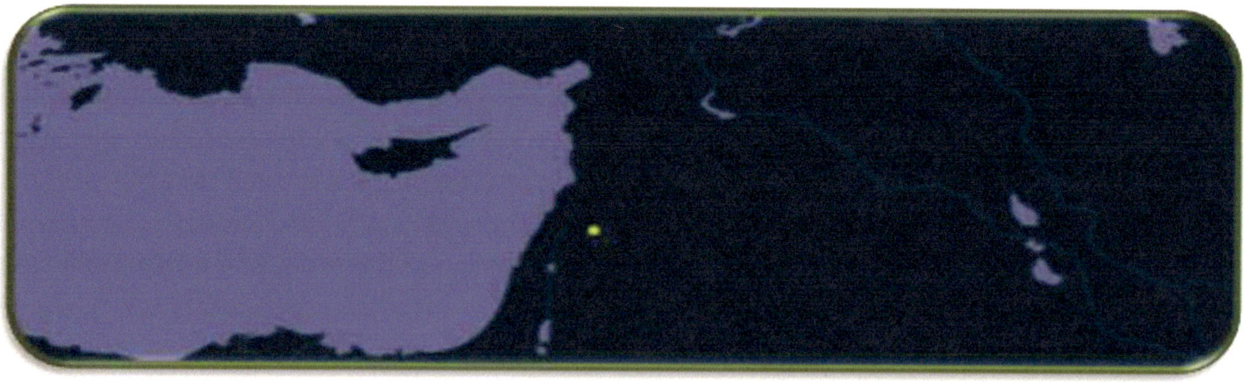

Botanical description:

A small shrub, with many branches, 30-50 cm high. Stems are erect, simple, covered with dense hairs, later becoming semi-growth. Leaves are narrow, linear, semi-pointed at both ends, covered with woolly gray hairs, short and often arched, deeply divided into very small parts, overlapping each other in a dense and transverse manner. Each part is divided into three ovate-rounded and serrated lobes.

The heads are gathered in compound comb inflorescences. The head contains tubular and radial flowers. The heads are long, twice the length of the head. The bract is 3-4 mm, sub-spherical, covered with grey, woolly hairs. The flower seat bears bracts. The lingual flowers are female, few in number, yellow, tridentate, from one-third to one-half the length of the bract, and are arranged in a single row on the periphery of the head. Central flowers tubular, hermaphrodite, pentamerous. Fruit compressed, narrow-base, broad and truncated at the apex, without ovules.

Flowering: April to September.

Habitat and geographical distribution: Western Iran - Turan.

History and Heritage:

Achilles is an Arabicized name derived from the Greek word achille, which is the name of the Greek mythological hero "Achilles", the hero of Homer's Iliad, who is said to have used species of this genus to heal his enemy after striking him with a sword. Soldiers also used it to reduce bleeding during the Trojan War between 1194 and 1184 BC. The story states that the wise man Chiron is the one who gave the secrets of this plant to his young disciples who later used it during the Trojan War. The name of the species falcata means "sickle."

Part used: Aerial parts.

Chemical components: Mono- and semi-terpene ketones, ketones including: achillin and achillifoline.

Favonoids: quercétagetine, pectolinarigenine. Coumarin compounds, and a small amount of tannin compounds. Volatile oils vary in their components depending on their source. In the oil of Lebanese origin, it is noted that its most important components are 21%, artemisia 5%, fragranol 17%, grandisol .ketone terpinen-4-ol, 1.8 -cineole 4%. In the oil of Jordanian origin, the most important components are: 17%, p-cymene 11%, 1.8-cineole 4%, camphor .terpinen-4-ol 5%, ß-thujone 10%. In the oil of Iranian origin, the most important main components are camphor 22.1% and 8-cineole 10%. The percentage of oxygenated compounds reached 79% of the total oil. In addition to trans-sapinol and its esters, butanoate, isobutanoate, 2-methylbutanoate and 3-methylbutanoate in both the aerial and terrestrial parts.

Properties and medical uses:

Studies have proven the properties of volatile oil in inhibiting the growth of some types of fungi and bacteria, especially gram positive.

The alcoholic extract of the plant has the ability to reduce the formation of arterial and venous clots. The plant has anti-inflammatory, antispasmodic, digestive and bile secretion stimulating properties, and helps in getting rid of liver toxins, due to its volatile oil and monoterpene ketones.

The decoction of the aerial parts is a natural source of antioxidants. The leaves and flowers are used to prepare a tincture or ointment that is used topically to treat wounds, stop external bleeding (hemorrhoids) and reduce rheumatic pain. Achillea falcata extract has anti-reproductive activity.

Environment:

It is widespread in dry deserts on poor, stony soils.

Cultivation and productivity:

The plant is propagated by seeds or by cuttings of vegetative and root growths, but seed propagation is the best economically. It is recommended not to store seeds for more than 3 years.

Achillea fragrantissima (Forssk.) Sch Bip.

Santolina fragrantissima Forssk.

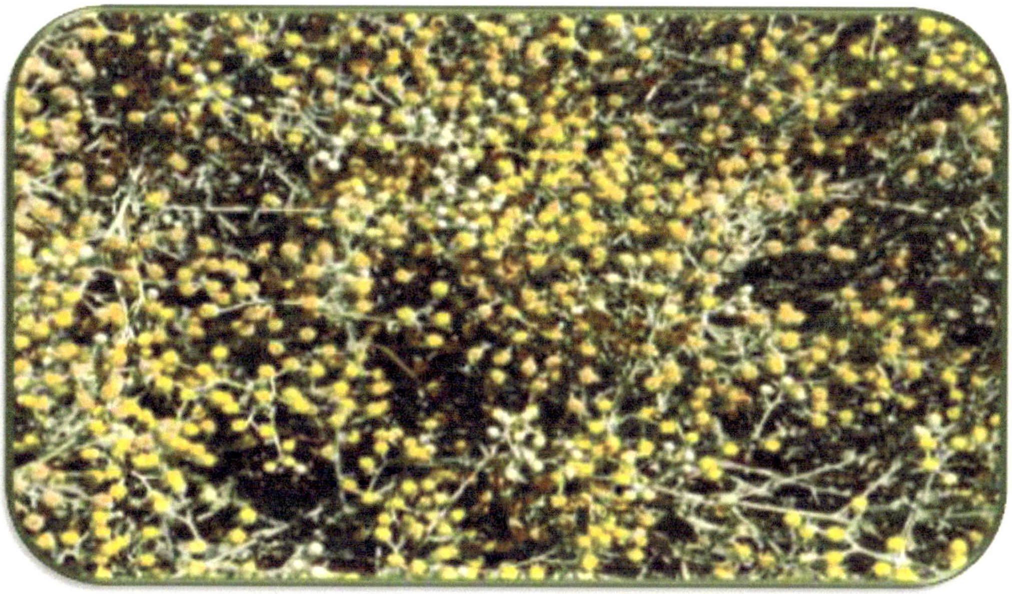

Family: Asteraceae (Compositae)

Common names: Asteraceae, Wild Aster

Foreign names: Santoline Fr., cotton Lavender Eng.

Occurrences : 1,767 occurrences

Distribution in the world

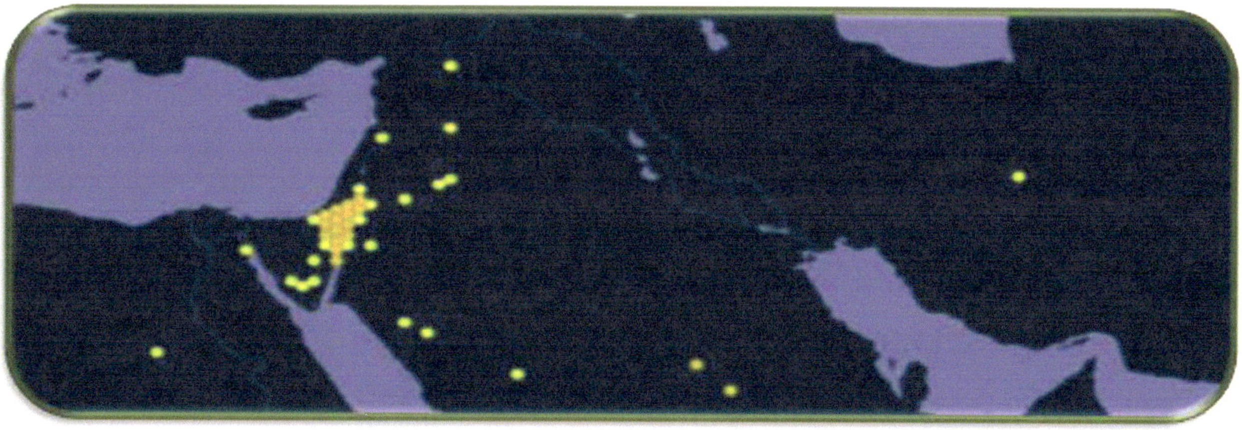

Botanical description:

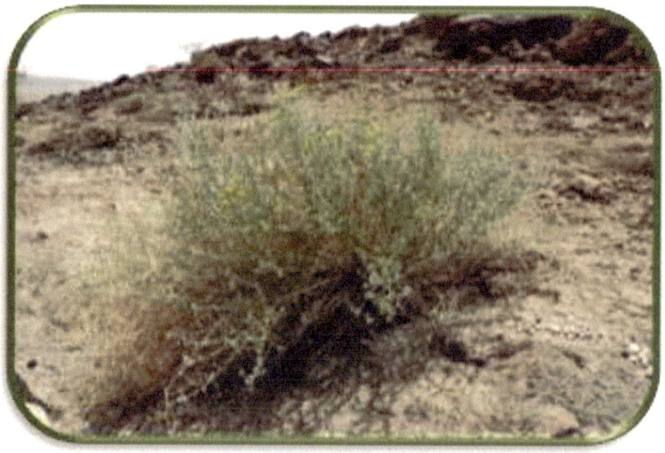

A small shrub, fragrant, woody at the base, 50-100 cm high, covered with woolly-white hairs.The branches are numerous, slender, stiff, ending in a group of small heads that gather in a racemose-branch inflorescence. The leaves are simple, small, oblong or oval, not divided, somewhat thick, serrated at the edge, gray in hair, becoming almost bare later. The flower heads are disc-shaped, gathered in a loose raceme. The bracts are overlapping, oblong-ovate, gray-haired, about 5 mm long. The peripheral, lingual flowers are yellow, small, and the central one is tubular. The fruit is an acinate, without ovules.

Flowering: March - October

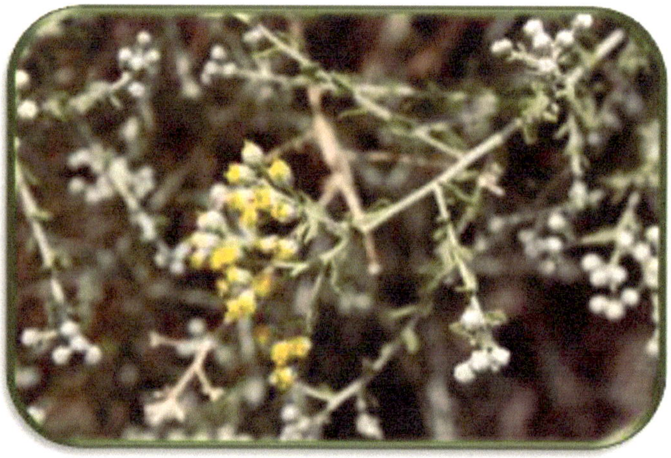

Habitat and geographical distribution: Western Iran - Turan, and eastern Arabian desert.

History and heritage:

The genus name was mentioned in the previous type, while the species name fragrantissima is from Latin and means "perfume. The species of the genus have been used for a long time in folk medicine to stop bleeding and treat wounds, and it was known in ancient times in the Far East, where it was mentioned on the grave of Confucius, and it was also used in India alongside rosemary in fumigation to treat fever. In Scotland, an ointment is made from it to treat wounds.

Part used: Flowering plant.

Chemical components:

The aerial parts contain 1% volatile oil, the most important compounds of which are: thujone, and para-cymene57. % p-cymene : The most important of which are 8% tannin compounds. terpinen-4-ol. , artemisia alcohol, 33% santolina alcohol, Phlroglucin, Resorcin. Favonoid compounds, the most important of which are: cirsilol, swertisine, vicenine. Many fatty acids, the most important of which are lauric acid, palmitic acid, myristic acid, bitter substances, and many other compounds. The roots contain some of the aforementioned favonoid compounds. Seven monoterpene ketones (Achillolide-A), two flavonoids, chrysosplenol-D, chrysosplenetine, and four alkamides (including pellitorine) were identified. The plant also contains various phenolic compounds such as: protocatechule, santolina alcohol, eugenol, artenimole, salicylic acid ester, and ferulic acid, which is one of the most abundant phenolic compounds found in the cell walls of seeds and leaves.

Properties and medical uses:

The volatile oil of the flowering tops has antibacterial properties, especially against Gram-negative Echerichia coli and Candida albicans fungi, and it stimulates the secretion of bile juice.

Research indicates To the effectiveness of the aqueous extract of the plant in stopping the growth of malignant melanoma cells (anti-tumor), and showed the properties of the wormwood in treating diabetes. The sage is popularly used as a hot digestive drink that is useful in treating gastrointestinal disorders, malabsorption (celiac disease), headaches resulting from digestive disorders, and some types of nervous headaches (nerve sedative), and to expel worms, treat dysentery, chronic diarrhea, and tonsillitis, and is useful in treating nerve pain in the ear (tinnitus). A decoction of its aerial parts or its volatile oil is used as a fat to treat nerve inflammation and skin diseases in Scalp (alopecia), to treat hair follicle weakness by massaging, opens and strengthens hair pores, relieves rheumatism pain, chronic arthritis and gout, stops bleeding, treats wounds and skin allergies, treats hemorrhoids, spring conjunctivitis, and eye infections.

Herbal hyssop is used as a herbal bath to relax the nerves and give the body a pleasant scent. Polyphenols have anti-allergic, anti-inflammatory, anti-cancer and anti-bacterial properties. Its ethanolic extract is effective in wound healing. Essential oils were obtained from the hyssop, and these oils and their nanoemulsions showed effective bactericidal activity against the mold mite Tyrophagus putrescentiae, and suitable nanoemulsions containing these oils can be developed to eliminate it. The phytochemicals present in the plant are useful in neurodegenerative diseases in which neuroinflammation is part of the pathophysiology.

Use warnings:

It should not be used internally before meals because it harms the stomach, and the herb is a menstrual stimulant, so pregnant women are warned against using it.

Environment:

It is spread in the valleys of dry areas, the edges of small valleys and water bodies. It prefers non-saline calcareous lands.

Cultivation and productivity:

Similar to what was mentioned in the previous type

Achillea millefolium L.

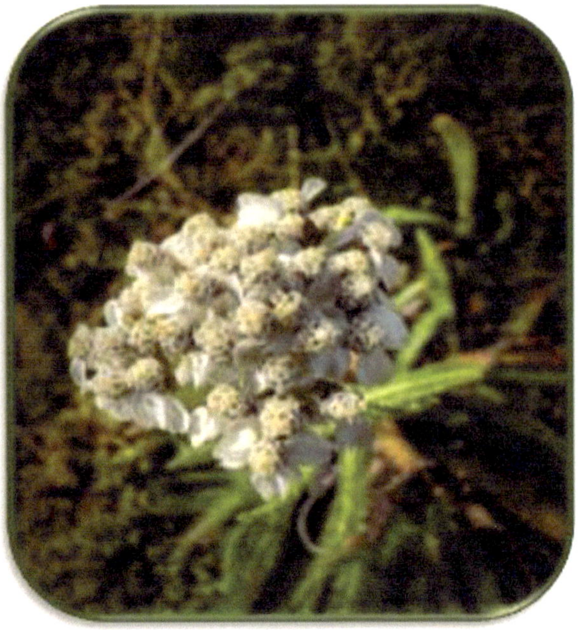 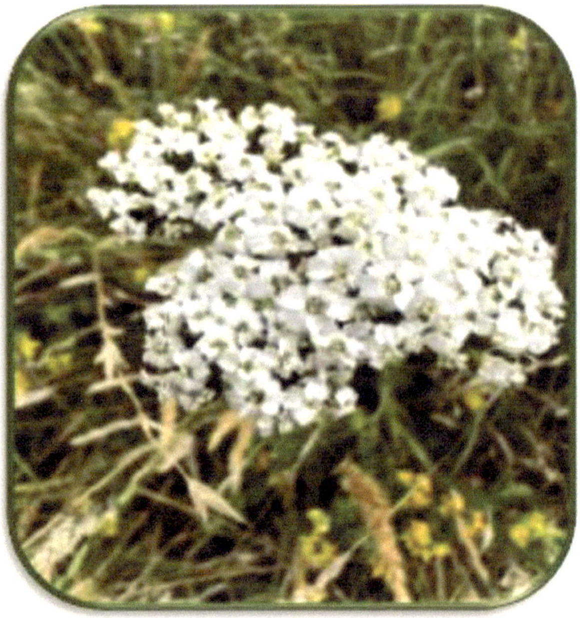

Family: Asteraceae (Compositae)

Common names: Achillea millefolia

Foreign names: feuille Mille Fr. Yarrow, Eng

Occurrences : 1,438,185 occurrences

Distribution in the world

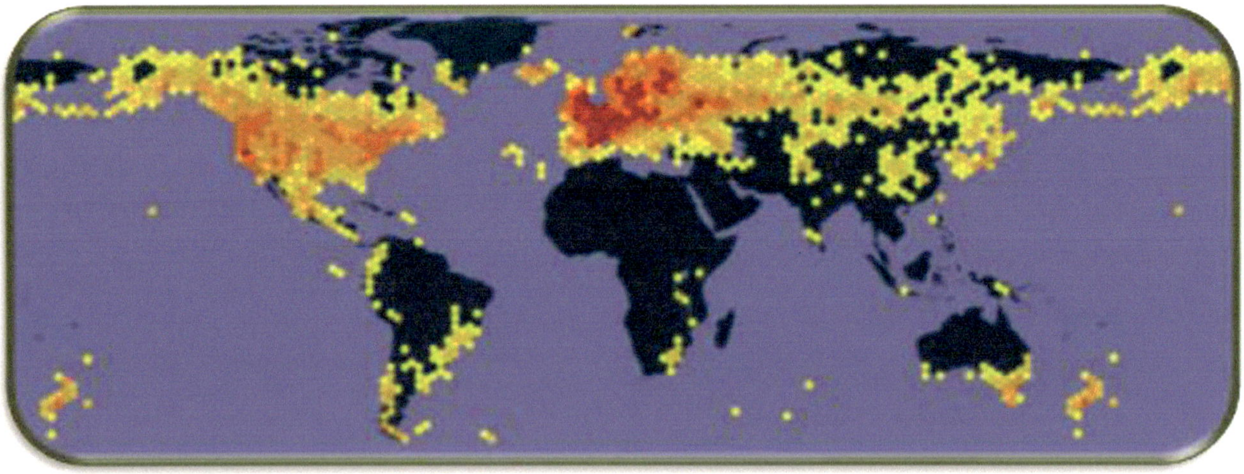

Botanical description:

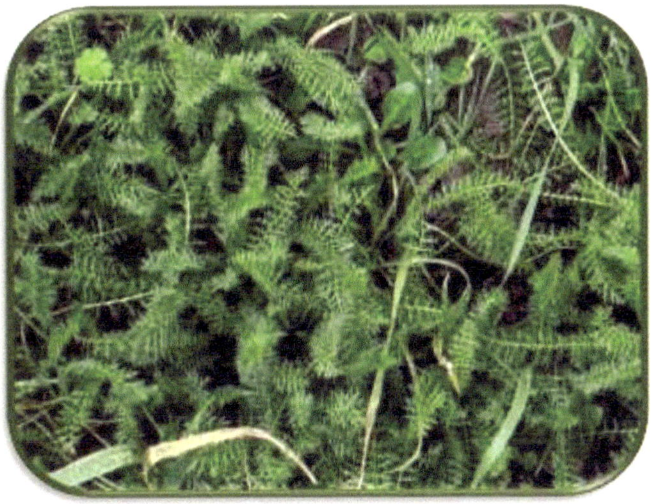

A perennial aromatic herb, reaching a height of about a meter. The stem is simple, branching at the level of inflorescence formation. The leaves are compound, pinnate, and petiolate, from several centimeters to about 20 cm long, and 1-4 cm wide. Its leaflets are deeply lobed, and its lobes are ribbon-like, and are located on the axis in an oblique manner. The inflorescences are primary, and in turn are gathered in apical, semi-comb-like inflorescences. The flower head is small, about 5 mm long, 3 mm in diameter, containing about 5 white, pink or red lingual flowers and numerous yellow tubular flowers. The bract is three-rowed. The inflorescence seat bears narrow scales. The fruit is almost oval, its apex is truncated to a length of 1.5-2 mm. The species is taxonomically very heterogeneous in form and tissue chemistry, and many subspecies are known, difficult to identify, due to the presence of many hybrids among them.

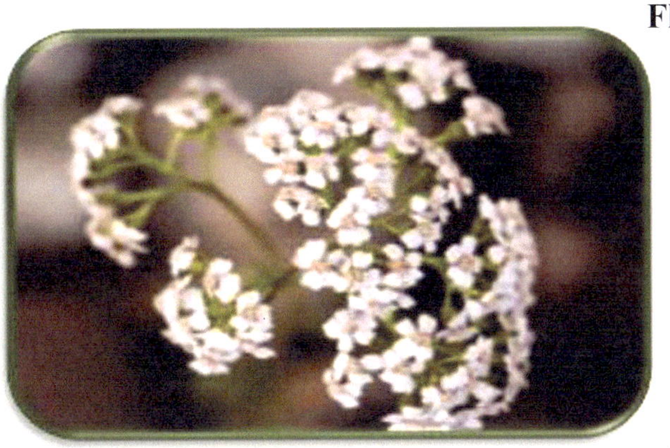

Flowering: From March to October.

Habitat and geographical distribution:

Southern Europe is likely to be the natural origin of the species of the genus. It is cultivated in America, Canada and China, and is also cultivated in many European countries.

History and heritage:

The genus name was mentioned previously, while the descriptive name for the species millefolium means "the plant has hundreds of leaves" (one thousand leaves).

Part used: Flowering aerial parts.

Chemical components:

The flowering aerial parts contain 1-0.2% volatile oil, the most important compounds of which are chamazulene 40%, camphor 20%, beta-pinene 23%, cineole 1,8-, and others.

Monomeric and semi-terpene ketone compounds, including: guaianolides, germacranolides, and alpha achillicin , and peroxyachfolid Flavonoids, including apigenine, luteolin, rutin. Pontica epoxide: polyynes. L-hydrostachydrine, L-stachydrine: betaine The aerial parts of the plant contain volatile oil, and forty-three compounds have been identified in it, the most important of which are germacrine 12%, Nerolidol 7.3%, sabinin 6.7%, p-mentha-2,8-dien-1-ol 4.5%, and 1.8-cineole 4%.

Properties and medical uses:

Aromatic herb, with anti-inflammatory and anti-allergic effects. Its aqueous property can be used to benefit from the products Secondary to obtain antioxidants. It is used to treat respiratory diseases, diabetes, and high blood pressure, and has antibacterial and antifungal activities. The plant has stimulant and cholagogue properties (guaianolides), germacranolides, spasmolytic (flavonoids), and anti-inflammatory (chamazulene). It is used to treat anorexia, liver, gallbladder, and digestive system diseases. The decoction of the plant is used topically to treat wounds, hemorrhoids, and varicose veins.

The aqueous extract of A. millefolium inhibits the growth of cancer cell lines, and the hexane extract of the flowers showed a significant decrease in systolic and diastolic blood pressure, mainly due to the presence of leucodin and achillin (epimers) compounds. The organic extracts showed vasodilatory activity. Screening of three lactone monoterpenes (isosectotanaphartolide, artelodoisinolide A, and millefolium A) isolated from Achillea millefolium showed inhibitory effects on lung cancer cells (possibly by inducing apoptosis). Most of the antioxidant and anti-inflammatory properties of this herb are attributed to its flavonoid content.

Precautions for use: Achillea is not prescribed for pregnant women.

Environment:

The plant grows in pastures and meadows, on roadsides, and in fields. It is mainly spread in cold areas where it tolerates cold during its vegetative growth and flowering, and can tolerate frost up to 25. Its cultivation in high mountainous areas where low temperatures and high humidity lead to a deficiency in the amount of the active ingredient. Cultivation is successful in silty and sandy silty soils, and it can grow in poor soils. It tolerates soil salinity and pH up to 8.8.

Cultivation and productivity:

The plant is propagated by seeds or by separating vegetative and root growths, but seed propagation is the best economically. Seeds are planted in the nursery in the fall, and germinate after one to two months, then transferred to the permanent soil when they reach a height of 8-10 cm. One hectare needs 43-48 thousand seedlings, resulting from 3 kg of pure seeds. It is recommended not to store seeds for more than 3 years. The plant is watered moderately, and can tolerate thirst during its growth and development. Fertilization, especially nitrogen, increases the amount of active ingredient. The inflorescences are picked when they bloom once every two weeks until the end of autumn, and it is important to pick in the early hours of the morning, and to focus on collecting the half-opened inflorescences. The hectare yields 6-7 tons of dry inflorescences in the first year, and production increases by 10% until the fourth year, then gradually decreases after that, when it is recommended to renew the cultivation in another place.

Achillea santolina L.

Achillea tenuifolia Lam.

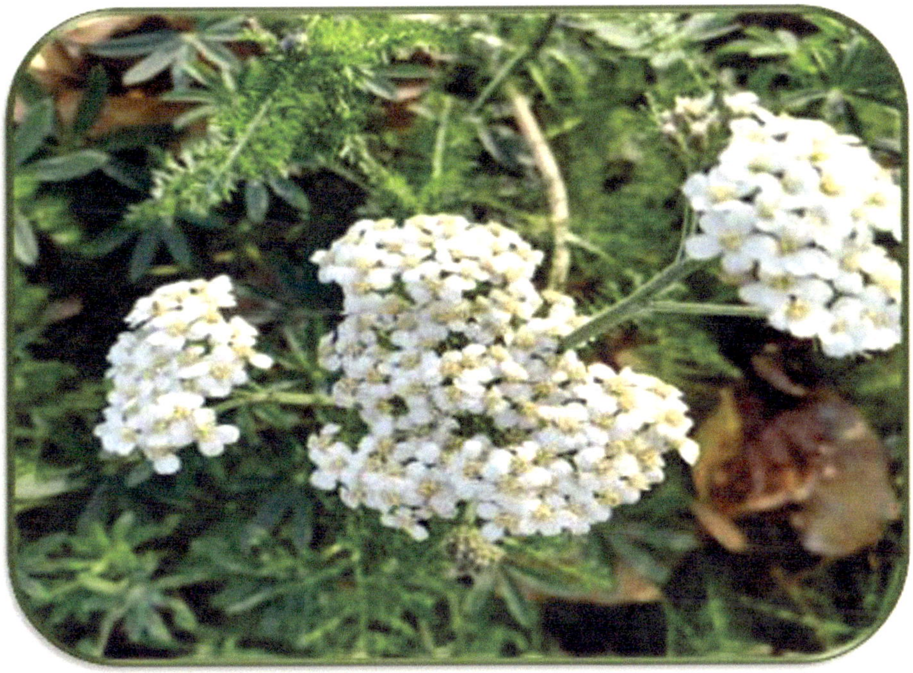

Family: Asteraceae (Compositae)

Common names: Holy sneezewort, Holy sneezewort

Foreign names: Eng. Santoline-leaved sneezewort, Fr. Achillee santoline

Occurrences : 679 occurrences

Distribution in the world

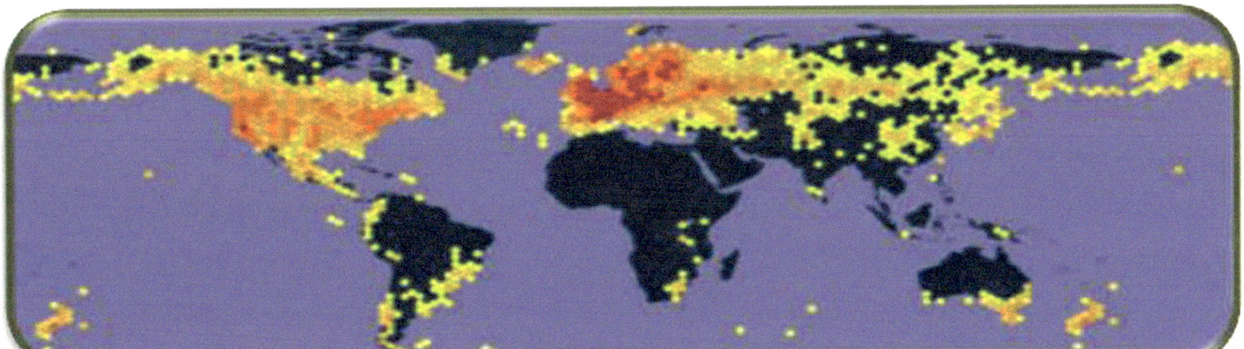

Botanical description:

A perennial herb, 15-30 cm tall, covered with grey woolly hair. Stems are erect to ascending, simple or branched, leafy, especially in the upper section below the flower heads. Leaves narrow, linear, green, deeply divided into very small parts, overlapping transversely, but not compact (loose). Each part is divided into 3 rounded lobes, with a serrated and thorny margin. The heads contain tubular and lintel flowers, and are gathered at the end of the stem in compound racemes. The peduncle is 4-5 mm, semi-spherical to spherical, with hairs that are compact and woolly. The lintel flowers are yellow, terry. The lobes are wider than they are long, and are shorter than the hemp. The fruit is akin Very compressed, narrow at the base, wide, and cut off at the top. Fertile.

Flowering: From March to April.

Habitat and geographical distribution:

Iranian-Turanian, and is widespread in Syria, Lebanon, Palestine, and Iraq.

History and heritage:

The genus name was mentioned previously, but the species name santolina is from Latin, and means "sacred.

Chemical components:

The aerial parts contain volatile oil, the most important compounds of which are: terpineol, fragranyl acetate, fragranol, cineole, camphor, trans carveol Favoneoids, crystalline materials, the most important of which are: santolin, and santolinol. 24 were separated The compounds and their percentages in Achillea tenuifolia are the most important: limonene (28.6%), α-cadinol (12.7%), borneol (6.7%), caryophyllene oxide (3.2%), borneyl acetate (4.3%), and para-cymene (2.3%).

Properties and medical uses:

The volatile oil has antibacterial properties against both gram-positive and gram-negative bacteria. Research on mice has shown the anti-inflammatory effectiveness of volatile oil, and demonstrated the ability of the plant, with its antioxidants, to stimulate the pancreas and reduce blood sugar levels. The decoction of the plant is popularly used as a general tonic, stimulant, expectorant, digestive, carminative, and intestinal worm repellent.

Environment: It is widespread in dry areas and on poor, stony soils.

Cultivation and productivity:

The plant is propagated by seeds or by cutting off vegetative and root growths, but seed propagation is economically better

Artemisia absinthium

Absinthium oficinale Brot., *Absinthium vulgare* Lam., *Artemisia pendula* Salisb.

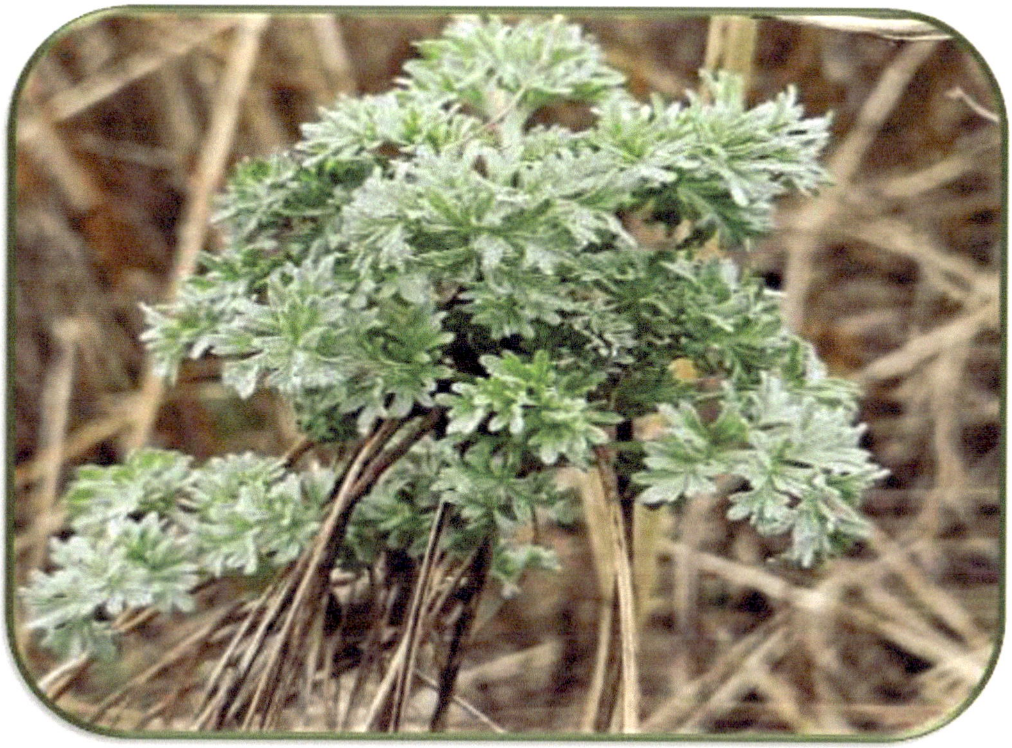

Family: Asteraceae (Compositae)

Common names: Wormwood, Absinthe, Grey

Foreign names: Green ginger, Wormwood, Absinthe, Fr. Absinthe, Vermouth

Occurrences : 81,834 occurrences

Distribution in the world

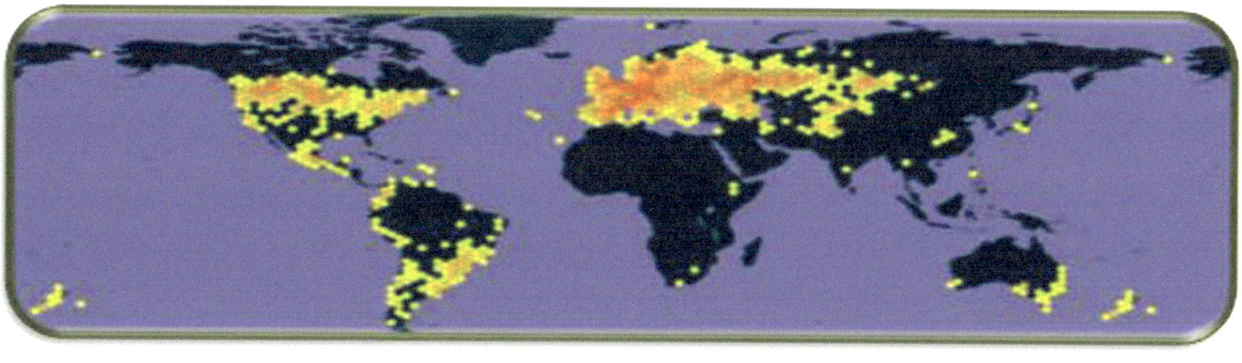

Botanical description:

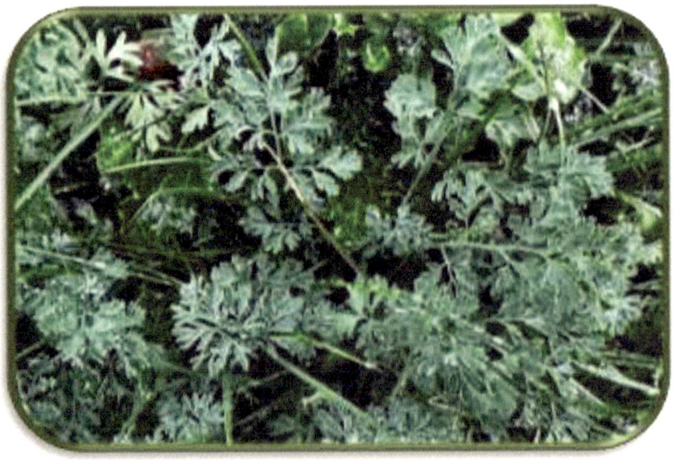

A perennial, aromatic herbaceous plant, covered with dense silky hairs, reaching a height of about a meter (or more), with a horizontal, woody underground stem and an erect stem. The stem is notched, dotted, glandular, gray in color, abundant in leaves, and highly branched in the upper part. Lower leaves long-pinnate (up to about 10 cm long), ovate, blade 8-15 cm long, 4-8 cm wide, deeply divided 2-3 times into linear-ovate lobes, 4-10 mm long, 2-4 mm wide. Middle and upper leaves short-pinnate to semi-pinnate, lobes fewer in number. Floral leaves pinnate, three-lobed or entire margin. The flowers are gathered in small, almost spherical, short-stemmed, drooping, head-shaped inflorescences (2-4 mm in diameter), which in turn form fragrant, pyramidal-shaped paniculate inflorescences, characterized by an aromatic odor and a bitter taste, reaching a length of about 30 cm. The bracts are linear, oblong, hairy, arranged in 3-4 rows, the inflorescence seat is flat, densely hairy. Flowers are yellow, the outer ones are fertile female, and the disc ones are fertile hermaphrodite. The two stalks are prominent. The fruit is a very small berry (1-0.8 mm), oblong to cylindrical, smooth, without pubescence.

Flowering: From June to September.

Habitat and geographical distribution:

The plant grows wild in central and southern Europe and northern Africa. It is currently cultivated in many temperate regions of the world, Algeria, Italy and France are the main areas for cultivating Damsis.

History and Heritage:

The genus name Artemisia is named after Artimis, the wife of the Carian King Mausolus (c. 377-353 BC). considering that she was the first to take the plant to treat some women's diseases. Some other sources attribute the name to the goddess Artimis. Hippocrates highly valued it, and gave it the name of the goddess Artemis (goddess of hunting and sister of Apollo in Greek mythology) in appreciation of its benefits. As for the name of the species, its source is Greek and Latin from the word absinthion, which means "unpleasant", i.e. the plant is unpopular because of its bitter taste. The plant has great importance in the East and the West, mentioned In ancient Egyptian writings, the Romans planted it on the sides of the roads, and put its soft parts in their shoes to protect them from foot pain during long journeys.

It was used to expel worms, and it was customary to offer its drink to horse racing champions in the Roman era as a guide to thieves.

Part used:

Dried fresh aerial growths including the leaf bases, volatile oil. The plant is collected in the summer during the flowering period.

Chemical components:

Absinthium A. contains many compounds Chemicals such as: lactones, essential oils, consisting of 34 compounds (Artemisinin, alpha and beta thujone 29.39%), β-Thujone, β-pinene 07.32%, γ-Terpinene, 4-Terpineol, Myrcene, Bornyl acetate, Cadinene, Camphene, trans-Sabinyl acetate, Guaiazulene, Chamazulene 39.2%), Camphor, Linalool, organic acids Organic, Resins, tannins, and phenols. Bitter mono- and semi-terpene compounds: artabsine, matricine, anabsinthine, absinthine Favonoids: artemitine (derived from quercetol) contains flavonoid compounds (quercetin), flavonoid glycosides (such as isoquercetin, quercetin -3-O-rhamnoglucoside, and isorafentin-3-O-glucoside), phenolic acids (such as coumaric, salicylic, chlorogenic, and vanillic acids) that contribute to scavenging free radicals.

Properties and medical uses:

Volatile oil and bitter compounds have digestive properties through their effect on the taste receptors in the tongue, which triggers a reflex that stimulates the stomach and digestive secretions. Volatile oil also has anti-inflammatory properties. Research has proven the effectiveness of bitter compounds (monoterpenes and a half) against tumors. The drug is used in cases of loss of appetite, disorders of the functions of the liver, gallbladder, stomach and digestion (increased digestive secretions in the stomach and liver). It is used to treat Crohn's disease (intestinal inflammation). The drug helps rid the body of toxins, especially lead and mercury compounds. The decoction of the plant is used popularly in cases of depression, liver diseases, menstrual disorders, anemia, and to expelWorms such as Ascaris worms. The plant extract is used topically as a poultice to treat ulcers, wounds and insect bites. The plant is traditionally used for diseases, digestive disorders and microbial infections. The ethanolic extract has a high antifungal capacity. Polyphenolic analysis revealed the presence of twenty-one different components, to which the observed activities can be attributed. A. absinthium extracts showed antibacterial activity against both Gram-positive and Gram-negative bacteria, but no activity against yeasts. It has been used in traditional Asian and European medicine as an effective general remedy for diseases of the digestive system, and in the treatment of parasitic worms, anemia, insomnia, bladder diseases, difficult-to-heal wounds, and fever. Antiulcer, cytotoxic, analgesic, antidepressant, neurotrophic, cell membrane stabilizing, and antioxidant. Azulene and its derivatives have been widely used in anti-allergic, anti-bacterial, and anti-inflammatory treatments, including anti-inflammatory for peptic ulcer, anti-tumor for leukemia, anti-diabetic, and antiviral.

Side effects and warnings:

Damsa is a very effective medicine, which requires caution when taking it because it contains the toxic compound thujone, as large doses of it (more than 3 g per day) cause vomiting, stomach and intestinal cramps, headaches, and epileptic seizures.

Environment:

It grows in dry and neglected lands, arid slopes, and roadsides. It tolerates drought. It thrives in all types of soils, and grows best in poor, dry soils on Warm slopes, where it lives longer, and the percentage of essential oil is greater in this case, as well as in alkaline soils with good drainage.

Cultivation and productivity:

It is propagated by seeds that are scattered in greenhouses from the end of winter until the beginning of summer, and they germinate after 2-6 weeks at a temperature of 15 ° C. The seedlings are removed and placed in bags, and they can be transferred to the permanent ground in the summer or kept in a refrigerated greenhouse It can be propagated by semi-woody cuttings in summer or by division in spring or autumn.

Artemisia herba-alba Asso.

*Seriphidium herba-album (*Asso.) Soják, *Artemisia aragonensis* Lam., *Artemisia billardiereana* Besser., *Artemisia gallica* subsp. *maroccana* Pau.

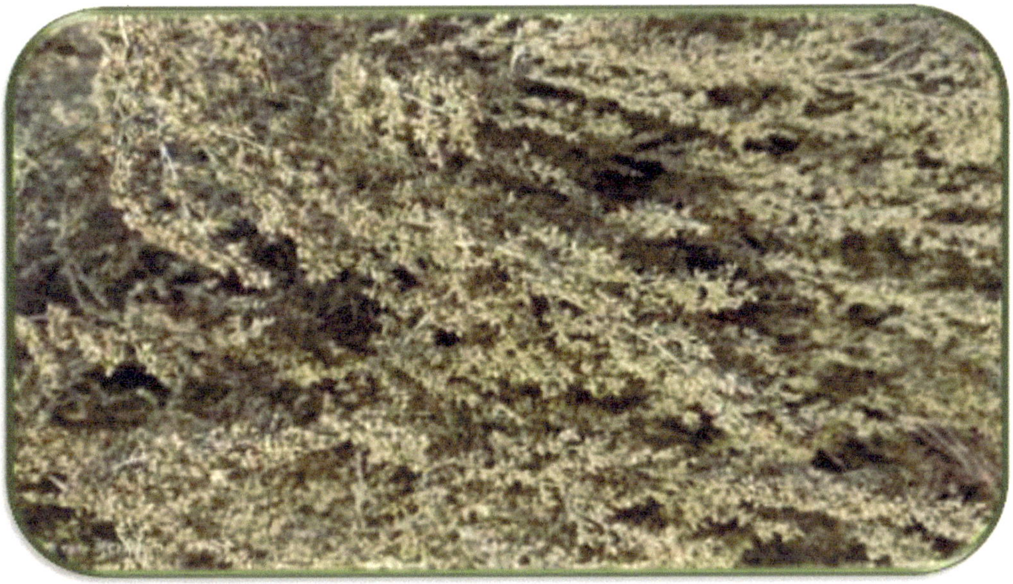

Family: Asteraceae (Compositae)

Common names: White wormwood.

Foreign names: Arabian wormwood, Fr. Armoise blanche

Occurrences : 6,121 occurrences

Distribution in the world

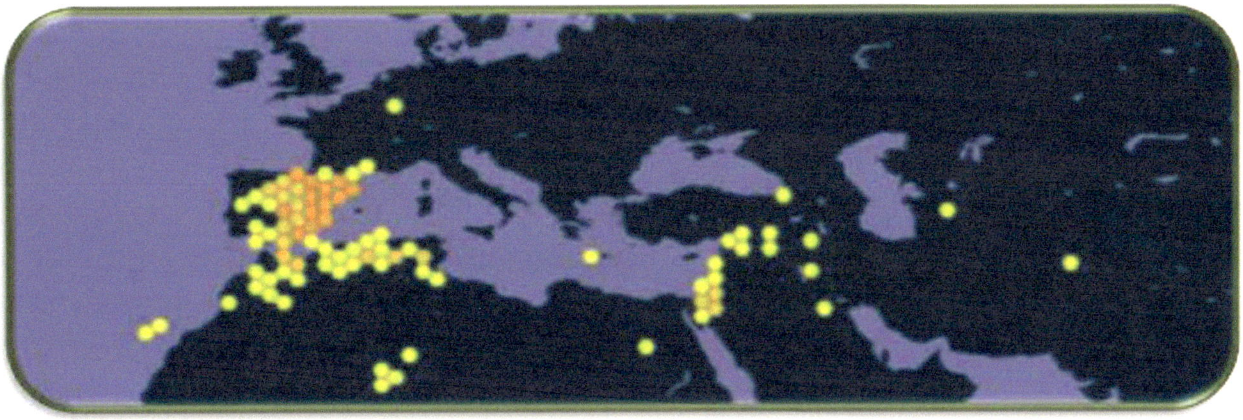

Botanical description:

A small shrub, 20-40 cm high, fragrant, densely hairy, later becoming bare, grey to silver in colour, with many stems, shallow roots. Stems erect, solid, each ending in an erect, branched, clustered inflorescence. Leaves of sterile branches, especially the lower ones, are obtuse, oval to circular in general appearance, deeply divided more than once (twice) into elongated parts. The floral stem leaves are shorter, few-lobed, and the leaves of the short branches are gathered in groups. The peduncles are oblong, gradually shortening towards the base, 3-4 mm long, and contain 2-4 flowers. The hemp pieces are overlapping, folded, the outer ones are small, rounded and fleshy and herbaceous in texture, while the inner ones are longer, oblong, rounded at the apex, and membranous and shiny. The fruit is an oblong, glabrous and smooth berry.

Flowering:

September to December.

Habitat and geographical distribution:

The Mediterranean basin, and is found in the Middle East and North Africa in particular.

History and heritage:

The genus name Artemisia was mentioned previously, while the species name means "white herb."

Part used:

The entire flowering plant except for the roots.

Chemical components:

The flowering vegetative parts contain: 1.7-1% volatile oil, yellow in color, its chemical components differ clearly according to the plant's geographical source and chemical pattern, and in general, monoterpene compounds, especially oxygenates, constitute about 40% of its compounds: 1.8-cineol, camphor, thujones, camphor, 13% santolina alcohol, 12% artemisia ketone, and monoterpene ketones: artemisinin, santonin, and dehydroleucodine. Found in the aerial parts of wormwood, responsible for the medicinal properties of the plant, and flavonoids .cirsilineol, hispidulin

Properties and medical uses:

The volatile oil (togon, santolin alcohol) has antibacterial, antifungal and anti-inflammatory properties. The compound santonin has anthelmintic properties. Research has shown the antioxidant effectiveness of wormwood aqueous extract, and for the treatment of cutaneous leishmaniasis. Research indicates the effectiveness of the aqueous extract of the leaves in reducing blood sugar levels, and there is evidence of its importance in treating some neurological diseases (Alzheimer's). Artemisinin is used in the manufacture of malaria drugs. Wormwood, with its volatile oil and santonin, is one of the important species used in folk medicine. The decoction of the plant is used to treat coughs, phlegm, stomach cramps, digestive disorders, expel gases and worms, liver failure, and reduce diarrhea. Its infusion is also used to relieve diabetes mellitus. The infusion of the flowers is used topically in the form of antiseptic compresses against bacteria and skin fungi, scabies and syphilis, and to ripen pimples, skin ulcers and eczema, as well as in menstrual disorders. An external disinfectant for animals and an insect repellent. Wormwood oil is used in veterinary medicine

Use warnings:

It should not be used excessively or continuously, due to it containing the toxic compound santonin, and it should not be used by pregnant women.

Environment:

It is spread in dry and semi-dry bioclimatic layers on sandy and silty steppes and calcareous loamy plateaus that may be high sometimes. It is drought tolerant, lives on rainfall above 90 mm/year, and the decrease in temperature in winter does not seem to affect its presence within the bioclimatic zone in which it lives.

Cultivation and productivity:

Artemisia is propagated naturally by seeds that are collected after they mature, and can be sown later. It can be propagated by semi-woody cuttings or by cuttings.

Artemisia scoparia Waldst. Kit.

Oligosporus scoparius (Waldst. & Kit.) Less., *Artemisia gracilis* L'Hér. ex DC., *Artemisia capillaris* var. *scoparia* (Waldst. & Kit.) Pamp., *Draconia scoparia* (Waldst. & Kit.) Soják.

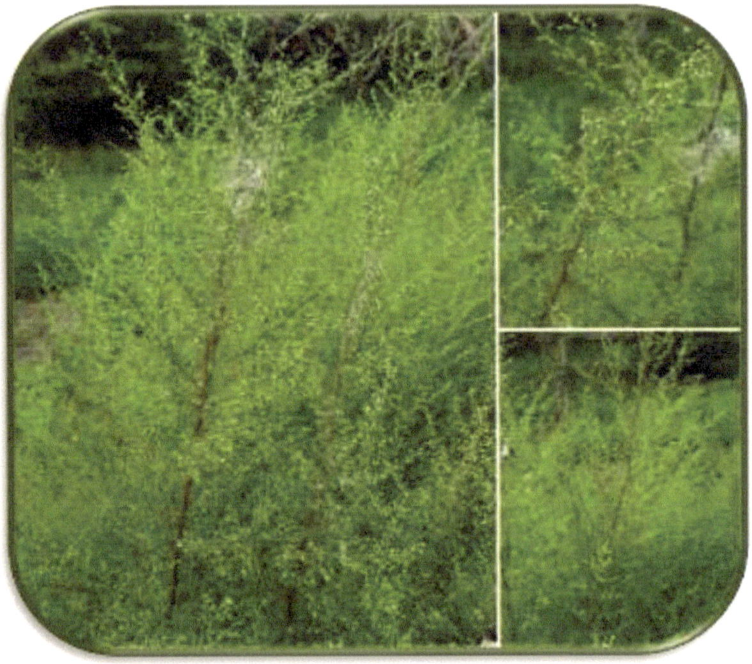

Family: Asteraceae (Compositae)

Common names: Salmas.

Foreign names: Armoise: Fr. wood, worm stem Red Eng

Occurrences : 6,911 occurrences

Distribution in the world

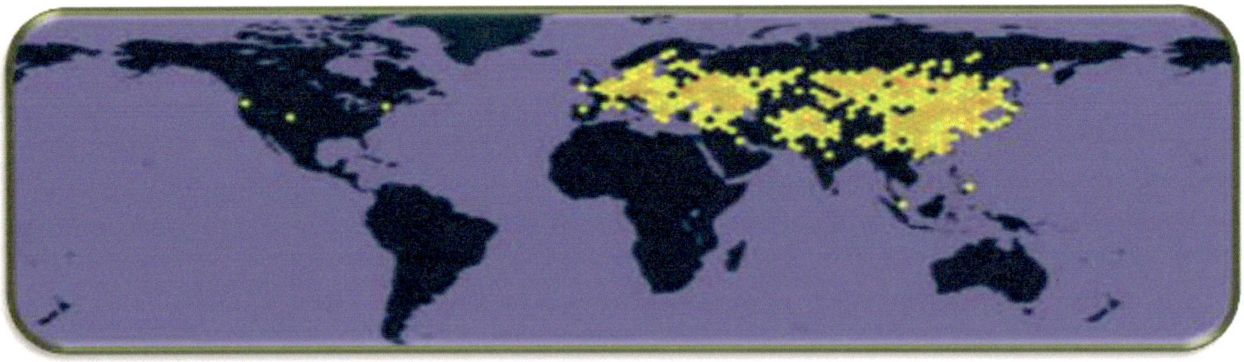

Botanical description:

A biennial herbaceous plant, 40-60 cm tall, glabrous except for the basal leaves which are covered with a grayish down. The stem is erect, branching along the stem, and forming broad, flattened clusters of branches. The basal leaves are obtuse, ovate or rounded in general shape, deeply divided twice into oblong-spoon-shaped lobes, blunt at the apex. The stem leaves are low, deeply divided into narrow, hard lobes. Inflorescences are capitate, numerous, spherical-ovate, small, about 3 mm in diameter, borne by short panicles, surrounded by bracts of unequal size, the outer ones being short and ovate, the inner one's oblong, with a relatively wide, dry, membranous margin. The peripheral flowers are female, arranged in a single row, the corolla is reduced, three-toothed. The central flowers are tubular, hermaphrodite. The fruit is an inverted oval, smooth berry.

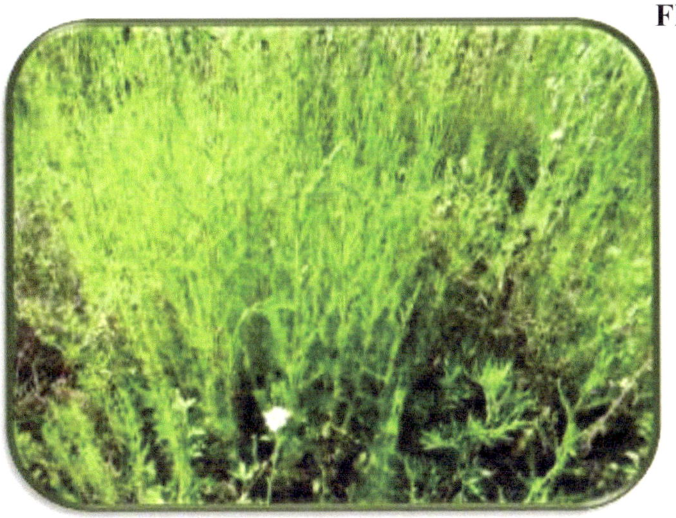

Flowering: September – November.

Habitat and geographical distribution:

The Mediterranean basin, and is widespread in North Africa.

History and heritage:

The genus name was mentioned previously, while the species name Scoparia means "broom-like", i.e. "its shape resembles a broom."

Chemical components:

The flowering stem and seeds contain volatile oil, which reaches 0.75%, the most important of which is Scoparone.

Medical uses:

The volatile oil has antibacterial properties (gram-negative and gram-positive) and antiseptic. It reduces cholesterol levels in the blood, is a diuretic, and dilates blood vessels. Recent studies have shown that it has diverse biological activities, especially with regard to liver protection and anti-inflammatory. The flavonoid compounds extracted from it show inhibitory activities against many strains of influenza virus. Salsam is popularly used to treat jaundice, liver and gallbladder infections (stimulates bile secretion), urinary retention, itching of wet sores, jaundiced hepatitis, influenza, and as a general anti-septic.

Environment:

It grows in steppe areas, prefers light, well-drained, sunny soils, and warm, dry places.

Cultivation and productivity:

It reproduces by seeds that are collected after they mature, and can be sown later. It can be propagated vegetatively.

Calendula officinalis L.

Caltha oficinalis (L.) Moench, *Calendula aurantiaca* Kotschy ex Boiss., *Calendula eriocarpa* DC., *Calendula hydruntina* Lanza.

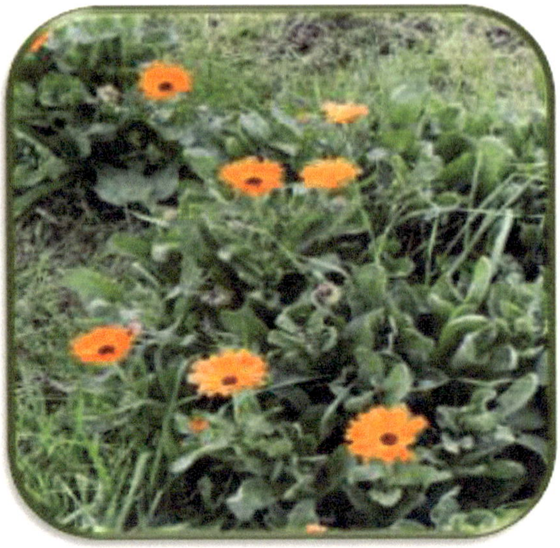
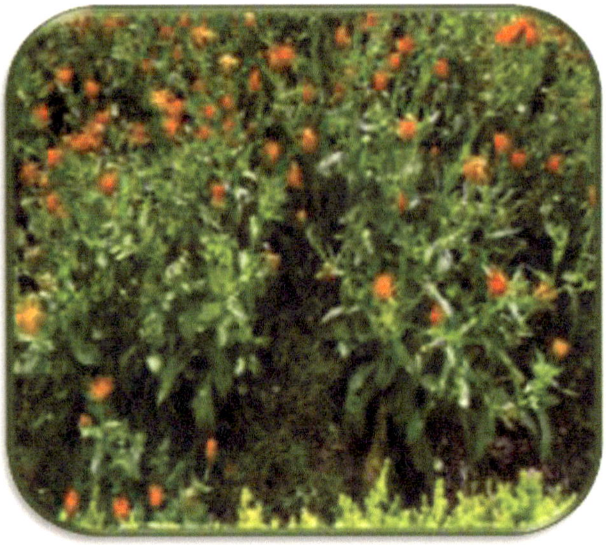

Family: Asteraceae (Compositae)

Common names: Daisy, Garden Calendula

Foreign names: jardins des Souci Fr. Marigold, Eng

Occurrences : 36,558 occurrences

Distribution in the world

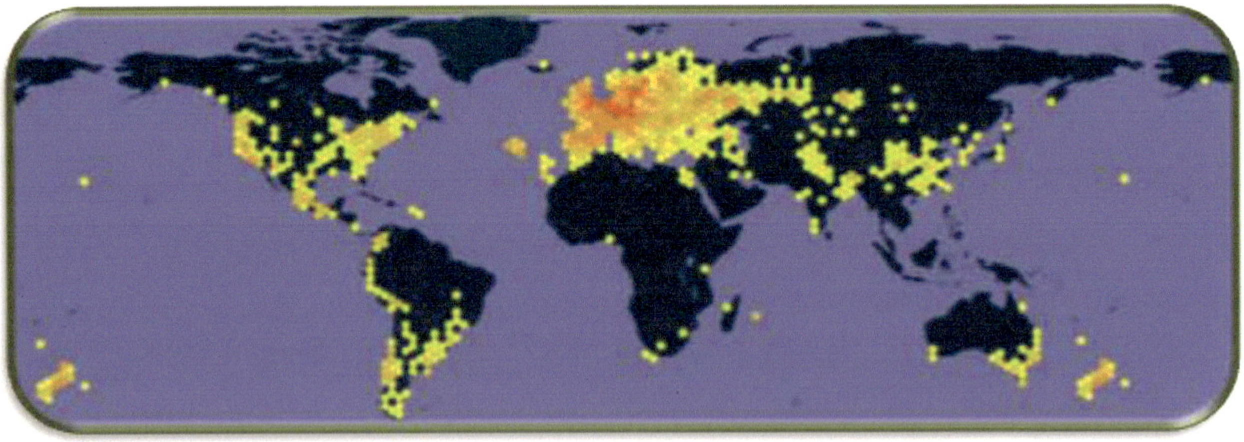

Botanical description:

An annual herb, 20-50 cm tall. Stem branched, hairy. Leaves alternate, ovate-lanceolate to lanceolate, lower obtuse, upper obtuse, blunt-edged, entire, base tapering gradually, 4-10 cm long. Inflorescences terminal panicles, 4-7 cm in diameter, composed of orange-yellow flowers, of two types: lintel and tubular. Bracts in two rows. The lingual flowers are located in the periphery, and are fertile female flowers. The corolla consists of the fusion of three segments to form a very short tube, which soon splits into a lingual shape 20-40 mm long and 5-7 mm wide, with three teeth at its apex. The central flowers are tubular, five-toothed, and hermaphrodite, but functionally male, yellow in colour, and smaller than the previous ones. The fruit is akin, arranged in 2-3 rows, curved to varying degrees and varied in shape, the outer part is scaphoid, its dorsal face bears short spines, and the inner part is strongly curved "semi-ringed", smaller in size, bears transverse wrinkles, the ovary is absent. It blooms during a long period of the year, especially in summer, and the plant has a strong unpleasant smell.

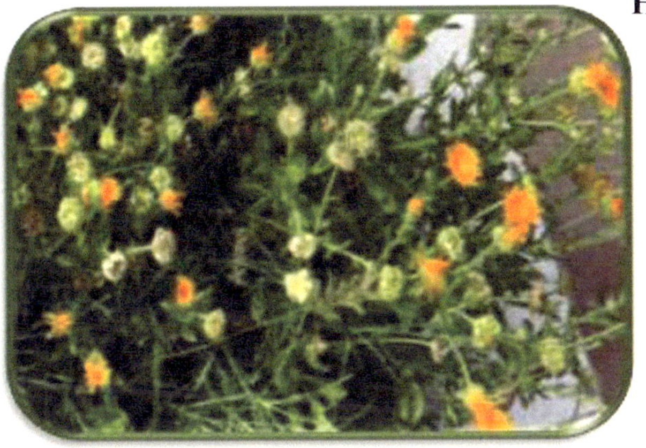

Habitat and geographical distribution:

Southern and central Europe and western Asia.

History and Heritage:

The Arabic name "Azure" is derived from the Persian word meaning "fire-colored", referring to the color of the flower. The scientific name of the genus is from the Latin calendae, meaning "first day of the month", perhaps referring to the English calendar (Calender), due to the repetition and continuity of its flowers. The species name oficinalis means "medicinal." The flowers have been used in folk medicine for a long time, and were considered an effective treatment for smallpox and measles. It was used by Greek, Indian and Arab doctors, and the first writings about the plant were found in Dioscorides, where he used the plant's infusion for liver diseases and to relax the intestines. The book of herbs written by Macer in the twelfth century also recommended the plant to improve eyesight, achieve clarity of mind, and bring joy and happiness to the soul. It was mentioned by Ibn Sina, Al-Ghasani and Ibn Al-Baytar.

Part used: Dried flowers.

Chemical components:

The flowers contain: Triterpene glycosides Terpenes 10-2%. Triterpene alcohols: including monooles triterpenes 0.8%, dioles triterpenes 4%, trioles triterpenes, taraxasterol, faradiol, and their esters, especially lauric acid and palmitic acid and others. Favones 0.3%-0.8%, the most important of which are isorhamnetin and quercetin. Volatile oil 0.2%, the most important of which is alpha-cadinol. Bitter compounds: calendin, phenolic acids: caffeic acids, salicylic acid.

Coumarins: scopoletin, esculetin, umbelliferone.

Carotenoids: the most important of which are zeaxanthine, lutein, fatty acids, polysaccharides. 15% Tannins, gums, and important substances. Green grass contains triterpene saponins, flavones, carotenoids, and volatile oil.

Properties and medical uses:

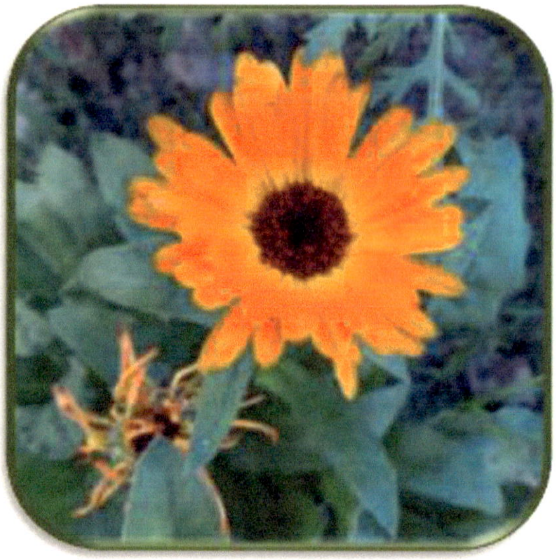

The flowers have volatile oil that has anti-inflammatory properties, helps in wound healing, treating burns, granulation-promoting, and treating inflammation of the skin, mouth, and pharyngeal mucosa. The flowers also have antimicrobial properties, such as Staphylococcus aureus and Candida monosa fungi. Initial experiments have shown its effectiveness against HIV, vesicular stomatitis, and rhinovirus. The infusion or decoction of the flowers is popularly used to treat gastritis and chronic ulcers, improve digestion, increase bile secretion, relieve intestinal spasms, and expel worms and parasites. The infusion of the flowers or their preparations are used in the form of a tincture or topical ointments to treat conjunctivitis, wounds, eczema, cracked hands, nipples, and fistulas. It has also been used in the form of an ointment for hemorrhoids. Calendula is often used in the form of injections, tincture, or ointment to treat dermatitis, burns, insect bites, and leg ulcers.

Precautions for use:

It should not be used by pregnant women.

Environment:

Chrysanthemum grows wild in orchards, on roadsides and slopes, it likes exposed and humid places. It is widespread in semi-humid, semi-arid and dry environments in warm and moderate regions, the ideal temperature for its growth is 25-30°C, frost and cold limit its growth and harm the flowers. The inflorescences respond to changes in temperature and humidity, as they open on sunny and dry days, and close on cloudy and rainy days. It is considered a light-loving species, but it can grow in shady places. It is planted in all types of soils, preferring hot gravelly or calcareous clay.

Cultivation and productivity:

It is planted for medicinal and ornamental purposes. Seeds are planted in the spring in rows in pits or basins, 2-3 seeds are placed in the hole, covered with a light layer of soil, and watered directly. It can also be planted in lines with a distance of 30 cm between each plant. Seeds germinate 7-15 days after planting, and vegetative growth continues 15-30 days until the first flower bud appears. The inflorescences bloom 5-15 days after the flower buds appear. Appropriate service operations are carried out, including pruning, weeding, fertilization, irrigation (taking care not to deprive the plant of water during the flowering period and not to dry out the soil) and removing the withered lower leaves. The plant blooms throughout the year in warm areas, but stops blooming in winter in cold areas. The inflorescences are harvested in sunny weather, when the outer linseed flowers are in a horizontal position, and are dried in the shade without piling them on top of each other. As for the leaves, they are collected in Morning after dew drops have evaporated. Production under good conditions: 1-1.5 tons/hectare of dry flowers, and about 300-400 kg/hectare of seeds.

Carthamus persicus **Willd. Desf. ex Willd.**

C. flavescens sensu Boiss., *C. palaestinus* Eig., *Atractylis armena* (Willd.) Poir., *Atractylis armena* Poir.,*Carthamus armenus* Willd., *Carthamus flavescens* Willd., *Carthamus palaestinus* Eig ex Rech.f., *Heracantha armenia* G.Don ex Loudon., *Kentrophyllum aureum* Boiss.

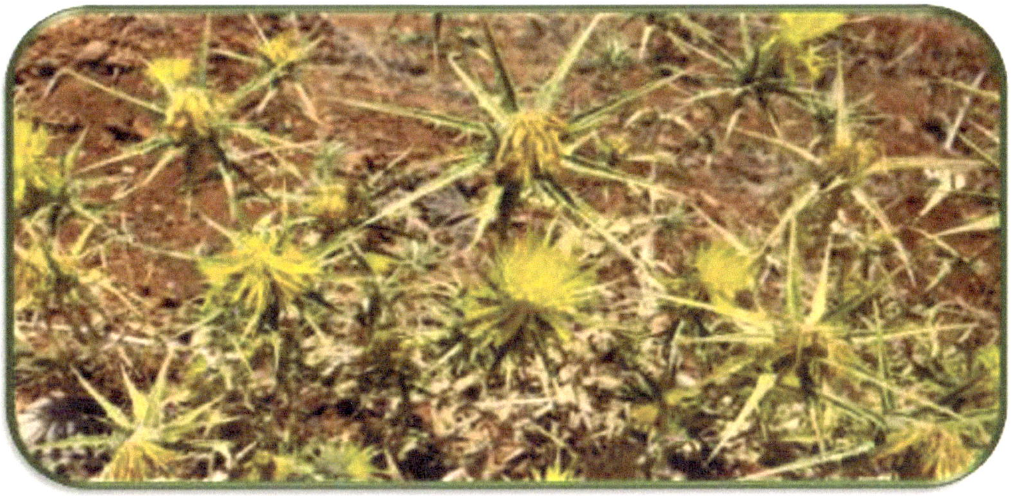

Family: Asteraceae (Compositae).

Common names: Yellow safflower, Amber.

Foreign names: Wild safflower, Fr. Carthame de Perse

Occurrences : 207 occurrences

Distribution in the world

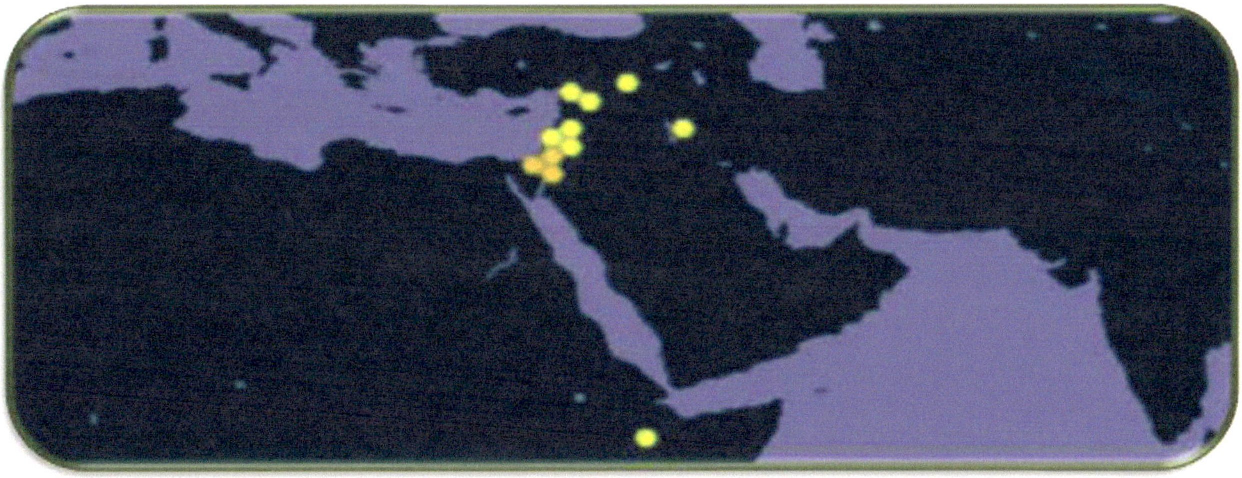

Botanical description:

Annual herb, 30-50 cm high, semi-growth. Stem is white, solid, branched in a panicle. Leaves are simple, alternate, lanceolate, with some short yellow spines on the margin. Basal leaves emerge in the form of a rosette, obtuse, wither when flowering. Stem leaves are low and almost embracing the stem. Flower heads are homogeneous, branched in a panicle, surrounded by a double bract. The outer bract is almost as long as the flowers, its bracts are lanceolate, serrated, thorny, resembling stem leaves in shape, the inner bract is broadly oval, 2.5-2 cm in diameter, its bracts are lanceolate, entire, ending in a weak spine, shorter than the outer bracts, straw-like, semi-waisted at the bottom. The inflorescence seat is semi-fleshy in texture and covered with scales resembling hairs. The flowers are all tubular, equal, and yellow in colour. The fruit is a smooth, inverted conical, quadrilateral echinoderm, bearing a serrated ring at its apex, the navel is lateral, the marginal fruits are devoid of pubescence. The echinoderm of the inner echinoderm is perennial, its hairs tend to be purple, feathery, arranged in more than one row, its length exceeds by about one and a half times the length of the echinoderm.

Flowering: From April to May.

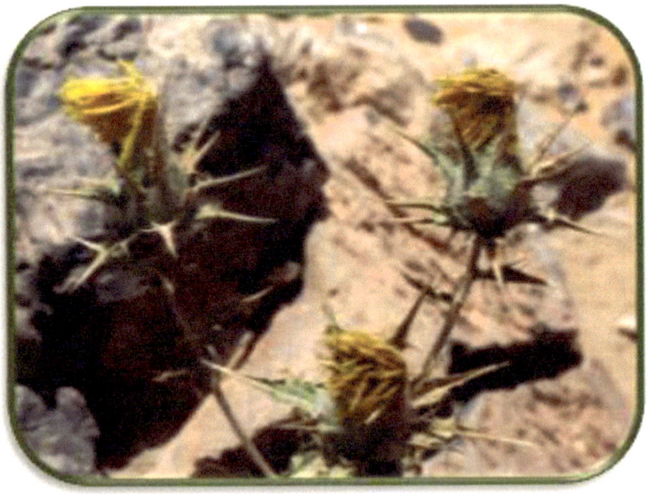

Habitat and geographical distribution:

Western Iran-Turania region, grows wild in Iran, Syria, Palestine, Lebanon, northern Iraq, and Turkey.

Other species include:

Safflower, native to the western Mediterranean. C. lanatus, which is a woolly safflower, a medicinal plant , C. caeruleus, which is blue, and is widespread in the Mediterranean.

Safflower or dyer's safflower, the herman, Carthamus tinctorius L.) is grown in the United States, Europe, and the countries of the eastern Mediterranean for its flowers used in food coloring, and its seeds, which give edible oil.

History and heritage:

It is believed that the scientific name of the genus is derived from the Arabic karthom or karthum, while Nahal (2009) states that the scientific name is of Aramaic origin, taken when one of its species was introduced from the East to Europe in the sixteenth century, and planted to extract a red dye that is used to dye silk, and from which blush is made. The descriptive name of the species tinctorius means "dye", and the descriptive name of the species persicus means "Persian", referring to the original homeland of Iran.

Part Use:

Seeds and the oil extracted from them, flower bits (collected in the morning, and dried in the shade, because the sun's rays break down the pigment present in them)

Chemical components:

The seeds of both species contain: A fatty oil rich in fatty acids such as oleic acid, linoleic acid a. linoleic 88-55%, and linolenic acid a. linolenic acid. The flower bits contain flavonoid compounds such as carthamidin (tetrahydroxyflavanone), carotenoids, glycosides, red pigment (Red) Carthamin, and carthamone Flavonoids (Orange red). Flower petals contain protein, crude fibers and ash. It also contains alkaloids, lignanoids, organic acids, polyacetylene, ribofafine, steroids, and quinochalcone C-glycosides. Other quinochalcone components isolated from aqueous extracts of flower petals include cartormin, safflomin B, safflomin C, isosafflomin C, precarthamine, yellow safflor B, tinctormin, and flavonoids (azaleatin, saffloroside, and cinaroside). The aqueous extract of the flowers also contains On: isocartormin, semiquinonechalcone C-glycoside, is an isomer of cartormin. There is a relationship between the content of active ingredients and the intensity of flower color. The more colorful flowers (bright red, light yellow or bright orange) were characterized by a higher content of anhydrosafflor B, kaempferol, quercetin, and safflomin C, compared to the less colorful flowers. Studies have shown the presence of 20 to 29 compounds in safflower essential oil. Hydrodistillation of safflower bits gives a pale yellow oil (0.175% v/w). Twenty compounds were identified, representing 99.81% of the oil, the most important of which are: undecanoic acid, octane, heptacosane, a. nonanoic acid, a. tetradecanoic acid, and hydro1-naphtol tetra.

Properties and medical uses:

The Persian saffron C. persicus is similar in its uses to the cultivated saffron or false saffron C. tinctoria. Saffron seed oil is used to prevent arteriosclerosis, reduce blood pressure, improve blood circulation, and reduce the formation of blood clots. The plant is popularly used to treat high cholesterol (LDL), and the decoction of the seeds is popularly used for its laxative and facilitating properties to treat constipation, and to treat wounds, vitiligo, melasma, and itching. Saffron flowers are used as an emmenagogue, abortifacient, expectorant, and anti-pneumonia. In addition to its use in treating internal and external wounds. Eating saffron oil helps in losing weight, maintaining and renewing muscle mass, and has a Antioxidant.

Pharmaceutical forms:

Safflower is available in the form of tea, especially, and in preserves, and liquids, sold under names such as Saffron oil, Safflower.

Drug interactions and precautions for use:

Safflower should not be taken with medications that may affect the immune system, such as: IImuram Prograf, . The flowers, oil, or seeds should not be used by pregnant and lactating women. It should be used with caution in the case of burns, blood infection, organ transplantation, or any other condition that suppresses the immune system. It should also not be received Any vaccine when eating saffron.

Other uses:

Two dyes are extracted from saffron flowers, one is red carthamon, which dissolves in foundations, and the other is yellow carthamin, which dissolves in water. Red lipstick and blush are made from the red dye, and saffron dye is also used to dye cotton and silk fabrics. A fatty oil is extracted from the seeds that can be used as food. Safflower flowers are known for many food uses (flavor and food dyes). The colors of crushed safflower petals are similar to saffron stigmas, which makes fraud easy due to the huge price difference between the two drugs.

Environment:

Safflower is a plant of sunny, hot and dry areas, characterized by its high resistance to drought and hot weather. Its seedlings tolerate a temperature drop of up to -6°C. Its humidity requirements are very low, the seeds may rot in the inflorescence, and fertility is weakened in conditions of high humidity.Lives in various types of soils except for the well-drained. It tolerates poor soils, tolerates salinity, and gives a high yield in well-drained, fertile or fertilized soils.

Cultivation and productivity:

The plant is propagated by seeds. Organic and mineral fertilizers are added to the soil, then it is prepared by plowing it to a depth of 30 cm, leveling it and smoothing it. Seeds are planted by picking behind the plow or in holes in lines so that the distance between the lines is 50-60 cm and between the holes inside the line is 20-25 cm. It is also possible to follow the planting method in square holes at a distance of 45 cm with several seeds placed in each hole. Planting is done in winter. The processes of individualization and patching are carried out two weeks after germination in irrigated agriculture in particular, and the service processes of fertilization, irrigation and weeding continue. The petals are collected in the morning and spread out in the shade to dry. The plant is uprooted and the seeds are collected in late summer. One hectare yields 30-70 kg of shoots and 750-1500 kg of seeds.

Centaurea cyanus L.

Centaurea segetalis Salisb., *Cyanus segetum* Hill.

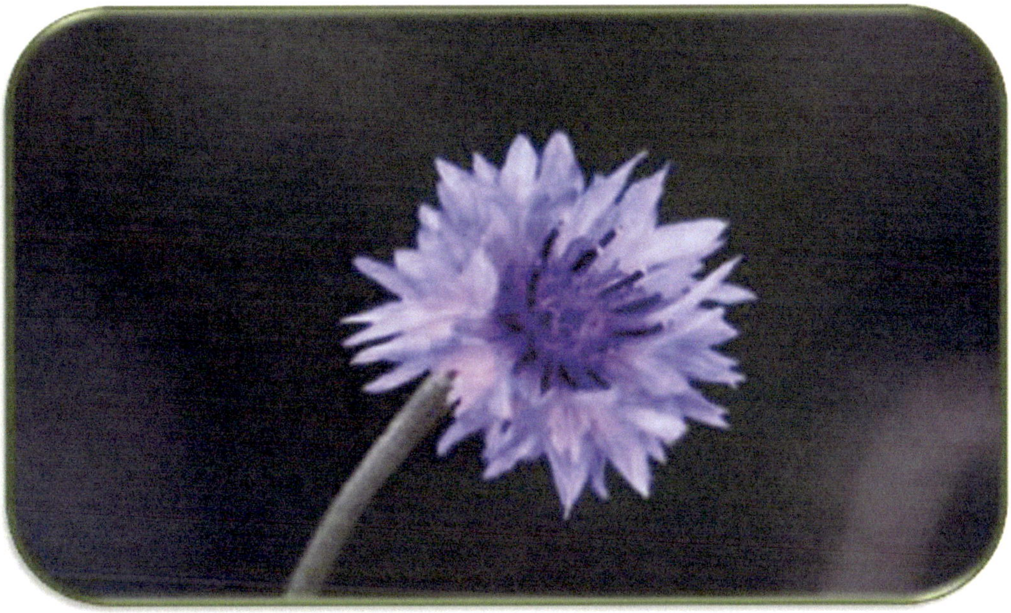

Family: Asteraceae (Compositae)

Common names: Bitter, bitter, centaury, amber centaury, tsar nasha, amber dew.

Foreign names: Eng. Cornflower, Red starthistle, Fr. Bleuet des champs

Occurrences: 172,709 occurrences

Distribution in the world

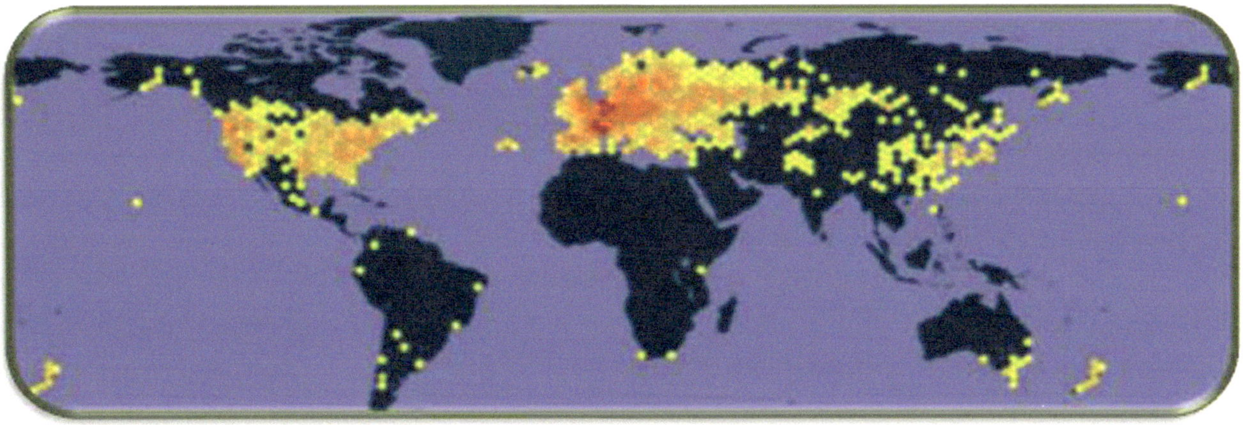

Botanical description:

A biennial herbaceous plant, erect, dichotomously branched from the base, 40-60 cm high. Leaves are simple, Long, soft, lower leaves form a rosette, serrated or lobed to varying degrees, 1-6 cm, and papillary The lobes are lanceolate, the oblique is winged. Stem leaves are long, linear, acute, feminine, their lobes are few in number; terminal leaves have entire margins. Flower heads lateral and terminal, short-stalked or sessile, solitary. The bract is ovate-conical, 12-15 mm long, 5-7 mm wide (without spines). The bracts are glabrous, leathery, with a narrow membranous margin, bearing a flattened, sword-shaped bract, 10-20 mm long in the median bracts, and provided at their base with 2-3 pairs of lateral spines 2-3 mm long. The inner bracts are thornless, membranous at the apex. The flowers are pink, all tubular. The bracts are small, smooth, 3-4 mm long, without pubescence.

Flowering: May to July.

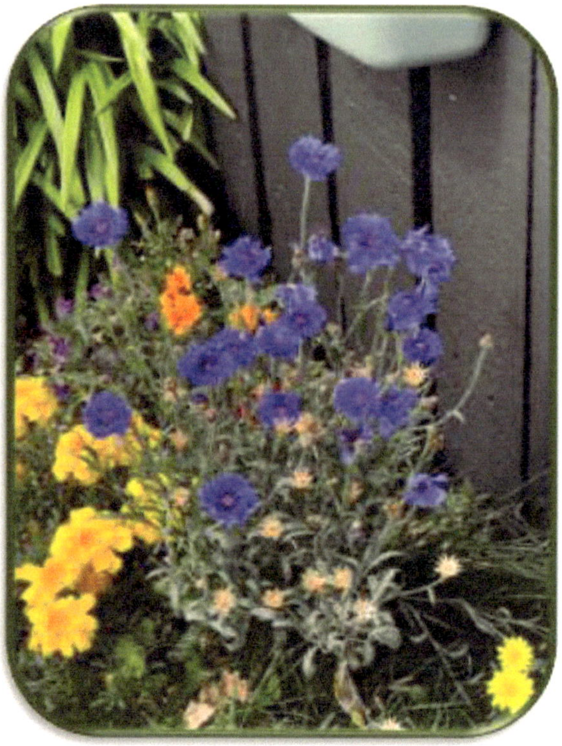

Habitat and geographical distribution: Europe, North Africa, Egypt, Syria, Lebanon, Palestine, Turkey, Greece

History and Heritage:

Centaurion is an Arabic name derived from the Greek kentaurion, which is the name of a number of medicinal plants dedicated to Centaure Chiron, a mythical creature half man and half horse, who according to Greek mythology lived in Thessaly, and it was believed that he discovered the species of these plants.

Part used: Flowers.

Chemical components:

Anthocyan pigments, the most important of which are succinylcyanin (centaurocyanin), cyanidine, flavonoids and bitter compounds. 55 phenolic compounds were identified in the leaf extracts: 30 phenolic acids and their derivatives, 25 glycosides, favonoids and aglycones. In addition to the presence of centauridine, gasidine, camphoride, nepetin, and phenolic acids and their esters. Six simple favonoids were isolated: Eupatorine, Eupatiline, Jaceosidine, Cirsiliol, Hispiduline, Apigenin, and lactones in addition to only one compound derived from mono- and semi-terpenes (sesquiterpenes): kenesin. Cnicin

Medical uses:

The drug has antibacterial properties (centaurocyanin). The Centaurea genus is used in folk medicine for its anti-inflammatory, antipruritic, antitussive, laxative, and astringent properties. Bitter is used in folk medicine to treat fever, vaginal discharge, menstrual disorders, and as a liver tonic,cleanses the body of toxins, treats headaches (all types of headaches), is a diuretic, and dissolves urinary stones. The infusion of its fresh or dried flower powder is used as a topical compress to treat wound infections, eyelid infections, itching, scabies, and skin eczema, especially chronic ones. Its leaves are appetizing when they are fresh, raw or cooked. Studies indicate that all tested extracts are non-toxic and can be of great importance in combating pathogenic strains of plants and humans.

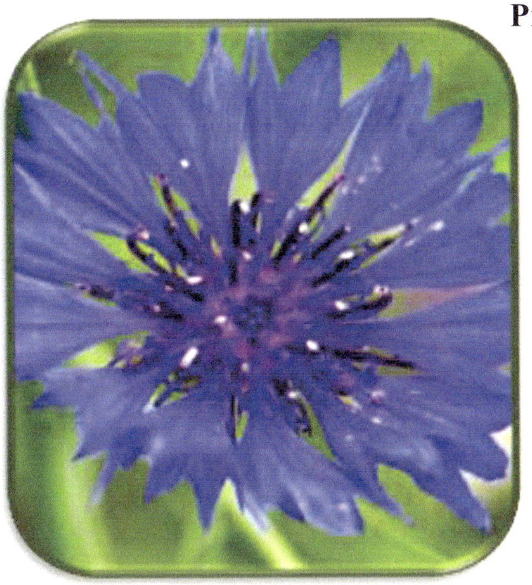

Precautions for use:

It is not recommended to use it in patients with calculous and tumorous bile duct obstruction.

Environment:

It grows wild in wheat fields, and also grows on the sides of roads, water channels, and neglected places on sandy and stony soils. It tolerates cold, and grows in different types of soils from sandy to heavy, provided that they are well drained, and it can grow in poor soils. It tolerates high levels of alkalinity in the soil, and it can tolerate soil dryness well. It cannot grow in the shade.

Cultivation and productivity:

The plant is propagated by seeds that are planted in a cold greenhouse, and when the seedlings grow, they are transferred individually to pots, and transferred to the permanent land in the summer. If there is a sufficient quantity of seeds, they are scattered directly in the permanent land at the end of summer and the beginning of autumn. It blooms in mid-summer and the beginning of autumn, and the seeds ripen at the end of summer and the beginning of autumn

Cichorium intybus L.

Cichorium rigidum Salisb.

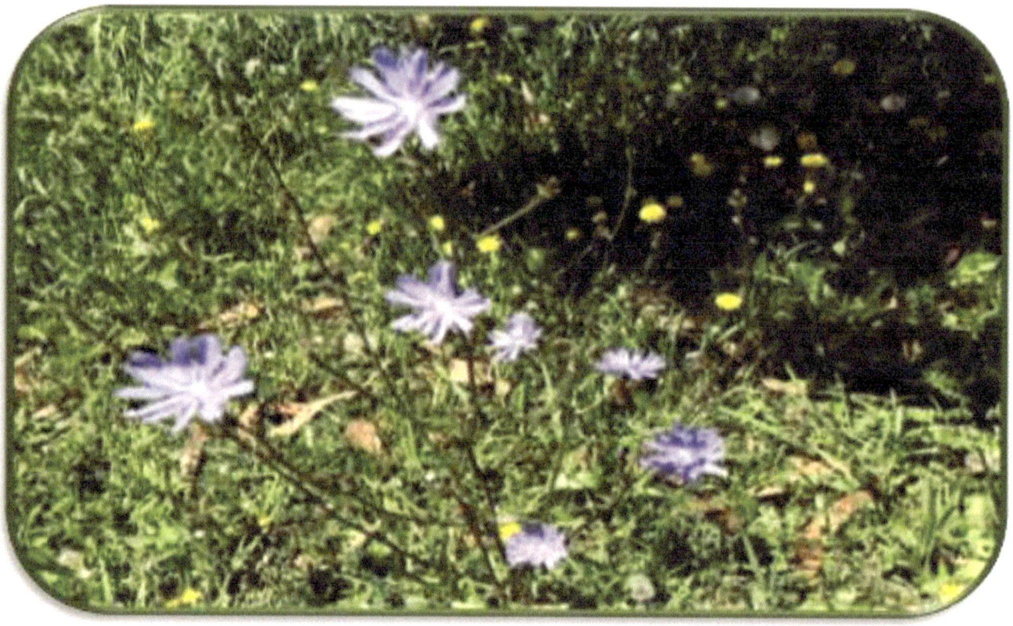

Family: Asteraceae (Composite)

Common names: Wild chicory

Foreign names: Wild chicory

Occurrences : 296,744 occurrences

Distribution in the world

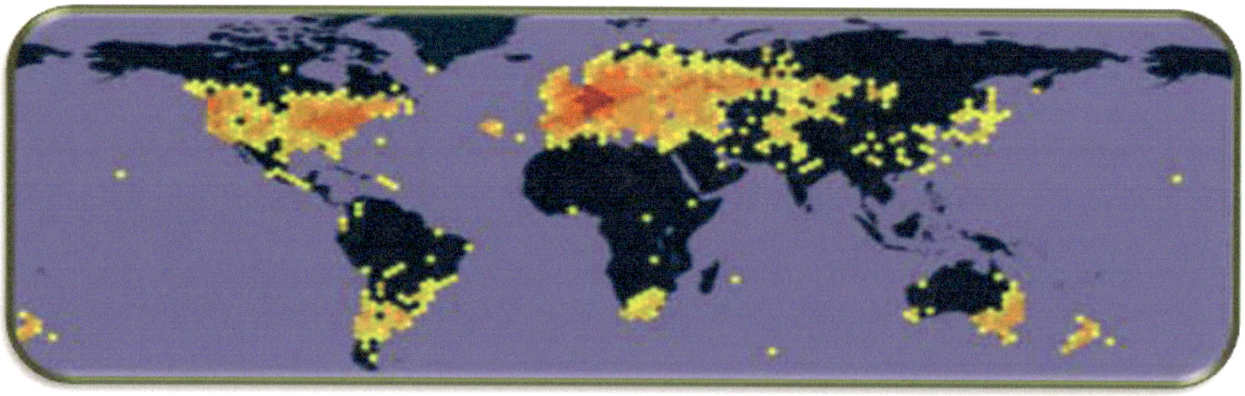

Botanical description:

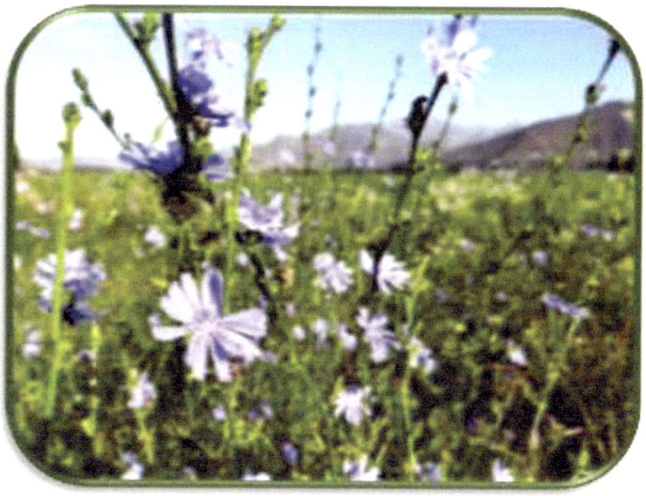

Perennial herb, with deep roots, 30-100 cm high. Stem erect, branched, thin. Leaves simple, covered with hairs, especially on the median nerve. Lower leaves are obtuse, lobed, lobes directed towards the base, and the terminal lobe is the largest. Stem leaves are lanceolate, semi-pinnate, and the upper ones are entire. The heads contain only lintel flowers. Lateral heads are low, found in pairs or in bundles, apical heads are solitary and spiked. The bract is double. The outer bracts are oval, forming a cup-like shape, while the inner bracts are linear and longer, all glandular and ciliated. The flowers are linolecular, blue in colour, about 3 times longer than the bract. The fruit is a short achene, the bract is perennial, short, consisting of a number of small scales, 8-10 times shorter than the body of the achene itself.

Flowering: May to June.

Homeland and geographical distribution:

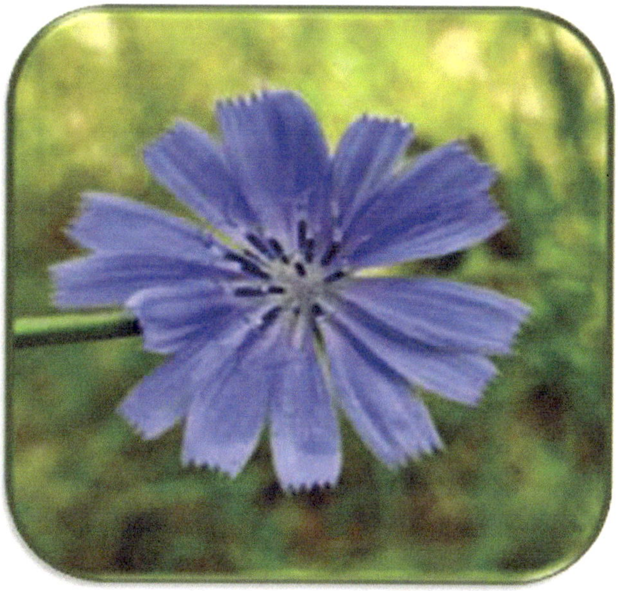

It is believed that the original homeland of the plant is the eastern Mediterranean regions, from where it moved to Europe, America and many other regions of the world.

History and heritage:

The word chicory is derived from Syriac, and the scientific name is the Greek and Latin name for this plant, and it is the name of a medicinal and edible species since a long time. The plant was known in ancient times to the Egyptians, Greeks and Romans. The Romans called it IIntubus or IIntubum, and the Arabs called it in folk medicine for its use in liver diseases.

Part used:

The entire flowering plant (with the roots) fresh and dried.

Chemical components:

Sesquiterpenlactone compounds, including: lactucin, and lactucopicrin Flavonoids, including: chicoroisides, sonchuside, and hyperosideCaffeic acid derivatives: cinnamic acid, a. chicoric acid, a. chlorogenic acid, a. isochlorogenic acid, and a. tartaric acid Coumarins, including: umbelliferone. Bitter substances. Amaroid leaves are rich in vitamins A, B, C.

Properties and medical uses:

The plant has properties that reduce blood pressure, cholesterol, anti-edema, diuretic, and digestive stimulant. It is used in cases of loss of appetite and digestive disorders. Wild chicory is popularly used to treat loss of appetite, indigestion, liver diseases, constipation, fluid retention, and hemorrhoids. Dandelion juice is used as a laxative for children.

Pharmaceutical forms:

Wild chicory is available in the form of a raw herb, roasted or unroasted root, and specialties, and is sold under the name chicory.

Side effects and warnings for use:

It should be completely avoided in case of sensitivity or skin irritation to the components of chicory or in case of heart disease, because it may affect the heart.

Other uses:

Roasted chicory roots are sometimes used as a substitute for coffee due to their coffee-like flavor and aroma, although they have a sedative effect, so some people add them to coffee to counteract the stimulation caused by caffeine.

The young leaves of the plant are used as a seasoning for food. The old leaves of the plant are dried and eaten like celery. The roots can be boiled and eaten with butter.

Environment:

The plant grows wild in farms, vegetable and ornamental gardens, on roadsides and irrigation canals. It is successfully grown in dry and semi-dry environments in hot, warm and temperate regions. It tolerates relatively cold, and a temperature of 15-17°C is suitable for growth. It can be grown in places with poor lighting. It is successfully grown in most lands, especially medium and light yellow, well-drained lands. Its cultivation in heavy soils leads to the formation of irregular roots. Suitable pH 5.5-6.5

Cultivation and productivity:

The plant is propagated by seeds that are planted in early autumn in special beds, scattered or in rows, with a distance of 10-15 cm between them. Service operations of weeding and irrigation continue until the seedlings are 12-15 cm long, where they are uprooted and planted in the permanent soil within channels or lines. It takes about 100g of seeds to plant one acre, which yields about 8000-10000 seedlings. The field is irrigated immediately after planting, and the service operations of patching, weeding and fertilization continue. The plant matures after 3-4 months to obtain the vegetative mass, and after 6-7 months to obtain the enlarged roots.

Cnicus benedictus L.

Centaurea benedicta L.

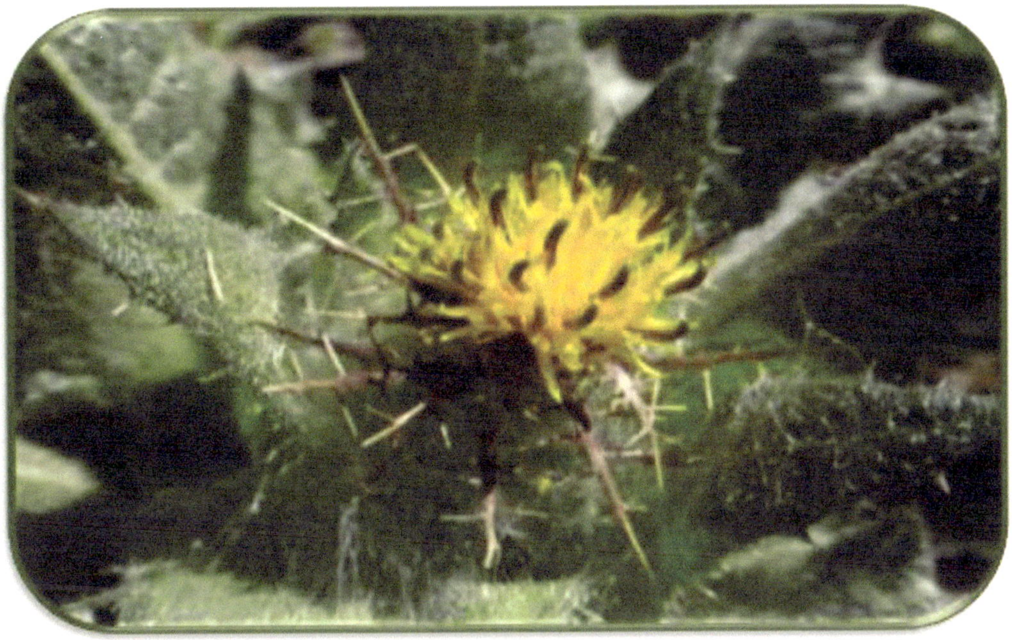

Family: Asteraceae (Compositae)

Common names: Blessed thistle, Holy thistle, Spotted thistle, Flowering thistle

Foreign names: beni Chardon Fr. thistle, Holy Eng.

Occurrences : 5,032 occurrences

Distribution in the world

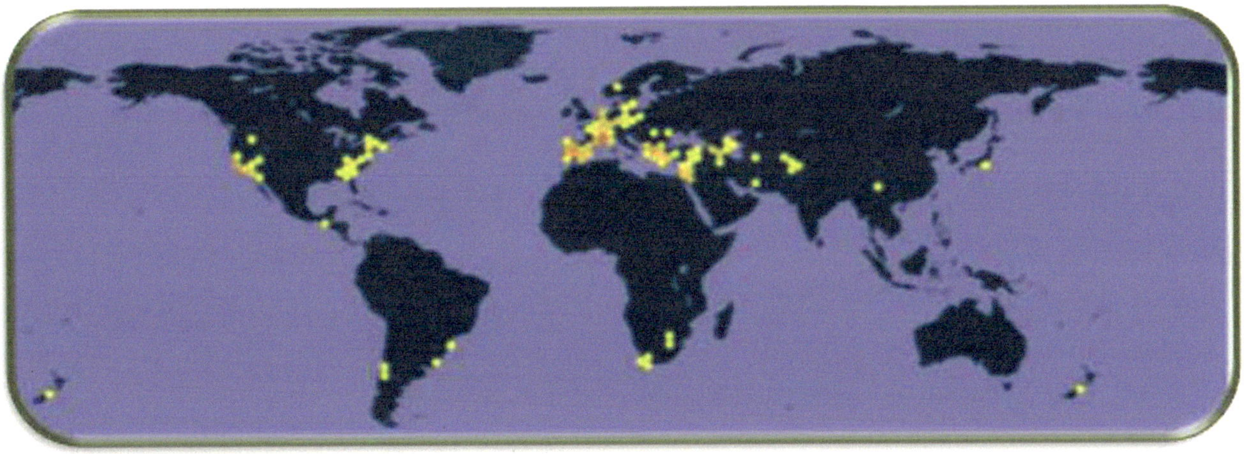

Botanical description:

An annual herb, 10-30 cm high, hairy to spidery. Stem short erect, bearing a terminal head, dichotomously branched from the base, branches supine. Leaves light green, leathery, oblong-lanceolate in general shape, nerves prominent on the lower surface, lobes oblong-triangular, edges serrated-thorny. Basal leaves short-pinnate.

Stem leaves hugging the stem, slightly echinodermic. The floral leaves are ovate to broadly oblong, thorny, surrounding and covering the head. The head is solitary, ovate. The outer bracts are membranous, folded, ending in a long needle, with thorns on both ends, and the inner bracts also end in needles. The flowers are tubular, yellowish, with violet veins, shorter than the bracts. The fruit is an acorn, oblong to cylindrical, bare, shiny, with prominent ribs, ending at its top with a serrated edge, its length is 7-10 mm, the acorns are in two rows (10+10) and of two different lengths, its petioles are 20 and longer than the acorns.

Flowering: From March to April.

Habitat and geographical distribution:

The Mediterranean and Iranian Turanian regions, and it is spread in large areas of the world, including North America. It is cultivated in many countries (especially European) as a medicinal plant. To obtain oil from its seeds.

History and heritage:

A medicinal and edible plant, known for a long time. It was used in folk medicine as a hot drink to treat digestive and liver disorders in particular. Monks planted it in Europe to use it as a treatment for several diseases. Early herbalists believed that it treated "all diseases", as it was prescribed for headaches, to strengthen the heart and stomach, and to treat external tumors. The plant was described in the nineteenth century as a tea or flowers prepared from the tops Developed to treat fever, liver problems, and breathing.

Part used: Aerial part of the plant.

Chemical components:

Monomeric and semi-terpene ketones, bitter taste, including: cnicin, salonitenolide, and artemisiifolin. Lignans (bitter compounds), including: trachelogenin, arctigenin, and nortracheloside. Volatile oil, its most important components: nonane, undecane, tridecane, paracymene, fenchon, citral, and cinnamaldehyde. Favonoids: apigenin, luteolin, and astragalin. Triterpenes: alpha-amyrin, multiflorenol. Minerals (potassium, magnesium, calcium), and tannins.

Properties and medical uses:

The bitter substances stimulate the salivary glands to secrete saliva, as well as gastric (cholesterol) and intestinal juices, which improves appetite and relieves indigestion. The plant has bitter compounds, especially cnicin, which have antiseptic and antimicrobial properties. Experiments on laboratory animals have shown the cytotoxic effect of the plant (cnicin). The decoction of the plant is popularly used as an expectorant, appetite stimulant, digestive and digestive stimulant, and diuretic of bile and urine. The plant is used topically in the form of a tincture or ointments to treat rheumatism and hemorrhoids, and to disinfect bacterial infections of all kinds, ulcerated wounds and boils, and breast infections and abscesses associated with breastfeeding.

Other uses:

The roots, flowers and stem of the plant are eaten raw or cooked. The bark of the plant is widely used in the tanning industry.

Drug interactions and precautions for use:

Excessive doses cause vomiting. It should be taken with caution by those who are being treated with antacids such as Maalox, or medications containing aluminum hydroxide, and ulcer medications such as H2 blockers such as ranitidine, and other proton pump inhibitors such as omeprazole and its family, as the plant increases gastric acid secretion, thus reducing the effect of these medications. It is not prescribed for pregnant women, as it is a stimulant for the uterine muscle, and may cause miscarriage. Not to be used by people with Crohn's disease and chronic intestinal infections, as it may cause irritation and irritation in the stomach and intestines.

Environment:

The plant grows in agricultural lands, quarries and neglected lands. It prefers dry soils in sunny locations, and grows best in fertile and well-fertilized soils.

Cultivation and productivity: The plant is propagated by seeds that are scattered directly in the permanent soil in early autumn or spring in beds or in rows with a distance of 50 cm between each plant. The seeds germinate after 2-6 weeks usually at a temperature of 10 ° C.

Cynara scolymus L.

*Cynara carduncul*us *subsp. scolymus* (L.) Hegi., *Cynara carduncul*us subsp. *Carduncul*us.

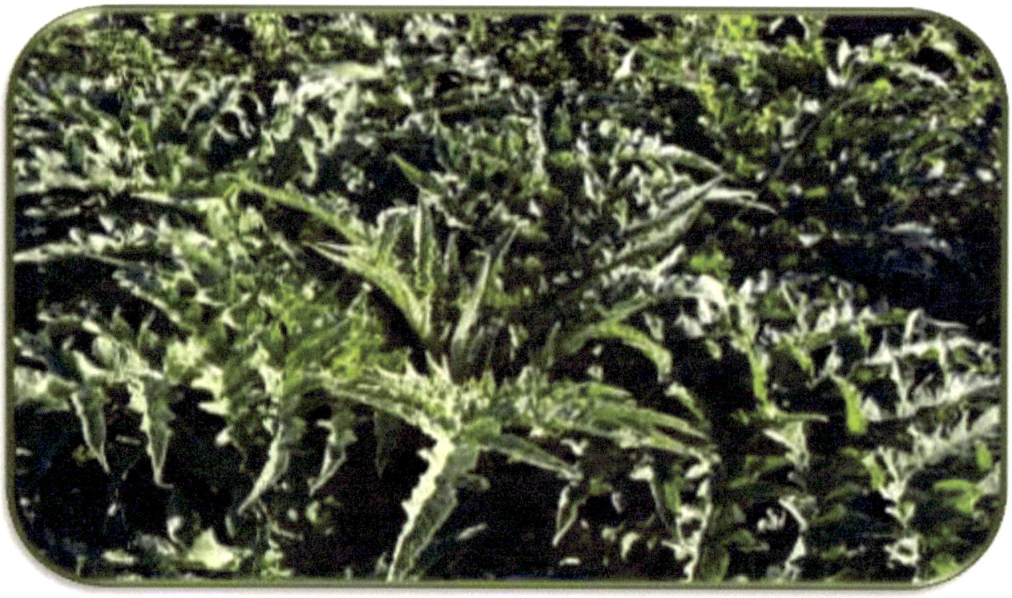

Family: Asteraceae (Compositae)

Common names: Artichoke, Anker, Ankenar, Artichoke

Foreign names: Artichaut Fr. Artichoke, Eng

Occurrences : 938 occurrences

Distribution in the world

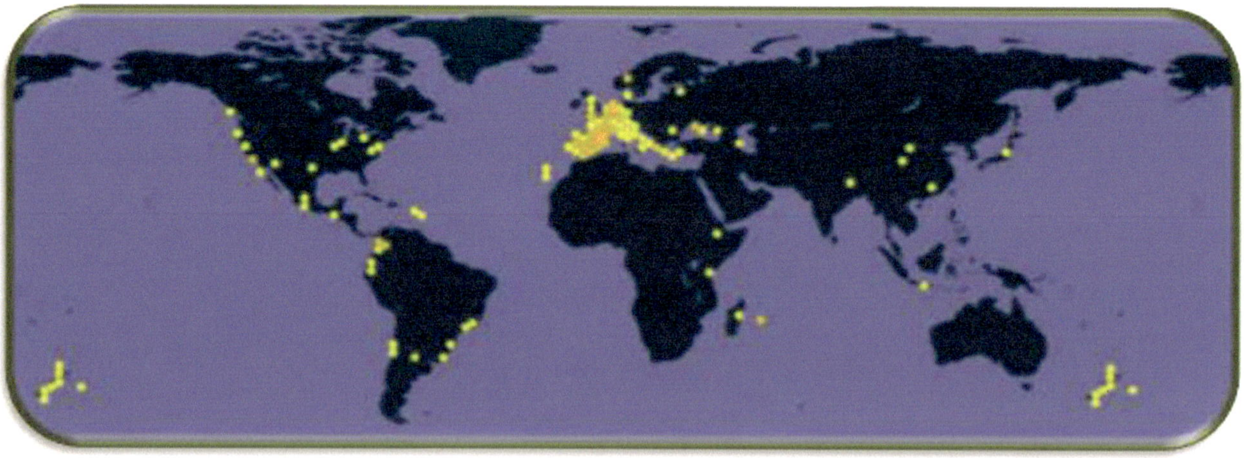

Botanical description:

Perennial herb, with a short root. Stem is thick and strong, erect, little branched, can reach a height of 2 m. Leaves are long, large, pinnate, compound, lanceolate, hairy, thorny, upper surface is bare and light green, lower surface is gray with abundant hairs. The main inflorescence is large, spherical, thorny. The bracts are arranged in several rows, overlapping, fleshy in texture, their bases are swollen, and can be eaten raw or cooked. The inflorescence seat is thick and fleshy, pitted, and contains within these pits long white coarse hairs. The flowers are tubular, five-lobed, blue or lilac or white in colour. The fruit is acorn, glabrous, inverted oval-oblong, almost quadrangular. The hairs of the aphid are in several rows, fused to their bases in a short ring.

Flowering: From July to August.

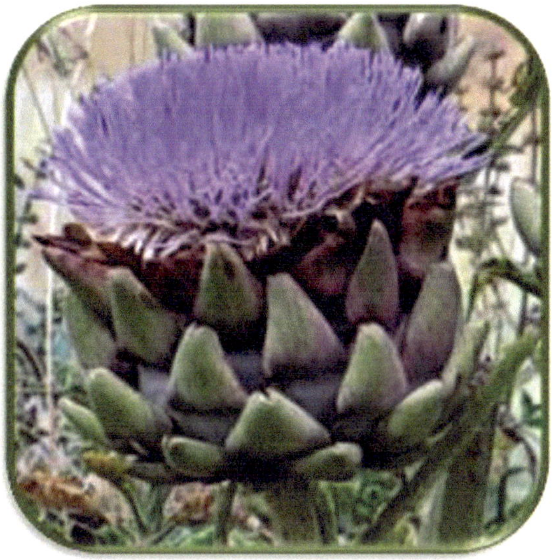

Habitat and geographical distribution:

Its homeland is the Mediterranean basin, and its cultivation is widespread in many countries of the world for food and medical purposes.

History and heritage:

The scientific name of the genus is derived from the Greek Kynara or Kinara, which is the name of the plant from the Greeks. The plants that humans have cultivated since ancient times, and its knowledge dates back to the era of the Pharaohs, where they drew it on the walls of temples alongside hieroglyphic writings, and from them the Arabs took it and knew its benefits and cultivated it, as the Greeks and Romans knew it. The artichoke entered England in the early sixteenth century as a vegetable for cooking and as an ornamental and decorative plant in the gardens of monasteries.

Part used: Leaves (bitter taste), roots.

Chemical components:

The leaves contain: caffeic acid derivatives, including: cynarin, chlorogenic acid, neochlorogenic acid, and cryptochlorogenic acid. 0.5% flavonoids, the most important of which are rutin, cynaroside, and scolymosides. Lactones sesquiterpene 4%, cynaropicrin (bitter compound), dehydrocynaropicrin, grossheimin, and cynaratriol. Enzymes (oxidase, scorpinase). Minerals potassium, calcium, and magnesium, vitamins A and B. The roots contain caffeic acid derivatives, including chlorogenic acid.

Properties and medical uses:

Coffee acid derivatives and the bitter compound cinnarin are the most important active compounds in artichoke leaves, and their usefulness in treating liver disorders and stimulating its digestive bile secretions has been proven. Studies have confirmed the properties of artichoke that lower cholesterol and fat levels, and are useful in reducing atherosclerosis. It is also used in treating digestive system disorders. It is popularly used for its appetite stimulating, diuretic, digestive, and liver stimulating properties to protect it from toxins and diseases, especially jaundice, and to prevent gallstones. Artichoke leaf extract contains many compounds that have antioxidant and anti-inflammatory effects against many diseases, including liver cirrhosis. It also contains many biological activities, including inhibition of NF-B activity, anti-hepatitis C activity, and anti-trypanosomiasis activity.

Side effects, interactions and precautions for use:

It may cause allergic reactions in the hands. Artichoke is prohibited for those suffering from rheumatism, arthritis, gout, urinary tract diseases, and allergies. Artichoke roots and leaves are not given to patients suffering from obstruction of the bile duct, because the compounds present in the leaves and roots of this plant are cholagogic compounds. It is not used in cases of pregnancy and lactation.

Environment:

At the beginning of its growth, the plant needs temperatures of -14-16 degrees Celsius, and moderate air and soil humidity, as increased soil humidity leads to root rot. The plant is sensitive to temperatures below 4°C, but the presence of sufficient moisture in the soil increases its resistance to cold. The growing season extends from 150 to 170 days, and it loves light in all stages of its life.

Cultivation and productivity:

It is propagated by offshoots, which are small-sized plants (having a root system and a green system). A third of the green system is pruned, the roots are trimmed, and then planted in permanent soil in the presence of water so that the root and a small part (about 1 cm) of the base of the stem are buried under the soil surface. The land is well plowed, leveled, and divided into terraces 1 meter wide after adding a mixture of local fertilizer, superphosphate, and potassium sulphate.

Irrigation Depending on the type of soil, the surrounding environmental conditions and the age of the plant, in general, the period between irrigations should be close during the first stage of the plant's life, and the plants should not be deprived of water during this period, then the period between irrigations gradually increases starting from the onset of winter and the decrease in temperature, while in the spring when the temperature begins to rise, the period between irrigations is reduced. The flower heads are cut with 5 cm from the holder before the appearance of Purple flowers are at their peak in late summer and early fall.

Gundelia tournefortii L.

Gundelia tournefortii var. *araneosae* DC., *Gundelia glabra* Mill., *Gundelia tenuisecta* Freyn & Sint., *Gundelia tournefortii* var. *glabra* (Mill.) DC., *Gundelia tournefortii* var. *tenuisecta* Boiss.

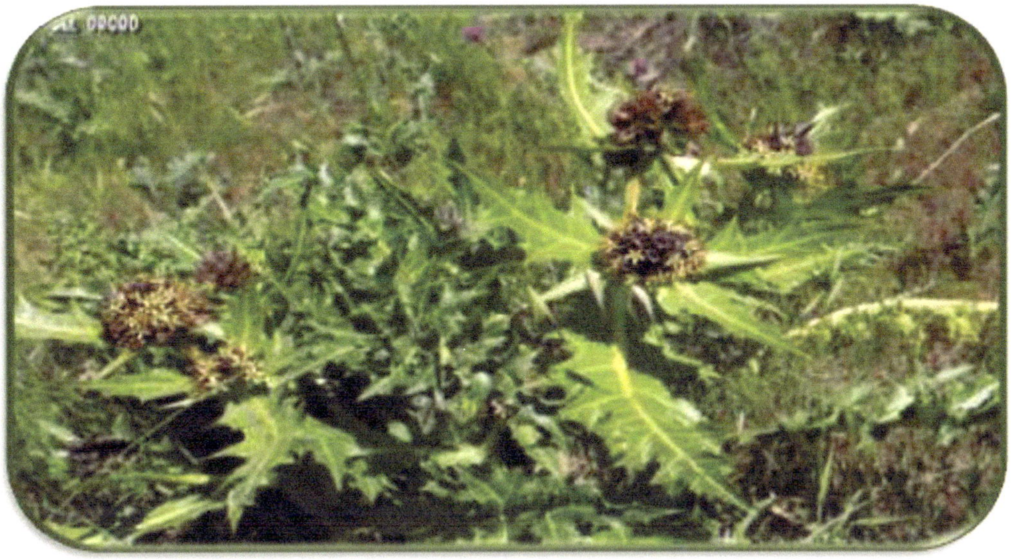

Family: Asteraceae (Compositae)

Common names: Tumbleweed, Gundelia, Akoub

Foreign names: Eng.

Occurrences : 4,301 occurrences

Distribution in the world

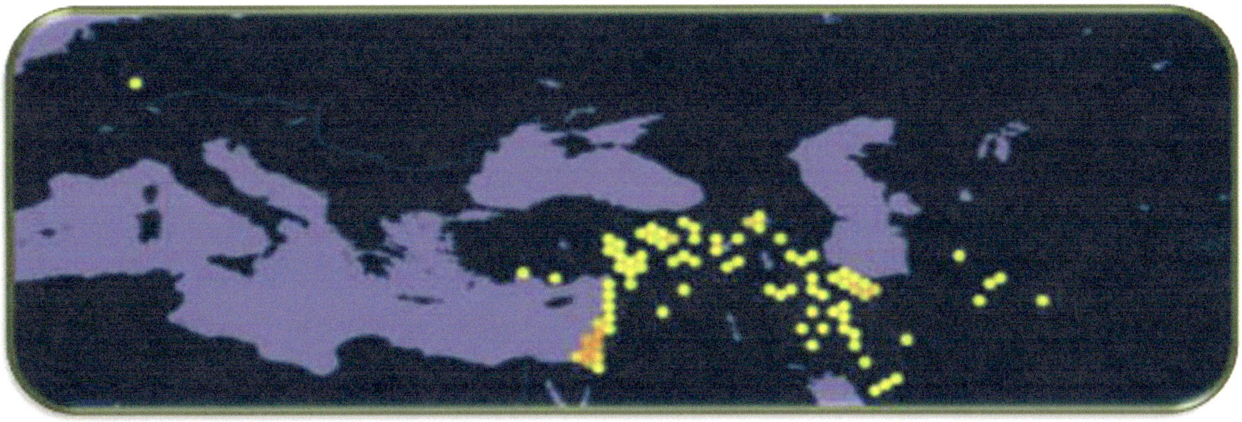

Botanical description:

A perennial, thorny, coffee-producing herb, 30-50 cm high, covered to varying degrees with spider-like hairs, and may be almost hairless. The stems are thick, notched, simple or branched at the top. The stems break near the base when ripe, and roll in the wind. The leaves are large, fleshy in texture, oblong to oblong-lanceolate, their nerves are very thick, their lobes are serrated and thorny. The lower leaf blade gradually tapers, while the rest of the leaves are low. The flower heads are broad, oval in shape, compound, containing many heads densely clustered, each of which is supported by a thorny bract. The single head contains 5-7 flowers, the central flower is fertile (hermaphrodite) and the peripheral ones are sterile. The diameter of the compound head is 4-8 cm, surrounded and covered by the upper leaves. The bracts are lanceolate, leathery in the lower part, covered with spidery hair, and terminate in a strong spine. The flowers are dark crimson outside, yellow inside. The anthers are yellow. The fruits are achenes, contained singly in somewhat woody cones, Resulting from the fusion of the bracts of the individual heads. The acanthus is topped with a serrated crown.

Flowering: From March to May.

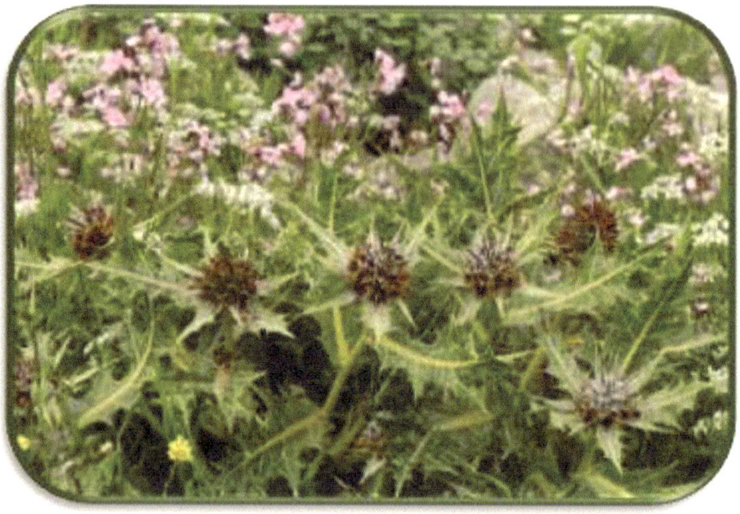

Habitat and geographical distribution:

Eastern Mediterranean regions, the akoub is spread wild in Syria, Palestine, Jordan, Iraq, Iran, Azerbaijan, Armenia and Anatolia, and is cultivated in some countries as a type of vegetable.

History and heritage:

The scientific name of the genus Gundelia goes back to the German scientist Gundelsheimer Andreas (1668–1715 AD). The Latin name of the plant species goes back to the French scientist Tournefort (1656-1708), while the name "Akub" is of Aramaic origin.

The plant has good nutritional value and multiple medical uses. The species was highlighted after 1998 in particular, after the discovery of abundant dust from its pollen on a linen fabric believed to be an ancient shroud, which is currently preserved in the Cathedral of Saint John the Baptist in Turin, Italy.

Part used: Aerial parts and seeds

Chemical components:

Aerial parts contain coumarin compounds, the most important of which are: scopoletin, esculin, and many sterol compounds, including stigmasterol, sitosterol, and molluscidal saponins. Caffeic acid derivatives (phenolic compounds), the most important of which are: gallic acid, a. caffeic acid, a. neochlorogenic acid, a. cryptochlorogenic acid, and a. chlorogenic acid. Volatile oil, its main components: eugenol, methyl eugenol, alpha-terpinyl acetate, caryophellene

Properties and medical uses:

Heel is traditionally used to treat chest pain, stroke, stomach pain, vitiligo, diarrhea, and bronchitis. It has laxative, analgesic, anti-inflammatory, antiparasitic, antibacterial, antiseptic, and emetic effects. The leaves, stems, and young flower buds, as well as the roots and seeds, are popularly used to treat digestive system diseases, especially liver disorders, and in cases of low blood pressure and allergies. Research has shown the antioxidant properties of the plant (especially the seeds), and has also demonstrated the effect of the plant extract on several enzymes such as glutathione-S-transferases, which contribute to the treatment of cancer cells.

Research has shown the antifungal and antibacterial effectiveness of scopoletin. It has also shown its ability to reduce blood uric acid levels, and its methanol and hexane extracts have antidiabetic activity. It has a moderate effect in preventing platelet aggregation. The extract of scopoletin combined with milk cream is effective in healing second-degree burns in the skin of mice, and can be a complementary or alternative medicine in wound healing. The effectiveness of sitosterol, stigmasterol, lupeol, gitoxinin, alpha-amyrin and artemisinin against cancer cells has been verified.

Other uses:

Leaf bases, stems and young flower buds are part of the dietary habits of some people in Syria, and immature flower inflorescences are used in Syrian cuisine after cooking as an alternative to artichokes.

Environment:

Akoub is a plant of dry, semi-dry and sunny areas, and is widespread in mountainous, fallow, and stony lands and hills. It prefers well-drained sandy soils.

Cultivation and productivity:

The plant is subject to intensive collection during the spring, in order to obtain its tender parts for food consumption, which puts great pressure on the species and threatens it, so it is recommended to adopt appropriate methods for its cultivation in order to compensate for the deficiency resulting from these practices. It has been observed through experiments that its seeds are difficult to germinate, and research is currently directed towards finding a suitable way to stratify its seeds or attempt to propagate it vegetatively using modern methods. The plant is propagated by seeds that require appropriate hormonal treatment with gibberellic acid. Stratification at a temperature ranging between -4 and +4 °C for a period of 2-4 weeks increases the germination rate.

Matricaria recutita L.

M. chamomilla L.,

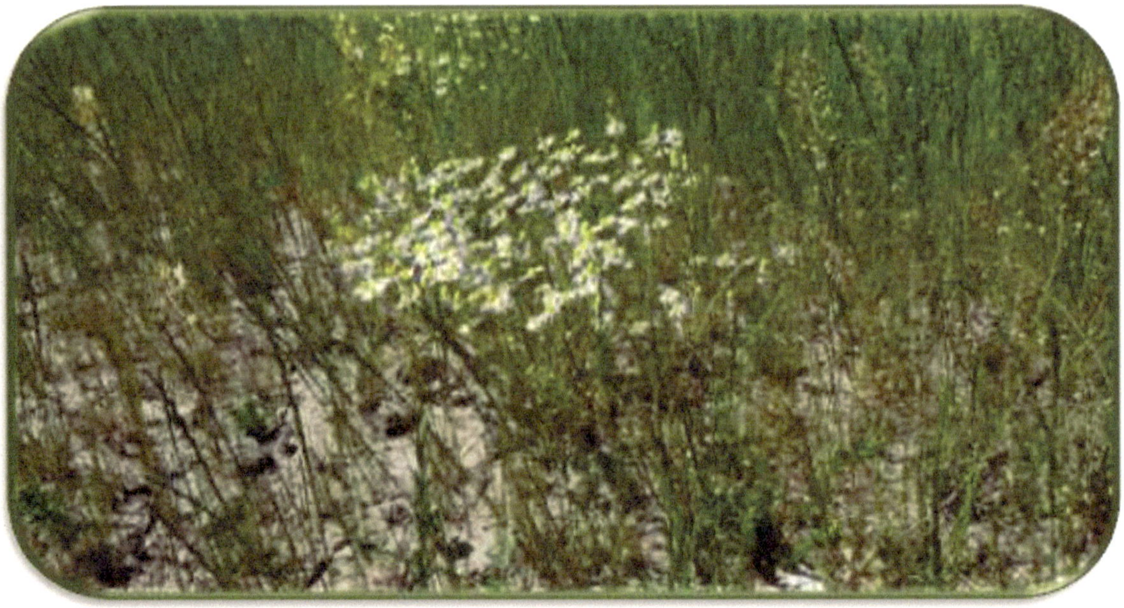

Family: Asteraceae (Compositae)

Common names: True chamomile

Foreign names: Camomill Fr. German, Chamomile Eng

Occurrences : 63,071 occurrences

Distribution in the world

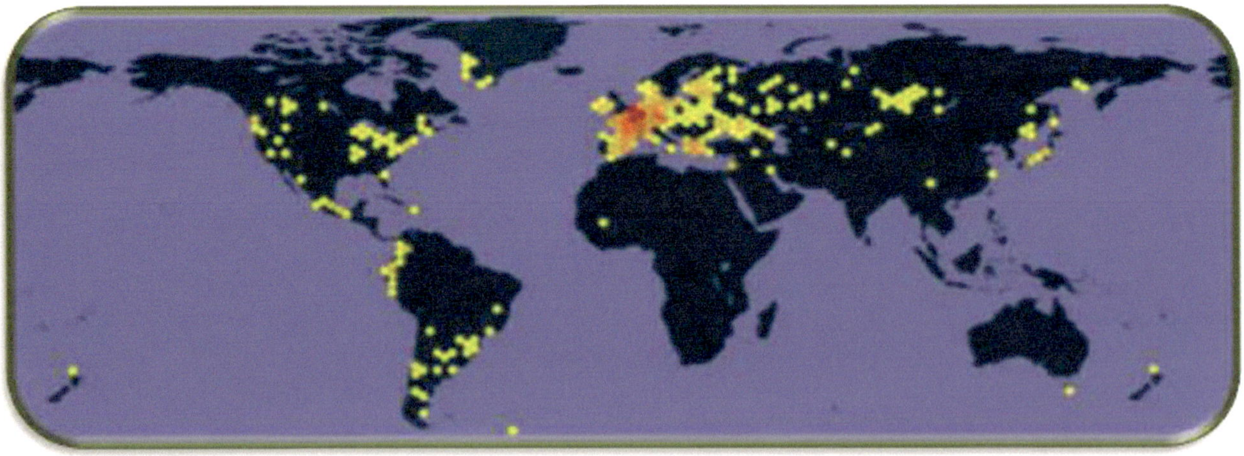

Botanical description:

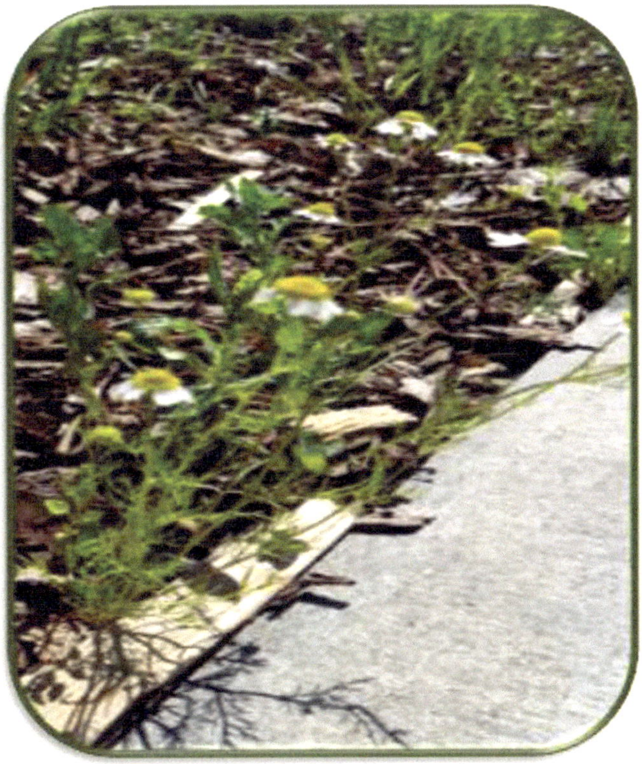

An annual, glabrous, aromatic herb, 10-40 cm tall. Stem simple or branched from the base, erect or ascending, branching from the top in a panicle. Leaves deeply divided into narrow, entire-edged lobes, ending in stigmas. Heads 1.5-2 cm in diameter, long-stalked, composed of lintel-shaped flowers on the periphery, and tubular flowers in the center. Bracts Elongated, glabrous, with a broad, membranous margin, entire. The inflorescence is long conical. The lingual flowers are white, elliptic, and bend downwards after flowering. The central tubular flowers are yellow. The fruit is a small acorn, about 1 mm long, slightly arched, bearing 3-5 lobes on the ventral side.

Flowering: April to May.

Habitat and geographical distribution:

European - Siberian, Mediterranean, and Iranian - Turanian. Also among its species: Golden chamomile aurea M. An annual herb with Mediterranean distribution, with multiple medicinal benefits.

The species chamomilla Matricaria is known as the true or German chamomile, and the species nobile chamomile (Anthemis) is called the Roman or English chamomile.

History and heritage:

The origin of the word chamomile goes back to the Persian language (babunk). The scientific name of the genus is translated from the ancient Latin for the genus The name was assigned Parthenum, which was originally given to the genus Chrysanthemum, which is the chrysanthemum, and then it was assigned to this genus, while the descriptive word for the species recutita is from Latin, and means "standing."

Part Used: Flowering heads, and the volatile oil extracted from them.

Chemical components:

The organic extracts of flowers and stems contain 43 and 45 compounds respectively, including bisabolol oxide A, tonghaosu from flower extract, and apigenin-7-β-d-glucoside from stem extract. As for the volatile essential oil, its percentage reaches 1.5%, and it contains more than 15% of the chamazulen compound (resulting from the transformation of matricin by saponification), monoterpenes, monoterpenes and sesquiterpenes, including α-bisabolol and bisabolol oxide derivatives, and their percentage in the volatile oil reaches 33%. The percentage of farnesen reaches 45%. .% Polyene derivatives, coumarins such as herniarin and umbelliferone and acetylenic compounds. Flavonoids in the form of monoglycosides of apigenin, the percentage of which in the petals reaches 5% Aromatic organic acids: anisic acid and vanillic acid a. .vanilic and polysaccharides 10%, simple hexagonal sugars, and starch.

Properties and medical uses:

The flowers and essential oil have anti-inflammatory properties, are antispasmodic for smooth muscles, and help heal wounds and skin ulcers. Antibacterial and growth inhibitor. The drug is used internally to treat digestive spasms and inflammatory diseases of the digestive system. It is also used to treat irritation of the mucous membranes in the mouth, throat, pharynx, and upper respiratory tract, and to treat coughs, fever, colds, wounds, and burns. Chamomile is used topically as a gargle to treat gingivitis, as an inhalation to treat inflammatory respiratory diseases, as washes or baths to treat genital infections, skin and mucous membrane infections, bacterial skin diseases, and for supportive treatment of wounds and skin ulcers. Chamomile preparations are used in the form of baths or soaks to relieve hemorrhoid pain, especially after hemorrhoid surgeries, and to treat anal eczema, fistulas, and inflammatory gynecological diseases. It is popularly used to treat insomnia, digestive disorders, eye irritation, menstrual disorders, bleeding, skin ulcers, hemorrhoids, acne, and in baby baths.

Chamomile extracts have shown clear effectiveness in inhibiting the growth of cancer cells and reducing the migration of colon cancer cells, and have also shown effectiveness in reducing the infection of viruses that cause upper respiratory tract infections.

Other uses:

Chamomile oil is used in the preparation of many cosmetic products, and is available in the form of preserves, liquids, creams, and ointments. Its preparations are sold under the names flowers Chamomile, organic Chamomile, chamomile and others.

Side effects, interactions and precautions:

Possible side effects of chamomile include allergic conjunctivitis (inflammation of the eye), skin irritation, severe allergic reaction (shortness of breath, wheezing, itching and rash) and vomiting.

Chamomile should not be taken with blood thinners such as coumarin or any other medications, because chamomile reduces their effectiveness. It should also be avoided by pregnant or breastfeeding women, because it induces abortion. Caution should also be exercised because some of its components Chamomile has caused harm to some animal fetuses. It is preferable to use the plant with caution for those who are sensitive to the components of the essential oil, or have previous skin irritation.

Environment:

Chamomile is a light-loving plant, it grows in moderate and semi-hot climates as long as the humidity is moderate and water is available. It tolerates cold, but warm weather stimulates and increases the concentration of active ingredients. It is best grown in yellow and light clay soils that are well-drained, with slight to moderate alkalinity, and is relatively tolerant of salinity.

Cultivation Productivity:

Chamomile is propagated by seeds, which are planted in the nursery. One acre needs about 150g of seeds. The seedlings can be transferred to the permanent land about 40 days after planting, taking into account adding fertilizer to the land before preparing it for planting.

The plants are watered directly after planting every 3-5 days in the first stage, then watered at a rate of watering every 10-15 days, noting that the chamomile plant needs 10-12 waterings during its life cycle. Weeding is done about 3 weeks after planting and is repeated when necessary. One hectare yields 750-1000 kg of dry white inflorescences. One ton of dry inflorescences yields about 3-3.5 kg of aromatic oil.

Pulicaria arabica (L.) Cass.

Inula arabica L., *Conyza kotschyi* Sch.Bip. ex Schweinf., *Erigeron inuloides* Poir., *Inula paludosa* Link ex DC., *Inula palustris* Link, *Inula planifolia* Link ex DC.

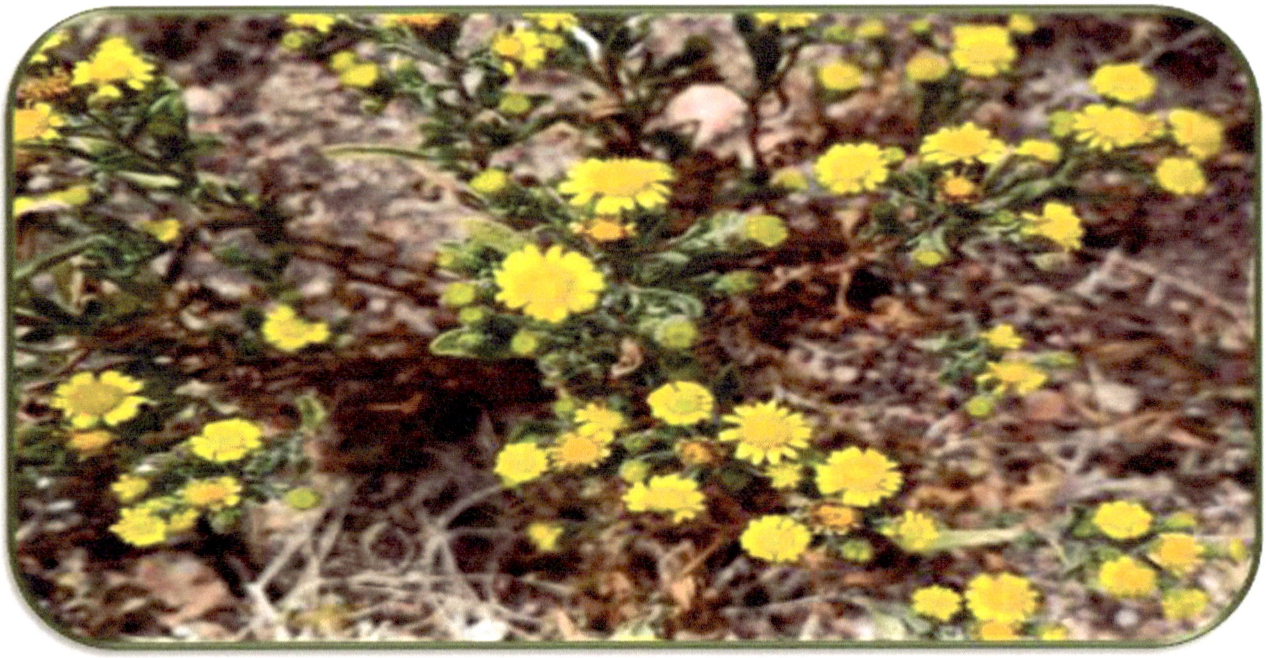

Family: Asteraceae (Compositae)

Common names: Arar, Jathjath, Sabt, False Flea Weed

Foreign names: Pulicaire Fr. fleabane, false Ladies' Eng

Occurrences : 7,592 occurrences

Distribution in the world

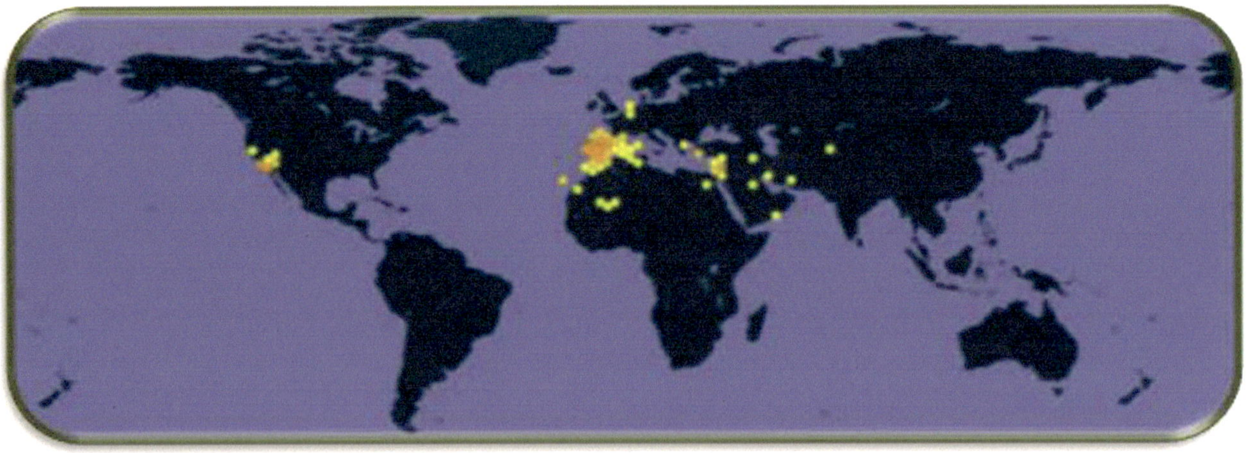

Botanical description:

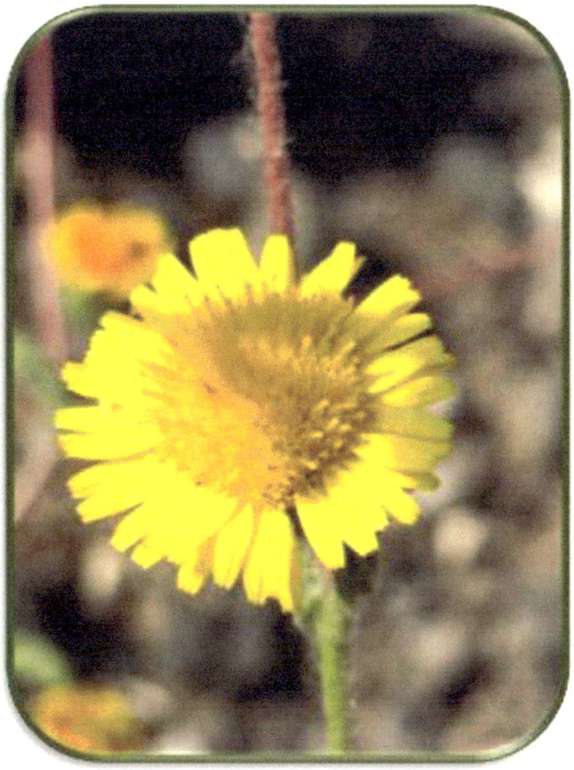

An annual herb, 30-80 cm high, Graw. Stem erect, branched dichotomously from the base or midrib. Leaves simple, soft, oblong to lanceolate, complete or almost complete, stalk low, almost embracing the stem. Leaves of floral branches 5 mm wide or more. Flower heads 1-2 cm, containing sphenoid and tubular flowers, located singly at the ends of branches. The bracts are linear, conical, hairy, the outer ones are herbaceous. The flowers are yellow, the lanceolate ones are slightly longer than the tubular ones. The ovules bear stiff hairs. The bracts are in two rows, the outer row is short, composed of fused short scales forming a dish-like shape, serrated, and persisting with the fruit. The petioles of the inner row are 10-12, thin, and their length exceeds about 3 times the length of the ovule.

Flowering: From April to September.

Habitat and geographical distribution:

Eastern Mediterranean region, and western Irano-Turanian region.

History and heritage:

The scientific name of the genus is believed to be derived from the word pulex, meaning "flea", referring to the use of the plant in repelling insects. Most species of this genus are used in folk medicine. It is rarely grazed by camels or sheep. It is used as an insect repellent, as it is placed under and on dates before transporting and storing them, and it is also placed under sleeping pillows to repel insects. It gives a pleasant smell. Arab poets have always mentioned it in their poems.

Part used: The whole plant.

Chemical components:

The plant contains a volatile oil rich in mono- and semi-terpene compounds (sesquiterpenes): germacrene, α-cadinol, δ-cadinene, borneol, α-terpineol, thymol, p-cymene. Favonoids (glycosides quercetin, chrysosplenol, and sterols).

Properties and medical uses:

A popular aromatic medicinal plant in the Arabian Peninsula, widely used for its digestive and carminative properties. The plant powder is used as a sneezing suppressant. Studies have shown the plant's antibacterial properties against some types of bacteria and fungi such as yeast and Candida, and it has been noted that it causes mild inhibition of the central nervous system and is a powerful pain reliever, antipyretic, and anti-inflammatory with liver and kidney protective activity due to its antioxidant activity.

Other uses:

Volatile tamarisk oil is used in the perfume industry.

There are several types:

The first type, glutinous Pulicaria, called Gall, is a famous plant in the United Arab Emirates. The second type, Pulicaria orientalis, is famous in Saudi Arabia, and is used as a worm repellent and a strong decongestant. It is also used to stimulate appetite, treat digestive disorders, reduce fever, and as an anti-malarial. The third type, Pulicaria undulate, is used to treat hemorrhoids. The fourth type, known as Ayoub's thorn Pulicaria dysenterica, is famous for repelling insects and resisting dysentery.

Environment:

It is widespread in desert areas on slopes and rocky valleys. It tolerates all difficult environmental conditions, and lives on harsh, sandy, and salty soils.

Cultivation and productivity:

Uncultivated, propagated by seeds and vegetatively by cuttings wild plant

Silybum marianum L. Gaertn.

Carduus marianum L., *Carduus lactifolius* Stokes, *Carduus versicolor* Salisb., *Mariana lactea* Hill

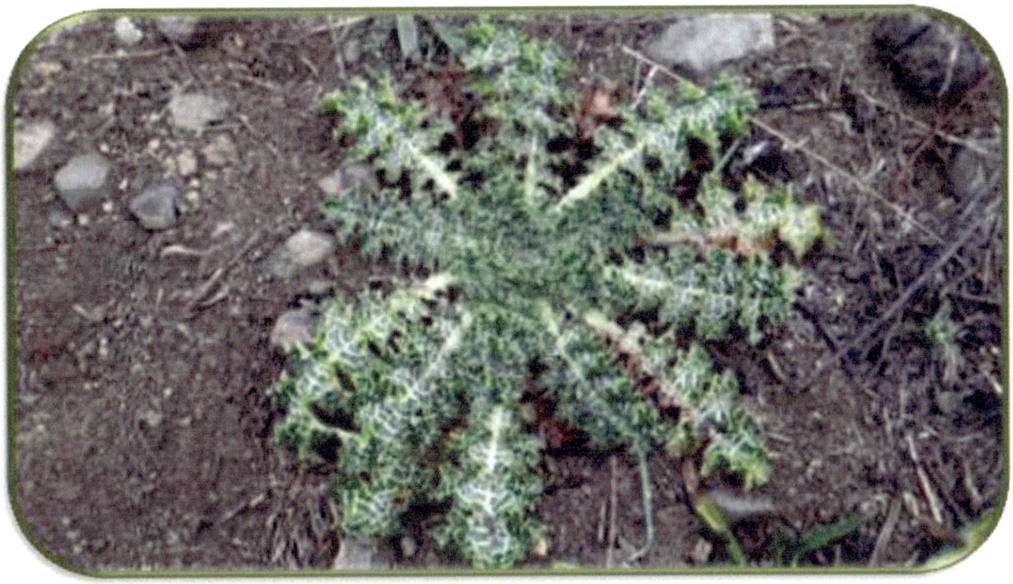

Family: Asteraceae (Compositae)

Common names: St Mary's thistle, Milk thistle, Fr. Chardon-marie

Foreign names: St Mary's thistle, Milk thistle, Fr. Chardon-marie

Occurrences : 64,436 occurrences

Distribution in the world

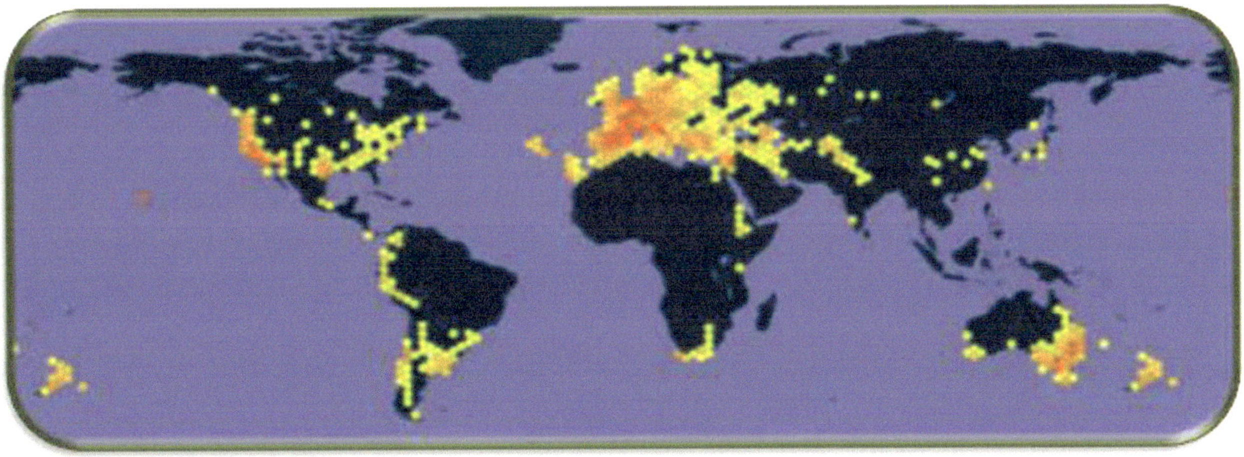

Botanical description:

An annual herb, 25-100 cm high, semi-growth, thorny. Stem cylindrical, grooved, strong, simple or sparsely branched. Leaves large, green, speckled with white, especially at the ends of the nerves, shiny, lobed. Lobes ovate-triangular, tips strongly toothed. Basal leaves very large, gradually tapering at the base, upper leaves auricular, hugging the stem. Flower heads solitary, 6-10 cm in diameter. The bracts end in a triangular appendage, with a strong, thorny head, curved downwards. All flowers are tubular, purple or white. The fruit is aconite, 6 mm long, black spotted with yellow, bearing a white bract.

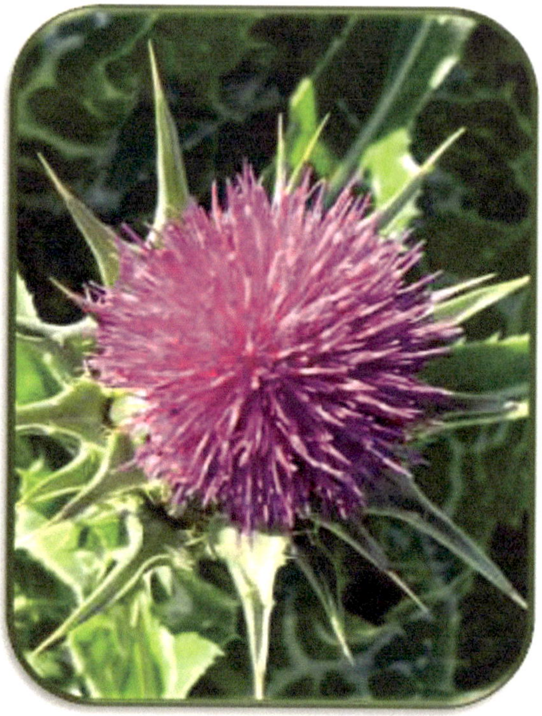

Flowering: March to May.

Habitat and geographical distribution:

Mediterranean and Irano-Turanian, extending to southern Europe, northern Africa and the Euro-Siberian region.

History and heritage:

The scientific name of the genus is derived from silybon or sillybon, which is the name of one of the edible thorny plants, then it was chosen to name this genus. The descriptive name of the species marianum is in reference to the Virgin Mary.

Part used:

The green plant and mature seeds.

Chemical components:

The green plant contains flavonoids: apigenin, luteolin, kaempferol chrysoeriol, eriodictyol, quercetin, naringenin and taxifolin and their glycosidic compounds. Steroids: beta-sitosterol and its glycosides.

Polyynes compounds, organic acids, such as fumaric acid 3.3%. Ripe seeds contain: silymarin mixture (flavonolignan), 1.5-3%, silybin A, silybin B (silibinin), silychristin, silydianin, and isosilybin B, A. Fixed oil 20-30% fatty oil, proteins and sugars. Silymarin is a standardized extract, a mixture of flavono-lignans.

Properties and medical uses:

The plant has been shown to have anti-cancer properties (cervical cancer, liver cancer, lung cancer), lactation stimulating, neurotoxic, and immune system-balancing properties. Studies indicate that silybinin is a candidate for the treatment of Parkinson's disease. The plant seeds have liver-protective properties due to the presence of silymarin, silychristin, and silydianin. .silydianin

Silymarin encourages the liver to produce glutathione, which helps to get rid of liver cell toxins, and inhibits the production of leukotriene, thus it has anti-inflammatory properties. Silymarin activates the synthesis of ribosomal protein, activates the process of liver cell renewal, and treats hepatic cirrhosis. Research has shown that silymarin contributes to reducing liver fibrosis in individuals suffering from conditions Inflammatory liver disease resulting from chronic viral hepatitis (C-B), or cancer patients undergoing chemotherapy. It is considered a sugar, blood pressure, and lipid lowering agent and is an anti-obesity and anti-atherosclerosis agent. Silibinin inhibits the production of superoxide, nitric oxide, and free radicals, and the formation of leukotriene. Glutathione also protects against hepatic and mitochondrial oxidation. The plant has properties that protect the kidneys from damage caused by acetaminophen, cisplatin, and vincristine.

The seeds of the silymarin plant are used to protect the liver from diseases associated with alcohol consumption, gallbladder disorders and stones, and kidney inflammation. It also reduces the growth of cancer cells in breast, cervical and prostate cancer. The plant is currently widely used in Europe and the United States to treat liver diseases, where the drug silymarin is extracted from the plant and is prescribed for patients with viral hepatitis.

Precautions for use:

A doctor should be consulted before use in children, pregnant and lactating women, as diarrhea may occur in rare cases, and therefore use is under medical supervision and in specific doses, due to the presence of high concentrations of nitrates that are converted in the body to nitrites, leading to nitrite poisoning, the symptoms of which are difficulty breathing and cramps.

Environment:

It lives in neglected places and on the edges of fields, roads and railways. It thrives in sunny, calcareous, well-drained agricultural soils. It tolerates temperatures as low as -15°C.

Cultivation and productivity:

It is grown as a vegetable in many countries of the world. It is propagated by seeds that are scattered in early spring. The plant can bloom in the summer and complete its life cycle during one growing season. It is possible to delay the seeding, but in this case the plant behaves like a biennial plant and does not bloom until the following spring.

Tanacetum densum (Labill.) Sch.Bip.

Pyrethrum densum Labill.

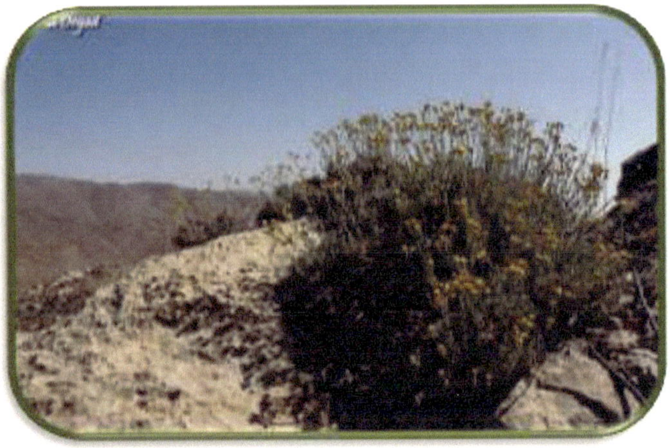

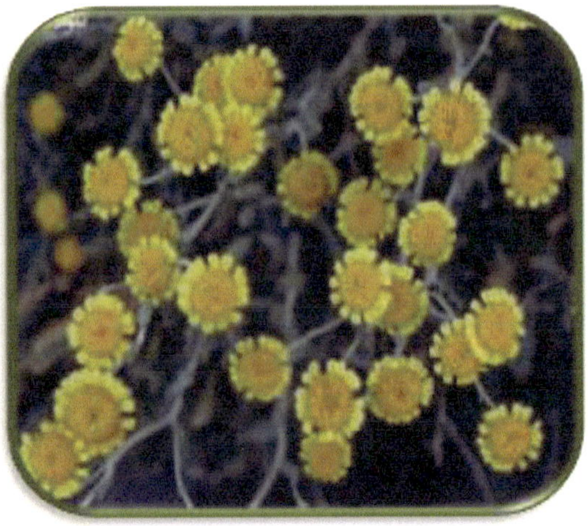

Family: Asteraceae (Compositae)

Common names: tansy.

Foreign names: Prince-of-Wales feathers, Silver tansy, Fr. Tanaisie

Occurrences : 170,122 occurrences

Distribution in the world

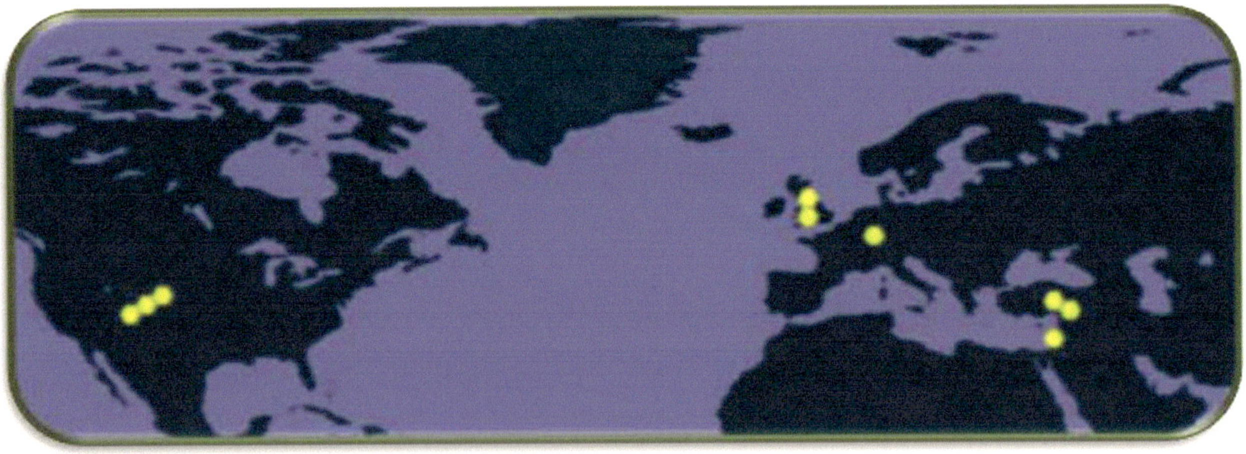

Botanical description:

A small shrub, 30-40 cm high and sometimes more. The stems are numerous, not climbing, and arise from a very woody root, densely covered with velvety-wool hairs, green or yellowish-white in colour. The branches are of two types: sterile (bearing no main inflorescences) and fertile. The sterile branches bear a greater number of leaves. The leaves are dull green, covered with woolly hairs, their outer circumference is oblong, their length is 2-5 cm, their ends gradually taper, they are obtuse to semi. the leaf blade is deeply divided into linear lobes that are closely spaced. As for the upper stem leaves, they are more reduced. The tip of each fertile branch bears a small number of heads, They are gathered in a comb-like inflorescence. The head inflorescence is longer than the head. The head is semi-spherical to oval, about 5 mm in diameter. The bracts are covered with woolly hairs, are tightly closed. The inner bracts have a membranous, torn apex. The lingual flowers are three-lobed, oblong-spoon-shaped, pale yellow. The fruit is acorn topped by a very short crown.

Flowering: From July to August.

Habitat and geographical distribution: Eastern Mediterranean, in Syria and Lebanon.

History and heritage:

Some references mention that the scientific name The genus Tanacetum is derived from the Latin Tanzita, which in turn is derived from the Greek athanasia, "immortality." The species name densum is from the Latin dens, meaning "dense," and may be a reference to the density of the velvety hairs that cover the numerous stems.

Part used: Flowering aerial parts

Chemical components:

Studies on a number of species of the genus, including T. densum, have shown that the aerial parts contain flavonoid compounds and mono- and semi-terpene ketones (guaianolide = carlaolide A) in addition to a volatile oil, the most important of which are: β-patchoulene 17%, camphor 15.5%, and cineole 11.5%.

Medical properties and uses:

The plant has anti-inflammatory properties due to the ketone compounds it contains. And bacteria, and reduces pressure, and there are positive indicators of its effect in treating some types of cancer.

Environment:

The plant grows in sunny high areas, and on slopes and high limestone and rocky plateaus at altitudes exceeding 2000 m above sea level in Syria and Lebanon within the eastern Lebanon mountain range, It tolerates drought relatively, and lives on neutral and medium alkaline soils PH = 8.5-6.6.

Cultivation and productivity:

The plant is propagated by seeds, Or vegetatively by dividing the plant in the spring. The plant is watered once a week and when needed.

Tanacetum parthenium (L.) Sch.Bip.

Matricaria parthenium L., *Chrysanthemum parthenium* (L.) Bernh., *Pyrethrum parthenium* (L.) Sm., *Chamaemelum parthenium* (L.) E.H.L.Krause, *Chrysanthemum*, *Dendranthema parthenium* (L.) Des Moul., *Leucanthemum odoratum* Dulac, *Leucanthemum parthenium* (L.) Godr. & Gren.

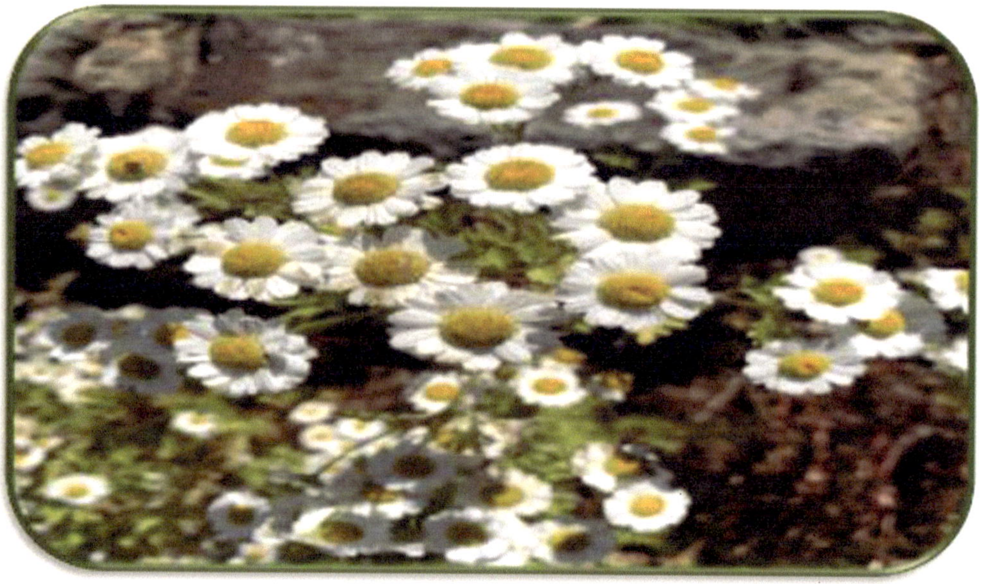

Family: Asteraceae (Compositae)

Common names: Feverfew, Fr. grande camomille.

Foreign names:

Occurrences : 103,196 occurrences

Distribution in the world

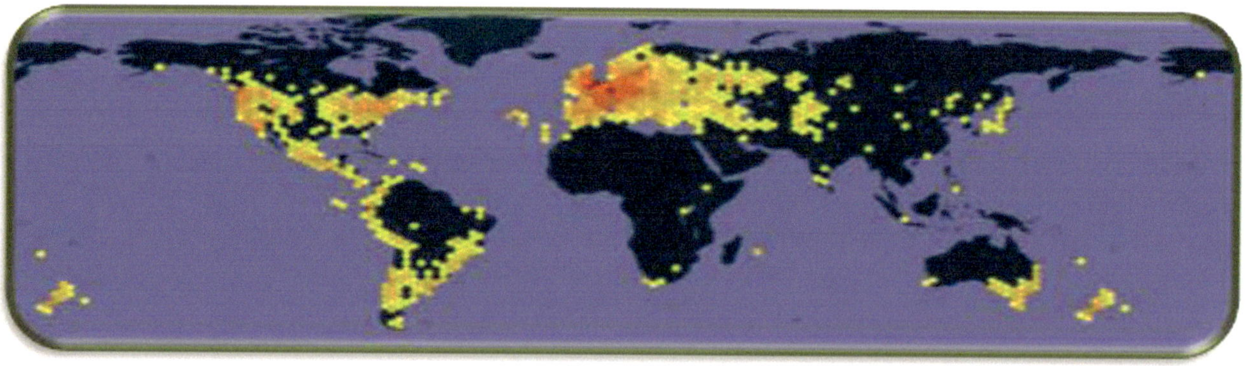

Botanical description:

Glossy to bare, 20-60 cm high. Stems erect, densely leafed, notched. Leaves oblique, Perennial herb, Soft, general shape ovate, deeply divided into elliptic or oblong lobes, the upper lobes are convergent. The heads are gathered in a comb-shaped inflorescence, 5-8 mm in diameter, short-branched, containing two types of flowers, white linoleum on the periphery, and yellow tubular in the center. The cannab is arranged in several rows. The lingual flowers are inverted oval, equal in length to the cannab, and are female. The fruit is a very small, white, acorn, topped with a very short, wavy-edged crown

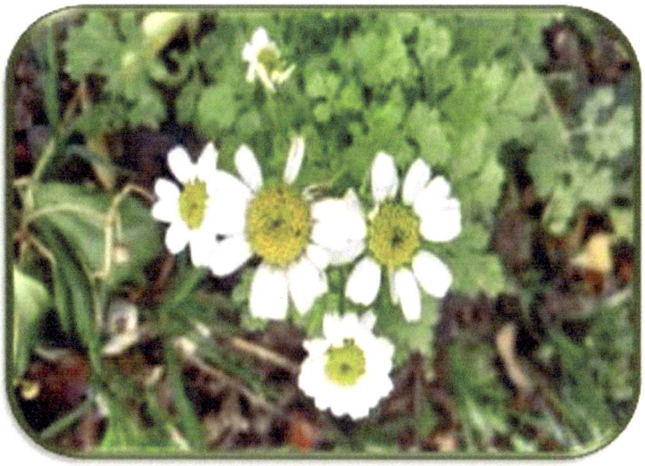

Flowering: From May to July.

Habitat and geographical distribution:

It grows in the eastern Mediterranean and southeastern Europe.

History and heritage:

The scientific name of the genus was mentioned in the previous species. Sources mention that the name describing the species is derived from the Greek parthenion. It was thought that its classic taste The plant was used in the past to relieve headaches only externally, because it was too bitter to be used internally.

Part used: The flowering plant.

Chemical components:

The plant, especially the leaves, contains: 0.75% volatile oil, the most important components of which are camphor, camphene, transchrysanthyl acetate, p-cymene, linalool, gamma-terpinene, delta-germacrene, and borneol. Monoterpene and a half lactones, the most important of which are: parthenolide, costunolid, canin, artecanin, transparthin-alpha-peroxide, and beta-hydroxy Parthenolide 3-beta-hydroxy-parthenolide, reynosin, and secotanapartholide A. Favonoids, including: apigenin, luteolin, and tanetin. The aqueous ethanol extract of the aerial parts consists of phenolic acids (chlorogenic acids).

Properties and medical uses:

The plant has anti-inflammatory properties due to its mono- and semi-terpene ketones (parthenolide). It is used as a pain reliever, and to treat rheumatism, arthritis, and allergies. The plant-derived compound parthenolide has properties that inhibit the growth of cancer cells, including human lung cancer. Parthenolide (a traditional Chinese medicine) has shown antitumor, anti-inflammatory and anti-malarial activity, and promotes programmed cell death of thyroid cancer cells (TPC-1). The aqueous ethanolic extract of the aerial parts of the plant has anti-herpes simplex virus activity, and is safe for oral and topical use. The decoction of the plant is used popularly as a general tonic, in the treatment of stomach spasms and indigestion, as a blood purifier, intestinal worm repellent, and as a menstrual stimulant. The decoction or volatile oil of the plant is also used topically as a pain reliever, anti-inflammatory, and antiseptic for wounds and burns, and is used as a gargle to disinfect the gums and mouth. It is also suitable as an insecticide (Colorado potato beetle) (Leptinotarsa decemlineata)

Use warnings: It is not used by pregnant women.

Environment:

It grows as a harmful weed on rocky slopes, walls, neglected places and ruins. It is suitable for most types of soil, but it fears acidic soils.

Cultivation and productivity:

The seeds are scattered in the spring in containers (or bags). The seeds are covered and watered, and the soil is kept moist. The seedlings are transferred to the permanent ground at the end of spring and the beginning of summer. If a sufficient quantity of seeds is available, they can be scattered directly into the permanent soil in beds or basins in the spring. It is sufficient to sow the seeds once, because the plant itself spreads its seeds in the following years.

Taraxacum officinale F.H.Wigg.

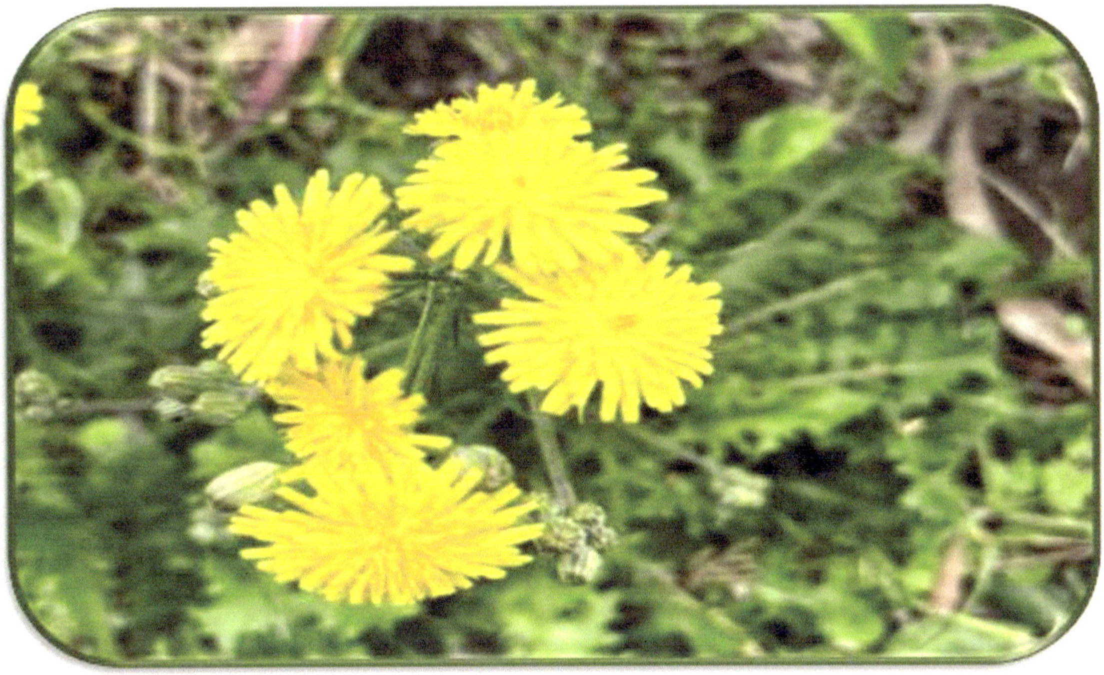

Family: Asteraceae (Compositae)

Common names: Dandelion, Dandelion, Dandelion, Dandelion.

Foreign names: Pissenlit Fr. Dandelion, Eng.

Occurrences : 395,684 occurrences

Distribution in the world

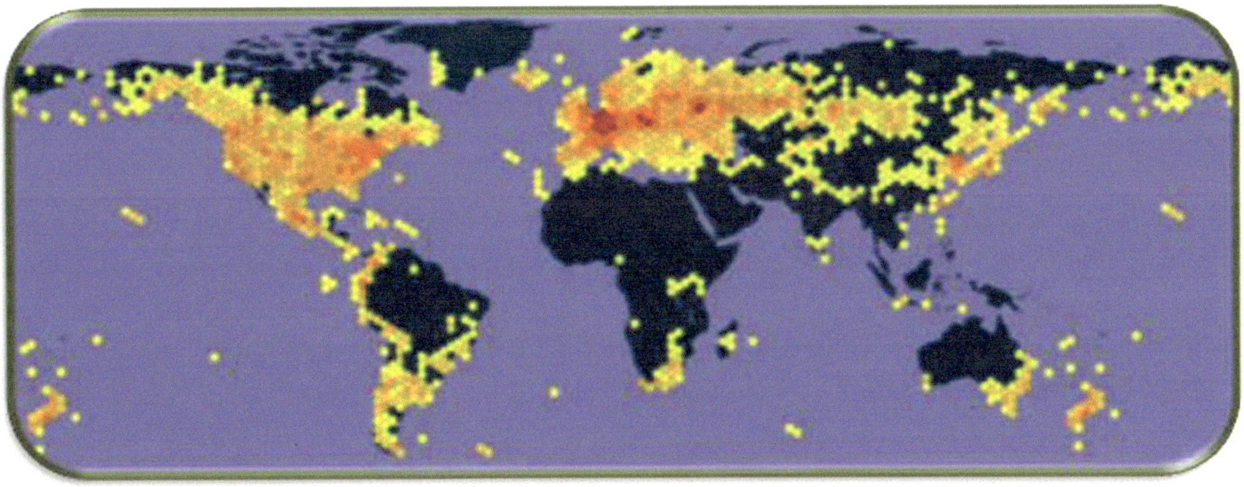

Botanical description:

A small perennial herb, stemless, with a thick and strong taproot. All leaves are basal, located on the surface of the soil forming a rosette-like shape, deeply lobed into lanceolate lobes. One or more stalks emerge from the center of the leaves, about 20 cm long, hollow, leafless, ending in a single main inflorescence. The head is homogeneous in flowers, containing only sphenoid flowers, yellow in color. The bracts are arranged in several rows, and are unequal in length, the outer ones being shorter, and curved backwards during and after flowering. The calyx is represented by a group of hairs, surrounding the base of the corolla, whose parts are joined together in the form of a small tube that soon splits to form a lingual ending in five teeth. The fruit is round, striped, thorny at the top, ending in a slender beak, brown to greenish-brown in colour (not red or reddish), topped with a dusting of white silky hairs in the shape of a funnel, which helps in dispersing the fruits by the wind. The species shows great morphological diversity, whether at the level of the leaves, fruits or the main inflorescence bracts, which has allowed the distinction of many subspecies and varieties.

Flowering: From November to May.

Homeland and geographical distribution:

European-Siberian. Widely distributed in the world, cultivated in many countries of the world such as Japan, India and America.

History and heritage:

The name Taraxacum goes back to the old Persian meaning "bitter purslane." Some believe that the scientific name of the genus is derived from the Arabic word: Tharakhchakon, while others believe that it is derived from the Greek: taraxis, meaning "eye disease" and akeomai meaning "I treat" or "I heal." Dioscorides mentioned it in his writings, and Arab doctors used it in folk medicine to treat liver diseases and cleanse the kidneys of deposits. The English name dandelion was coined by a surgeon who lived in the fifteenth century, who likened the leaves of the plant to the teeth of the seven or leonis dens in Latin. The leaves and roots of the plant are used in France to treat liver diseases, and the plant has been considered an elixir of life in Russia since ancient times, and it has been widely used in folk medicine to treat digestive disorders and jaundice. The whole plant is used in Chinese medicine to remove the effect of poison and increase milk production.

Part used:

Roots (pulled in autumn), whole plant (collected before flowering).

Chemical components:

The roots contain: sesquiterpenlactone, including taeraxinic acid glycoside. Triterpene compounds, such as campesterol, cycloartenol, sitosterol and stigmasterol. Flavonoides, such as apigenin glycoside, Vitamins, especially vitamin C, tocopherol, B vitamins, and beta-carotene, especially in the green leaves. The leaves also contain vitamins A-D, minerals, the most important of which are potassium and manganese. Amino acids such as asparaginic acid, glutaminic acid, and proteins. Mineral elements Fe, Ca, P, Na, K, Cl Cu, Mg, Zn, Carbohydrates, oxalic acid, and hydroxyacetic acid para.acid. Salivary substances, inulin.

Properties and medical uses:

The root has diuretic and digestive properties, by increasing digestive secretions in the upper part of the digestive system. It is used in the treatment of chronic colitis. It is also used to treat urinary tract infections, loss of appetite, indigestion, feeling of fullness and flatulence, liver and jaundice problems, and viral hepatitis. The roots are popularly used to treat constipation, indigestion, fluid retention resulting from premenstrual syndrome, heart failure, high blood pressure, to stimulate bile production, and to treat gallbladder problems and liver disorders. The leaves have a blood purifying effect. Natural products of dandelion leaves and root extracts can inhibit the development of liver cancer and reduce insulin resistance. Dandelion root extracts promote satiety and increase fat metabolism thanks to their content of chicoric acid, chlorogenic acid and sugars. The milky sap extracted from the leaves and stems of the plant is used topically to treat warts.

Pharmaceutical forms:

The plant preparations are available in the form of capsules, specialties, and tea. They are sold under names such as Dandelion.

Other uses:

Some roast the roots of wild dandelion and use them ground instead of coffee, and they make a heavy Dutch musk called Scnapps from its flowers, or add the leaves to soups and salads in food.

Precautions for use:

The plant is not prescribed in cases of obstruction of the bile ducts, or in cases of pyothorax and intestinal obstruction. The use of the plant may cause acidity, due to the plant containing compounds that stimulate digestive juices.

Environment:

A light-loving plant, it grows in abandoned places, on the sides of roads, inside bushes, and in fields. It tolerates low temperatures up to -29°C, and grows well in the presence of moisture and humus-rich soil, with a pH that is moderate to slightly acidic.

Cultivation and productivity:

It is propagated by seeds that are scattered in the spring in small areas, in a homogeneous manner and covered with a thin layer of soil, and its surface is sprayed with water after planting. Mineral nitrogen and phosphorus fertilization increases the amount of production. The seeds ripen shortly after the flowers open and the petals fall, and are collected at the beginning of summer before they dry out and fall. The roots are collected in autumn or spring, cleaned and placed under the sun until the milky liquid dries, then dried. One hectare yields 4-5 tons of dry roots.

Xanthium strumarium L.

Xanthium natalense Widder., *Xanthium abyssinicum* Wallr., *Xanthium antiquorum* Wallr., *Xanthium arenarium* Lasch,, *Xanthium brasilicum* Vell., *Xanthium inaequilaterum* DC.

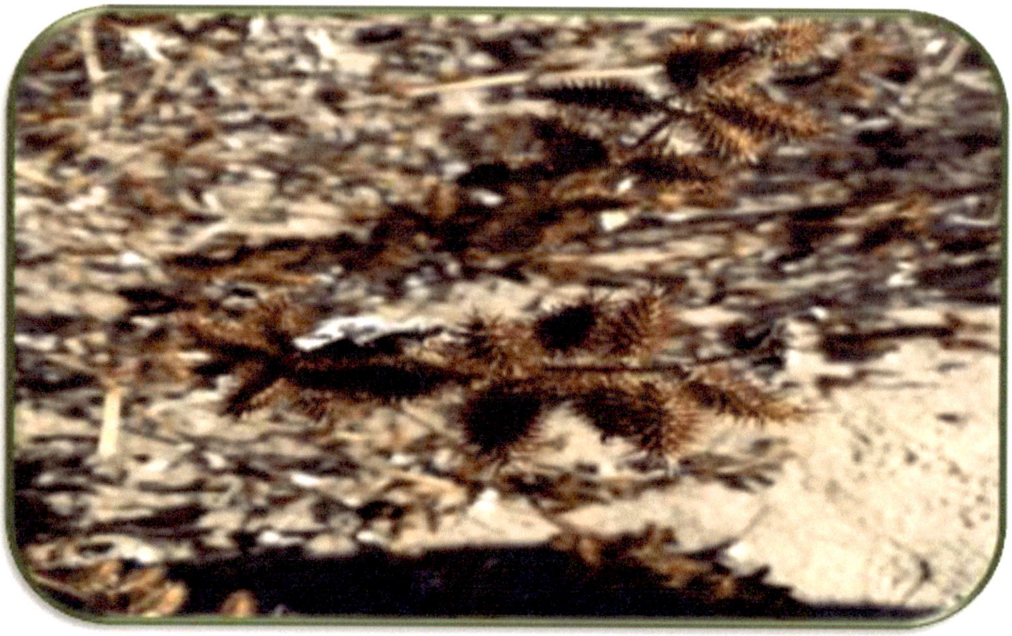

Family: Asteraceae (Compositae)

Common names: Yellow, Burrweed, Sticky

Foreign names: Lesser burdock, Burrweed. Fr. Cachurrera

Occurrences : 52,254 occurrences

Distribution in the world

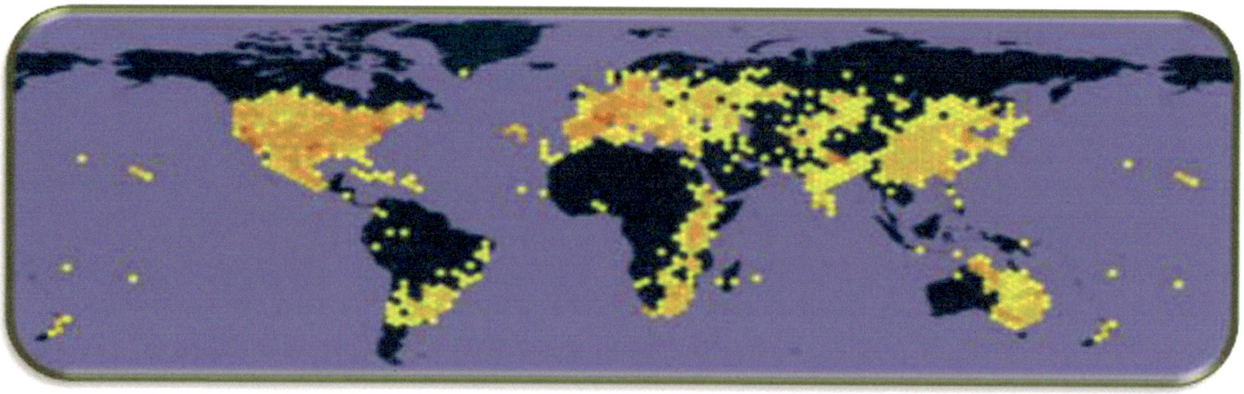

Botanical description:

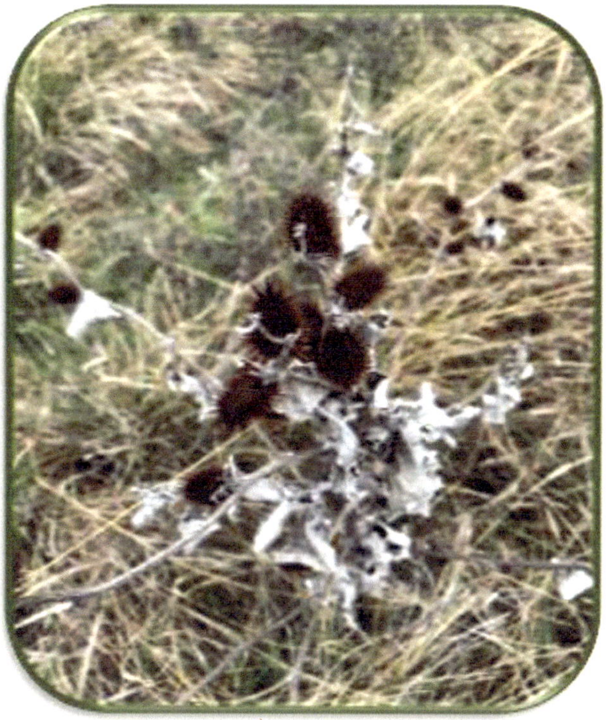

An annual herb, 30-100 cm tall, covered with short, dense hairs. Stem thick, erect. Leaves simple, alternate, spineless, triangular in general shape, margin lobed and irregularly serrated, base cordate or pedunculate, length of petiole approximately equal to length of leaf blade. Flowers unisexual, gathered in unisexual, monoecious heads. The male heads are spherical, its flowers are numerous and tubular, surrounded by free bracts, and are located at the ends of the branches. As for the female heads, they are located below the male heads in the axils of the upper leaves, individually or in small groups. The head contains two flowers without calyx or corolla, each consisting of a pistil only, and both flowers are surrounded by a leathery bract that is fused with the fruit, surrounds it, and ends with one or two straight, thorny teeth, equal in length to the thorns. The fruit is an acinate, compressed, each bract is surrounded by a hard, oval to oblong bract, 1.5-2 cm long, covered with spines that are hooked at the end, and its lower two-thirds are covered with short hairs and glands.

Flowering: May to September**.**

Habitat and geographical distribution: Spread throughout most parts of the world.

History and heritage:

The Latin name for the genus is derived from the Greek xanthos, meaning "yellow," due to the use of the leaves and roots in the preparation of dye. The name of the species strumarium is derived from the Latin struma, meaning "swine disease," due to its ancient use in the treatment of swine flu. The plant was used in the past to treat diseases of the thyroid gland and urinary system, diarrhea, and cholera.

Part used: Leaves, fruits and roots

Chemical components:

The leaves contain tannins, including xanthatin, and monoterpenes and ketones. The fruits contain sterol compounds (phytosterol), and glycosides: atractyloside (a toxic compound, causing a decrease in blood sugar). The seeds contain 36% proteins, volatile oil, and 38% fatty oil, which includes several unsaturated fatty acids (olive acid, linoleic acid), and glycosides similar to those found in the fruits, and resinous materials.

Properties and medical uses:

The plant is a traditional herbal medicine, widely used to treat many diseases, such as: rhinitis, sinusitis, headachc, stomach ulcers, bacterial rheumatism, fungal infections, and arthritis. The sticky is considered a poisonous and dangerous plant, especially the seedlings and young plants that contain a high concentration of toxic components. Research indicates that the compound xanthatin has properties that prevent cell division, and therefore its potential effect in reducing the proliferation of cancer cells. The fruit extract has antiseptic and antibacterial properties against some types of bacteria and fungi, and references indicate its antispasmodic and sugar-lowering properties. The decoction of the leaves and fruits is popularly used for its analgesic, diaphoretic, and diuretic properties, and in treating inflammation of the nasal mucosa. The infusion of the leaves is used topically to get rid of some types of parasites, and as an astringent in treating wounds and rheumatism. The decoction of the seeds is used internally to get rid of tapeworms, and the ground seeds (in the form of an ointment or alcoholic extract) are used topically as an anti-inflammatory, and in treating ulcerated wounds. The decoction of the roots is also used for its emetic properties, and in treating fever and swine flu. Recent research shows that the extracts and compounds of the liquorice have a wide range of activities, including anti-allergic rhinitis (AR), insecticidal, antiparasitic and antiviral activities, antioxidant activities, and lipid-lowering activities.

Precautions for use:

The plant is poisonous in all its parts. Symptoms of poisoning are irritation of the digestive system, respiratory and behavioral disorders, and general weakness.

Other uses:

A yellow dye is extracted from the leaves and is used in dyeing cotton fabrics.

Environment:

Grows The plant grows on the sides of roads, rivers, canals, fields and abandoned lands. It prefers sunny places. It grows in most soils, preferring poor, dry soils. It tolerates low temperatures of up to -15°C.

Cultivation and productivity:

The plant is propagated by seeds that are scattered directly in the permanent soil in the spring or autumn, and it can renew itself later, as its seeds are transmitted by the wind. The plant is considered a harmful weed in many countries of the world, and has become An invasive plant in many areas. Its invasion can be limited and eliminated by collecting, chopping, mixing it with fresh compost and fermenting it aerobically to produce compost, but its addition delays the maturity of the compost, which may be related to its antibacterial effect.

***Berberis vulgaris* L.**

Berberis racemosa Stokes.

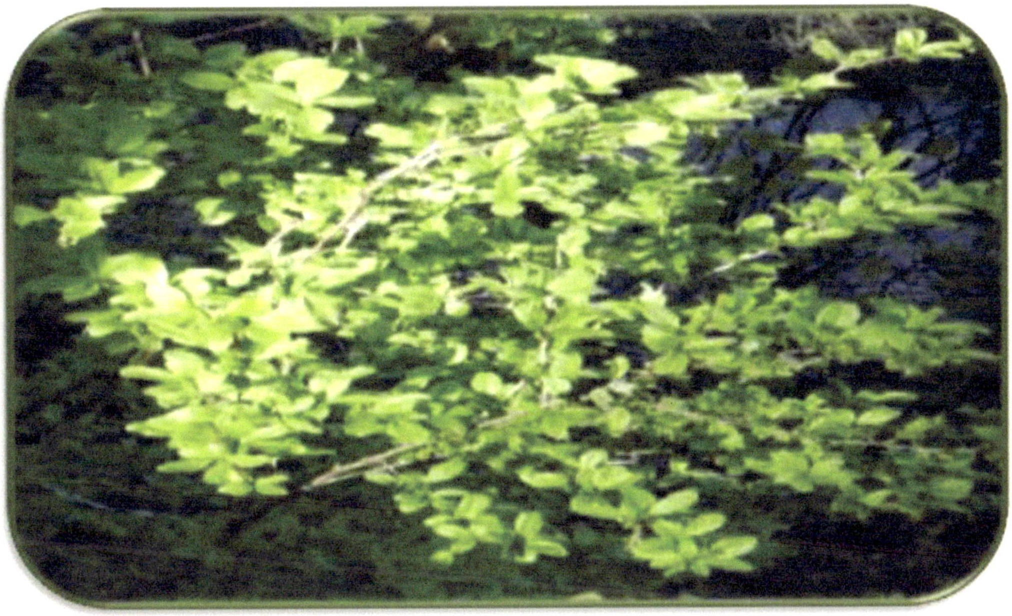

Family: Berberidaceae

Common names: Wind stick, common barberry, common zarshak, its knot

Foreign names: vinette Epine Fr. barberry, Common Eng.

Occurrences : 124,802 occurrences

Distribution in the world

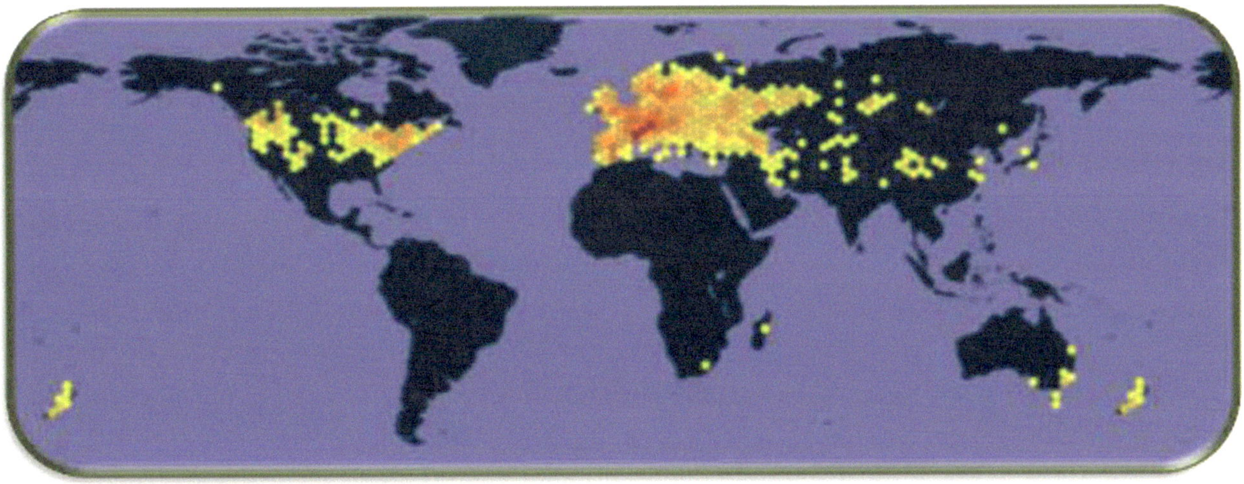

Botanical description:

A much-branched shrub, up to 2 m high. Branches are woody, erect, thorny, angular, initially yellowish-brown, then white to grey. Thorns are simple, dichotomous or trichotomous, strong, yellow, 1-2 cm long, located horizontally on the branches. Leaves are simple, leathery, inverted ovate to elliptic, 2-4 cm long, blade narrows to a stalk about 1 cm long, serrated edge, some of which turn into thorns. Flowers are gathered in short, drooping racemes, 5-7 cm long. Sepals 6, yellow. Sepals 6, orange. Male 6 stamens. Ovary superior, topped by a flat, flat stigma, perennial with the fruit. The fruit is a pink grape, oblong-cylindrical, 10-12 mm long, and about 6 mm thick, its outer fruiting shell is membranous-leathery to the touch, and contains 2-3 seeds.

Habitat and geographical distribution:

The genus Berberis includes about 500 species, and grows commonly in Europe, northern Africa, parts of America, central and southern Asia, and some northern regions of Pakistan and Iran.

History and heritage:

Fournier 1961, (in Nahal, 2009) believes that the word Berberis is derived from the local Arabic name in North Africa for the fruits of this shrub, while vulgaris means "common." Barberis was known in ancient times to the Indians and Babylonians, and was mentioned on Assyrian clay tablets dating back to 650 BC, and the Red Indians used it in ivory. The roots of the plant have been used for a long time in folk medicine to relieve spasms. The roots, bark, leaves and fruits were used in traditional Indian, Iranian and Chinese folk medicine, and its history dates back to at least 3000 years.

Part used: Fruits and root bark.

Chemical components:

The root bark contains 2-3% isoquinoline alkaloids, the most important of which are: berberine, berbamin, berbamunin, magnoflorine, and jatrorrhizin. In addition to containing tannins, resins and organic dyes. The fruits contain a high amount of alkaloids, tannins, phenolic compounds, oleanolic acid, gum, pectin, oleoresin, organic acids such as ascorbic acid, anthocyanins, carotenoids, vitamins, and proteins. The volatile oil of the fruits contains several compounds, including benzaldehyde, benzyl alcohol, 1-hexanol and II-2-hexenal. The volatile oil of flowers and leaves contains the following compounds: p-cymene, limonene, and ocimene. The most important alkaloids in the plant: berberine, oxycontin, palmatine, bervulcine, columbamine, jatrorrhizine, coptisine, and berbamine. The most important organic acids: chelidonic acid, and citric acid a. citric, and malic acid

Properties and medical uses:

The roots have properties that stimulate the circulatory and cardiac system, discharge bile, stimulate bowel movements, are antipyretic, antibacterial and antifungal, and are also used in the treatment of morphine addiction. It is popularly used to treat liver diseases (jaundice) and bile (gallstones), infectious gastrointestinal infections, in addition to treating cases of diarrhea and digestive disorders, and kidney diseases (sand and kidney stones), and it is also used to treat malaria and leishmaniasis, especially Leishmania tropica, and L. infantum. Barberry helps in treating chronic skin diseases, such as eczema and psoriasis. Its decoction is used as a gentle and effective wash to treat conjunctivitis and eyelid infections due to its berberine content. Berberine sulfate found in the root barks and bark of various types of barberry has antibacterial and antifungal properties. Ethanol stem extract inhibits the growth of bacteria with synergistic effects with ciprofloxacin such as Acinetobacter enteritidis, Salmonella coli, E. baumannii, and Ethanol stem bark extract inhibits the growth of gray mold Botrytis cinerea. The ethanolic fruit extract rich in alkaloids has anticancer activity, especially liver cancer cells (Hepg2), human breast cancer cells (MCF-7), and prostate cancer. Barberry rich in polyphenols can reduce the risk of Berberine (BER) has shown antioxidant, antitumor, antibacterial, liver-protective, and anti-inflammatory properties. Digestive, cardiovascular, nervous, neuropathy resulting from chemotherapy, diabetes, and pain resulting from sciatic nerve injury. It also has antioxidant, anti-anxiety, anti-depression, anti-anxiety, anti-Alzheimer's, anti-cancer, anti-viral, and anti-bacterial activities. Its extract is used to treat bacterial vaginitis. Berberine reduces cholesterol and triglycerides in the blood, improves liver enzyme function, and inhibits alpha-glucosidase, thus acting as an anti-obesity agent.

Other uses:

Barberry fruits are consumed fresh and dried, and are used in the production of various beverages, sweets, and fruit juice.

In addition, the leaves and fruits are used in the production of food flavors and tea. Cold-pressed seed oil helps delay the oxidation of soybean oil. Barberry water is used in preservatives in food industries.

Use warnings:

It should not be used during pregnancy. The barberry plant should only be used under the supervision of a medical doctor.

Environment:

The plant grows in rugged mountainous areas with calcareous soils, in sunny forest lands and on the edges of waterways and fields. It prefers light, acidic or moderate sandy and clay soils.

Cultivation and productivity:

The plant is propagated by seeds or vegetatively by stem cuttings and young root cuttings that are planted in late summer, and are preserved in fine sand with plastic cover to encourage them to form roots and be planted in early spring. Important species of this genus include: Lebanese barberry & Berberis libanotica Ehernb. A mountain shrub that grows in the highlands of the Syrian-Lebanese mountains (the eastern Lebanon mountain range) between 1400 and 2000 m and more. Stem erect, 15-150 cm, branches reddish-black, bearing yellow thorns Three-branched, often longer than the leaf clusters, fruit is an oval black or red berry.

Part used: Fruits and root bark.

Chemical components:

Fourteen compounds have been identified, belonging to different chemical classes in the extracts of roots and fruits. The root barks contain 2-3% isoquinoline alkaloids, the most important of which are: Berberine, Berbamin, Berbamunin, Magnoflorine, and Jatrorrhizin, in addition to containing tannic and resinous materials and organic dyes.

Properties and medical uses:

The plant is rich in alkaloids that may have anti-cancer activity and a high potential to eliminate cancer stem cells. The ethanolic extract of the Lebanese barberry root has shown anti-inflammatory and anti-cancer activity. It is used in folk medicine to treat malaria and cancer. A pink dye is extracted from the fruits and is used to dye silk, wool and cotton fabrics. A permanent yellow dye is extracted from the bark of its branches and roots.

Environment:

The plant grows wild in sunny, high forest areas 2200-1400 m, and on the sides of watercourses. It is tolerant of cold, as well as the edges of fields, and prefers light, moderate or slightly acidic sandy and clay soils. It is relatively tolerant of drought.

Cultivation and productivity:

The plant is propagated by seeds, or vegetatively by stem cuttings, and by tender root cuttings 10 cm long, which are planted at the end of summer, and kept in fine sand with plastic covering to encourage them to form roots and plant them at the beginning of spring. It is planted in a soil mixture of sand, soil and fertilizer (1:1:1), planting is done at a distance of 2-1.5 m, and if the soil is highly acidic, lime is added to it at a rate of 1 kg per plant.

Bongardia chrysogonum (L.) Griseb.

Leontice chrysogonum L., *Bongardia rawolfia* C.A.Mey., *Bongardia olivieri* C.A.Mey.

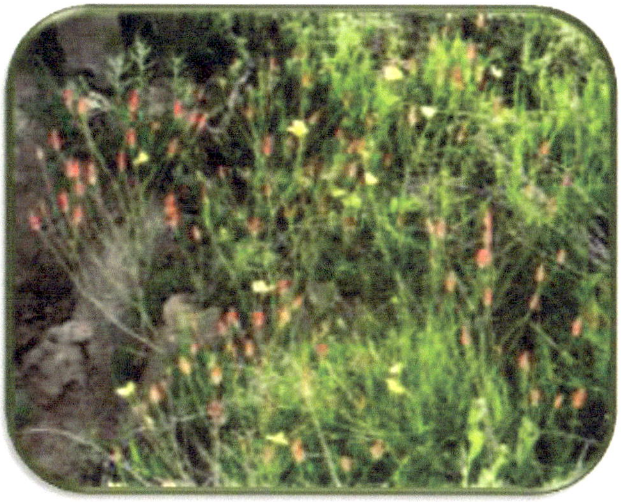

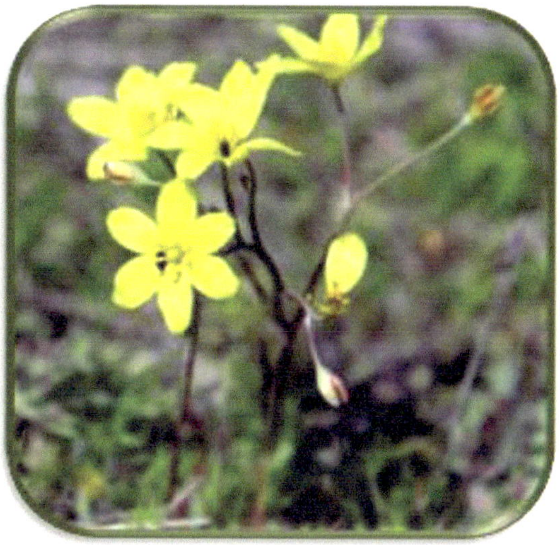

Family: Berberidaceae

Common names: Bongardie, Golden rod

Foreign names: Bongardie Fr. rod, Golden Eng.

Occurrences : 547 occurrences

Distribution in the world

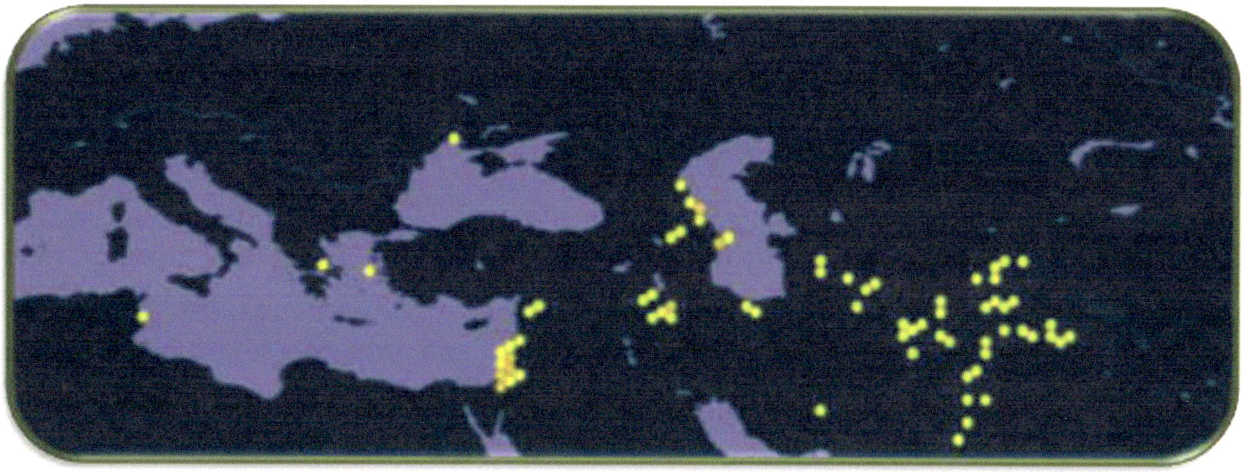

Botanical description:

A perennial herb with tubers found deep in the soil, spherical, compact in shape, large in size, 4-10 cm wide, bearing multiple leaf buds. It produces a bare, reddish-white, erect, branched aerial stem from the middle, leafless, 20-60 cm high. All leaves are basal, lying on the surface of the soil or slightly rising, deeply divided into opposite lobes, petiole, thick, serrated to lobed at the margin (3-6 lobes), ovate, inverted to pedicel at the base, often bearing a dark, dark purple spot at its base, and the length of the lobe is 2-4 cm. Flowers hermaphrodite, radiately symmetrical, yellow (including the stamens), long-stalked, gathered in a panicle, dichotomous, bearing semi-scale leaves below the branches. The calyx is petiolate, hexagonal. The corolla is 6-petaled, the petal length is about 1 cm. The male is hexagonal. The ovary is unicellular, containing 5-6 ovules, ending in a short style and a broad stigma. The fruit is a membranous capsule, swollen, oval to sub-spherical, reddish in color, with an irregularly torn end, 1.5-1 cm long, oval to oblong in shape. The seeds are few. (4-1)

Flowering: From February to March.

Habitat and geographical distribution:

The original habitat of the plant is North Africa and Western Asia, where it is naturally distributed in Syria, Turkey, the Caucasus, Iraq, Iran and even eastern Pakistan.

History and heritage:

The scientific name of the genus is attributed to the German botanist HG Bongard, who first named it. Linnaeus mentioned it in his book "Varieties Plantarum" 1753 as Leontice chrysogonum, and he took this name from earlier authors including Tournefort & Rauwolf. Rauwolf collected this plant near Aleppo in 1573, while Tournefort collected the plant during his trip The name was modified in 1700-1702 in the Aegean region, and the genus was later changed to Bongardia. It is known as a medicinal and edible plant in its natural areas of spread. Its leaves are used to treat eye inflammation in horses, and its tubers are also eaten cooked. Part used: tubers

Chemical components:

Tubers contain triterpenoid saponins (sapogenols) 12%, alkaloids 0.011%, including: lupine, bongardamine, bongardine, and isoquinoline.

Properties and medical uses:

The decoction of the tubers is popularly used to treat urinary tract infections, enlarged prostate, and hemorrhoids, as an antispasmodic, and is used to treat some cases of epilepsy. Several encouraging studies have been conducted on Rats, showed the effectiveness of soap compounds present in tubers in treating obesity, high blood pressure and diabetes. Tuber extracts have antioxidant, free radical scavenging and antispasmodic properties.

Other uses:

The leaves are consumed raw or cooked as the leaves of the sorrel plant Rumex sp.

Environment:

It grows in neglected lands, deserts and degraded pastures, on sunny stony slopes, and in agricultural areas between crops. The plant needs hot and dry conditions in the summer. It can grow in poor and dry soils, but it prefers light sandy soils, and requires well-drained soils. It does not prefer wet soils, and is affected by excessive humidity in winter, which may lead to rotting of tubers. Cultivation and productivity: It is propagated by seeds, and it is preferable to plant them in greenhouse conditions before transferring them to permanent soil. Seeds are planted immediately after they are ripe, in relatively deep pots, as the seedlings give roots that pull them down at a rate of 10-15 cm before their first leaves sprout. 3-4 seeds are placed in one pot.

***Borago officinalis* L.**

Borago advena Gilib., *Borago aspera* Gilib., *Borago hortensis* L., *Borago oficinalis* var. *alba* Gray, *Borago oficinalis* var. *coerulea* Alef.

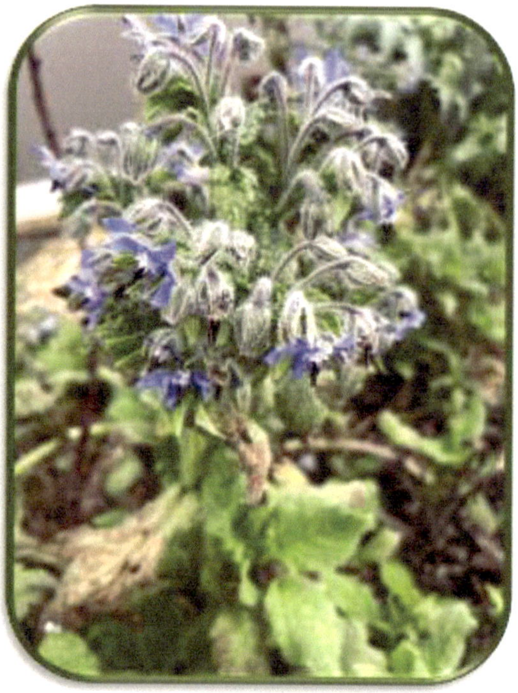

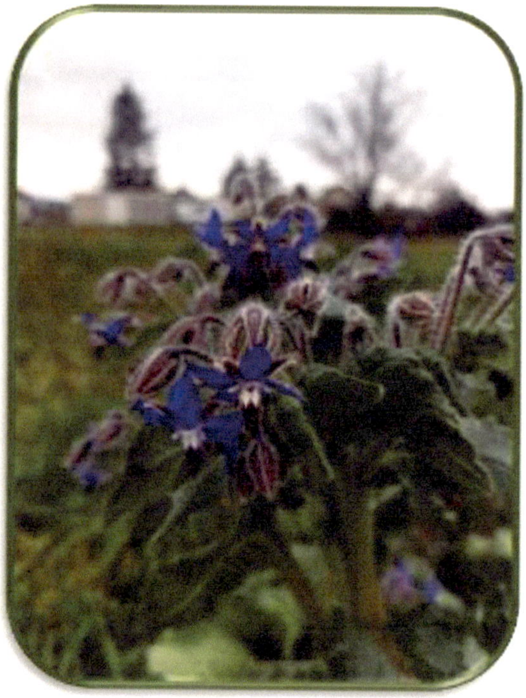

Family: Boraginaceae

Common names: Ox tongue, Borage, Bee bread, Abu Arq, Abu Arj, Harsha

Foreign names: Bourrache la Fr. Borage, Eng.

Occurrences : 150,164 occurrences

Distribution in the world

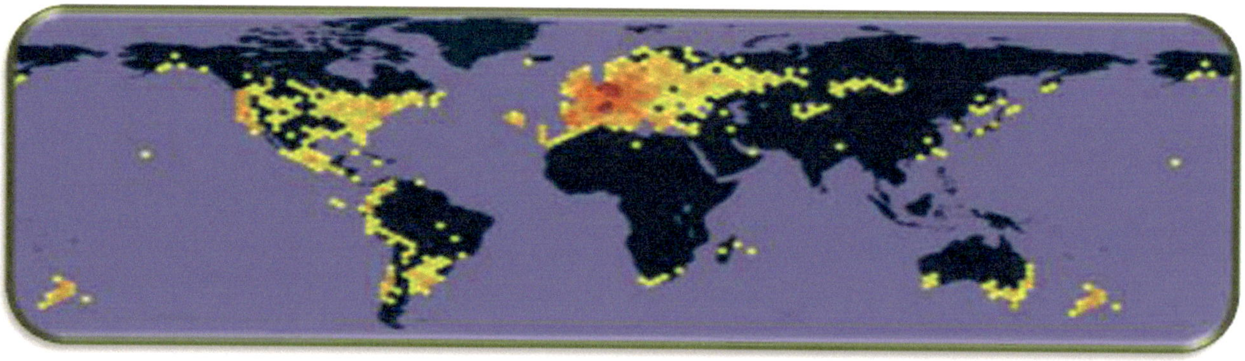

Botanical description:

Annual herb, stem erect or ascending, thick, branched, height 30-100 cm. All parts of the plant are covered with long, hard, flat hairs. Leaves are simple, alternate, lower ones obtuse, oval in shape. Floral leaves are low, Short, oblong in shape. Calyx 5 sepals, fused, lobes linear. Corolla 5 Pets fused, blue, wrinkled (folded) from below, somewhat velvety. Tube very short, lobes ovate, acute, flattened and star-shaped. Corolla scales bare, truncated. Stamens 5, filaments short, broad at base, extending near the apex to form the peduncle, anthers pedunculate, confluent, forming a black cone in the centre of the flower, distinguishing the flower of this species. Fruit 4 Pellets, erect, rough – Somewhat tuberous.

Flowering: March to September.

Home and geographical distribution:

The Mediterranean region, where it is spread in Syria, Lebanon, Palestine, Jordan, Iraq, Egypt, Libya, Tunisia, Algeria and Morocco. It is currently cultivated in many Eastern European countries such as Romania, Serbia, Bulgaria and Turkey.

History and heritage:

The scientific name of the genus is derived from the Latin bourra, which is the name of a coarse fabric with long piles, referring to the coarse nature of the plant, and oficinalis It means "medicine."

Hamham is a plant known as a medicine and food since ancient times. It was described as the herb of happiness. Its leaves and flowers were used since ancient times to improve the psychological state and increase the courage of Roman warriors. Dioscorides mentioned its properties that generate feelings of joy and happiness. Its flowers were used in the fifteenth century to soothe the soul and relieve worries and troubles. The great herbalist John Gerard quotes in one of his writings dating back to 1597 AD the old expression (I am the hyssop, always bring courage), and John Evelyn mentions in 1699 that it is "known for its effectiveness in encouraging and cheering the diligent student." The young leaves were used as greenery, and the Arabs used it for sweating, and it was mentioned by Ibn Sina and Ibn al-Baytar.

Part used:

Flowering plant and seeds, the plant is collected during the flowering period (the leaves have the smell and taste of fresh cucumber).

Chemical components:

A fatty oil called Borage oil is extracted from the seeds, rich in unsaturated fatty acids (linolenic acid -17-25%), and linoleic acid a. The oil also contains fatty acids: palmitic 10-11%, oleic 16-20%, linoleic 35-38%, eicosinoic 3.5-5.5%, erucic acid 1.5-3.5%, and nervonic acid 1.5%. The leaves contain pyrrolizidine alkaloids, including: supinin, lycopsamin, intermedin, amabiline, and thesinine. (They are toxic and carcinogenic alkaloids for the liver in their pure state.) They also contain salivary substances (important). Mucilages: Allantoin 30%, tannins 3%, and salicylic acid 1.5-2%. The flowers contain anthocyanin compounds, including: delphinidol, cyanidol, and flavonoids, including: kaempferol, quercetol, vitamin C, and minerals such as calcium and potassium. Medical properties and uses: The drink made from the flowers relaxes the heart and calms the insane. It is now known that the plant stimulates and activates the work of the The adrenal gland, which enhances the secretion of adrenaline, which is the "fight" hormone that prepares the body to work and act in critical and stressful situations. Borage oil is used topically in the form of cream, ointments or capsules for its emollient and softening properties for dry skin. It also maintains the vitality of the skin, reduces wrinkles, and is used to treat inflammation, skin ulcers, eczema, skin redness, rheumatism and arthritis. This is done in the form of boiled leaves. It is also used as a laxative in chest diseases (expectorant, cough, bronchitis), and as a diuretic, and in treating urinary tract infections (kidneys and bladder).

The plant has been used traditionally to treat digestive system disorders (colic, cramps, diarrhea), respiratory system, heart and blood vessels.

Environment:

The plant grows in fields and neglected fertile lands, as well as on the sides of valleys, river banks and salt marshes. It fears winds, so it is found on the edges of places Protected from winds. Prefers dry, semi-dry and semi-humid environments. Needs direct lighting for at least 6-8 hours per day, and weak lighting causes long and weak growth of the plant. Cultivation and productivity: It is propagated by seeds that are planted directly in the permanent soil if the area is moderate, but if the area is cold, the seeds are germinated in special nurseries in late winter, then the seedlings are transferred to the permanent soil in early spring to be planted Dimensions 40x40 cm. It is recommended to replant it at different intervals to provide its tender leaves for the longest possible period. It is planted in all types of soils, even heavy ones, provided that there is good drainage, the ground water level is not high, and it does not contain a high percentage of nitrates, because they cause rapid growth of leaves. The plant is collected before the flowering stage and left to dry, then the leaves are separated from the stems because the stems retain moisture for a longer period after drying, and thus become susceptible to rot.

Anastatica hierochuntica L.

Anastatica littoralis Salisb., *Myagrum hierochunticum* (L.) Crantz

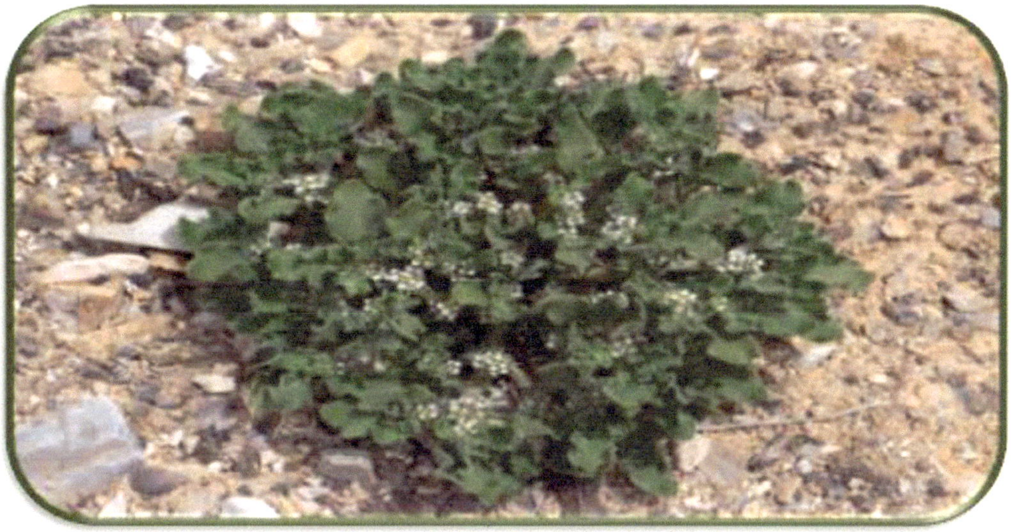

Family: Brassicaceae (Cruciferae)

Common names: St. Mary's flower, white mustard flower, rose of Jeric, rose of Jericho, palm of God Fatima bint al-Nabi, talq herb, kamsha, Aisha's palm

Foreign names: Fr. Rose de jericho

Occurrences : 1,492 occurrences

Distribution in the world

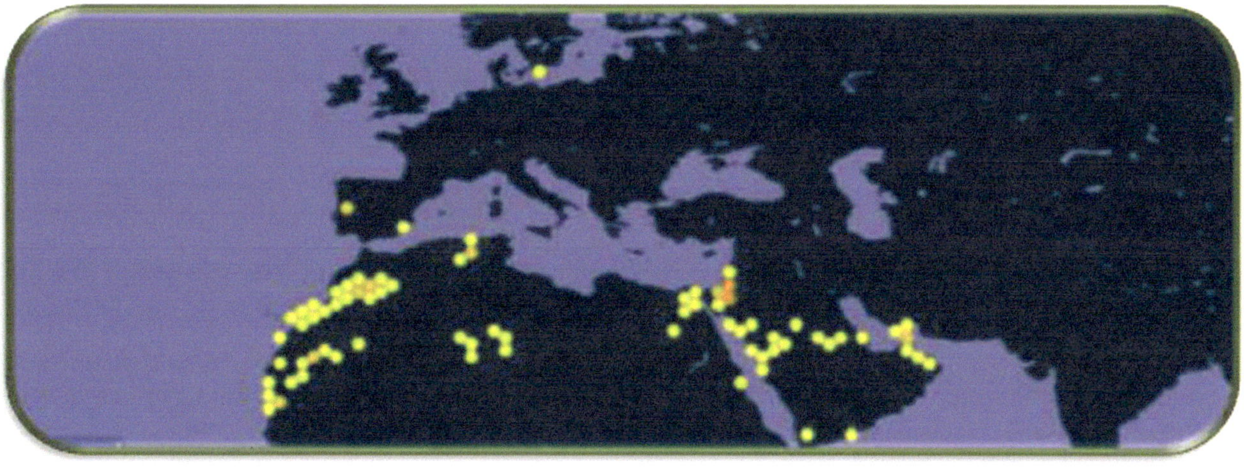

Botanical description:

Annual herb, covered with gray-star hairs, 3-20 cm high, becomes woody at the end of growth. Stems are lying or ascending, dichotomous. Leaves are simple, spoon-shaped - inverted ovate, gradually tapering to form the leaf petiole, blunt or acute, toothed, but the teeth are spaced apart, up to 1.5 x 3.5 cm, and are often smaller than that. Inflorescences are semi-spikelet, branched, short, located between the branches, covered with leaves, elongating after fruiting. Flowers are small, white, sessile to semi-sessile. Sepals are four erect, about 2 mm long, covered with star-shaped hairs - hard. Corolla is four-petaled, twice as long as the sepal. Petal consists of a nail and a blade. Male 6 stamens in two whorls (4+2). Female bicarpal, superior ovary, bicameral as a result of the formation of a false septum. The branches of the fruiting inflorescence are woody, arched, forming a spherical body containing the fruits. When moisture is present, the branches separate and the fruits spread far apart. The fruit is a mustard, hard, unopened, oval, covered with star-shaped hairs, its dimensions are 4-3×6-5 mm, the two valves are convex, each of them widens towards the apex to form a stalk that has a shape The spoon, its length is equal to or less than the length of the pen The hard perennial, which is 2-5 mm long, the false septum is thick. The seeds are oblong, wingless, compressed, ovate, in each chamber one seed.

Flowering: From February to April.

Habitat and geographical distribution: Desert-Arabian, and extends to the neighboring Sudanese regions. It grows naturally in The Sahara Desert, North Africa, Jordan, Palestine, Iraq and Iran.

History and heritage:

The genus name Anastatica is derived from The Greek word anastasis means "resurrection" or "resurrection", referring to the ability of the plant to grow after its death when water is available. It was mentioned by Ibn al-Baytar, al-Antaki, and Abu al-Qasim al-Ghasani under different names. The Arabs used the plant, especially the leaves and fruits, for medical purposes as an emmenagogue, and to treat epilepsy, headaches, and colds. It was used in the past as an indicator to predict the weather. In dry weather, the plant remains completely closed, while in wet weather, it begins to open at a high or low speed depending on the proximity of rainfall.

Part used: The dry plant, especially the leaves and seeds.

Chemical components:

The entire plant contains : Flavonoids, the most important of which are: luteolin, isovitexin, lucitin, quercetin, and kaempferol. Glucosinolates, including: glucoiberin, glucocheirolin Sterols. The fruits also contain glucose, galactose, fructose, sucrose, and raffinose.

Properties and medical uses:

A decoction of the plant powder is popularly used to reduce colds and labor pains and facilitate childbirth (talq herb), to lower blood sugar, and as a strong laxative, and is useful in treating jaundice, as an antioxidant, and to protect the liver. The tincture prepared from the herb is used topically to treat hemorrhoids, leprosy and vitiligo, and the juice of the young leaves is used to treat eye diseases (conjunctivitis). Many studies have indicated that the methanolic and aqueous extracts of this plant have antioxidant, antifungal and antimicrobial activities, and it has been proven that it has the ability to activate phagocytic cells and is antibacterial, which causes increased resistance to infection. The methanolic extract showed significant hypolipidemic activities in diabetic rats. It also showed anti-inflammatory, anti-melanin and gastroprotective activities.

Environment:

The plant grows in dry areas on stony slopes and plateaus in desert areas and on sandy- loamy soils in valleys with annual rainfall of less than 100 mm. After the rainy season, the plant dries up, its leaves fall, the branches bend inward, and the plant dies curled up in a ball. The fruits remain inside the ball, suspended and closed to protect the seeds and prevent them from dispersing prematurely. When the ball carried by the wind reaches a humid area or in the rainy season, the ball absorbs the water and the fruits open to scatter their seeds. If the amount of water is sufficient, the seeds germinate within hours. Part of the seed is dispersed near the mother plant by raindrops. The seed coat helps it stick to the soil, and the seeds can be carried by rainwater to greater distances, but their chances of survival are less. The plant can repeat this mechanism more than once, whenever conditions permit. Seeds can sometimes germinate while still in the fruit and within the dead, curled plant, giving the impression that the dead plant itself has come back to life

Cultivation and productivity:

The plant is propagated by seeds. Seeds are characterized by their high tolerance to extreme environmental conditions, and can remain dormant for years. It is recommended to collect seeds and scatter them in nature to propagate them.

Brassica nigra (L.) Koch.

Rhamphospermum nigrum (L.) Al-Shehbaz., *Sinapis nigra* L.

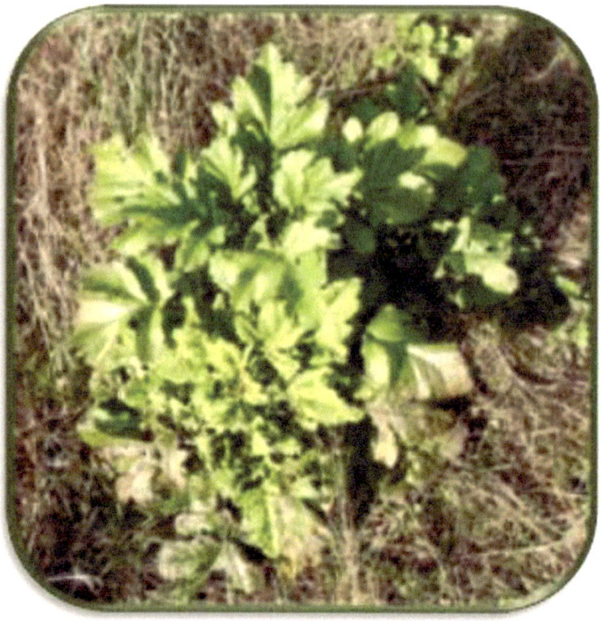 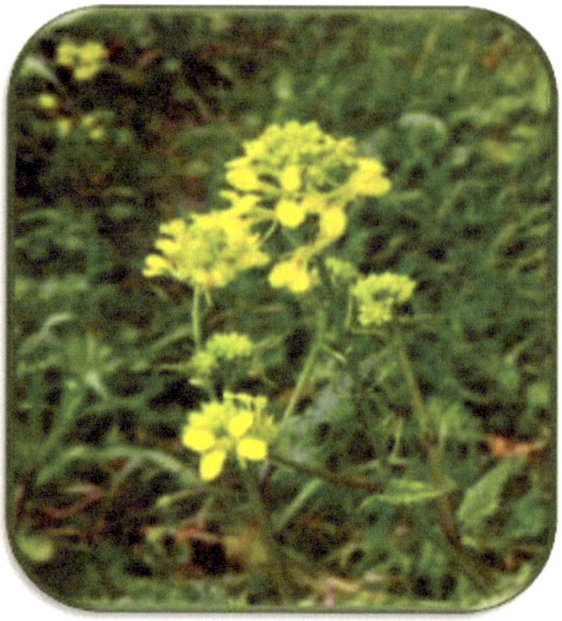

Family: Brassicaceae (Cruciferae)

Common names: Black mustard, Qarla, Qarra mustard

Foreign names: Black mustard, Fr. Moutarde noire

Occurrences : 53,106 occurrences

Distribution in the world

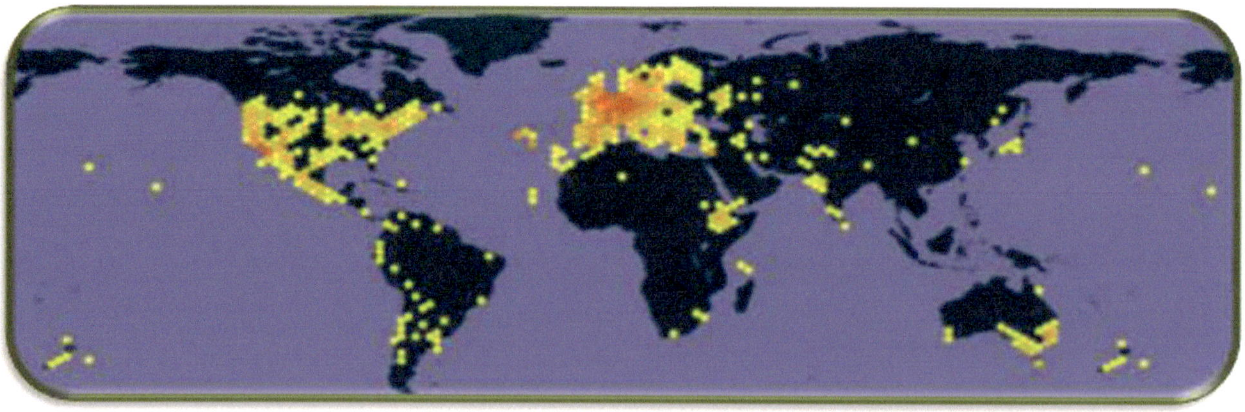

Botanical description:

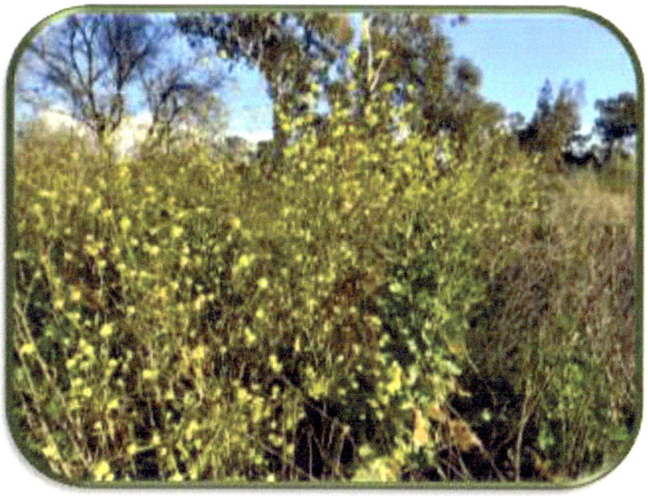

An annual herb, erect, 50-150 cm tall, slender branches, the lower part of it bears coarse hairs. The roots are fusiform. The lower leaves are long-pinnate, hairy, 15-40 cm long, deeply lobed, and the terminal lobes are larger. The upper leaves are short-pinnate, smaller, their base is toothed, lanceolate, glabrous, slightly serrated, the terminal leaves are often flat and have entire margins. Flowers in terminal or axillary panicles, condensed to form semicircular racemes. Sepals 4, 3.5-4.5 mm long. Petals 4, yellow, twice as long as calyx. Male 6 stamens of different lengths (4+2). Ovary bicarpel divided into two chambers by a false septum. Fruit: erect mustard, attached to the stem, 8-25 mm long, 1-3 mm wide, 2-6 mm long, cylindrical, straight, head seedless, narrow, 2-5 mm long. Seeds spherical, brown, 1-2 mm. Flowering: May to September. Similar to white mustard (White Rabenh (L.) alba B. Black mustard in its chemical components and uses.

Home and geographical distribution:

European, Siberian - and Mediterranean. It is naturally distributed in southern and central Europe, and parts of Asia. It is cultivated in temperate climate regions of Europe, Asia and northern Africa.

History and Heritage:

The scientific name of the genus is derived from the Celtic bresic or brassic, meaning "cabbage," which is the ancient Latin name for these plants. The species name nigra means "black." The species name alba means "white." Both black and white mustards have long been used medicinally and nutritionally. In the United Kingdom, the plant has been used in "hot mustard baths" to help people with colds. The ground seeds of the plant mixed with honey are used in Eastern Europe as a cough suppressant, and in Eastern Canada it was used to treat respiratory infections, by mixing the ground mustard seeds with flour and water, making a paste (compress), and placing it on the chest or back, and leaving it until the person feels a stinging sensation. Mustard compresses can also be used to relieve muscle pain. Part used: The seeds and their volatile oil.

Chemical components:

The seeds contain glucosinolate sulfur glycosides that vary depending on the type. White mustard (alba B.) contains the glycoside sinalbin, and black mustard contains the glycoside singrin. These compounds are hydrolyzed by enzymes, giving a volatile oil, the percentage of which reaches 1.3%. 90% of it includes the compound allyl isothiocyanate. The seeds also contain proteins (30%), mucilage, and fixed oil (27%), rich in sterols. And flavonoids, including: Vitin. It also contains phenylpropan derivatives (sinapin), which are bitter-tasting amino compounds. The predominant phenolic compounds are gallic acid, ferulic acid, and caffeic acid. Preparation of mustard oil: The volatile mustard oil used medicinally is prepared by distilling mustard seeds. Mustard oil is clear, colorless or yellowish, and has a sharp, tear-producing and irritating odor (it was used in wars as a tear gas).

Properties and medical uses:

The seeds and volatile oil have antiseptic properties and inhibit the growth of bacteria and fungi. Studies have confirmed its reddening properties for the skin. Black and white mustard oil are used to treat sinusitis, bronchitis, pleurisy and sciatica.

Popularly, the ground seed paste is used topically as a compress to treat pneumonia, respiratory congestion, fluid retention, intestinal gas, muscle pain, arthritis and soft tissue inflammation, rheumatism and gout. The decoction of the seeds is used in the form of water baths for the body and feet, in the form of local plasters to treat bruises, and in the form of gargles to treat inflammation of the mouth and throat. Mustard oil is also used topically to stimulate blood circulation, treat vascular diseases, heart failure, and ischemia.

Pharmaceutical forms:

Mustard is available in the form of mucilage, kiniments, tea, ground seeds (mustard flour), and oil. It is sold under names such as Musterole.

Other uses:

The seeds or paste are used in spices as an appetite stimulant. The young leaves, buds, and flowers are edible.

Side effects and warnings:

Using mustard oil as a compress leads to the evaporation of volatile sulfur compounds represented by the compound allyl isothiocyanate, which is irritating to the eyes, and may lead to respiratory problems and asthma attacks when inhaled. Mustard volatile oils should not be inhaled or tasted. A doctor should be consulted in the event of allergic conditions or any irritation of the skin and mucous membranes as a result of contact with mustard or its oil. Pregnant and breastfeeding women should avoid using the plant. Mustard oil should also not be used internally by people suffering from stomach ulcers or kidney infections, because mustard oil may irritate the mucous membranes in the stomach and kidneys. Hands should be washed well and eyes should be avoided after preparing medical products from mustard. Mustard oil compresses should not be used for more than half an hour.

Environment:

Black mustard adapts to different climatic conditions, tolerates cold, but prefers a moderate and dry climate, does not tolerate high humidity. Tolerant of lime, grows easily in many types of soil except heavy clay soils, and prefers light, deep, fertile, moist, and well-drained sandy soils.

Cultivation and productivity:

Black mustard is cultivated for its edible seeds. It is propagated by seeds that are scattered directly in the permanent soil or by seedlings 20 cm long. The seeds are scattered in 3X6 m beds or basins after rainfall in autumn or early winter. The seeds take more than a week to germinate.

The plants are fertilized only immediately after planting. The seedlings are transferred to the permanent soil in spring. They rarely need to be watered.

They are watered according to the plant's needs and soil conditions. The seeds fall from the pods when they open after full ripening, so it is preferable to start the collection process when the pods turn yellow and before they open, and it is important to collect in the early morning. One hectare produces the equivalent of 1.5-1 ton of seeds.

Capparis spinosa L.

C. sandwichiana DC.

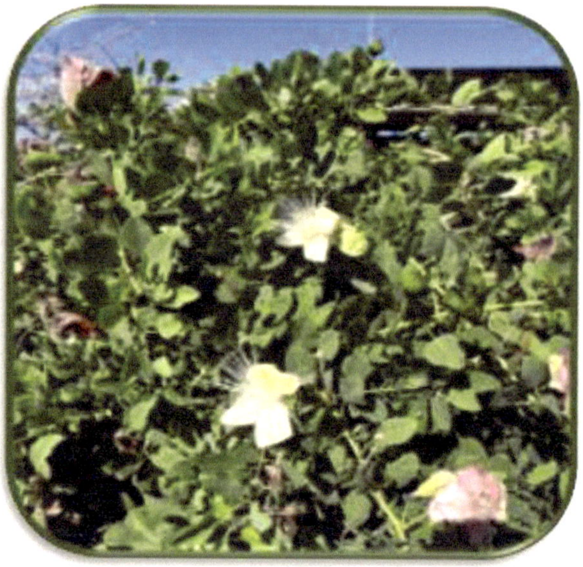

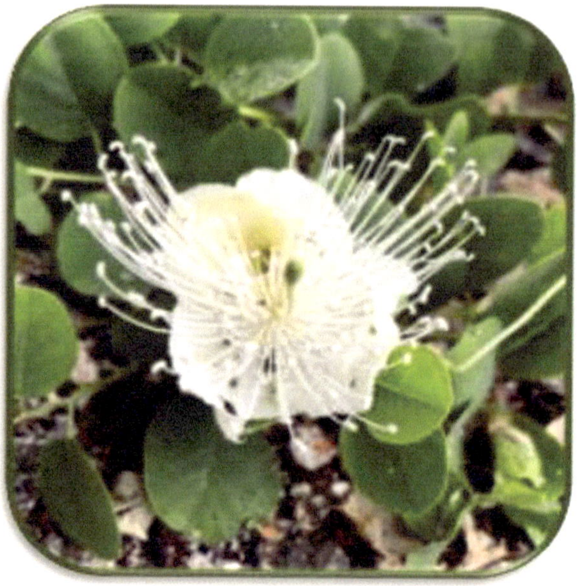

Family: Brassicaceae (formerly Capparisae)

Common names: Common caper bush, Caper, Fr. Caprier

Foreign names:

Occurrences : 17,182 occurrences

Distribution in the world

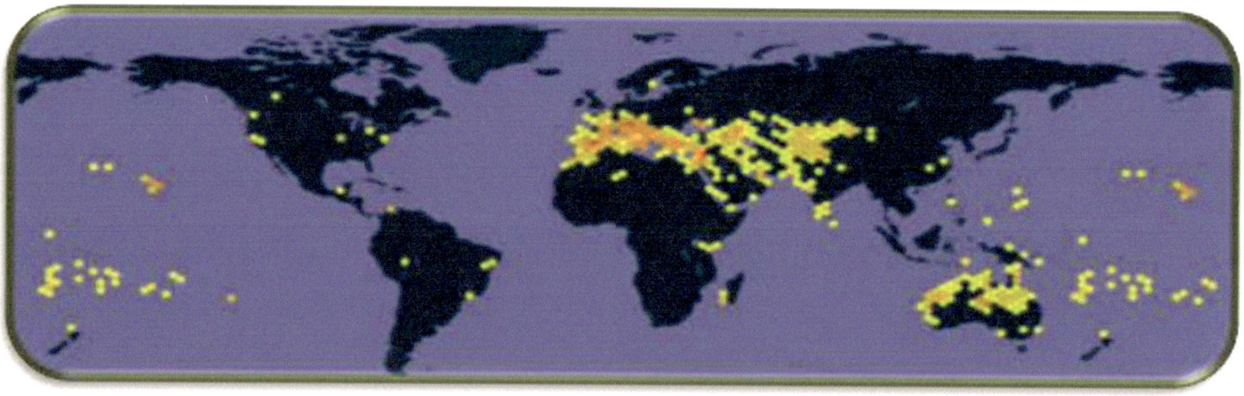

Botanical description:

A shrub with branches lying or ascending (at least two forms are distinguished from it, ascending and lying or creeping), smooth, glossless, with a colour tending to crimson or blue-green. The leaves are simple, long-petiolate, round or oval in shape, completely margined, glossless in the ascending form and larger, thicker, greener and bluer than in the lying form), the ears are transformed into strong, hooked-headed thorns that vary in length. Flowers solitary, axillary, long-stalked, bright white or tinged with pale pink, especially on the ascending form.) Calyx 4-lobed, glabrous, nearly equal in length, the posterior scaphoid. Corolla 4-lobed, inverted-ovate-rounded, nearly equal in size, the posterior scaphoid thick-edged, fused at the bottom, forming a nectar-protrusion. Stamens are numerous (80-120), their filaments are pink or bluish, usually shorter than the bare female carpel. Female carpels 2-8. Ovary superior, unicellular, ovules numerous. Fruit is a green berry, 2.5-4 cm long, opening through valves to produce black seeds and red pulp in the recumbent form, and its perianth turns outwards towards the carpel, or 3-6 cm long in the ascending form, opening through a single valve to produce black seeds and creamy pulp Colour.

Flowering: May to August.

Habitat and geographical distribution:

Mediterranean, extending to the Iranian-Turanian region. Widely distributed in Arab countries, including the countries of the Arabian Peninsula, and spread in the countries of North Africa, and cultivated in some countries of southern Europe.

History and heritage:

It is believed that the name of the genus came from the Arabic "Kabir" and spinosa means "thorny." It is mentioned that it was named Al-Qabar because it grows among graves, while the names "Asaf" and "Lasaf" are of Aramaic origin and are common in the Levant. The speciality of the caper was mentioned in the manuscript of Abi Jaafar bin Abi Khalid al-Mutatabb as a purifier of excess moisture in the stomach and an opener of liver blockages. King al-Muzaffar mentioned that its salted fruit, if washed and soaked until the hardness of the salt is gone, is beneficial in opening and purifying the blockages in the liver and spleen. It is one of the medicinal plants that have been widely used in traditional medicine throughout successive civilizations to treat various disorders and diseases. It was used in ancient Greece as a carminative.

Part used: Roots, fruits (whole plant.)

Chemical components:

Triterpenes, alkaloids such as stachydrine. Favonoids: glucocapparin, kaempferal, quercetin, isorhamnetin, rhamnetin, thomnocitirin. Sterols, terpenes, saccharides. The plant is rich in phenolic compounds and flavonoids, total phenols ranged from 24.21 to 62.27 mg gallic acid equivalent (GAE)/g dry weight (DW) in methanol extract of caper leaves taken from different locations in India. The aqueous extract of caper leaves (from Tunisia) recorded total phenols of 33.55 mg/g GAE/DW g, the aqueous extracts of buds contained 29.67 mg/g DW/GAE, while 27.427 mg/g DW/GAE was recorded in the methanol extract of caper leaves from Tunisia. g/GAE of total phenols in the aqueous extract of leaves. The aqueous extracts of roots and fruits (Iranian) contained 15.4 and 17.2 mg/g DW g/GAE respectively, less than the root ethyl acetate extracts containing 37.2 mg DW g/GAE, and the ethanol extract Fruit contains 34.2 mg/g DW g/GAE 100 g of capers contains: water 79 g, protein 5.8 g, fat 1.6 g, carbohydrates 6.5 g, fiber 5.4 g,

Properties and medical uses:

It is used for its analgesic and antioxidant properties, it is antifungal and anti-inflammatory, hepatotoxic and hepatitis B, antidiabetic and anti-leishmanial. It is popularly used as a diuretic, anthelmintic, digestive, antitumor, and treatment of arteriosclerosis. It is used topically to treat gout and scurvy, relieve leg pain, treat eye diseases, relieve headaches, treat cough, tearing and runny nose. A wide range of therapeutic benefits are attributed to caper extracts, such as antihypertensive, anti-obesity, anti-allergic, antihistamine, anti-inflammatory, or antibiotic. In India, the root bark is considered a laxative, tonic, diuretic, anthelmintic, emmenagogue, and sedative. Plant extracts are a common ingredient in hepatoprotective herbal medicines.

Other uses:

The use of capers in food has been approved by the Food and Drug Administration (FDA) in the United States of America. Its fruits are eaten pickled for their nutritional and spicy properties, and other parts of the plant are used in the manufacture of medicines and cosmetics.

Precautions for use:

May cause skin and digestive allergy symptoms.

Environment:

Capers grow on slopes, gravel lands, steppes, roadsides, near old walls and fences, around residential areas, and in abandoned places. The plant tolerates high and low temperatures. It is considered a drought-tolerant plant. It grows naturally in lands poor in nutrients, and is helped by its deep root system. It is found in deep, well-drained loamy soils. It tolerates salinity and lime.

Cultivation and productivity:

It is propagated by seeds or stem cuttings. Soft seeds germinate quickly, but at a low percentage, while dry seeds enter a dormant phase, and then need special treatment that extends for three months between Cooling and soaking in water. Dry seeds can be treated with sulfuric acid for 20 minutes, then washed with water and treated with gibberellic acid at a concentration of 1000 ppm for 24 hours to give the best results in the lying form, while the ascending form is more difficult to propagate. Seeds are planted at a depth of 1 cm. The plant begins to give flower buds in the fourth year of planting. Stem cuttings are taken at the end of winter and the beginning of spring with a diameter of 1 cm and a length of 8 cm, and are planted at a distance of 2.5-2 m after hormonal treatment for 10-15 seconds. The method of propagation by cuttings is fast and allows obtaining flower buds in the first year of transplanting. The plant blooms from the first year of planting by cuttings. Flower buds are collected manually in the early morning, and the collection process is repeated every 9-12 days. A 3-year-old plant produces 1-2 kg of flower buds.

Capsella bursa-pastoris (L.) Medikus.

Thlaspi bursa-pastoris L., Bursa bursa-pastoris (L.) Shafer, Nasturtium bursa-pastoris (L.) Roth, Rodschiedia bursa-pastoris (L.) G.Gaertn., B.Mey. & Scherb., Thlaspi bursa- pastoris subsp. pinnatifolia Ehrh.

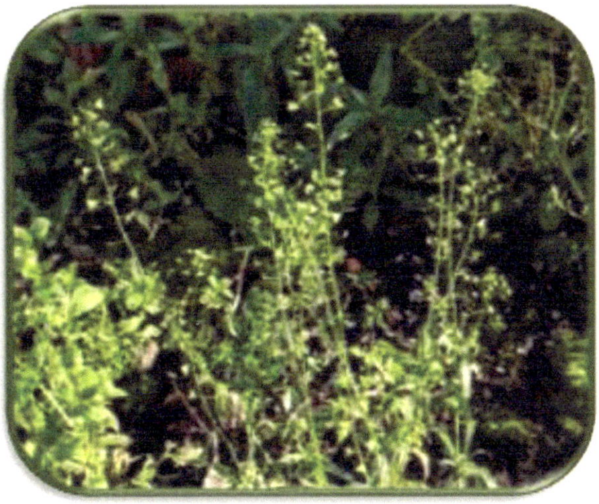

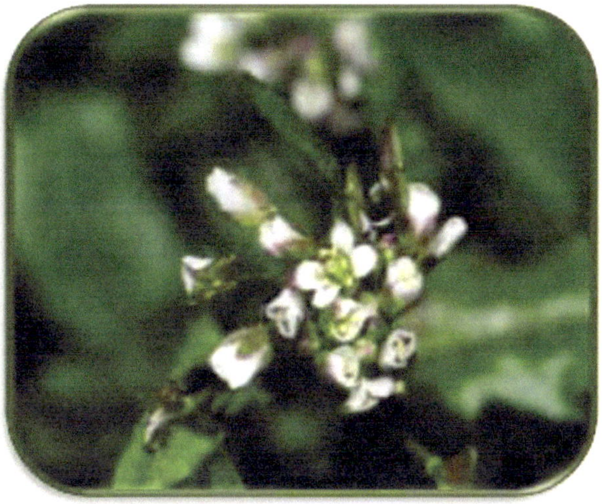

Family: Brassicaceae (Cruciferae)

Common names: Shepherd's tassel, Shepherd's purse.

Foreign names: Shepherd's burse, Fr. Bourse à Pasteur, Mother's heart

Occurrences : 588,482 occurrences

Distribution in the world

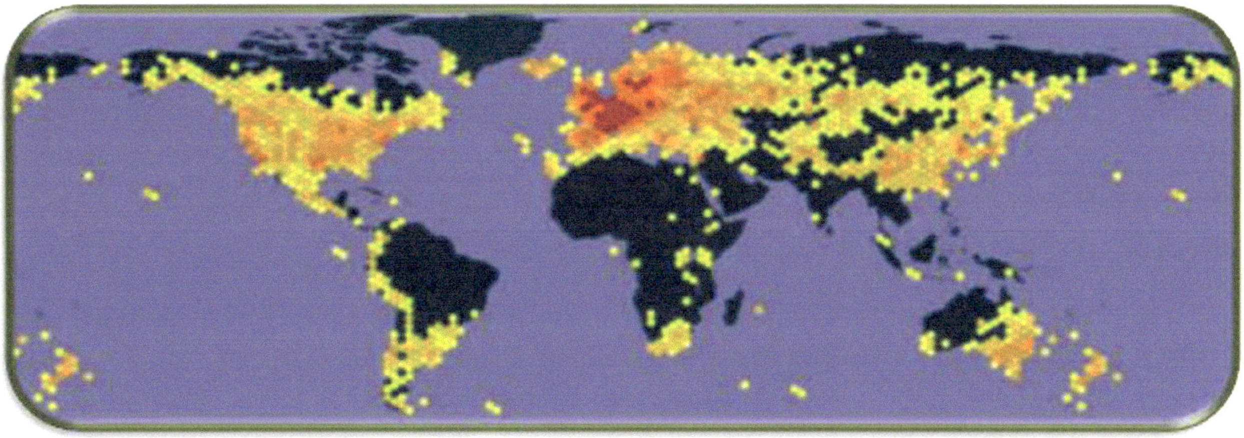

Botanical description:

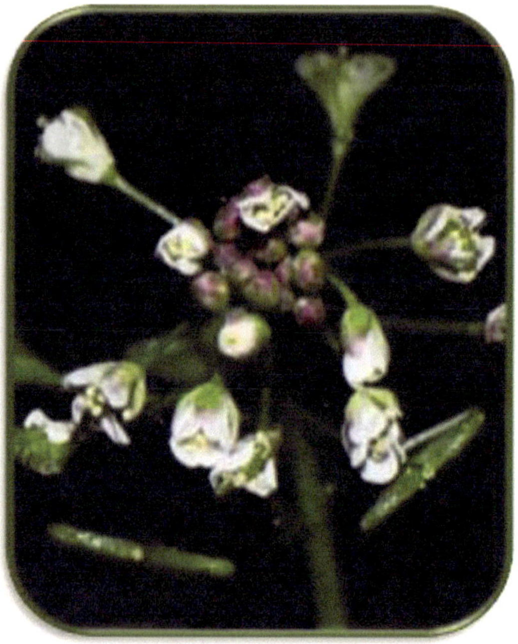

Annual herb, bare or sparsely haired, 10-50 cm high. Stem erect, simple or branched from below. Lower leaves 2-16 cm, forming a basal rosette, inverted lanceolate, gradually tapering to form a leaf stalk, entire or Serrated or lobed margin. Upper leaves 1-7 cm, Linear – Oblong, ovate, the base of its blade partially surrounds the stem, its edge is serrated or complete. Flowers are small (2-4 mm), gathered in densely flowered terminal racemes. Calyx 4 free sepals. Corolla 4 petals, white. Male 6 stamens of different lengths (4+2). Female bicarpal. Ovary composed of one chamber divided by a false septum into two chambers. Fruit inflorescence elongated, its panicles flattened (semi-horizontal position), Slender-threaded. Peduncle 4-8 mm, triangular, notched at the top (heart-shaped). Seeds up to 12 in each chamber

Flowering: December to April.

Habitat and geographical distribution: A semi-global plant.

History and heritage:

The scientific name of the genus is derived from the Latin capsa or capsula, meaning "box" or "sack", alluding to the apparent similarity between its heart-shaped seed pods and the leathery sacks that shepherds used to carry in the past. Shepherd's purse is a medicinal herb that has its place in both Eastern and Western traditions. The English name "Mother's heart" indicates its use in treating gynecological diseases. It is known as a tissue astringent in the first degree, which is why it is called the wound herb. The seeds of the plant have long been used in China to improve eyesight. Nicholas Kleber wrote in 1653 of the Shepherd's purse: "Few plants have more advantages than this, and yet it is so neglected."

Part used:

Aerial parts and seeds. Leaves are eaten raw or cooked, usually available year-round, and can be dried for later use. Leaves contain 2.9% protein, 0.2% fat, 3.4% carbohydrates, 1% ash. They are rich in iron, calcium, and vitamin C. Young flowering buds and seeds can be eaten raw or cooked. The seed contains 35% oil, which can be extracted and is edible. It has been proven that the plant capsule absorbs heavy metals in high concentrations, so caution should be exercised during long-term use.

Chemical components:

The aerial parts contain cardiac steroid compounds. Phavonoids, including: luteolin-7-rutinoside, rutin Singerine glycosides: nonyl-9 sulfinyl methyl glucosinolate and others Amino compounds, including: choline, acetylcholine, tyramine, bursin, Histamine. Caffeic acid and its derivatives, including chlorogenic acid. Potassium salts.

Properties and medical uses:

The plant, with its flavonoids and tyramine, has a positive effect on the contraction and timing of the heart muscle and vessels (improving blood circulation). It is used to treat epistaxis (nosebleeds), wounds, burns, and premenstrual syndrome, to reduce excessive menstruation, and to stop uterine bleeding. It is also a diuretic due to potassium salts. It is used to treat dysentery, boils, pyorrhea, and fever. Its compounds are used in the composition of medications for varicose veins, hemorrhoids, and burns.It is recommended to use it to reduce blood pressure and speed up labor (increases uterine contractions). The flavonoid compounds found in the plant are effective antiseptics and antibacterials in treating cystitis and high blood cholesterol (hypercholesterolemia). It activates liver enzymes (experiments on animal models). It is used in Chinese medicine to treat eye diseases, including glaucoma. It is also considered an antioxidant. It is worth noting that the green plant is more effective than the dried one. It can be used as a tincture, solution, or decoction like tea.

Drug interactions and precautions:

It should not be used with anticoagulants (aspirin and coumarin), diuretics and sedatives. Symptoms of palpitations, irregular heartbeat, difficulty breathing and muscle paralysis appear when taking excessive doses, and the components of its seeds cause skin irritation. It is not recommended to use it during pregnancy due to its uterine astringent effect. It is also recommended not to use it in cases of hypothyroidism (like the rest of the cruciferous family) and in cases of various heart diseases.

Environment:

The plant grows in meadows, orchards, on the sides of roads, abandoned fields and landfills. It also grows in most types of soil, even poor ones, but in this case its height does not exceed a few centimeters before it flowers and its seeds are scattered, while its height can reach up to 60 cm in fertile soil.

Cultivation and productivity:

It is propagated by seeds (quick-germinating) that can be planted at any time of the year. Spring is preferred as a suitable time to scatter them in shallow beds or lines with moderate soil moisture, taking care not to let the seeds leak randomly into crop and vegetable fields. The plant is cut completely when flowering and the beginning of fruit formation, and dried in the shade and in the open air without exposure to sunlight.

Diplotaxis harra (Forssk.) Boiss.

Sinapis harra Forssk.

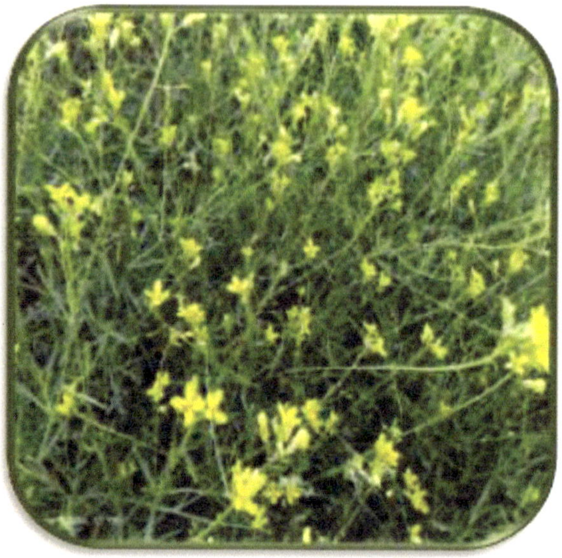

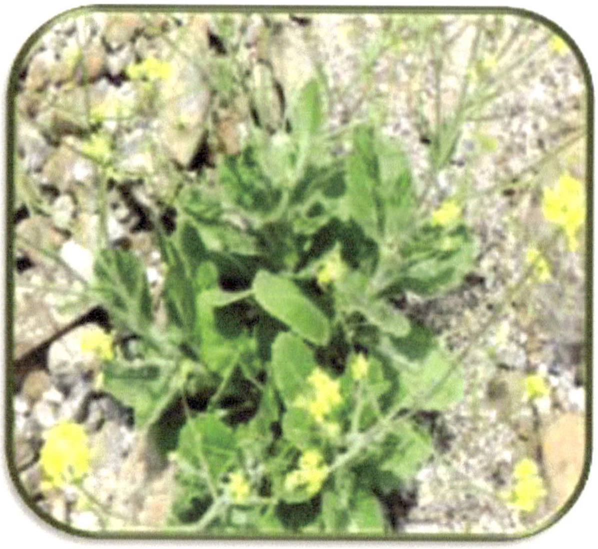

Family: Brassicaceae (Cruciferae)

Common names: Khoshian, Hara.

Foreign names: Diplotaxis Fr. Stink-weed, Eng.

Occurrences : 4,980 occurrences

Distribution in the world

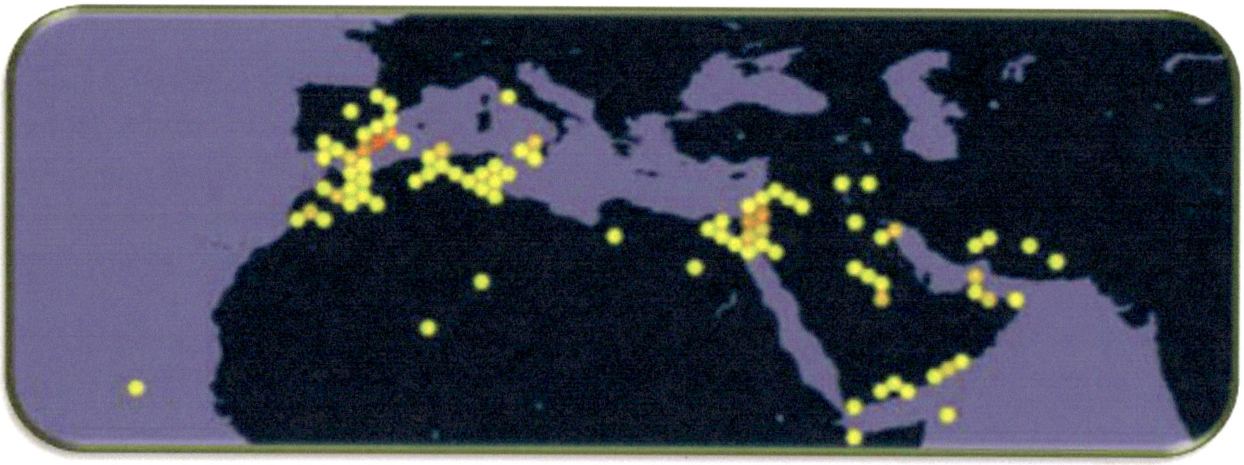

Botanical description:

A biennial or perennial herb, covered with hard hairs and sometimes almost hairless, 20-70 cm high. The stems are woody at the base and branched. The leaves are simple, mostly basal, 3-14 cm long, inverted ovate or oblong, gradually tapering to obtuse, serrated or lobed and sometimes entire at the margin. The stem leaves are lanceolate. The inflorescence is a loose cluster, containing 20-70 flowers. Flowers about 1 cm long, yellow, their pistils are equal to the length of the flower or shorter. Sepals

4, free, erect-flattened, hairy, 4-7 mm long. Petals 4, free, 8-10 mm long, yellow, their blade is inverted oval, gradually tapering to form a spike. Male 6 stamens in two whorls (4+2), and of different lengths. Female Bi-carpelic, ovary superior, divided into two chambers by a false septum. The fruit is a mustard, linear, 30-50 x 2-3 mm, pendulous, pedunculate. The valves are membranous, flat, twisted, the head is very short. The stigma is bilobed. The seeds are very small, arranged in two rows within each chamber.

Flowering: From February to May.

Habitat and geographical distribution:

Desert - Arabian, grows in the deserts of the Levant, Iraq, Iran, northern and eastern Arabia, Egypt, Libya, Tunisia, Algeria and Morocco.

History and heritage:

The scientific name is derived from the Greek diplous meaning "double", and taxis referring to the presence of two seeds in each chamber. And harra from Arabic meaning "hot." Part used: Aerial parts

Chemical components:

Glycosides, including sinigroside, which are hydrolyzed by the enzyme myrosinase, releasing volatile sulfur compounds including: isopropyl isothiocyanate, 3-butyl isothiocyanate, in addition to the non-volatile compound hydroxybutynyl isothiocyanate 3-butenly hydroxyl-2-. The seeds contain fatty acids, including: arachidonic acid, palmitic acid (palm a). Sterol compounds: stigmasterol, and β-sitosterol. Phytochemical analysis of the aerial parts showed the presence of flavonoid compounds, glucosinolates, and sterols, and that flavonoid glycosides have promising cytotoxicity with the ability to inhibit the growth of cancer cells. It was also found that the methanolic extracts obtained from the aerial part were effective against Escherichia coli. Properties and medical uses: Sulfur compounds and their derivatives exhibit antibacterial, antifungal and anti-nematocidal properties. Fatty acids in the seeds show high effectiveness in reducing the growth of bacteria and fungi. The plant decoction is used in folk medicine in cases of constipation.

Precautions for use:

The plant extract has an "irritating" and "reddening" effect on mucous membranes.

Environment:

It is widespread in dry and very dry steppe areas on stony gypsum soils and light, transported soils. It is one of the species that indicate overgrazing.

Cultivation and productivity:

The plant is propagated by seeds, and is rarely cultivated. The optimal temperature for seed germination is 15°C, and the germination rate decreases with distance from this temperature, up or down. It is noted that the highest percentage of seed germination occurs in a medium completely free of salts, and an increase in the percentage of sodium chloride is accompanied by a decrease in the percentage of Germination gradually.

Eruca vesicaria (L.) Cav.

Brassica vesicaria L., Eruca sativa subsp. vesicaria (L.) Jahandiez & Maire
Velleruca longistyla Pomel, Eruca sativa var. vesicaria (L.) Coss., Euzomum vesicarium (L.) Link, Raphanus vesicarius (L.) Crantz.

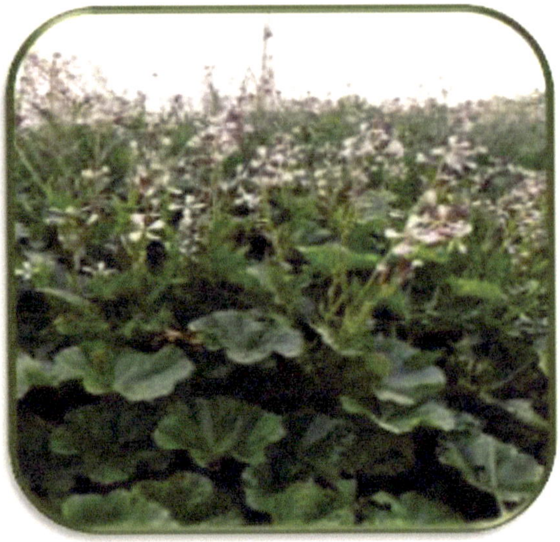

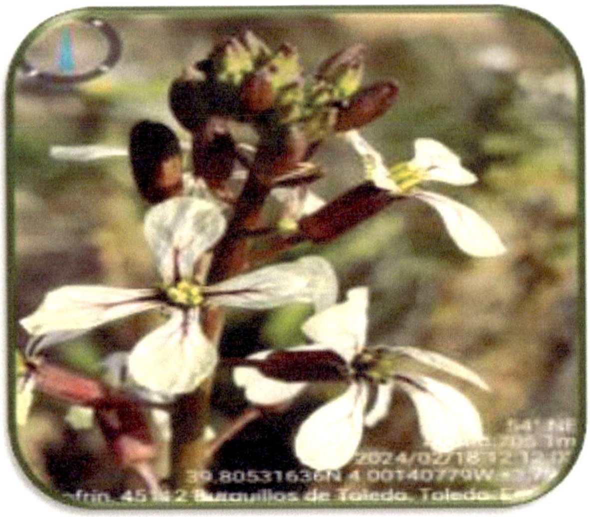

Family: Brassicaceae (Cruciferae)
Common names: Rocket
Foreign names: Roquette, Salad, Rocket Arugula, Rocket, Garden Eng. jardins de Roquette Fr.

Occurrences : 20,364 occurrences

Distribution in the world

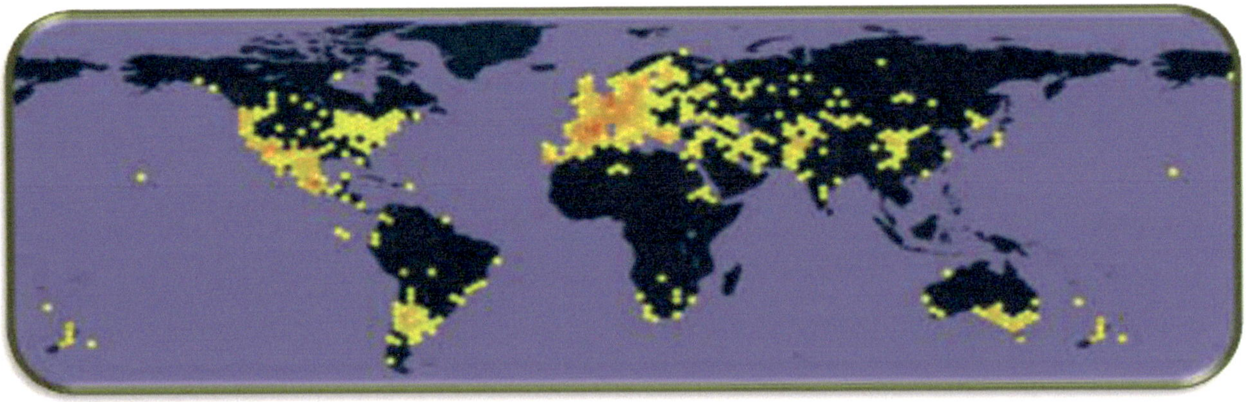

Botanical description:

Annual herb, 20-90 cm tall, usually single-stemmed, covered with hairs to varying degrees. Basal leaves are rosette-shaped, obtuse, lobed, terminal leaf larger. Lower stem leaves, upper leaves smaller, all somewhat fleshy. Inflorescence is clustered, leafless, compact to varying degrees, but not comb-shaped. Flowers are short-stemmed, then elongate later in the fruit. Calyx 4-septate, free, 7-11 mm long, erect. Corolla 4-petaled, free, 15-22 mm long, yellowish-white, veined with violet, consisting of a blade and a pinnate. Male 6 stamens in two whorls (4+2) and of different lengths. Female bicarpelous, ovary superior, unicameral, later divided by a false septum into two chambers. The fruit is a mustard, erect, swollen, adheres to the stem to varying degrees, oblong to semi-elliptic in shape, circular to semi-square in cross-section, its apex ends abruptly in a strongly compressed, sword-shaped beak. The beak is leathery in texture, rounded at the apex, semi-boat-shaped. The seeds are arranged in two rows, compressed, brown, with a reticulate surface.

Flowering: December to June.

Home and geographical distribution:

Mediterranean, Iranian-Turanian, spread in Syria, Palestine, Jordan and Lebanon, and cultivated in many countries of the world.

History and heritage:

The scientific name of the genus is the old Latin name for this plant. Watercress has been used since the Roman era in Italy, where raw watercress was added to salads. Arabs also knew the benefits of watercress since ancient times, and used it as an appetite stimulant and diuretic, and in treating burns and skin diseases.

Part used: Seeds, leaves.

Chemical components:

The seeds contain sulfur glycoside glucoerucin, which is hydrolyzed in the presence of the enzyme myrosinase and water, producing a volatile sulfur oil with a strong odor (irritating to the respiratory membranes.) 2.5% fatty oil, high percentage of vitamin C. The leaves contain sulfur glycoside similar to that found in the seeds. 100 grams of rocket contains 0.7 g fat, 3.7 g carbohydrates, 27 mg sodium, 2.6 g protein. It also contains calcium, iron, potassium, magnesium, vitamins A, C, K and folic acid. A study of the chemical composition and biological effectiveness of the essential oils of watercress (leaves, flowers, stems and roots) showed the presence of erucin isothiocyanate-4 methylthiobutyl at a rate ranging from 17.9% (leaves) to 98.5% (roots).

Properties and medical uses:

The seed powder has antioxidant and antibacterial properties. The leaves are popularly used for their appetite stimulant, expectorant, digestive, sugar-lowering and diuretic properties. It is also used to treat scurvy. It is used topically as a skin reddening agent, encourages hair growth, and is useful in treating burns.

The leaves are diuretic and stomach stimulant. The seed is stimulant. The dried seeds have antibacterial activity and have inhibitory properties for alpha-amyase and alpha-glucosidase enzymes. Watercress is rich in antioxidants and contains glucosinolates, which give it its bitter taste and strong smell, which protects the body from some types of cancer, including breast, prostate, lung and colon cancer. It contains a large amount of vitamin K and may help reduce osteoporosis.

Food uses:

The leaves are eaten raw, and a edible oil is extracted from the seeds, used as a substitute for turnip seed oil. The remains of the seeds after extracting the volatile and fatty oil are useful in the manufacture of mustard, which is known for its sharp smell. The flowers and young leaves are used as a seasoning in preparing salads.

Use warnings:

Attention should be paid to its irritating properties for the respiratory membranes.

Environment:

Cress grows wild in agricultural lands, fields, and on the banks of clean watercourses and streams in dry and semi-dry areas with moderate temperatures. The appropriate temperatures for vegetative growth range between 20 and 27 °C, noting that it can tolerate a temperature drop of up to -3.9 °C. Watercress needs full light in the early stages of growth, while it needs relative shade in the middle of the day when planted in the hot summer. The plant's ability to tolerate drought is weak, as it requires regular irrigation with clean water. It is planted in all types of soil, even poor ones, and gives good production in soils of medium fertility.

Cultivation and productivity:

It is propagated by seeds that are planted in early spring or autumn in rows or rows within basins. It is preferable to cover them immediately after planting with a thin layer of fine soil, and irrigate them immediately. Irrigation continues after germination at a rate of once every 10 days. The seeds begin to germinate at a temperature of 3-4°C and their germination is slow at this temperature, but it accelerates at a temperature of 18-20°C and is completed within 5-6 days. The plant needs organic and nitrogen fertilization in particular, as well as weeding and weeding.

Lepidium sativum L.

Cardamon sativum (L.) Fourr., Lepia sativa (L.) Desv., Nasturtium sativum (L.) Moench, Thlaspi sativum (L.) Crantz, Thlaspidium sativum (L.) Spach.

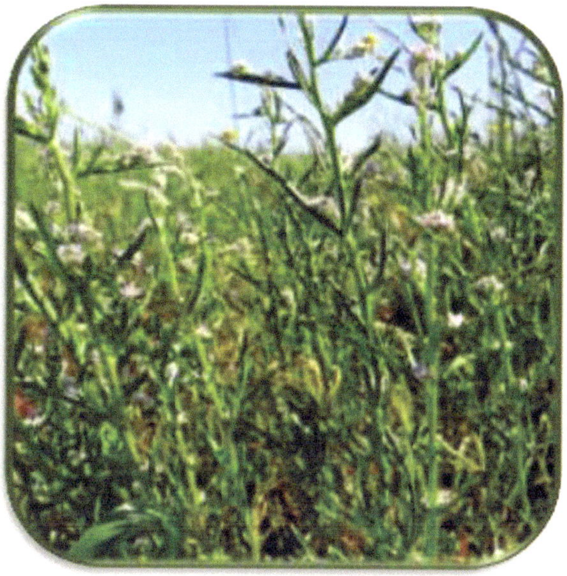

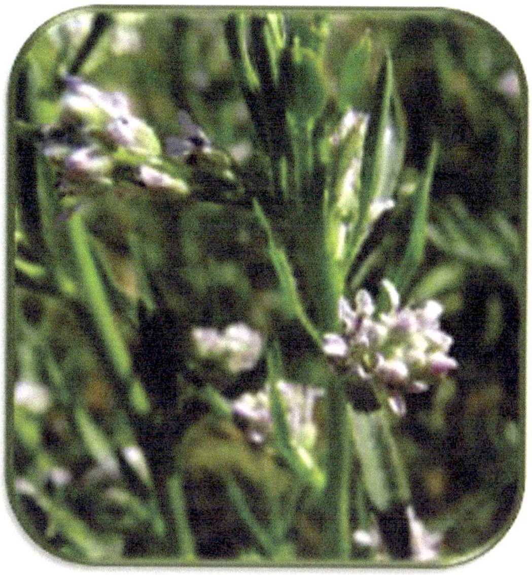

Family: Brassicaceae (Cruciferae)

Common names: Letter, Cress, Qarnoush

Foreign names: Garden Cress, Fr. Resson olenoise

Occurrences : 8,102 occurrences

Distribution in the world

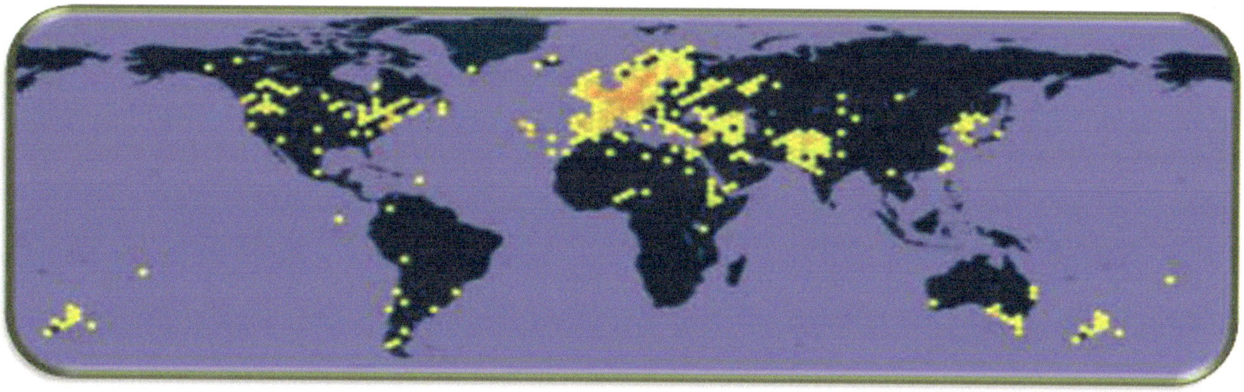

Botanical description:

Annual herb, glabrous, 25-60 cm high. Stem erect, branched. Lower leaves are pinnate, pinnately divided once or twice into irregular lobes. Stem leaves short, pinnate or sessile, upper entire, linear. Inflorescence Cluster, axillary and terminal. Flowers small about 2 mm, white. Calyx Its length is half that of the petals, A hair. The fruiting shamrock is erect, shorter than the fruit. The fruit is a mustard, its dimensions are 4-6 × 5-3 mm, ellipsoid to round, bare, the two valves are clearly winged;

The wing widens towards the apex to form a narrow pocket shorter than or equal to the pen. There is one seed in each chamber.

Flowering: March to May.

Habitat and geographical distribution:

Multi-regional in temperate and subtropical regions. It has spread to many regions of the world, and is widely cultivated.

History and Heritage:

The scientific name of the genus is a diminutive of the Greek word lepis, meaning "scale", alluding to the shape of the scallops, which is the ancient name for these plants. The descriptive name of the plant "sativum" means "planted." Watercress has been used since ancient times as an appetite stimulant and digestive, mentioned by Al-Antaki and Ibn al-Baytar, and Ibn Sina mentioned from Dioscorides that the best letter is the Babylonian red, and its strength is similar to that of mustard and radish seeds.

The presence of benzyl cyanide and benzyl isothiocyanate was detected. LC-MS results of the extracts of garden cress showed the presence of luteolin, quercetin, 7-hydroxy-4-, 6-,5-trimethoxyisofaphone, chlorogenic acid, sinapic acid, ascorbic acid, para-coumaric acid, 6-prenylnaringin.

Properties and medical uses:

Grass is widely used in folk medicine to treat respiratory tract disorders such as asthma, bronchitis and cough. The plant has antibacterial properties (depending on the age of the plant used). It has also been proven in experiments on mice to have an antiviral effect (against the encephalitis virus (SH)). The herb is popularly used for its appetite stimulant, digestive, vitamin C deficiency, expelling intestinal parasites, treating coughs, colds and chest diseases, and as a diuretic. The decoction of the seeds is used to treat diarrhea and skin diseases. The juice of the leaves is used topically to strengthen and activate hair follicles and stop hair loss. The paste of the leaves is used as a compress to treat Skin infections, ulcers, abscesses, hemorrhoids, eczema, spots and melasma on the face. The aqueous extract of the seeds is effective in reducing blood pressure and increasing water excretion, without any effect on the normal blood pressure or heart rate. Many studies have shown that garden cress extract is effective against bacterial strains and pathogens. Many preclinical studies using different parts of the garden cress have shown its potential in alleviating various disorders and improving health (such as antimicrobial, antioxidant, anticancer, antidiabetic, asthmatic and many other preventive activities.)

Precautions for use:

The plant should be taken as a fresh herb in oral preparations.

Garden cress should not be used by people with stomach allergies, indigestion and weak urinary tract. Large doses of mustard oil can cause skin blisters and necrosis.

Environment:

Grows wild in fallow lands, the edges of cultivated fields, the banks of irrigation canals and wetlands. It thrives in most soils, and requires moist, partially shaded soils during the summer to avoid rapid flowering.

Cultivation and productivity:

Propagation by seeds and cuttings. The soil is prepared for planting, and the land is divided into rows or lines. The seeds are scattered on the surface of the soil, and are not covered with soil, but are pressed with a piece of wood, then watered moderately. Planting is done at the beginning of spring, and can be done in batches at a rate of once every two or three weeks, so that the last crop is at the end of June. The seeds germinate in less than a week. The plant grows quickly, and mowing begins about 2-3 weeks after planting. Mowing is done at a height of 6-8 cm.

Nasturtium officinale R.Br.

Arabis nasturtium Clairv., Baeumerta nasturtium G.Gaertn., B.Mey. & Scherb.

,Cardamine aquatica Nieuwl., Cardamine fontana Lam.,Cardamine nasturtium Kuntze.,Cardamine nasturtium-aquaticum Borbás., Cardaminum nasturtium Moench, Crucifera fontana E.H.L.Krause., Nasturtium aquaticum Wahlenb.

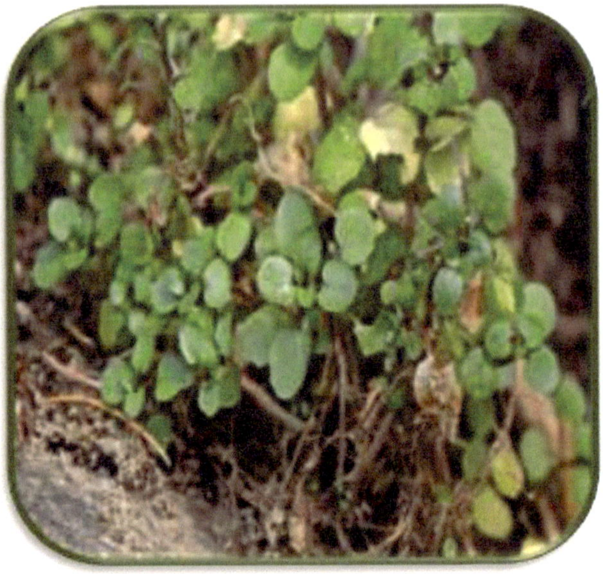

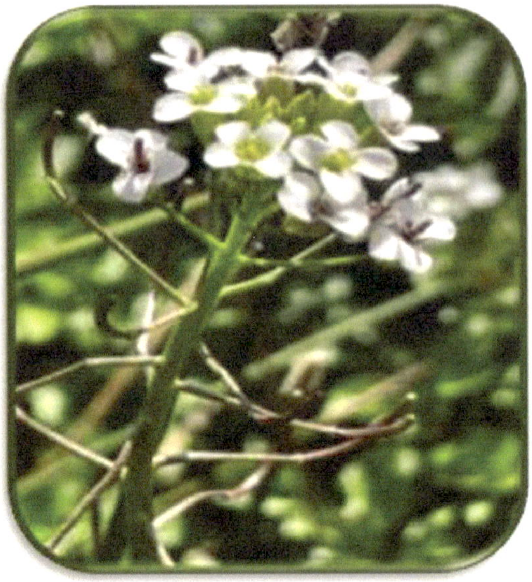

Family: Brassicaceae (Cruciferae)

Common names: Watercress, Qurat al-Ain, Harf, Nasturtium, Pasha's Tartur, Cress

Foreign names: Water cress, Fr. Cresson de fontaine

Occurrences : 105,966 occurrences

Distribution in the world

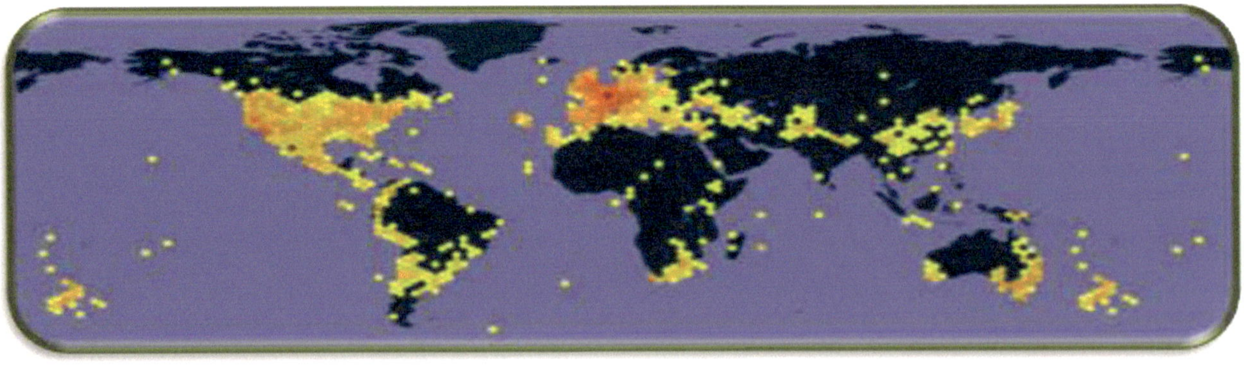

Botanical description:

A perennial, bare herb, 15-70 cm high. The stem is hollow, angular, spreads over the ground, and produces adventitious roots. Leaves Astringent, composed of 3-7 pairs of leaflets, 4-18 cm long; the lateral leaflets are oval or Pinate compound Elliptical in shape, and the leaflet The terminal ovate to ovate, all wavy to serrated, the peduncle fleshy and thick. The inflorescence is racemose. The sepals

4, linear, about 2 mm long. The petals 4, twice as long as the sepals, white. The fruit is mustard, oblong-linear, often arched, 1-3 cm long, 1-2 mm wide, its stalks horizontal or slightly drooping, the peduncle clearly shows the median nerve, while the lateral nerves are not clear. The seeds are ovate, Brown, pitted, arranged in two rows within each chamber.

Flower: From February to September.

Habitat and geographical distribution:

Grows in Europe, the Mediterranean Basin and Western Asia, has become widespread worldwide.

History and Heritage:

The scientific name of the genus is derived from the Latin nasus meaning "nose", and torque, meaning "I kill", referring to the spicy taste of this plant and the strong smell of its flowers. It was called "body health" due to its properties as a tonic, appetite stimulant, and anti-anemia and scurvy. The plant was traditionally eaten as a vegetable or salad, and the leaves were widely used as a blood purifier, diuretic, expectorant, blood sugar and lipid lowering agent, and to treat lung diseases, high blood pressure, and heart and blood vessel diseases. It was also used to treat stomach pain, as an anti-ulcer, and in the treatment of scurvy, tuberculosis, bronchitis, influenza, and asthma.

Part used: The tender flowering aerial parts.

Chemical components:

The flowering plant contains thioglucosides (0.9% of the wet weight), the most important of which are: gluconasturtiin, which decomposes by enzymatic hydrolysis to give a volatile, pungent-tasting sulfur compound (mustard oil), ethyl phenyl isothiocyanate (PEITC), which is an anticarcinogenic agent, and glucotropaeolin, and other sulfur compounds. Flavonoids, mineral salts, iron, calcium, magnesium, zinc, and many important vitamins, especially vitamin C and the precursor to vitamin A and B. Sugars 2%, proteins 1.5%, amino acids, especially lysine, fats 0.3%, and fibers 2%. Chemical analysis of the plant showed the presence of alkaloids, flavonoids, saponins, terpenoids, protein, essential and volatile oils, tannins, folic acid, vitamins C, A, E, and K, iodine, iron, potassium, and sodium. Calcium and Copper.

Properties and medical uses:

The plant is traditionally used fresh and cooked as food and for medical purposes such as respiratory diseases. The freshly harvested plant is used, because the dried plant loses its ivory properties. It is added to foods, appetizers and types of salads in the form of fresh green leaves, as they are appetizing and digestive.

The plant has the characteristic of external and internal use according to the type of disease and treatment. It is used to treat bronchitis and cough. The decoction of the leaves, rich in iron and vitamins, is used in cases of anemia, treating scurvy, getting rid of kidney stones, and reducing liver disorders. The juice of the leaves is used for its diuretic properties, antibacterial (gingivitis, tuberculosis bacilli), treatment of tumors, detoxification of the body, expelling worms and internal parasites, and lowering blood sugar levels. The decoction of the leaves is used topically in the form of compresses to treat skin ulcers, rheumatism, gout, and arthritis, and as a rub on the scalp to strengthen hair follicles and reduce hair loss.

Warnings for use:

High doses of mustard oil or the young plant cause irritation to the mucous membranes. It is not used in cases of stomach and intestinal ulcers and kidney infections. It is not recommended for pregnant women and children.

Environment:

Cress grows on the sides of streams and canals, and in shallow, slow-flowing water. It can be grown in moist soils if it is provided with suitable lighting and temperature conditions. It tolerates low temperatures but prefers moderate winters. The plant is sensitive to pollution, so it needs clean water.

Cultivation and productivity:

Giving new roots on the leaf nodes, which a fast-growing plant, its stems grow on the ground or float on the water Makes the plant easy to propagate vegetatively. It can also be propagated by seeds near lakes and water bodies. Plants are harvested 40-45 days after planting.

Boswellia sacra Flueck.

Boswellia carteri Birdwood, Boswellia bhaw-dajiana Birdw., Boswellia undulatocrenata Engl.

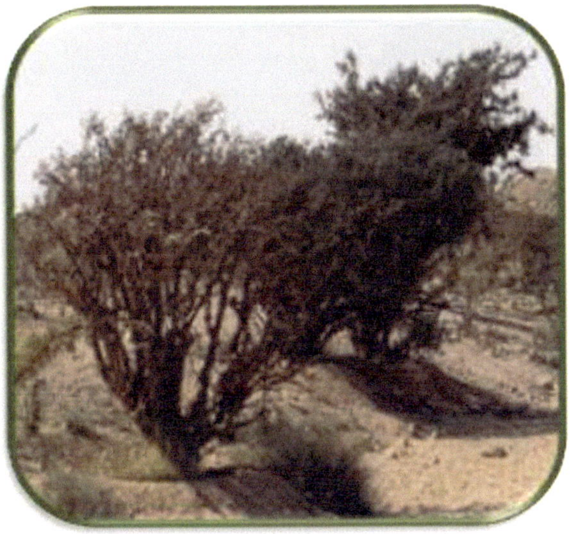

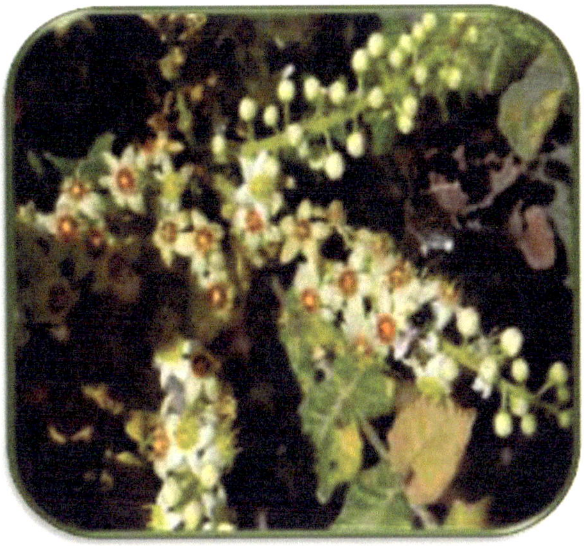

Family: Burseraceae

Common names: Frankincense, Frankincense, Bastaj, Roller.

Foreign names: Eng.Oliban, Olibanum, Fr. arbre à encens

Occurrences : 258 occurrences

Distribution in the world

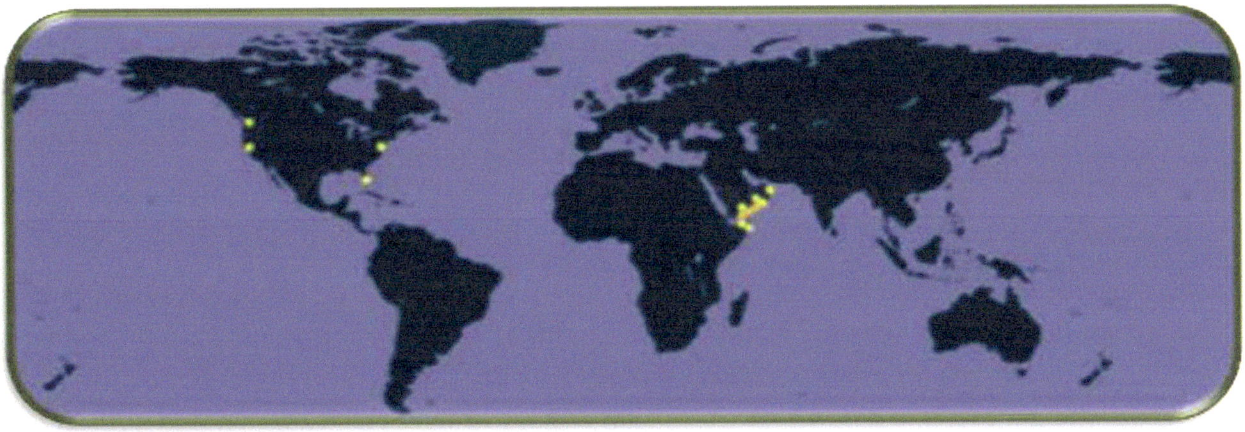

Botanical description:

A small tree, deciduous, 2-8 m tall, with one or more trunks, dense branches. It is noted that in trees that grow singly on steep slopes, the base of the trunk grows in the form of a cushion, sticking to the rocks, and contributing to the stability of the tree. The bark has a papery structure that barks off easily. Leaves are compound, pinnate, alternate, gathered in bunches at the ends of the branches. Leaflets are alternate, petiolate, 6-8 pairs, oblong, to crenulate in shape, wavy at the edge, 15-40 mm long, 8-

20 mm wide. Flowers are small, yellowish-white, gathered in racemose inflorescences in the leaf axils, about 10 cm long. Calyx is composed of 5 teeth, about 2 mm long. Corolla is 5 petals, 3-4 mm long. Male 10 stamens. Ovary surrounded by a fleshy disc. Fruit is a capsule, inverted oval, about 1 cm long, with 3-5 angles or wings in section, and opens into 3-5 sections, each containing a single seed.

Flowering: September to November.

Habitat and geographical distribution:

Southern Arabian Peninsula (Yemen and Sultanate of Oman in particular), along the northeastern coast of Somalia, and in India.

History and Heritage:

The scientific name of the genus Boswellia is derived from the name of John Boswell, and the species name sacra is from the Latin cra, crum meaning "pure" or "holy." It is called the sacred tree, because of its religious uses, mentioned in the Bible, and it is believed that the name frankincense came from milk (tree milk) or what is sometimes called bitter gum, which is a type of tree gum like frankincense, chewed and sometimes used as incense due to its sweet smell. Frankincense has been known since pre-Christian times. The Arabian Peninsula was once the only source of frankincense, and ancient civilizations such as ancient Yemen and the Nabataeans relied on its trade. It is believed that the center of the frankincense trade was the "lost" city of Iram of the Pillars in the southern Arabian Peninsula. The frankincense trade was linked to the Incense Route, a trade route linking India to the Arabian Peninsula and Egypt. The ancient records concerned with collecting and trading it were surrounded by many legends, and its use was linked to many religious rituals and medicines among many peoples, such as the ancient Egyptians. Greek and Roman doctors used frankincense to treat a large number of diseases, and the prices of frankincense in the markets of the Roman Empire were sometimes equal to the prices of gold. The therapeutic methods that depend on frankincense were mentioned in Syriac medical books, in medical texts that Muslim doctors relied on in the Middle Ages, and in Indian and Chinese medical manuscripts. Some people mistakenly call it male frankincense and female frankincense, which are scientifically incorrect names, because the flowers of the frankincense tree carry both the feminine and masculine organs (hermaphrodite).

The part used:

Frankincense, which is a resinous gum secreted by the bark of the tree trunk after it is cut. It has a distinctive smell and a bitter taste. Frankincense is classified according to color, purity, time of collection, and the place where the frankincense tree grows. The farther the tree is from the area where rainfall falls, the more it produces. Where quantity and type are better, milk that is white with a bluish tinge and free of impurities is considered the best and most expensive type of milk, and the quality decreases the more the color of the milk tends to red or is mixed with other impurities.

Chemical components:

Milk is composed of a homogeneous mixture of resin, gum, and volatile oil (60%), of which resins are soluble in water (the resin is in the form of a milky liquid before it hardens when exposed to air), 25% of which is gum containing boswellic acids (which has antimicrobial properties), 10-15%

volatile oil, the most important of which are monoterpenes, of which: 50% alpha-pinen, 20% limonene, and 4% sabinen. 4% myrcèn, phellandren, etc. Omani frankincense is characterized by its high content of volatile oil, reaching 15%, in addition to a high percentage of gum, and it is also characterized by the absence of the incensole compound in the volatile oil.

Properties and medical uses:

Boswellic acid is highly effective in treating asthma, rheumatism, arthritis, lowering blood fats, and reducing some types of blood cancer such as leukemia. It has also been shown to be a pain reliever, strengthens the body's immune system, enhances liver activity, and is a useful anti-inflammatory in treating coughs, bronchitis, and sinusitis. It is also used in treating colitis. Mucous ulcers, eye and gum inflammation. The essential oil has antiseptic properties for the respiratory system, and is used as a topical massage to treat rheumatism and joints, and to treat external wounds. It is a carminative and diuretic. Frankincense is popularly used to remove phlegm (expectorant), relieve abdominal and chest pain, and treat eye inflammation. It is also used as an antitoxin, and helps heal fractures in the form of plasters and waxes. Frankincense is a new candidate for treating degenerative diseases Neurological, Alzheimer's disease, and milk extract has a therapeutic effect in type 2 diabetes (T2D), and a small to medium dose of milk extract may be useful in enhancing the adaptive immune response in mild to moderate symptoms of COVID-19 virus infection. The promising effect of milk extract and boswellic acid B is attributed to their antioxidant, anti-inflammatory, immunomodulatory, cardioprotective, and antiplatelet aggregation activities. Antibacterial, antifungal and antiviral.

Other uses:

It is used in religious occasions as fragrant incense. The essential oils extracted from frankincense are used in the manufacture of perfumes and face and dry skin care creams.

Precautions for use:

Topical use of frankincense can cause skin irritation. Note: Frankincense may be adulterated with pine gum or gum arabic. Adulteration can be easily detected, as gum arabic does not ignite in fire, pine gum smokes and frankincense inflames.

Environment:

The frankincense tree grows in valleys, streams, rocky crevices, on the slopes of highlands and plateaus, and on low slopes in dry areas. It rarely grows in high areas with high atmospheric humidity. The tree's stem takes a cushion shape at the base of the trunk, which allows it to adhere to rocks and gives it greater stability. The tree tolerates the most difficult environmental conditions on rocky slopes and at altitudes of up to 1200 m.

Cultivation and productivity:

It is propagated by seeds. It was observed that the germination rate of seeds taken from trees that were severely wounded to produce frankincense is less than those taken from trees that were not wounded at all. However, the easiest method of propagation is woody cuttings, which root easily if suitable conditions are available. The tree begins to produce frankincense at the age of 8 to 10 years. Frankincense is obtained by making a vertical wound on the stem with a sharp tool, about 10 cm wide, and the collection may continue for 3-4 months. The growth of the tree and the quantity and quality of the frankincense produced vary according to the conditions in which the tree grows. It is known that the frankincense trees found in the narrow valleys of the arid regions that lie beyond the range of the seasonal rains in the Dhofar region in the Sultanate of Oman produce the finest types of frankincense.

Commiphora myrrha (NEES) ENGL.

Balsamodendrum myrrha Nees)basionym(, C. molmol)Engl.(Engl.

C. myrrha var.molmol Engl., Balsamea myrrha Baill.

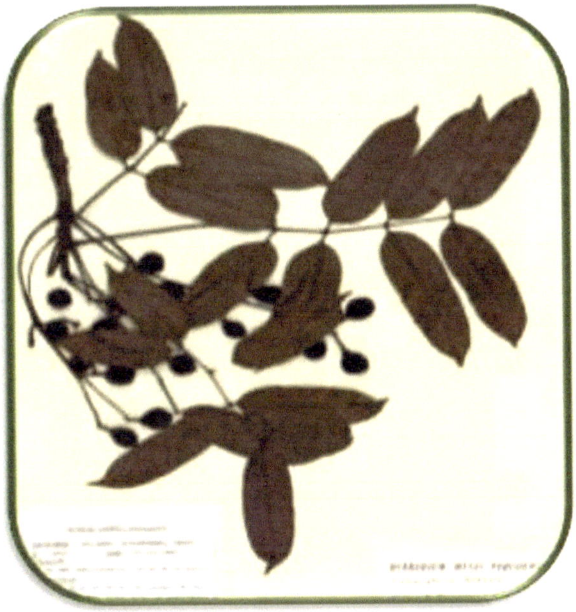

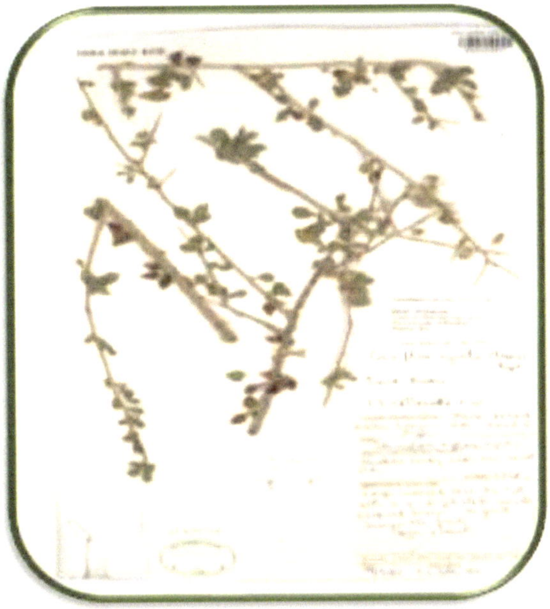

Family: Burseraceae

Common names: Myrrh, Myrrh, Ethiopian lock

Foreign names: Myrrhe Fr. Gum, Myrrh, Myrrh Eng.

Occurrences : 832 occurrences

Distribution in the world

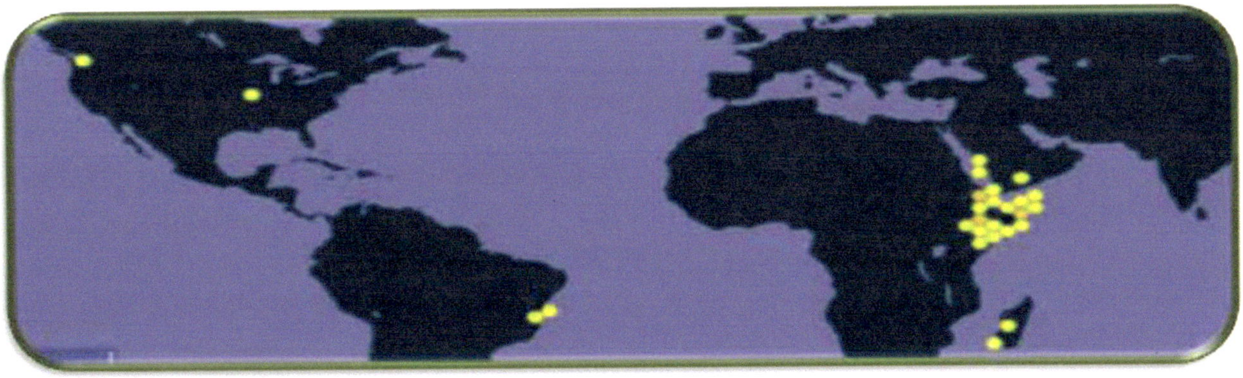

Botanical description:

A shrub or shrub, thorny, deciduous, 2.5-4 m tall. The bark barks off in silvery to white or gray plates. It is harvested from the bark of the branches when they are wounded, a thick, white-yellowish liquid, which turns into spherical, opaque, reddish-brown masses upon contact with the air. Leaves alternate, pinnate, compound of 1-3 leaflets of varying sizes, terminal leaflet larger, entire or serrated, lateral leaflets small, 2-3 mm wide, ovate, entire. Flowers in panicles of one or two flowers. Flowers are paniculate, 3 mm wide. Calyx 2.5-5 mm long. Petals white to dull brown or purple, 3-4 mm long. Male 8 stamens (4 long and 4 short). Fruit nuclear, compressed, oval to elliptic, blunt to sharp, thick, smooth.

Flowering: From March to June.

Habitat and geographical distribution:

It is spread in the southern Arabian Peninsula and eastern tropical Africa from the shores of Somalia, Eritrea, Ethiopia, Sudan, and Kenya.

History and Heritage:

The name of the genus Commiphora is derived from the Greek, where "kommi" means gum or "resin", and "phoros" means "bearer", mentioned by Nahal (2009) as "Kemphora" or "Balsan" and the first is an Arabization, as mentioned by Al-Shihabi (1982) as "Balsan", and some indicate that the name describing the species myrrha is from the Arabic: "Mur". A resin is extracted from the plant, known for thousands of years, and used to treat sore throats and gums, and it is a natural body perfume. Description The Greek physician Hippocrates (470-377 BC) described it as a balm for ulcers. The Pharaohs used it in mummification, and ancient Egyptian women burned it to repel household insects. It has been known since ancient times in Asia for its benefits and uses in treating wounds and other ailments. It has had a commercial status for more than a thousand years. Myrrh has been used in China, called "Mo Yao", since 600 BC, specifically to heal wounds.

Part used:

Myrrh (gum) is a resinous substance similar to frankincense or mastic beads, secreted by the stems of the plant after wounding them. Its consistency is thick, its color is light reddish brown, its smell is distinctive aromatic and its taste is pungent and bitter. Good gum is collected from myrrh directly from the tree trunk after it freezes. As for bad gum, it tends to be blackish brown in color, as a result of its age, or it appears as if it has sand in it, as a result of its collection after it flows into the sandy ground. Under the tree.

Chemical components:

Myrrh is composed of a homogeneous mixture of resin, gum and volatile oil resin - gum – Oleo Resin 25 – 40%: alpha-amyrenone alpha-amyrin, volatile oil 10-2%: It is mainly composed of monoterpene compounds and a half d-elemene, b-eudesmol, alpha-copaene, and monoterpene compounds and a half furanic compounds .curzenenone, furanoeudesma curzeren the most important of which, furanosesquiterpenes

Properties and medical uses:

The three elements of myrrh contribute to its therapeutic properties. The volatile oil and resins have antiseptic properties that are antibacterial, antifungal and antiviral. Its liquid preparations are used in the form of a diluted tincture or gargle in cases of inflammation of the tissues of the mouth, gums, and mucous membranes of the pharynx and bronchi. Myrrh tincture is used to treat athlete's foot (fungal growth between the toes). Myrrh has analgesic, astringent and antiseptic properties, and treats wounds, even infected ones, due to its volatile oil, which is rich in monoterpene compounds. Myrrh is popularly used as an appetite stimulant, digestive stimulant, and gas expeller. It is useful in cases of intestinal inflammation. In addition, taking myrrh capsules in cases of chronic respiratory inflammation accompanied by a lot of thick white mucus, as myrrh expels phlegm and dissolves mucus or sputum. Myrrh is used topically in the form of powder, tincture, or gargle liquid for its astringent and antiseptic effect in treating acne, skin infections, pimples, ulcers, anal wounds, hemorrhoids, gingivitis, rheumatism, and joint sprains. It is useful in treating schistosomiasis, diabetes (the aqueous resin solution has a direct stimulating effect on insulin), and stomach bloating.

Pharmaceutical forms:

Myrrh is available commercially either in its original form or as a volatile oil, capsules, dry powder or tincture.

Other uses:

Myrrh gum is used in the composition of many perfumes. Precautions for use: Myrrh is used internally with caution and under medical supervision, and it should not be overused because it causes problems in the colon. Myrrh gum should not be used during pregnancy, as it is a uterine astringent and may cause miscarriage. It is also not recommended to take myrrh gum for more than two weeks, as it may negatively affect the kidneys.

Environment:

The plant grows on the slopes of basalt rocks in high-temperature areas with an altitude ranging between 250 - 1300 m above sea level, and rainfall of 230 - 300 mm / year. Sensitive to frost. Does not like excessive humidity, as winters with heavy rains lead to rotting and death of trees.

Cultivation and productivity:

Propagated by seeds or cuttings. The branches give roots easily. They do not develop a main taproot, but a network of small roots, so they can be planted in containers successfully.

Opuntia ficus-indica (L.) Mill.

Cactus ficus-indica L., Cactus opuntia L., Opuntia ficus-barbarica A.Berge, Opuntia arcei Cárdena, Opuntia chinensis)Roxb.(K. Koch, Opuntia incarnadilla Griffiths, Opuntia vulgaris Mill.

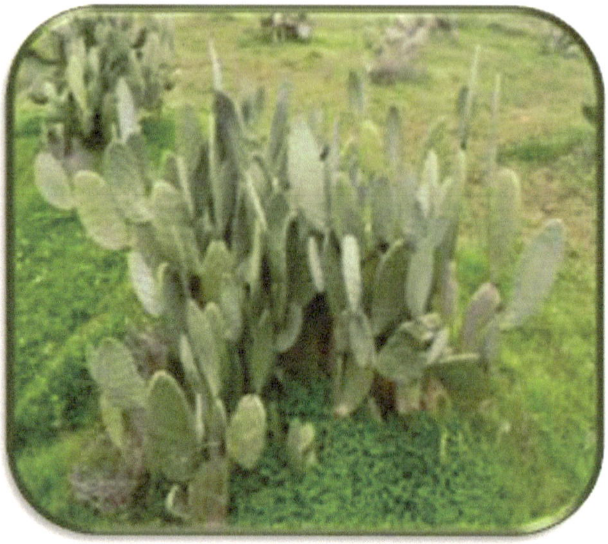

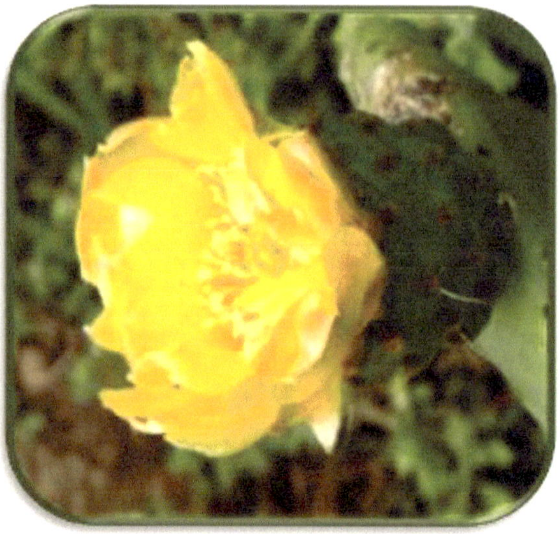

Family: Cactaceae

Common names: Cactus fig, prickly pear, cactus. Cactus Barbary

Foreign names: Eng. Prickly pears, Fr. figuier de Barbarie Foreign names:

Occurrences : 21,794 occurrences

Distribution in the world

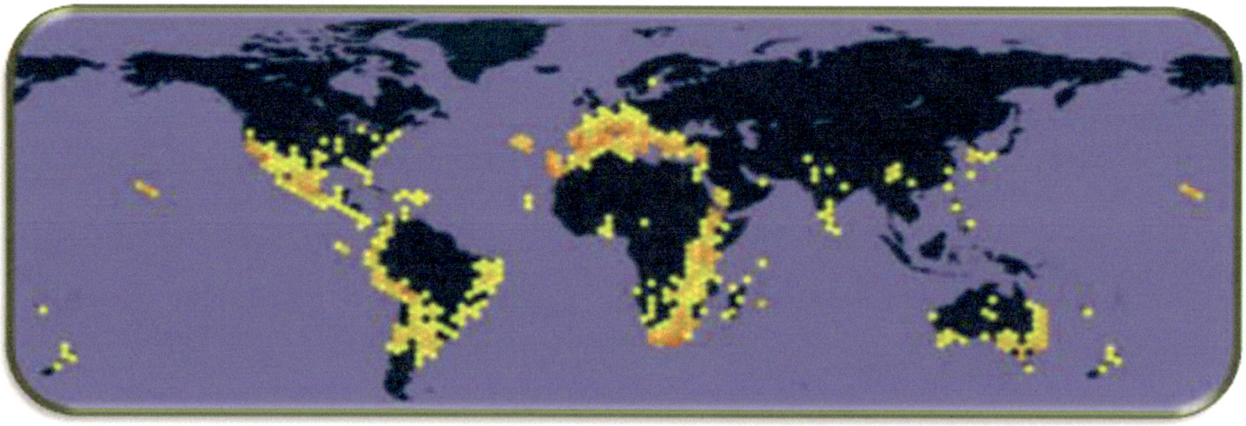

Botanical description:

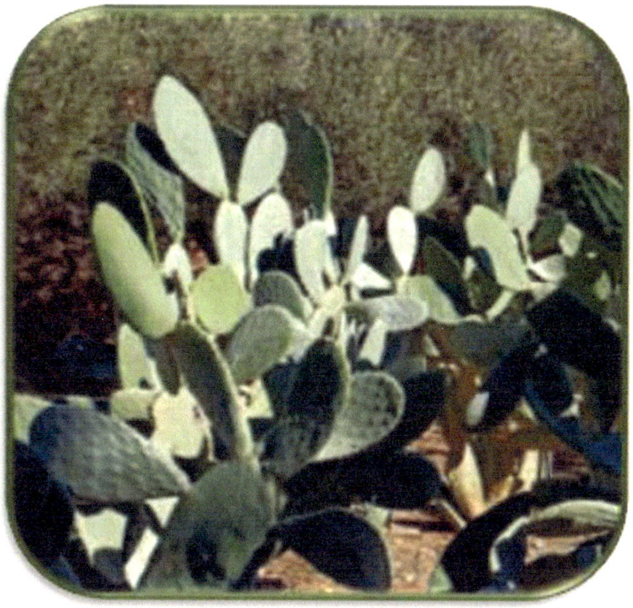

A shrub, which may reach several meters. The base of the old individual is woody, cylindrical to varying degrees, bearing a series of articulated plates that represent flat stems, each of which is tens of centimeters long, and has an oval to rectangular shape, with circular pads spread over its surface, from which emerge short and weak white or brown thorns and hairs, representing modified leaves, which are easy to separate from the plant and penetrate the skin. Flowers arranged in groups on the margin of the upper and upper lateral plates. The bracts are simple, composed of 8-10 or more segments, ovate to elliptic, 3-4 cm long, light yellow. Stamens are numerous, their anthers cylindrical. The style is thick, ending in several stigmas; the ovary has a thick outer wall, leathery to the touch, and bears a pad on its surface from which emerges thorny hairs, which continue to grow on the fruit. Fruit Sweet, eaten after barking.

Flowering: Late spring and early summer. Opuntia ficus-indica f. inermis is often grown, a cultivated form of the same species Opuntia ficus-indica f. Inermis

Homeland and geographical distribution:

Mexico, from where it was introduced to southern Europe, Africa, the Middle East, and India, and is cultivated in most Arab countries.

History and heritage:

The scientific name of the genus is derived from the name of an ancient city in Greece "Opus" or "Oponte." The descriptive name of the species "indica ficus" means "fig of India." The plant has been used since ancient times as a barrier fence, due to its highly palatable edible fruits.

Part used: Fruits, stems (plates).

Chemical components:

The ripe prickly pear fruit contains 14% of its weight as sugars, 1.5% as proteins, and a high percentage of vitamins A and E (alpha and beta tocopherol a-Tocopherol, β-Tocopherol), vitamin K, and vitamin C (25-30 mg per 100 g), as well as selenium and organic acids, the most important of which are glutamic acid, citric acid, malic acid, oxalic acid, and mineral salts: magnesium, sodium, potassium, calcium, and manganese. Iron Zinc, copper and phosphorus. The seeds contain 3-10% protein and 6-13% fatty acids, mainly linoleic acid. The red color of the fruits and juice is due to the presence of vacuolar pigments: betalains (betanin and indicanthin) which are antioxidants. Betalains are vacuolar pigments that include two classes of compounds: betacyanins (red-violet) and betaxanthins (yellow). The fruits contain flavonoids, such as: quercetin, isoramentin and campherol. The bark extract contains phenols.

The gum of the tablets provides many nutritional benefits (polysaccharides: arabinose, galactose, galacturonic acid, rhamnose, and xylose. It contains uronic acid at a rate of 10%). The juice of the fruits and barks contain many phenolic compounds: (hydroxycinnamic acids, hydroxybenzoic acids), flavonoids, lignin, and stilbenes.

Properties and medical uses:

Prickly pear has digestive properties, especially for fatty substances, stimulating, laxative, and cleansing the digestive system. Eating ripe prickly pear fruits is the best way to Prevention and treatment of indigestion and constipation. Studies have shown the positive effects of eating prickly pear fruits in combating cramps, dysuria and dysentery. Ancient Arab doctors advised their obese patients to limit their diet to eating prickly pear fruits for the purpose of losing weight.

The ancient Arabs used the prickly pear stems to treat the respiratory system, especially whooping cough. The stems are used after being split lengthwise as compresses to treat back and spine pain. The stem extract is anti-cancer and anti-oxidant, and reduces blood glucose and cholesterol levels. The methanol and ethanol extracts of aloe vera stems and fruit barks showed antibacterial activity. The seed emulsion showed anti-oxidant and anti-inflammatory activity, and enhanced the skin's hydroxyproline content, collagen properties, and blood vessel formation. It helps accelerate the healing of skin injuries. The stem extract showed antibacterial activity against Gram-positive bacteria compared to Gram-negative bacteria.

Environment:

The plant grows in various types of soil. Unlike many plants, it needs irrigation during the flowering period. It can be grown in wet areas. It may turn into an invasive plant in some areas.

Cultivation and productivity:

It is propagated by seeds, but the most common is to propagate it vegetatively by means of its panels or parts thereof, especially the side panels close to the soil surface. It is preferable to expose the parts to be rooted to the sun for 7 to 15 days before placing them directly in the permanent soil, in holes 2-3 m apart, and in lines 3-4 m apart, and irrigated with limited amounts of water. It is easy to establish and requires only a few agricultural treatments. Its growth is relatively fast, achieving dense soil coverage that prevents it from being eroded by wind and rain.

Cannabis sativa var. indica.

Cannabis sativa L.

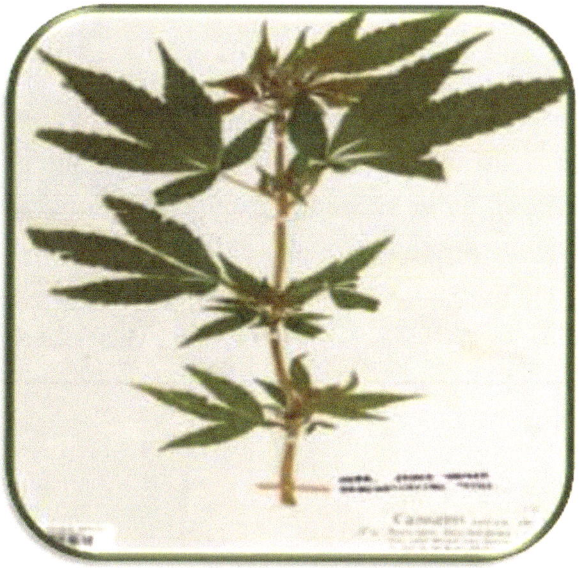

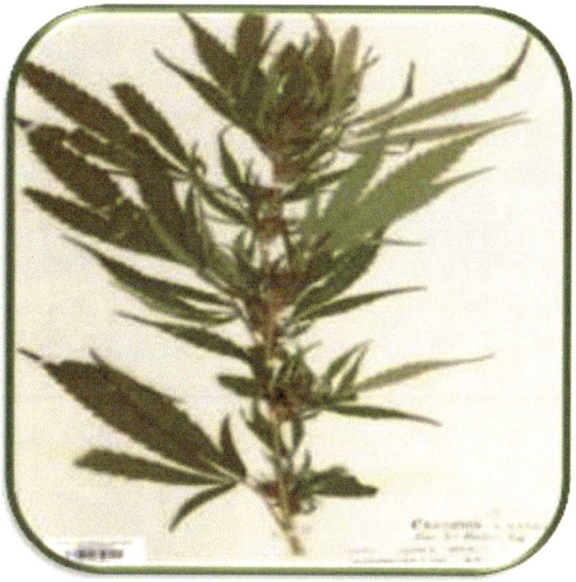

Family: Cannabinaceae

Common names: Marijuana, Hashish, Kif, Cannabis

Foreign names: Eng. Indian hemp, Marijuana, Fr. Chanvre indien

Occurrences : 33 occurrences

Distribution in the world

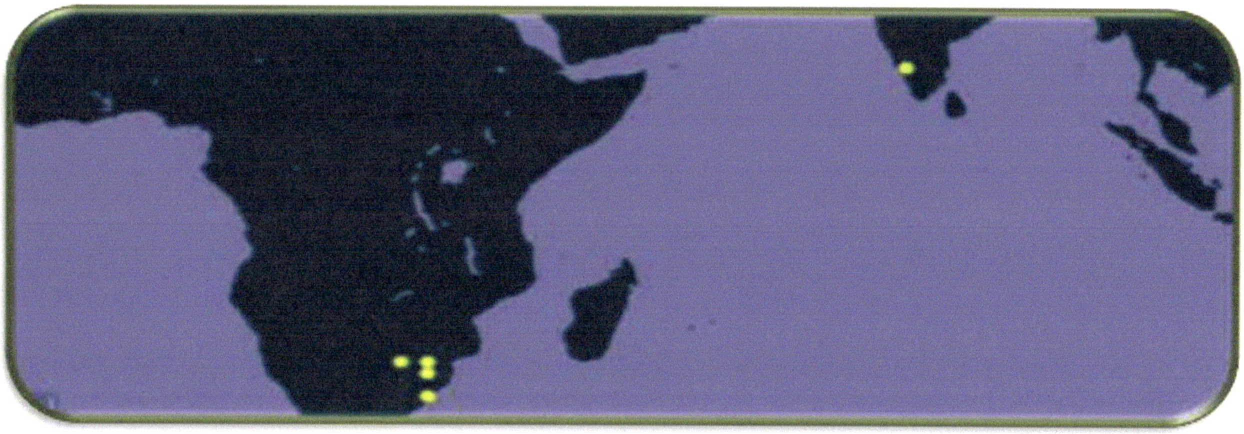

Botanical description:

Annual herbaceous plant, 75-200 cm tall. Stem erect, angular, covered with dense hairs. Leaves compound, palmate, consisting of 3-9 leaflets, spoons 2-8 cm. Leaves narrow lanceolate, serrated, apex pointed, 3-12 cm long, 3-15 mm wide, underside hairy and covered with resinous glands. Ears 4-6 mm long. Flowers unisexual, dioecious plant. Male flowers 4-6 mm, greenish, panicle 1-3 mm, gathered in paniculate inflorescences, petals 3-4 mm. Female flowers semi-subsistent, surrounded by leafy bracts, 4-13 mm long, covered with small glandular hairs, membranous bracts, folded at the base of the ovary, female bicarpal. (Male plant longer and stronger than female plant.) Fruit acorn, 3-4 mm in diameter, shiny, yellowish to brown, finely hairy to almost hairless, oval in shape.

Flowering: April to September.

There are two varieties belonging to the species. L sativa :Cannabis

The first is called fiber hemp: vulgaris var. sativa C., grown in temperate regions for its fibers and oil seeds. The second is called Indian hemp: indica var. sativa C., from which the drug known as "hashish" is extracted. It was known to the ancient Chinese, Indians, Mongols and Greeks, and was mentioned in ancient books. Homeland and geographical distribution: Central and Western Asia (the Caucasus, China, Iran and northern India), Indian hemp is grown illegally for use as a narcotic drug. Hemp fiber is grown in many countries of the world such as India, China, Japan, Russia, Korea, America, European countries (France, Romania, Bulgaria, Italy, Spain, Ukraine, Yugoslavia, Belgium) and North Africa, Iran, Turkey, and others.

History and heritage:

The scientific name for the genus kannabis comes from the name of the plant in Greek, and in Persian Kanb, and the word sativa means "cultivated", i.e. cultivated hemp.

It has been known in China since about 4000 BC. Marijuana is a Mexican term that was initially used to refer to cheap tobacco, but today it refers to the leaves and dried flowers of the cannabis plant.

Part used: The female flowering tops.

Chemical components:

Cannabinoid phenolic compounds: including cannabinol (inactive compound), tetrahydrocannabinol (physiologically active compound).

Non-cannabinoid phenols: spiroinane, dihydrostilben. Volatile oil -0.1 0.3%, rich in monoterpene and monoterpene (sesquiterpenes) such as β-caryophyllen, humulen, and caryophyllene oxide, α-pinene, β-pinene, limonene, and others. Alkaloids cannabisativin, cholin, and trigonelline. Flavonoids, including canniflavon. The fruits contain fatty substances (esters of unsaturated fatty acids), cannabinoids, and tetrahydrocannabinol. Cannabis can be classified into varieties based on the chemical content of the leaves of cannabidiol (CBD) and tetrahydrocannabinol (THC).

The first is called fiber hemp: vulgaris var. sativa C., grown in temperate regions for its fibers and oil seeds. The second is called Indian hemp: indica var. sativa C., from which the drug known as "hashish" is extracted. It was known to the ancient Chinese, Indians, Mongols and Greeks, and was mentioned in ancient books. Homeland and geographical distribution: Central and Western Asia (the Caucasus, China, Iran and northern India), Indian hemp is grown illegally for use as a narcotic drug. Hemp fiber is grown in many countries of the world such as India, China, Japan, Russia, Korea, America, European countries (France, Romania, Bulgaria, Italy, Spain, Ukraine, Yugoslavia, Belgium) and North Africa, Iran, Turkey, and others.

History and heritage:

The scientific name for the genus kannabis comes from the name of the plant in Greek, and in Persian Kanb, and the word sativa means "cultivated", i.e. cultivated hemp. It has been known in China since about 4000 BC. Marijuana is a Mexican term that was initially used to refer to cheap tobacco, but today it refers to the leaves and dried flowers of the cannabis plant.

Part used: The female flowering tops.

Chemical components:

Cannabinoid phenolic compounds: including cannabinol (inactive compound), tetrahydrocannabinol (physiologically active compound).

Non-cannabinoid phenols: spiroinane, dihydrostilben. Volatile oil -0.1 0.3%, rich in monoterpene and monoterpene (sesquiterpenes) such as β-caryophyllen, humulen, and caryophyllene oxide, α-pinene, β-pinene, limonene, and others. Alkaloids cannabisativin, cholin, and trigonelline. Flavonoids, including canniflavon. The fruits contain fatty substances (esters of unsaturated fatty acids), cannabinoids, and tetrahydrocannabinol. Cannabis can be classified into varieties based on the chemical content of the leaves of cannabidiol (CBD) and tetrahydrocannabinol (THC). Cannabidiol (CBD) is useful in a range of neurological and psychiatric disorders, including ASD Autism, psychosis, neuropathic pain, cancer pain, HIV, migraines, Huntington's disease and cerebral hypoxia. CBD oils have anti-insect effectiveness.

Side effects and warnings for use:

Severe addiction causes personality disorder, and cannabis that is traded illegally may be mixed with carcinogenic compounds and compounds Other very dangerous. Side effects of use in addition to addiction include dry mouth, skin irritation, headache, sensitivity, tachycardia, peripheral vasodilation, low blood pressure, vascular disturbance, low testosterone, and low sperm count. It is prohibited during pregnancy and lactation.

Environment:

This plant is a summer crop, tolerates temperature changes, and fears frost. Its cultivation is widespread in many environments, and is found in temperate climates Wet. Cannabis thrives in deep, moist, well-drained, fertile and non-acidic soils.

Cultivation and productivity:

Fiber hemp is grown for its fibers, which are used in a number of industries, and for its energy-rich seeds, which are used in bird feed, and in a number of medical and pharmaceutical industries. The plant is propagated by seeds, at a rate of 80-110 kg/ha. Cannabis is planted during the spring and early planting is preferred, when no frost is expected. Early planting helps in early harvest, weed resistance, and disease escape. Biotechnological research using plant tissue culture as a propagation system for cannabis and genetic engineering strategies for exploitation in the phytotherapy industries using medical cannabis strains has witnessed great activity in response to future demands for innovative cannabis products.

Herniaria hirsuta L.

Herniaria arenaria var. hirsuta)L.(Kuntze, Herniaria glabra var. hirsuta)L.(Kuntze, Herniaria vulgaris subsp. hirsuta)L.(Bonnier & Layens, Herniaria vulgaris var. hirsuta)L.(Griess., Paronychia hirsuta)L.(E.H.L.Krause.

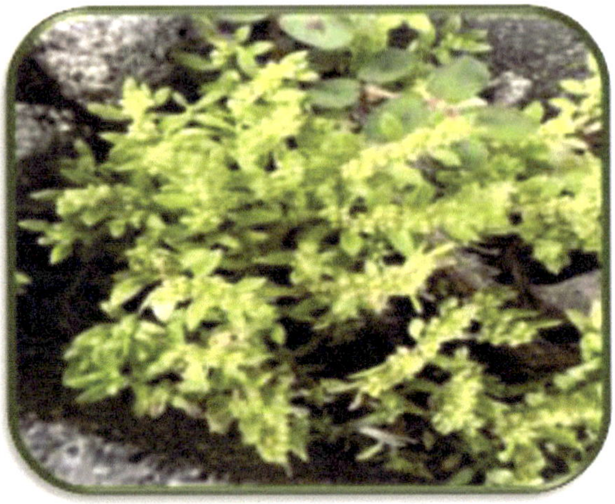

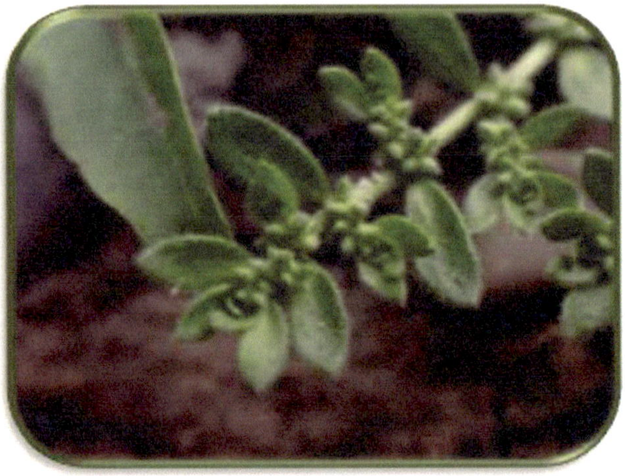

Family: Caryophyllaceae

Common names: Umm Labida, Umm Waj Kabd, Hernia weed, Nauman, Mokar, Suwaiqa

Foreign names: Fr. Turquette: , Hairyrupture wort Eng.

Occurrences : 16,098 occurrences

Distribution in the world

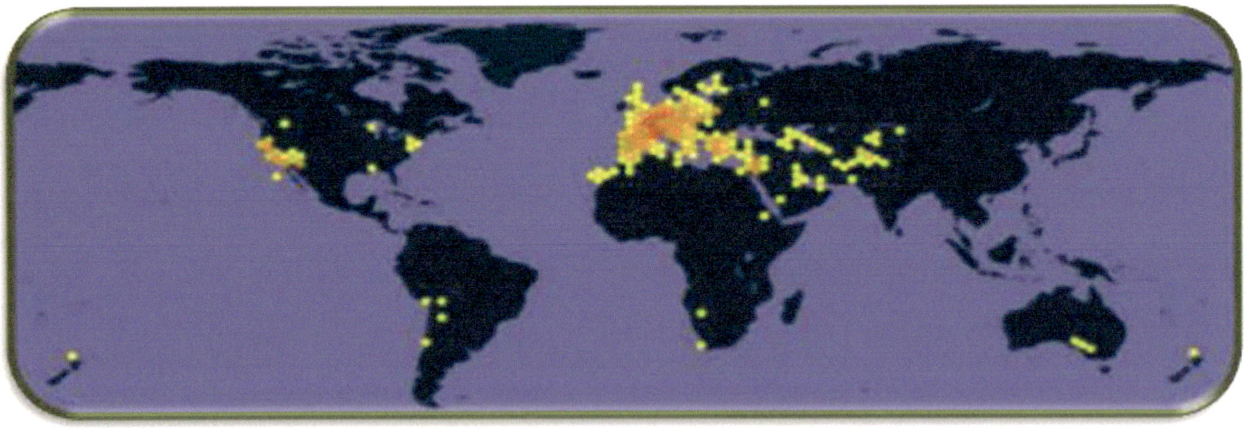

Botanical description:

An annual herb (sometimes tending to become perennial), covered with hairs, 4-15 cm tall. Stems are supine, sometimes growing in clusters. Leaves are simple, petiolate, 5-10 mm long, opposite lower ones, lanceolate-elliptic to oblong-linear, gradually tapering at the base, hairy at the edge. Ears and bracts are membranous, dry, fringed. Flowers are small, petiolate, gathered in what resembles capituli. Calyx 5, 1-2 mm long, oblong, covered with rough hairs Straight or hooked at the end, their length is almost equal to the width of the calyx. Petals 5, short, conical-filamentous. Stamens 5-2. Ovary monochambered and monoovule, ending in two stigmas. Fruit protuberant, sub-spherical, protruding from the calyx. Seeds spherical to lenticular, blackish, shiny.

Flowering: March to April.

Habitat and geographical distribution: Multi-regional.

History and heritage: The genus name is derived from the Greek hernia, meaning "hernia", alluding to its use in the past to treat hernia, and the species name hirsuta means "thorny", i.e. long and hard thorns.

Part used: Flowering plant

Chemical components: Triterpene saponins: nins saponins herniaria, containing in their structure the aglycones medicagenin, gypsogenin. The percentage of these compounds increases during the flowering period. Flavonoids include: hyperoside: hydroxycoumarins, umbelliferone, herniarin: 0.06% tannins, traces of volatile oil, and Paronychine alkaloid with a repulsive odor.

Medical properties and uses:

The plant has diuretic and antispasmodic properties due to its content of saponins, flavonoids, coumarins, and tannins. Research indicates the effectiveness of the plant extract in treating kidney, bladder and urinary tract infections, and reducing the formation of stones, by reducing the size and number of calcium oxalate crystals, and preventing their accumulation and adhesion to the epithelial cells of the kidney, thus facilitating their excretion through urine. The effectiveness of the plant extract in dissolving gallstones has also been proven. The decoction of the plant is popularly used as a mild astringent, in treating respiratory disorders, and in purifying the blood. The plant extract is used topically to treat neuritis, rheumatism, gout, wounds, pimples, skin ulcers, and to wash the eyes to clean and disinfect them. The aqueous extract of the plant can be used as an alternative to skin softening soap. The plant is used as an expectorant, is used to treat hernias, and has been used to accelerate ulcer healing. The ethanolic extract has antibacterial properties against Escherichia coli. The aqueous extract has significant antioxidant activity.

Environment:

The plant grows on the sides of roads, in fields and steppes in areas with semi-arid or arid climates. It likes sunny places in valleys with sandy loam soil, and on sandy slopes. It does not like excessive moisture, and grows well in gypsum soils, which it is an indicator of. It succeeds in poor soils.

Cultivation and productivity:

The plant is propagated by seeds. It is preferable to plant the seeds in bags or small pots under nursery conditions, and transfer them to the permanent ground after a year, at the beginning of spring.

Stellaria media (L.) VilL.

Alsine media L., Stellaria media subsp. typica Bég., Stellularia media)L.(Kuntze.

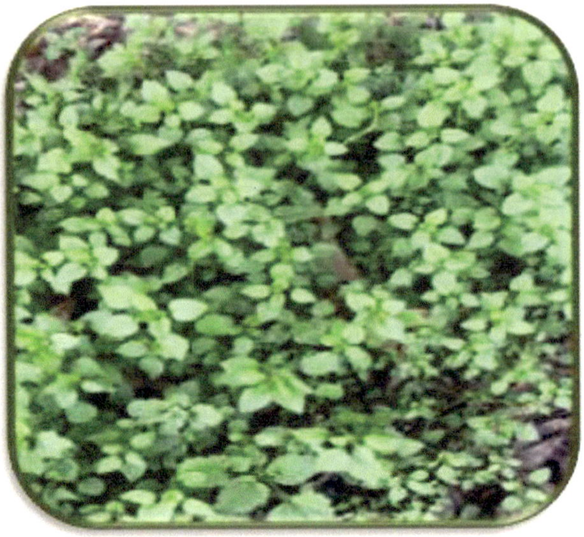

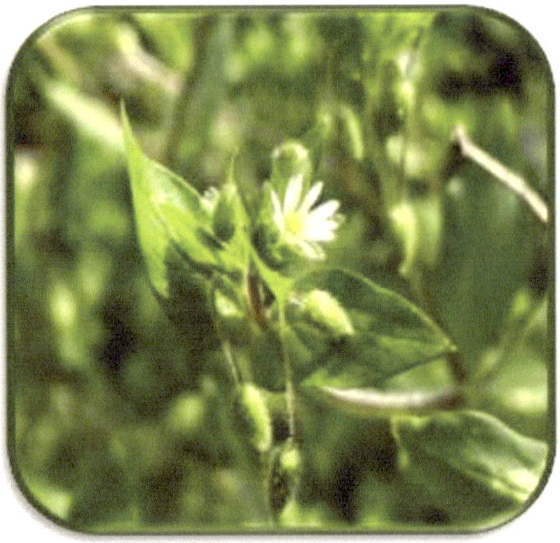

Family: Caryophyllaceae

Common names: Qazzaz weed, comb, rope, Qazzazah, star.

Foreign names: Stellaria Fr., Chichweed Eng.

Occurrences : 589,757 occurrences

Distribution in the world

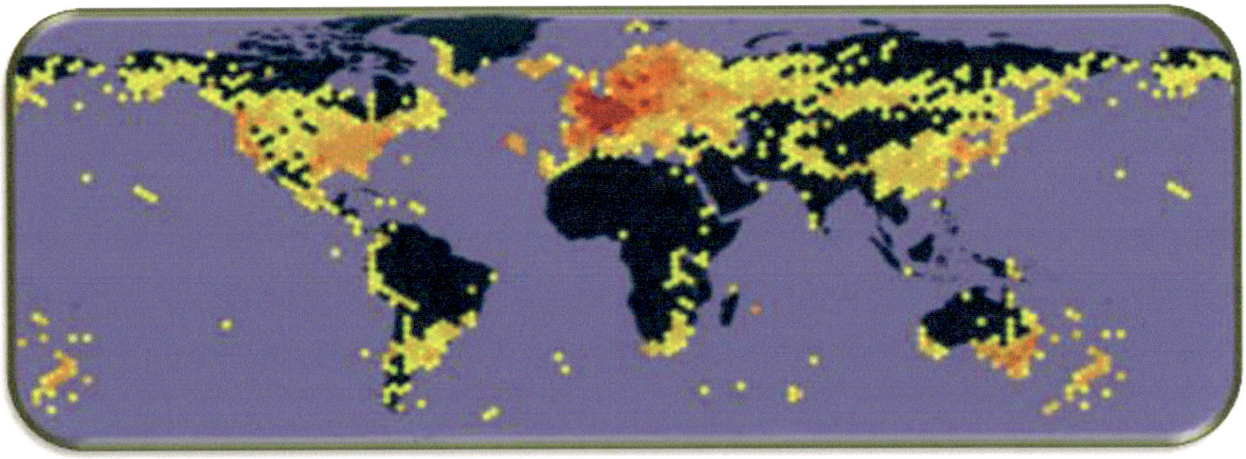

Botanical description:

Annual herb, 10-50 cm tall. Stems weak, lying or ascending, branched, glabrous to hairy or glandular, often bearing one or two lines of hairs. Leaves 0.6-3×6-1 cm, long-spined to petiolate, ovate to oblong to elliptical, glabrous or fringed.

Inflorescence semicyanotic, bifurcated. Sepals as long as calyx or longer, downy. Sepals 5, free, 2-7 mm long, ovate-lanceolate, margin white, downy to glabrous. Petals 5, longer or shorter than sepals, white, bilobed to sometimes bipartite. Stamens 3-5 (sometimes 5-10). Styles 3, very short, or up to 1.5 mm long. Fruit a capsule, larger than or equal to calyx. Seeds 0.7-1.4 mm, black to pale brown, with sharp or blunt tubercles on the surface.

Flowering: January to April.

Habitat and geographical distribution:

It is distributed in most parts of the world, and is cultivated in North America and Australia.

History and heritage:

The scientific name of the genus is derived from the Latin word "stella" meaning "star", referring to its petals arranged in a star shape, and media meaning "medium." The plant was given to birds as a tonic in the Middle Ages, and it was also collected as a type of vegetable.

Part used: Flowering aerial parts (collected from April to September.)

Chemical components:

Flavonoids: including rutin, ascorbic acid (vitamin C 0.1 – 0.15%), alkaloids. Chemical examination of aqueous, ethanolic, and methanolic extracts showed the presence of: alkaloids, saponins, cardiac glycosides, fatty acids, tannins, terpenoids, and phenolic compounds. The leaf extracts contain active flavonoids such as luteolin, vicenin, isoquercetin, genistein, and apigenin. Vanillic acid, caffeic acid, p-hy- droxybenzoic acid, chlorogenic acid, and ferulic acid were identified. Two triterpenoid saponins derived from aglycone were isolated: gypsogenin and oleanolic acid. Three metabolites were detected from the aerial parts: tetraterpenoid Tetramethyloctane, trimethyloctane, and heptyl-3′-hydroxy-2′6-methylpropanoate. These metabolites showed anti-obesity and anti-inflammatory activity. Several important compounds were identified in the plant leaf extract: methyl stearate, hexacosanyl palmitate, β-sitosterol, 6,7-dimethyl heptacosane, 3-methyl-6-hydroxy-heneicos-3-enyl acetate, tria-acid contanoic acid, tricontanol, hentriacontane and pentacosa-nol. Fresh and mature leaves contain a high percentage of ascorbic acid, carotenoids and tocopherol. It also contains important essential and non-essential amino acids such as glycine, alanine, lysine, thymine, uracil, aspartic acid, glutamic acid, serine, proline, thymidine, tyrosine, 2-histidine, g-aminobutyric acid and threonine. Phytochemical examination of the leaf extract revealed a high percentage of saponins. 1.19 (mg/g), phenol 45.5 (± 0.25 mg/g), and flavonoid 1.4 (mg/g). The main minerals in the plant: nickel, zinc, copper, sodium, cobalt, magnesium, lead, iron, manganese, cadmium and mercury.

Properties and medical uses:

The decoction of the plant is popularly used to treat rheumatism, gout, joint stiffness, tuberculosis and blood diseases. It is used topically in the form of compresses to treat skin diseases such as eczema, wounds and suppurations. It is used in the form of washes or baths to treat hemorrhoids and eye infections.

The biologically active metabolites have shown diverse pharmacological activities such as anti-obesity, anti-fungal, anti-bacterial, anti-oxidant, anti-proliferative, anti-inflammatory, anti-diabetic, and anti-anxiety. Different parts of the plant have been used to treat various digestive disorders, diarrhea, measles, jaundice, gastrointestinal and reproductive tract infections, respiratory tract infections and asthma. They also reduce swelling and are used as compresses for fractures. The isolated compounds have shown significant pharmacological activities such as anti-tumor and anti-cancer. In India, a decoction of the leaves is used to bandage deep wounds, stop bleeding and reduce swelling, and the ground leaves, stem and root are used as a plaster cast for dislocations and swelling. The decoction of the plant has unique moisturizing and soothing properties that encourage its use to relieve skin itching, menstrual pain and scabies. Flavonoids and beta-sitosterol compounds in the plant significantly inhibit the activity of lipase and amylase in mice and reduce total triglycerides and cholesterol.

Other uses: Its leaves and tender stems are consumed as salad.

Precautions for use: No accidents or side effects are known with the appropriate intake of the specified dose.

Environment:

The plant grows on walls and roadsides and in agricultural fields and humid places. It prefers moist soils in bright and semi-shaded places.

The plant grows and becomes strong in fertile soils, and blooms in poor soils when it is young. The plant grows up to 40 cm in moist, fertile soil rich in nitrogen, especially in meadows.

Cultivation and productivity:

An easy-to-cultivate plant, propagated by seeds that are scattered in early spring in basins isolated from neighboring fields so as not to invade agricultural lands. The seeds germinate and grow quickly, and require moderate humidity.

Catha edulis (Vahl) Endl.

Celastrus edulis Vahl, Catha forskalii A.Rich., Catha inermis J.F.Gmel., Celastrus tsaad Ferreira & Galeotti ex Walp., Dillonia abyssinica Sacleux.

Occurrences : 692 occurrences

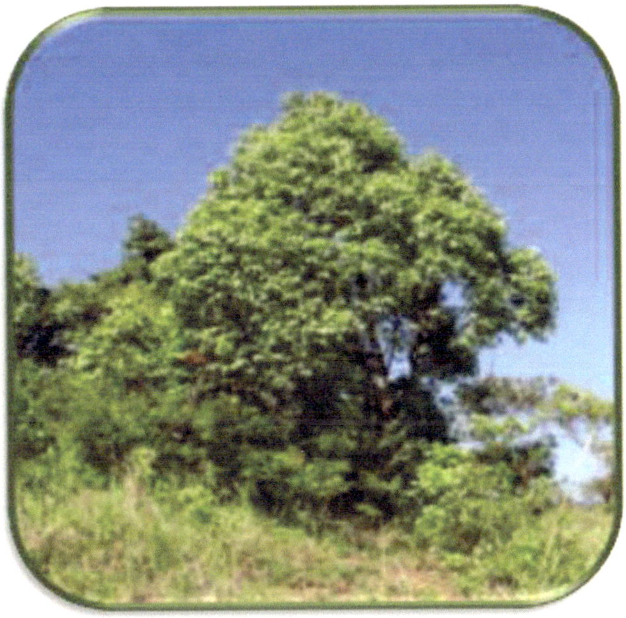

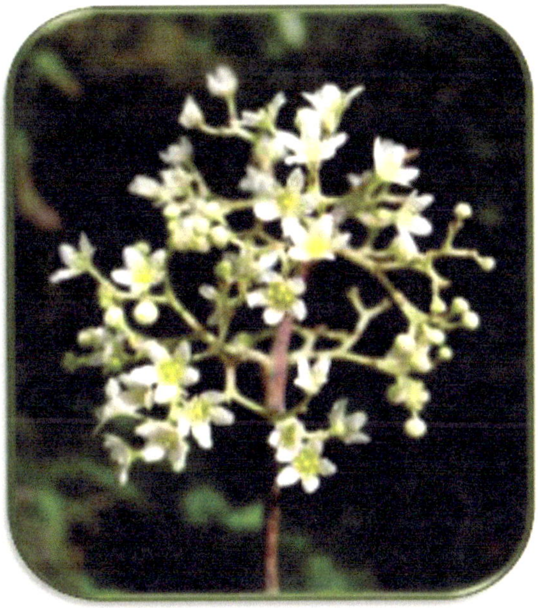

Occurrences : 692 occurrences

Distribution in the world

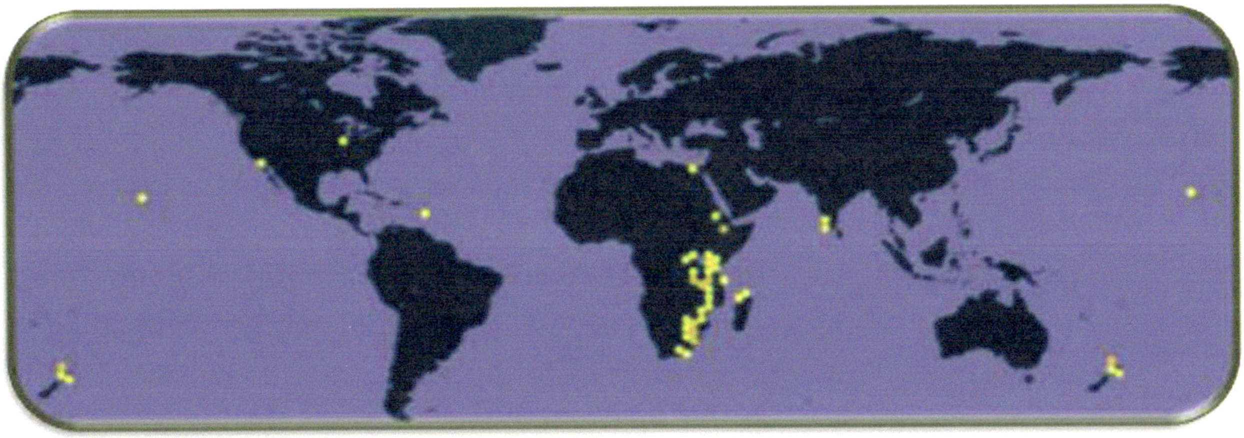

History and Heritage:

The genus name Catha is believed to be from the Arabic "qat", and the species edulis from the Latin, meaning "edible." Al-Shahabi (1978) mentioned that he did not find the word qat in the vocabulary, nor in the mothers of the dictionaries, and he believes that it is of Ethiopian origin Tchat moved with that plant that grows naturally in Ethiopia. The part used: The leaves (they have a distinctive aromatic smell, and their taste is sweet and astringent.) The young leaves are harvested in the morning from the bushes, and kept moist. The leaves remain fresh for about four days, after which they change from green to yellow. It loses a large amount of its active ingredients.

Chemical components:

Young leaves contain catechin tannins (astringent properties), volatile oil, vitamin C and alkaloids - 0.3-0.9%, phenyl amines (alkyl) Phenyl, the most important of which is: cathinone alkaloid, which is the main active compound, characterized by instability, and quickly turns in old or aged leaves into cathine alkaloid (norpseudoephedrine), in addition to another alkaloid An analogue of cathine called norephedrine The quality of khat leaves depends on the percentage of cathinone alkaloid in them, because it is the compound that gives khat the stimulating effect it produces, and its effect is ten times that of cathine. Cathinone is an unstable compound, and its content decreases in the few days following the harvest of the leaves, which shows the importance of using young leaves. The concentration of alkaloids in old or aged leaves is much lower than it is in young, tender leaves. The plant also contains tannic acid.

The main minerals in the plant: nickel, zinc, copper, sodium, cobalt, magnesium, lead, iron, manganese, cadmium and mercury.

Properties and medical uses:

The decoction of the plant is popularly used to treat rheumatism, gout, joint stiffness, tuberculosis and blood diseases. It is used topically in the form of compresses to treat skin diseases such as eczema, wounds and suppurations. It is used in the form of washes or baths to treat hemorrhoids and eye infections.

The biologically active metabolites have shown diverse pharmacological activities such as anti-obesity, anti-fungal, anti-bacterial, anti-oxidant, anti-proliferative, anti-inflammatory, anti-diabetic, and anti-anxiety. Different parts of the plant have been used to treat various digestive disorders, diarrhea, measles, jaundice, gastrointestinal and reproductive tract infections, respiratory tract infections and asthma. They also reduce swelling and are used as compresses for fractures. The isolated compounds have shown significant pharmacological activities such as anti-tumor and anti-cancer. In India, a decoction of the leaves is used to bandage deep wounds, stop bleeding and reduce swelling, and the ground leaves, stem and root are used as a plaster cast for dislocations and swelling. The decoction of the plant has unique moisturizing and soothing properties that encourage its use to relieve skin itching, menstrual pain and scabies. Flavonoids and beta-sitosterol compounds in the plant significantly inhibit the activity of lipase and amylase in mice and reduce total triglycerides and cholesterol.

Other uses: Its leaves and tender stems are consumed as salad.

Precautions for use: No accidents or side effects are known with the appropriate intake of the specified dose.

Environment:

The plant grows on walls and roadsides and in agricultural fields and humid places. It prefers moist soil in bright and semi-shaded places. The plant grows and becomes strong in fertile soils, and blooms in poor soils when it is young. The plant grows up to 40 cm in moist, fertile soil rich in nitrogen, especially in meadows.

Cultivation and productivity:

An easy-to-cultivate plant, propagated by seeds that are scattered in early spring in basins isolated from neighboring fields so as not to invade agricultural lands. The seeds germinate and grow quickly, and require moderate humidity.

Qat cultivation requires unstoned, well-drained land. The land is prepared in the dry season and before the rains fall, and the necessary fertilizers are added to it. Vegetative propagation of qat is relied upon, and seed cultivation is not preferred, due to the low germination rate. The productive life of the qat shrub begins after 2-3 years of cultivation. Productivity is 1-2 tons/hectare.

Properties and medical uses:

The process of chewing the leaves releases the alkaloid cathinone, which stimulates physiological effects in the body, represented by activating the central nervous system, which is manifested by a general feeling of euphoria and increased mental and muscular alertness and activity, accompanied by loss of appetite and emaciation, high blood pressure, and increased body temperature with decreased urination.

Qat is used to reduce weight and treat obesity, because the hormone serotonin leads to loss of appetite and suppresses the feeling of hunger. It is also used to alleviate the symptoms of asthma, due to its effectiveness in expanding the bronchi. It has antibacterial and antidepressant effects. Chewing the plant may cause other symptoms such as gingivitis, tooth decay, gastritis, and acute myocardial infarction.

Side effects and precautions for use:

1. Its effect on the digestive system: Qat is a major cause of loss of appetite, emaciation, and indigestion. The tannins present in it, due to their astringent effect, cause inflammation of the stomach and pharynx and chronic constipation, which leads to the formation of hemorrhoids and malnutrition, in addition to the appearance of chronic ulcers in the mouth and gums. And the tongue.

2. Its effect on the heart and circulatory system: The chemical compounds of qat lead to an increase in heart rate, constriction of blood vessels, and an increase in blood pressure.

3. Its effect on the urinary and reproductive system: It causes difficulty in urination and involuntary semen secretion after urination, due to the effect of qat on the prostate and seminal vesicles and the congestion and contraction it causes, which helps in prostate enlargement and sexual weakness.

4. Its neurological and psychological effects: It is noted that qat chewers tend to be mentally lazy hours after addiction, followed by a feeling of anxiety accompanied by a sharp temperament and nervousness and then depression.

5. Qat and diabetes: Qat addiction leads to an increase in the blood sugar level, which makes its user more susceptible to diabetes.

6. Qat chewing during pregnancy leads to a decrease in the birth weight of the newborn. It has also been noted that qat is secreted with the breast milk of a nursing mother.

7. Long-term use of qat disrupts the human biological clock, causes digestive and intestinal ulcers, liver and kidney cirrhosis. Environment: Qat grows wild on the highlands of some areas in Ethiopia, Yemen and Somalia. The qat tree is planted on mountainous heights and plateaus with an altitude of about 800 m, within a wide spectrum of annual rainfall between 1000 - 1500 mm/year, and is often planted mixed with coffee bushes. Qat shrubs prefer dark red, well-drained soils rich in minerals and organic matter, and a pH between 6 and 8.2.

Cleome droserifolia (Forssk.) Delile.

Rorida arabica J.F.Gmel., Rorida droserifolia)Forssk.(Thulin & Roalson, Roridula arabica Roem. & Schult., Roridula droserifolia Forssk.

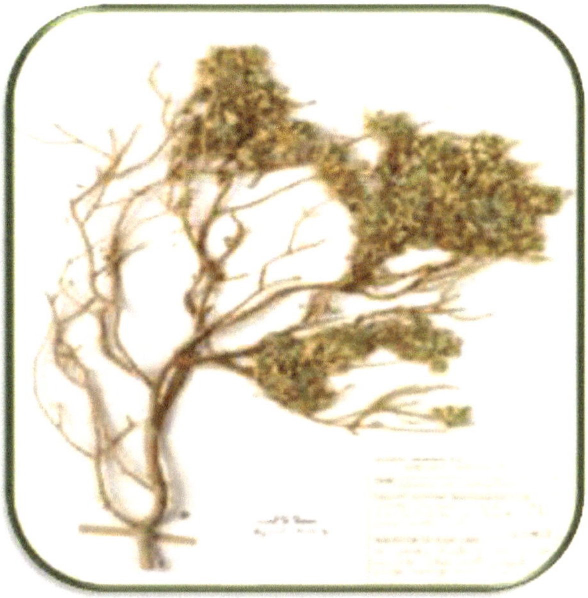

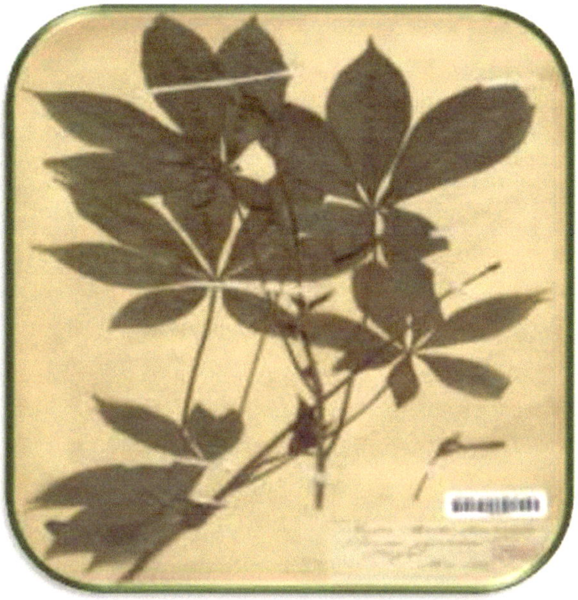

Family: Cleomaceae (formerly Brassicaceae, Cruciferae)

Common names: Al-Mashta, Al-Samwa, Reeh Al-Bard, Afin, Qarn Al-Ghazal, Abu Tarboush

Foreign names: Cleome Fr. herb, Cleome Eng.

Occurrences : 172 occurrences

Distribution in the world

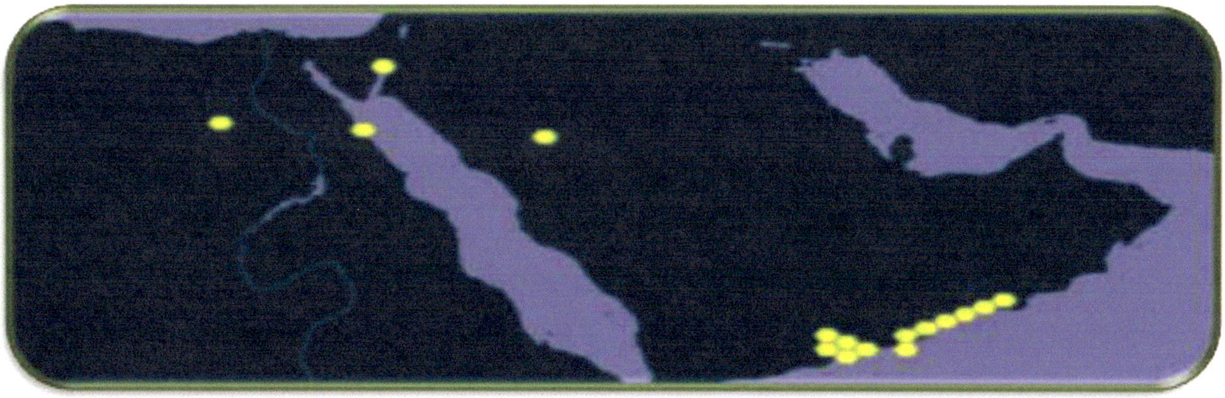

Botanical description:

A small shrub, resembling a pillow in its general shape, green to yellowish in color, abundant leaves, abundantly branched and overlapping, 25-50 cm high. Leaves are simple, long-spiked, rounded to kidney- or semi-heart-shaped, tri-nerve, covered with short simple hairs and long glandular hairs, diameter 0.5-1.5 cm. Flowers are solitary in the axils of the upper leaves, long-stalked, tending to double symmetry, width 1.2-1 cm. Sepals 4, glandular, oblong. Petals 4, reddish to yellow, bearing a thick, scaly-like appendage at its base, ciliated-glandular at its apex. Stamens 4, shorter than the style. Female bicarpel, ovary unicameral, semi-palatine, oblong or ellipsoid, glandular. Fruit capsule, pod erect or flattened, glandular, 1.5-1 cm long. Seeds compressed, renal to round, glandular.

Flowering: March to May.

Habitat and geographical distribution:

Eastern Sudan. It is found in Egypt, Libya and the Kingdom of Saudi Arabia.

History and Heritage:

The genus name Cleome is believed to be derived from the Greek Kleio meaning "enclose", and includes approximately 150 species of annuals and perennials. The species name droserifolia is from the Greek droseros meaning "dew or dewy plant", and may be an adjective for the glandular hairs that cover the leaves.

Part used:

Flowering aerial parts (the plant has a distinctive smell)

Chemical components:

0.4% sulfurous volatile oil. Its most important compounds: Benzyl isothiocyanate,Caryophylen, naphthyl-n-, Carotol, propyl ether, etc., Sulfur glycosides: glucocaparin,Flavonoids 0.3%, the most important of which are: kaempferol, isorharmnetin, rhamnosidem, quercetin and artemitin. Sterol compounds: beta-sitosterol band stigmasterol. Triterpene compounds, coumarins, alkaloids, and docosanioc acid.

Properties and medical uses:

The plant has sugar-lowering properties, in addition to its hepatoprotective effect and enzyme stimulating effect. The plant extract shows antibacterial properties against Staphylococcus aureus, Escherichia coli and Candida albicans fungi. The alcoholic extract also shows an effect similar to antihistamines, and it is a hypotensive, mild analgesic and diuretic. The plant is popularly used in cases of indigestion, to stimulate liver function, increase bile secretion, reduce blood sugar levels, and treat asthma and kidney diseases. The paste made from the juice of the leaves is used topically for its antiseptic properties in treating wounds and skin infections. The seeds are used as a worm repellent, gas reliever, stimulant and astringent.

Precautions for use:

The plant is poisonous, toxicity manifests itself in symptoms of convulsions, tremors, sweating, respiratory disturbance, then loss of consciousness and death.

Environment:

It is widespread in hot deserts, among rocks and in valleys, and grows in stony and sandy valleys and plains

Colchicum autumnale L.

Bulbocodium antumnale)L.(Lapeyr., Colchicum commune Neck.

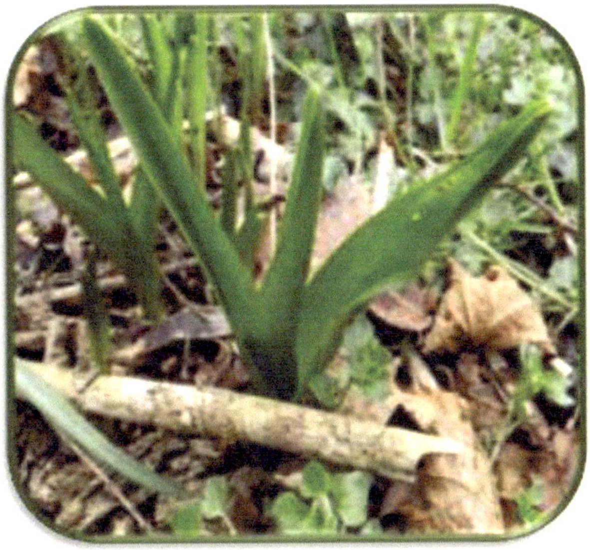

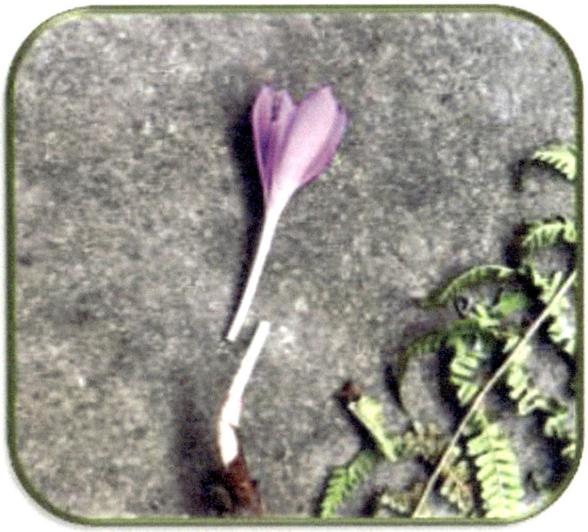

Family: Colchicaceae

Common names: Autumn saffron, Autumn saffron, Autumn saffron, False saffron.

Foreign names: Colchique Fr. Colchicum, Eng.

Occurrences : 13,120 occurrences

Distribution in the world

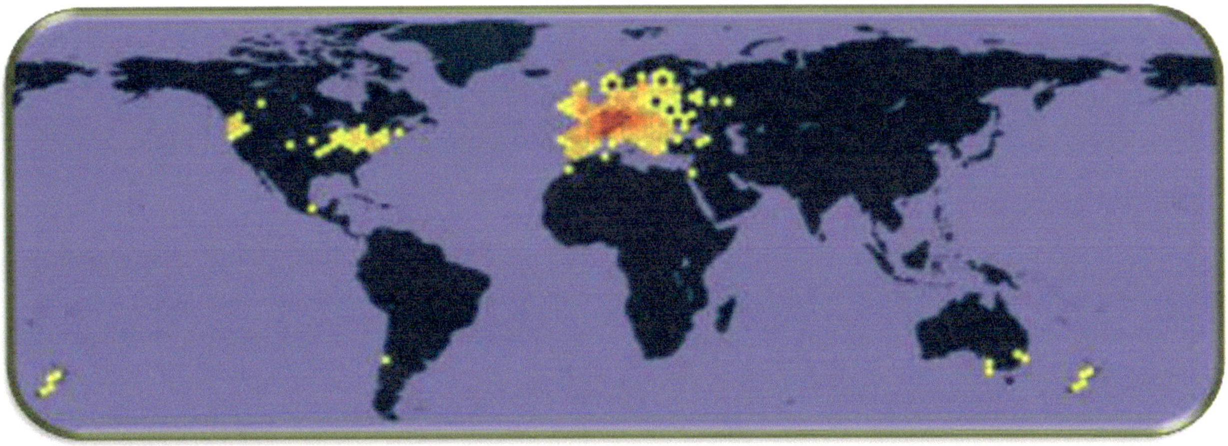

Botanical description:

A perennial herbaceous plant with corms. The corm is oval in shape, covered with dry leaves (sheaths) brown, convex on one side, flat and elongated downwards on the other side, replaced every year by a new corm that develops alongside the corm of the previous year at the base of the flowering branch. Leaves and flowering shoot enclosed in a white tubular sheath, turning brown the following year. Leaves 2-9, at base of plant, linear to lanceolate, appear with or after flowering, outer leaf base tubular.

Flowers solitary or in short racemes, 2-5 brightly colored hermaphrodite flowers. The scutellum is simple, pubescent, pink or purple or white (rarely yellow), funnel-shaped, consisting of a long tube and a hexagonal blade. Stamens 6, shorter than the lobes of the scutellum, situated at the mouth of the tube, the inner whorl slightly longer than the outer. The ovary is situated below the soil, three-chambered, each chamber containing several ovules. Styles 3, free, filiform, long, protruding beyond the scutellum tube. The fruit is a capsule, oval to ellipsoidal, triangular, tapering to form a beak, carried on a long stalk, ripening near the surface of the soil. The seeds are spherical or angular. Flowering: Most species flower in late autumn and early winter. Habitat and geographical distribution: Areas bordering the Black Sea. It is believed that the word Colchicum is derived from the province of Colchis overlooking that sea. Mediterranean, Iranian-Turanian and Saharo-Arabian. The species is found in the cold and humid regions of Central Europe, on the coasts of European countries overlooking the Mediterranean Sea, and in the countries of the Eastern Mediterranean.

History and heritage:

The scientific name comes from Colchis, the homeland of Medee, the poisonous plant known to the ancient Greeks, alluding to the toxicity of the plant. The descriptive name for the species, automnale, means "autumn", indicating that it blooms Surangan was known to Surangan is of Persian origin, and was mentioned in Ibn al-Baytar's vocabulary. In autumn. Name Ancient physicians considered it a poisonous and medicinal plant

Part used:

Flowers, ripe seeds (collected in early summer), corms.

Chemical components:

A poisonous plant in all its parts, the seeds contain tropolone group alkaloids -0.25-1.2%, the most important of which are colchicine, a compound with a glycosidic structure, colchicoside, and a fatty oil. The corms contain a lower percentage of tropolone alkaloids, the most important of which are colchicine, demeco-line, colchicoside glycoside, many organic acids, and the flavonoid pigment apigenin, in addition to starch. The flowers contain alkaloids similar to those found in the corms.

Properties and medical uses:

Colchicine alkaloid is very toxic, has properties that inhibit cell division in mitosis and meiosis, and inhibits chromosome migration. It is used to inhibit cell division (some types of cancer). It is given orally only to treat acute rheumatic attacks, joint pain, gout, and Mediterranean fever (F.M.F). Colchicine is used topically to treat rheumatism and joint pain, and to treat skin tumors, psoriasis, chronic eczema, and ocular inflammation. It has been used to treat asthma, gout, and dysuria. It is anti-inflammatory and anti-fibrosis. Its leaves contain components that kill ticks. Cormat powder It can be an ant killer. RIFA

Pharmaceutical preparations:

It is available in the form of juice, ampoule, pills, tincture, dry extract. Side effects and warnings for use: Highly toxic, its use without medical supervision can cause paralysis of smooth muscles, abdominal pain, diarrhea, nausea, vomiting, and digestive bleeding. And liver and kidney irritations, anemia, neuritis, myopathy, and bone marrow damage. It is not used in the elderly. Its preparations are not used in cases of diseases Heart, kidney, digestive system disorders and liver diseases. Prolonged use leads to hair loss, do not give to pregnant and lactating women. Environment: Surangan tolerates cold and frosty climate conditions for long periods without any significant damage thanks to the hardness of the internal tissues. It is suitable for all agricultural lands, and prefers sandy and silty soils that contain lime and organic materials to obtain large-sized corms. It tolerates soil acidity (pH), which helps protect the buried corms from fungal and bacterial infection.

Cultivation and productivity:

Surangan is planted in temperate regions in late summer and early fall, using seedlings or corms, while in cold regions it is planted in spring using corms. °C) When planting seedlings, it is important to take the seeds from fresh fruits and soak them in hot water (45°C) for several minutes, then in water Normal for 24 hours to facilitate the embryo's exit from the hard seed pod. The seeds are planted in covered nurseries during the fall, and left until small seedlings with small corms are formed. The corms are transferred to be planted in the permanent ground early the following fall. The seedlings or corms are placed in lines spaced 60-65 cm apart and at a rate of 25 cm between one corm and another on the same line, then the land is irrigated immediately after planting. The plant is irrigated at a rate of once a month as Increased soil moisture leads to rotting of the corms, and irrigation is stopped when the leaves turn almost yellow. It is recommended to add some trace elements (copper and manganese) when adding traditional fertilizers because of their importance in the formation of active ingredients. Corms are collected during the flowering period, when the leaves wither and before the formation of the new bulb, and seeds are collected after the fruits ripen in late summer, depending on the region. After collecting the corms, they are washed, cleaned and cut into transverse slices Aired, away from moisture, thin, then spread out to dry under the sun, then collected, packed and stored in a cool place. One hectare yields 2.5-2 tons of dry corms

Terminalia chebula Retz.

Myrobalanus chebula Gaertn)Retz.(, Myrobalanus gangetica Kostel)Roxb.(, Terminalia gangetica Roxb., Terminalia reticulata Roth B.Heyne ex., Buceras chebula)Retz.(Lyons.

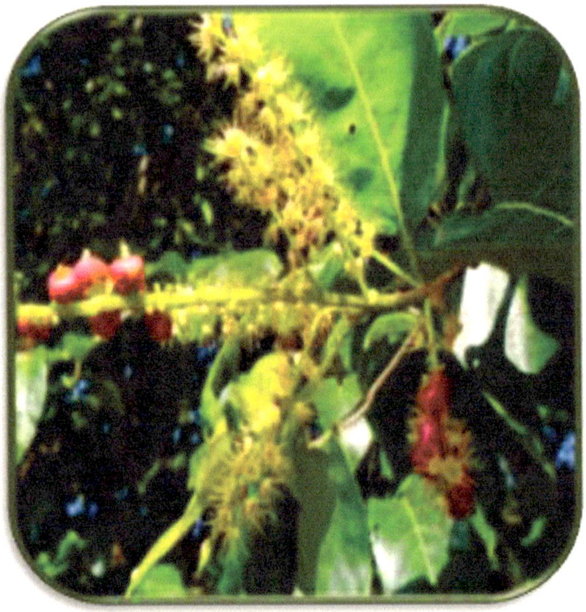

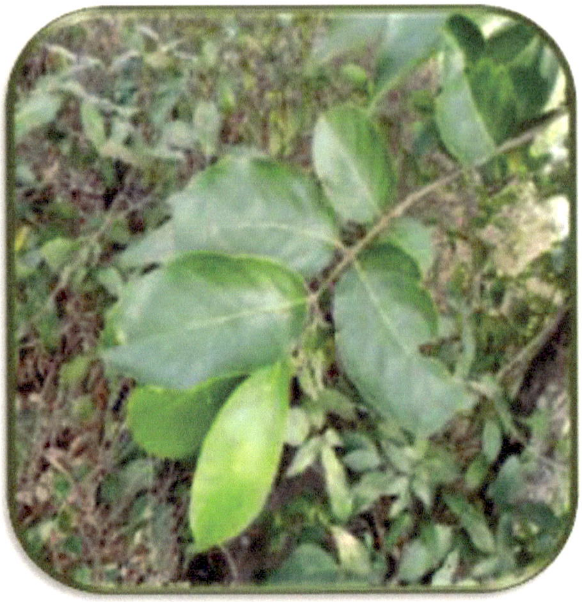

Family: Combretaceae

Common names: Ahlij, Balij, Indian barley (Levant), Lob, Dates of Obaid, Heglig

Foreign names: Chebule Badamier Fr., myrobalan Black almond, Eng.Indian

Occurrences : 1,302 occurrences

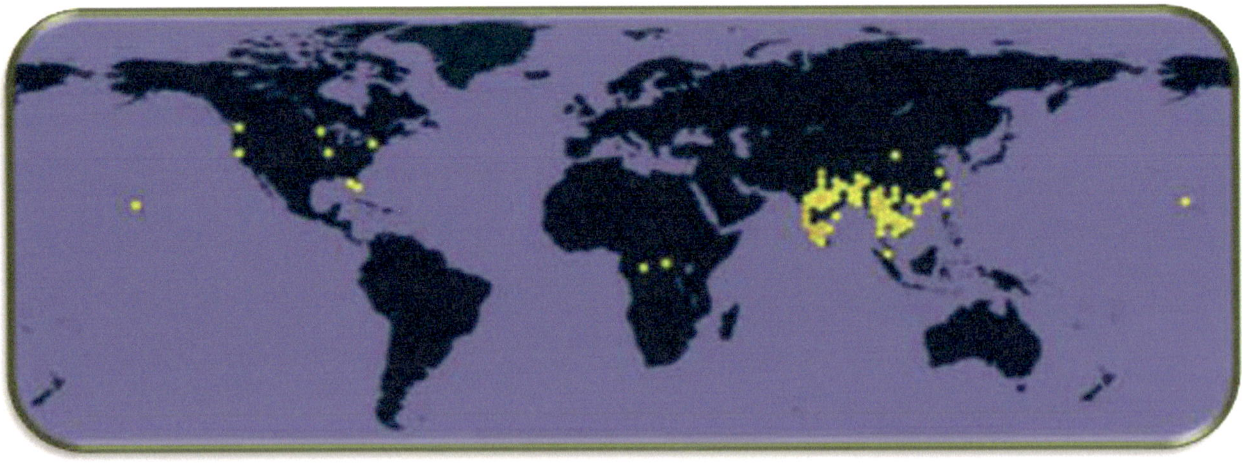

Botanical description:

A tree that reaches a height of 25-30 m. Its branches are flat, pale green in color; the bark is gray and smooth. Leaves alternate to semi-opposite, 10-15 cm long, 4-8 cm wide, elliptic or oblong, round or cordate at the base, leathery to the touch, covered with silky hairs when young, later becoming bare.

The spadix bears two glands at its apex, 1-4 cm long. The inflorescence is a terminal spike, 5-15 cm long, with a hairy axis. Flowers hermaphrodite, about 5 mm wide, yellowish, bracts linear, hairy, 5-6 mm long, pendulous. Calyx tube 3-4 mm, glabrous outside, hairy inside, teeth 5, very short, triangular. Petals absent. Male 10 stamens. Ovary unicameral. Fruit nuclear, ellipsoid or inverted ovate, 2-4 cm long. Flowering: April to June.

Homeland and geographical distribution:

India, Malaysia, Pakistan, Iran, Sudan, and It is grown in many other countries.

History and heritage:

The genus name comes from the Latin terminus, meaning "terminal - upper - apical." Al-Shihabi (1978) states that the name is from Persian and of Sanskrit origin.

Part used:

Ripe fruits and leaves.

Chemical components:

The fruits contain tannins (gallotan-nins) 45–20%, including: chebulic acid, chebulinic acid a., terchebulin, terflavin, punicalagin.

Sugars including:

glucose, fructose, and sucrose. Fruit acids 2% including: quinic acid a. Quinic, Shikimic a. .shikimic. The seeds contain proteins and 40% fatty oil. The hydroalcoholic extract of the myrobalan fruit contains: gallic acid, methyl gallate, corialgin, shibulgic acid, and shibilenic acid

Properties and medical uses:

The fruits, due to their myrobalan acid content, have antioxidant, immunosuppressive, hepatoprotective, and alpha-glucosidase inhibitor properties.

The fruit extract is an antibacterial and antiviral (viral hepatitis). Studies have also identified many raw materials The chemical in the fruits is used in the synthesis of hormones and contraceptives. Research has shown the anti-toxic properties of the leaves and their effect in reducing liver cell damage resulting from inhaling harmful chemicals. The decoction or infusion of the fruits is popularly used for its cholesterol- and fat-lowering properties to cleanse the digestive system. It is also used for its laxative and astringent properties that are useful in treating constipation, diarrhea, cough, and asthma attacks, and in reducing the formation of mucus in the respiratory tract, and treating burning urination or cases of bloody urine. The decoction of the fruits is used topically to treat wounds, bleeding ulcers, and leprosy.

Myrobalan is an acetylcholinesterase inhibitor, and acetylcholinesterase inhibitors are used in neurodegenerative diseases mainly to treat the cognitive symptoms (mostly memory and learning deficits) of dementia. These symptoms are weakened by the role of acetylcholine in the central nervous system. Antidepressant, anti-anxiety and anti-inflammatory.

Other uses:

Ripped fruits are used in baking and soup preparation. The stem bark was previously used as a worm repellent and a substitute for soap. The pulp of the fruit is used in some countries to treat stagnant water and kill parasites in it.

Environment:

The plant tolerates high temperatures, but does not tolerate cold and dryness. It grows at altitudes of 400-2000 meters, preferring fertile soil.

Cultivation and productivity:

The myrobalan is propagated by seeds. After collecting and drying the seeds, the dry fleshy cover is removed. The hard shell can be broken without damaging the pulp, then soaked in cold water for 36 hours. This method gives a good germination rate.

Bryonia cretica subsp. dioica (Jacq.) Tutin

Bryonia dioica Jacq., Bryonia ruderalis Salisb., Bryonia scarlatina Dumort.

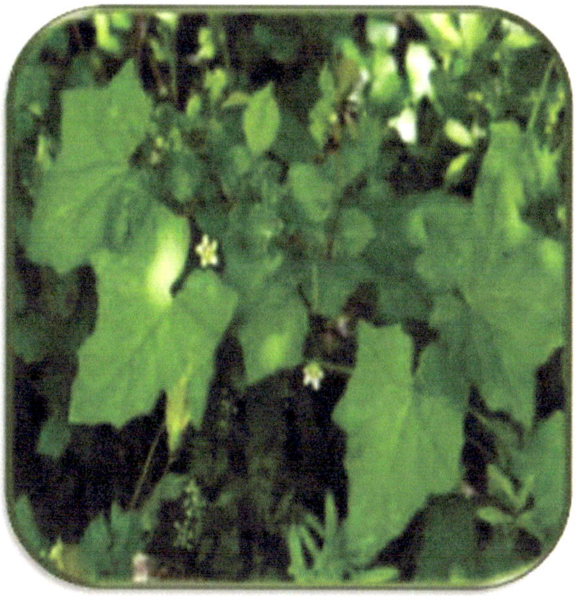

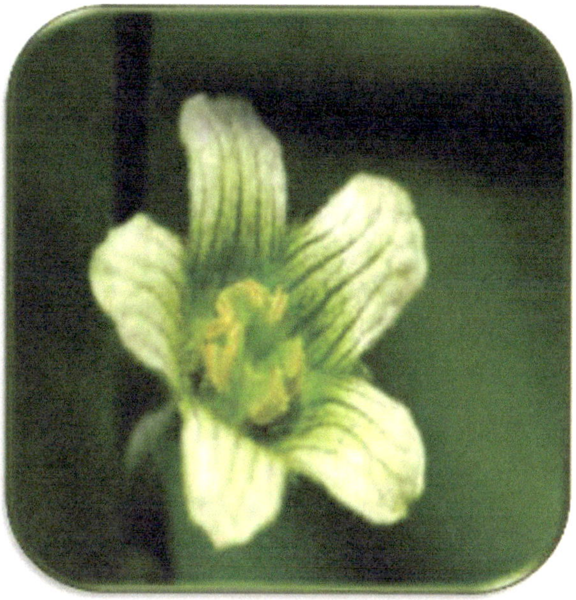

Family: Cucurbitaceae

Common names: El Fasher, Bitter Game, Snake Grape, Ardisha.

Foreign names: dioïque bryone Fr. bryony, red Eng.

Occurrences : 19,212 occurrences

Distribution in the world

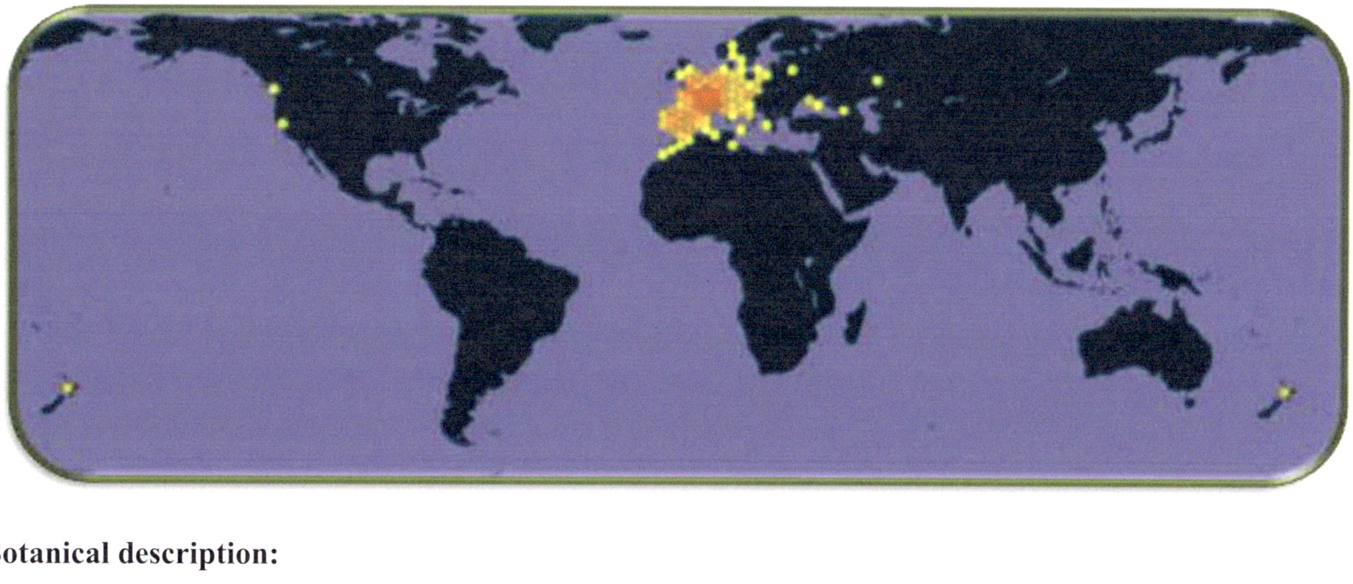

Botanical description:

A perennial dioecious herb. The root is fleshy and tuberous, storing nutrients. The stem is slender, glabrous, smooth, climbing, and the tendrils are long and unbranched. The leaves are glabrous, ovate to sub-round in general shape, cordate at the base, palmately lobed to 5-7 ovate-lanceolate lobes. The stalk is glabrous or bears scattered white tubers. Male flowers are gathered in racemes, 5-15 cm long, containing 12-30 flowers, with long, fine, threadlike inflorescences. Sepals 5, short, triangular. Corolla downy, yellow, bearing green veins, cycloid, five-lobed. Male 5 stamens, free, with dense hairy filaments. Female inflorescences are loose or dense, sometimes branched from the base, containing 4-25 flowers, ovary spherical, smooth, stigma almost prominent. Fruit is grape, red, spherical, diameter 7-9 mm. Seeds are semi-compressed, oval, smooth.

Flowering: March to May.

Habitat and geographical distribution:

Eastern Mediterranean countries, southern Europe and northern Africa.

History and Heritage:

The name is derived from the Greek bryein, meaning "growth", alluding to its growing green branches and the strength of its roots. The species name dioica is from the Greek and means "double-headed." The plant was used medicinally in Europe, and was written about in the English Constitutional Medicine in 1653. It was mentioned by Ibn al-Baytar, al-Antaki and Ibn Sina: "The root of the fashra with karsana and fenugreek clears the appearance of the body, purifies and refines it. It removes freckles and black marks that remain after ulcers."

Part used:

Roots (collected during summer and early autumn), young shoots (collected in spring and early summer). Chemical components: The plant, especially the roots, contains cucurbitacin (a toxic and irritating compound for the skin and mucous membranes), which is found in the young roots in the form of glycons and glycosides. And a small amount of glycosides: bryoamarid, bryoside, bryodiosides C, A. And triterpenic acids, including: bryonolic acid, bryocoumaric acid, and alpha-hydroxy-multiflora. multiflora

And on proteins that inhibit ribosomes, including: bryodine-L, and bryodine-R. And on fatty acids, starch, resin and alkaloids.

Properties and medical uses:

The drug (cucurbitacin) has laxative and laxative properties, and is used in cases of chronic constipation. It also has antiviral and anti-inflammatory properties, and lowers blood pressure. The drug is popularly used to treat diabetes, internal infections, such as duodenal ulcers, bronchitis, asthma, and whooping cough. It is a diuretic and is used to treat dropsy, joint inflammation, especially gout. It is primarily prescribed for painful rheumatic conditions. The root is diaphoretic, expectorant, irritant, and anthelmintic. The root is used internally in small quantities to treat peptic ulcers. Externally, it is used to treat muscle and joint pain and pleurisy.

Pharmaceutical preparations:

It is available in the form of tinctures, decoctions and powder (powder).

Precautions for use:

The drug is very toxic when used in high doses, and the plant should not be used except under medical supervision. It is warned against its use in children, pregnant women and breastfeeding women.

The drug is irritating to the skin, and can cause irritation, spotting, red spots and itching on the parts it touches. Can cause convulsions, hypothermia, and coma.

Environment:

A fast-growing, deep-rooted climbing plant, It grows in shady places in woodlands, forests, or on the banks of streams. It grows in most types of soil, provided it is well-drained and non-acidic.

Cultivation and productivity:

An easy-to-cultivate plant. It is propagated by mature seeds that are scattered in lines, or planted in greenhouses in special containers, and transferred to the permanent soil after a year, taking into account that the plant is dioecious when planted in order to obtain seeds.

Citrullus colocynthis (L.) Schrad.

Cucumis colocynthis L., Colocynthis vulgaris Schrad., Cucumis bipinnatifidus Wight ex Naudin, Cucumis colocynthoides Schult., Cucurbita colocyntha Link.

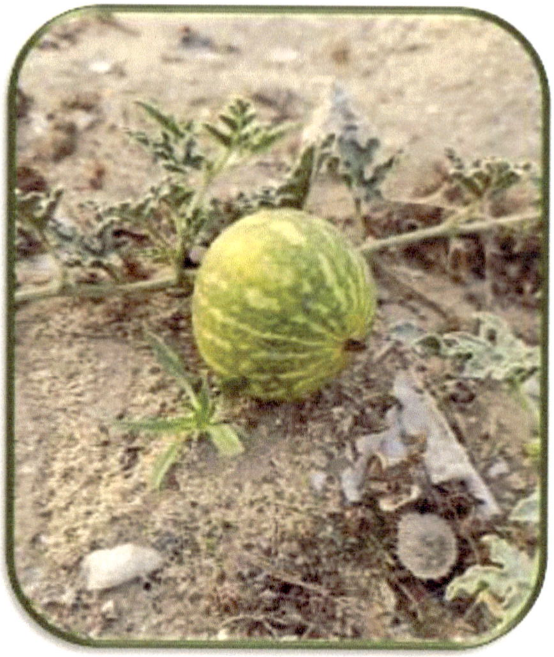

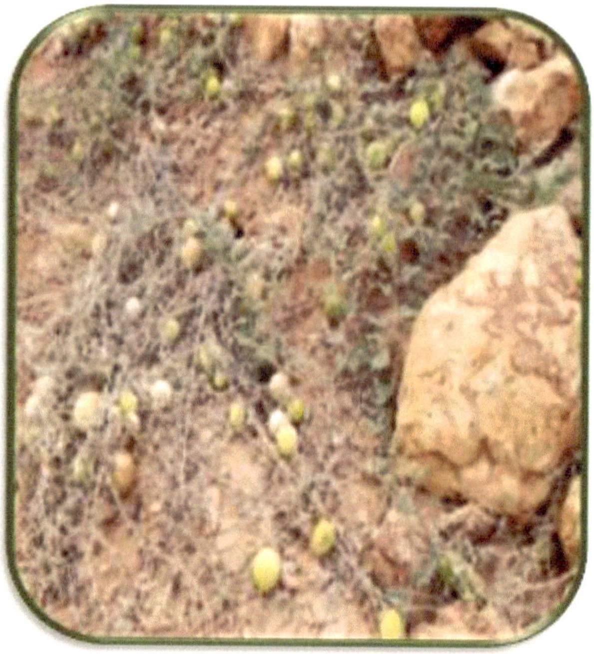

Family: Cucurbitaceae

Common names: Colocynth, wild sage, wormwood, bitter apple.

Foreign names: Colycynth, Bitter apple, Fr. Coloquinte

Occurrences : 1,819 occurrences

Distribution in the world

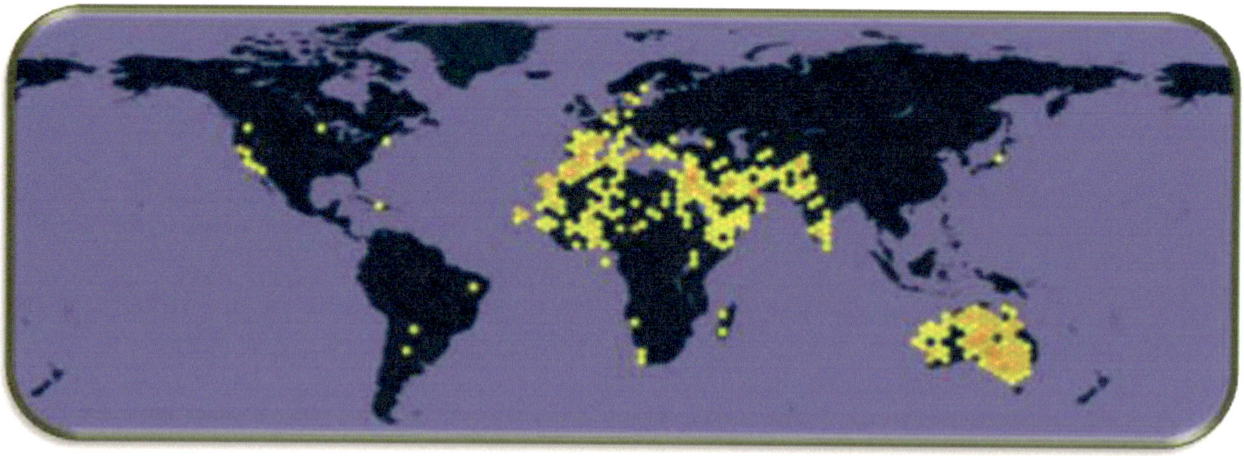

Botanical description:

A perennial herbaceous plant, green to gray in color, rough in texture, branched from the base. The stems are slender, ribbed, of varying lengths, covering the ground, covered with hairy hairs. The tendrils are short and slender, simple or branched. The leaves are hard, rough on both sides, the upper side is pale green, and the lower side is gray covered with hard hairs; Triangular - ovate, acute at the apex, cordate at the base, deeply divided into 5-7 lobes. Lobe blunt at the apex, sinusoidal - wavy at the margin, divided in turn into lobes. Flowers unisexual (monoecious plants), solitary, yellow in colour. Male flowers with short panicles, 5 narrow sepals, as long as the flower seat, corolla 5 petals fused in the form of a broad tube, ending in 5 acute-apex and stigma lobes. Male 5 stamens, short filaments. The quantity in female flowers is similar to that of male flowers, the ovary is inferior, hairy, and 3 sterile stamens (stamens) are seen. The fruit is fleshy, spherical, the size of an orange (about 10 cm in diameter), slightly hairy at the beginning of its formation, then becomes bare when ripe, green marked with wavy yellow stripes, turns yellow when dry, the inner fruit cover is spongy, white, and very bitter. Seeds are numerous, compact, smooth, shiny, tending to brown. Flowering: May to August.

Habitat and geographical distribution:

Arabian desert, grows wild on the coastal sands of northern. Africa, southern Europe and western Asia. It is widespread in the Levant desert. The most important countries exporting its fruits are Egypt, Sudan, Turkey and Spain.

History and heritage:

The scientific name of the genus is the diminutive of the name Citrus, meaning lemon, due to the similarity of the size and color of its fruit when ripe with the fruits of oranges (lemon), while the name of the species is from the Greek kolokynthis meaning "gourd." The Romans, Greeks and Arabs used it to treat constipation and cleanse the digestive system. Ibn Sina said about it: “Colocynth is of male and female type. The male has a fibrous pulp and the female is soft and smooth. The best type is the very white one, while the black one is bad. It should be harvested in the fall, and it should be harvested, rather it should be left as it is. If that is done, it will weaken it. It should not be harvested unless its fat is removed from its insides if it is yellow and the green color has not completely barked off, otherwise it is harmful and bad.”

Part used:

The spongy pulp of ripe fruits (colocynth), seeds, and leaves.

Chemical components:

The pulp of the fruits (colocynth) contains anthraquinone glycosides: cucurbitacins (Elater-in) and bitter compounds: colocynthin, colocynthetin and organic acids derived from coffee acid, including chlorogenic acid and alkaloids, resinous materials, and pectic compounds. The seeds (some call them hebeid) contain a fatty oil -15-20% yellow in color, rich in fatty acids (linseed oil 70 %, oleic acid 10-16%, palmitic acid, nutmeg acid), and compounds not yet identified, with a blood sugar-lowering effect, phytosterols, alkaloids, saponins and sugars. The leaves contain cucurbitacin glycosides E B, cucurbitacins.

Properties and medical uses:

Anthraquinone glycosides are generally known for their laxative and laxative properties. Until recently, colocynth was considered among the most powerful laxative herbal drugs that are widely used in the treatment of constipation. Chronic. Recent studies have shown the effect of leaf glycosides in reducing the proliferation of breast cancer cells, and the alcoholic extract of the leaves has shown anti-inflammatory activity.Research has shown the effects of the aqueous extract of colocynth seeds on lowering blood sugar levels, in addition to the effectiveness of the alcoholic extract of the seeds and leaves against some types of bacteria, such as Bacillus pumilus and Staphylococcus aureus. The aqueous infusion of the fruit pulp is popularly used in cases of chronic constipation, stimulating bowel and stomach movement, aiding digestion, reducing the resulting gases, and treating liver and gallbladder diseases (jaundice). The leaf extract is used as a diuretic and in treating asthma and jaundice. The seed oil is used to treat hemorrhoids, some skin diseases such as inflammation, ulcers and scabies, and is used in the form of compresses to relieve rheumatism and joint pain. The use of colocynth has declined at present, and its use is currently limited to veterinary indications in the treatment of skin diseases (scabies and ticks). The fruits are used to treat colds, parasitic worms, dropsy, ulcers, bronchitis, splenomegaly, neck tuberculosis, anemia, and elephantiasis. The root was also used against abdominal distension, coughing and asthma attacks.

Other uses:

The ground seeds (washed in water and salt to get rid of bitterness) and roasted, rich in fatty oils and proteins, are used in preparing some types of soup.

Precautions for use:

The pulp of the fruit, with its cucurbitacin content, causes irritation of the mucous membranes of the intestines, accompanied by severe bloody diarrhea. Generally, an overdose causes vomiting, gastroenteritis, bloody diarrhea, colic, kidney irritation, and liver damage. The lethal dose starts at 2 grams and leads to abdominal cramps, fatigue, weakness, dizziness, irregular breathing, cessation of blood circulation, and paralysis of the limbs, which can lead to death unless treated as quickly as possible. It is prohibited during pregnancy and breastfeeding.

Environment:

Colocynth is a sunny, dry and desert plant. Xyrophytic. The ideal temperature for flowering and fruit ripening ranges between 25-27 degrees Celsius. Poor lighting causes female flowers to appear later than male flowers. It prefers light soils, especially sandy and gravelly ones. It tolerates high levels of soil salinity and alkalinity. The appropriate pH is 8-7.

Cultivation and productivity:

The plant is propagated by fresh seeds. The seeds are planted during the spring and early summer in wide lines (150-180 cm) and within holes, with a distance of 30-25 cm between them, at a rate of 3-2 seeds per hole. The thinning process is carried out later, and two plants are left in the hole. Appropriate service of moderate irrigation, fertilization and pest control. The plant blooms during spring and summer depending on the region. The fruits are collected when they are ripe, and this is indicated by the yellowing and drying of the leaves and the yellow-green color of the fruits, and the hardening of their skin. After collecting them, the fruits are transferred to the drying place, and left in a shaded place for several days, then packed and stored in a ventilated place, away from humidity. The production of a hectare ranges between 1.5-1 ton of whole dry fruits or 1 ton of Segmented fruits.

Ecballium elaterium (L.) A. Rich.

Momordica elaterium L., Bryonia elaterium)L.(E.H.L.Krause, Ecballium agreste Rchb., Ecballium elaterium var. monoicum Batt.

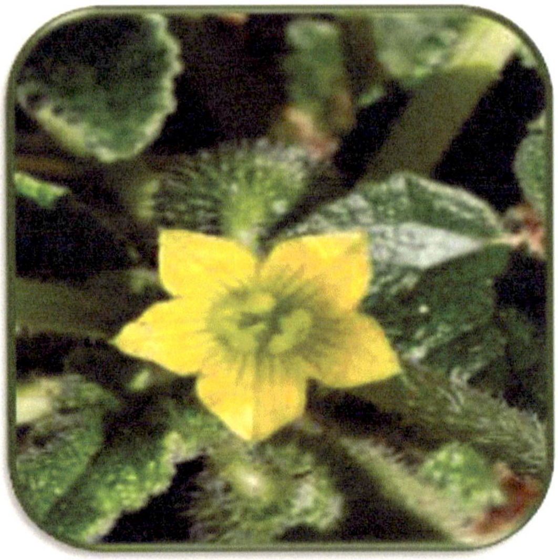
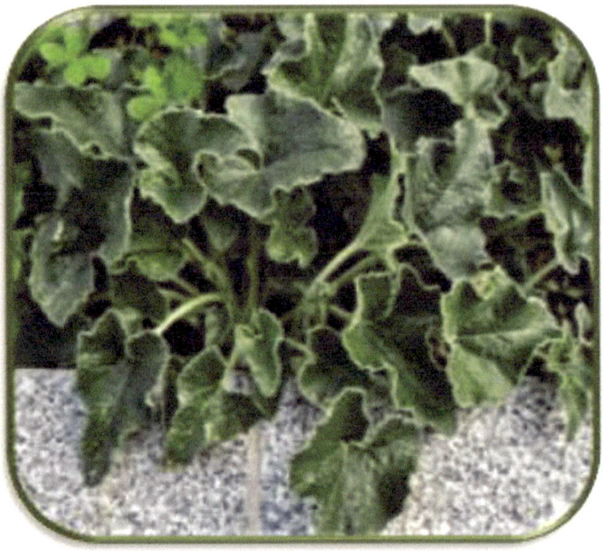

Family: Cucurbitaceae

Common names: Squirting cucumber, Donkey's squash

Foreign names: Squirting cucumber, Fr. Cocombre dane

Occurrences: 43,270 Occurrences

Distribution in the world

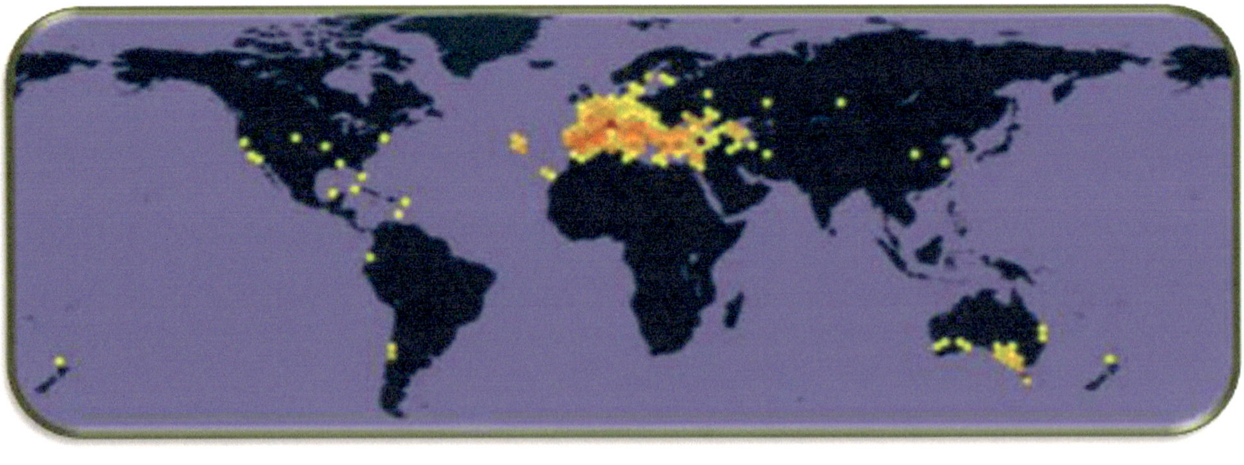

Botanical description:

Perennial herb, branched from the base. Stem thick, somewhat fleshy, rough, hairy, spreading on the ground, without tendrils. Leaves simple, oblong, cordate-ovate, blunt-topped, crest-shaped and wavy-edged. Flowers unisexual, and the plant is monoecious. Male flowers are gathered in racemes, the axis of which is shorter than the leaf spoons, downy. The corolla is yellow, composed of five petals and covered with rough hairs. The calyx has five linear-lanceolate sepals fused in the form of a bell-shaped tube, ending in five oval-oblong lobes, sharp at the tip. The male has five free stamens, short filaments. Female flowers are solitary, the inflorescence is similar to that of male flowers, and 3-5 stamens (sterile, anther-less stamens) are observed. The female is triplocarpal, the ovary is inferior, oblong in shape, covered with hairs. The style is short. The fruit is pendulous, oblong-elliptic, covered with thorny hairs, green, filled with juice that spurts with the seeds for a long distance (several meters) when the fruit separates at maturity, through a basal opening (the area where the fruit connects to its holder). The seeds are oblong, compressed, smooth, blackish-brown in color.

Flowering: From April to December.

Habitat and geographical distribution: Mediterranean and Iranian-Turanian. It has spread to many other regions of the world.

History and Heritage: The scientific name of the genus Ecbalium comes from the Greek ekballein, meaning "thrown out", referring to the fact that when the fruit ripens, it suddenly detaches from the stalk, and the resulting gap throws its juice and seeds with such force that it is carried several meters away. The descriptive name of the species elaterium comes from the Greek elatêrion, meaning "facilitator." Its medical benefits have been known for a long time, as it lowers blood pressure and is a laxative. It was mentioned by Ibn al-Baytar, al-Antaki, and Ibn Sina.

Part used: Fruits.

Chemical components:

Cucurbitacins, resin, carbohydrates, mucilage. The seeds contain high percentage of carotens. E. elaterium seed oil showed high iodine value 160.12 (± 0.14 g/100 g oil). The high saponification value 191.57 (± 0.034 mg KOH/g oil) of E. elaterium seed oil indicates high amounts of low molecular weight fatty acids. Elaterium E. seed oil is characterized by its high content of unsaturated fatty acids: linoleic acid (48.64%), punicic acid (22.38%) and oleic acid (15.58%), in addition to β-sitosterol and γ-tocopherol.

Properties and medical uses:

The drug has antioxidant, liver and bile stimulating, anti-inflammatory and antiviral effects.

It is popularly used in cases of liver and biliary diseases, and cases of prevention of liver cirrhosis or necrosis, and in diseases Colds and flu. Seed oil is a powerful inhibitor of cancer cell growth. Seeds contain a protease inhibitory polypeptide, which works specifically against trypsin, being one of the most effective trypsin inhibitors. The juice is antimicrobial, anti-inflammatory, and antirheumatic. It is used internally to treat edema associated with kidney and heart complaints and rheumatism.The plant is traditionally used to treat ear infections, sinusitis, malaria, headaches and rheumatism.

Other uses:

Seed oil can be used in the manufacture of shampoo, shoe polish, and skin cream.

Side effects and warnings:

The fruit extract has an irritating effect on the mucous membranes and causes skin allergies. Its use causes nasal allergies and coughing.

Do not use during pregnancy and lactation.

Excessive doses cause gastroenteritis and may lead to death.

Environment:

The plant grows on the sides of roads and railways, and in fallow and plowed lands. The vegetative system is sensitive to frost, but the root system can withstand cold winter conditions. It prefers moist and well-drained soils

In sunny places. It thrives in fertile soils, but can grow in poor soils. The plant can become a weed in some areas.

Cultivation and productivity: The seeds are scattered in early spring in fertile compost in a greenhouse or nursery. 2-3 seeds are placed in plastic containers or bags, and later thinned to the strongest plant. The seeds germinate in 10-21 days at a temperature of 25 ° C. The plants are transferred to the permanent ground when the temperature rises in the spring.

***Cupressus sempervirens* L.**

Cupressus elongata Salisb., Cupressus pyramidalis O.Targ.Tozz., Cupressus sempervirens subvar. pyramidalis Hayek, Cupressus sempervirens var. pyramidalis Nyman.

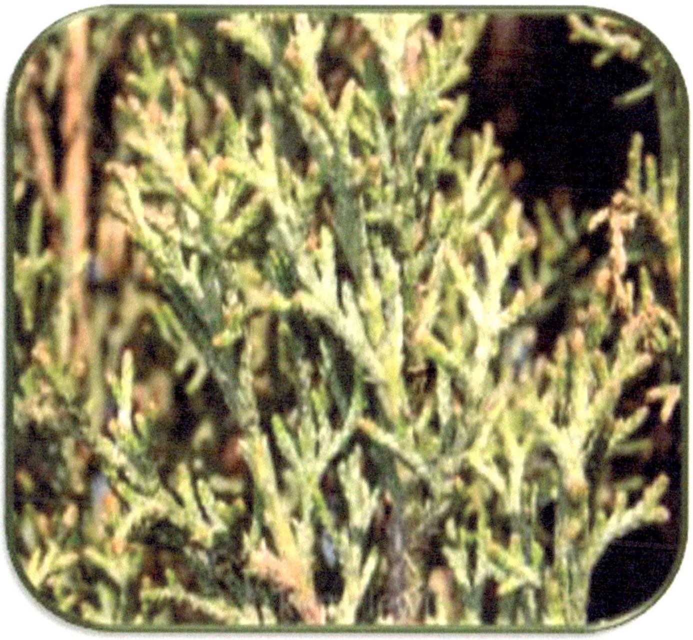

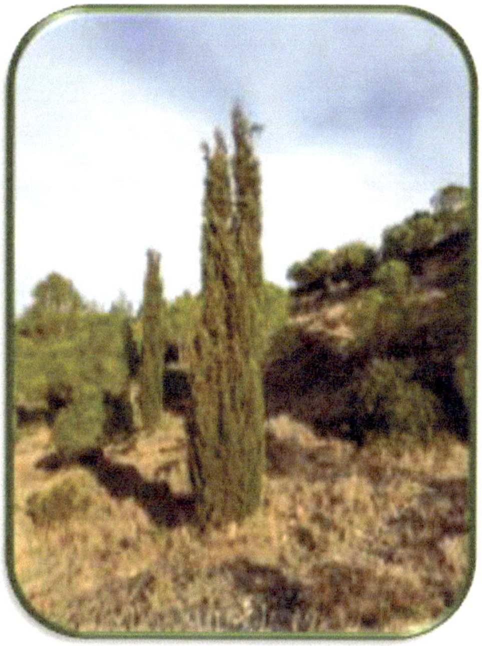

Family: Cupressaceae

Common names: Evergreen cypress.

Foreign names: Cyprès Fr. Cypress, Eng.

Occurrences: 17,561 Occurrences

Distribution in the world

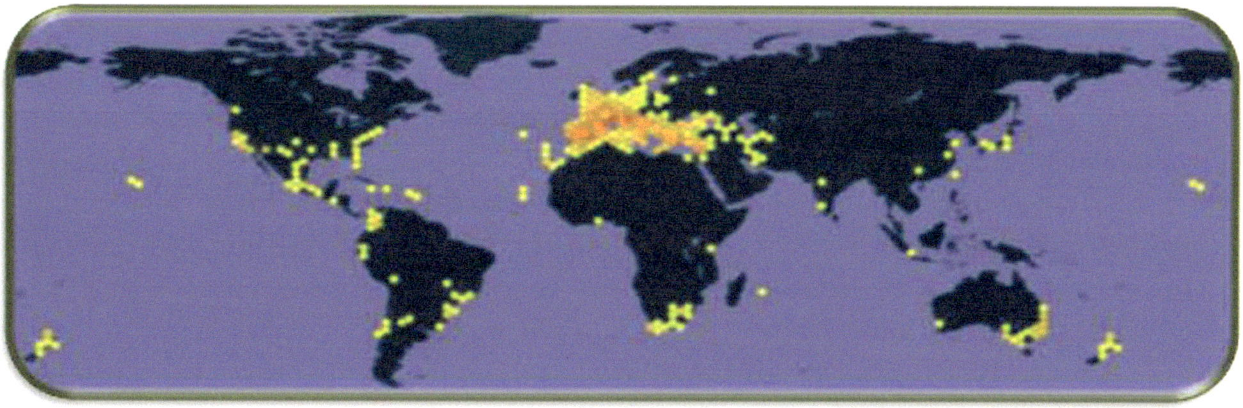

Botanical description:

Evergreen tree, 10-30 m tall, trunk diameter can reach about 1 m. The branches are very dense, erect or spread horizontally, the leaves are scaly, crossed and overlapping, triangular in shape, convex, and there is often a resin gland sunken in the back. Flowers are unisexual and monoecious, the male flowers are gathered in small cones, which arise at the ends of the branches. The female flowers are gathered in spherical cones, approximately 2-3 cm in diameter, and composed of 6-14 scales. Seeds are 5-7 mm, equipped with a wing-like edge. One kilogram of them contains approximately 120,000 seeds, which mature within a year after pollination. This species has the most important varieties: Horizontal evergreen cypress var. C.s. The evergreen columnar cypress pyramidalis var. C.s.

Flowering: March to May.

Habitat and geographical distribution:

The regions of the eastern Mediterranean and southwestern Asia Minor, from where it spread to the rest of the countries to occupy areas much wider than its natural distribution area. It is naturally distributed in Iran, Turkey, Syria, Lebanon, Jordan, Cyprus, Greece, Italy, Libya, Tunisia and Morocco. History and heritage: The Arabic name of the genus "Siro" is derived from the Sumerian origin Hasuru. The genus name Cupressus is the ancient name of the tree and sempervirens means "evergreen" in Latin. The Romans considered it a symbol of fertility. The ancient Greeks used it to treat some diseases such as dysentery, asthma and cough. The cypress was considered a funeral tree by the ancient Romans, and was frequently planted in their cemeteries. It was mentioned by Dioscorides, Ibn al-Baytar, Ibn Sina and al-Antaki. The part used: female cones (collected before they are fully ripe), young leafy branches. The volatile oil extracted from them.

Chemical components:

Female cones and young leafy terminal branches contain a volatile aromatic oil, composed mainly of terpene carbons and alcohols, the most important components of which are: alpha-pinene, camphene, silvestrene, p-cymene, cadinene, cedrol, and furfural alcohols furfurol, in addition to tannins (3-5%) and flavonoids.

Medical properties and uses:

The essential oil has antiseptic, antispasmodic, and vasoconstrictive properties. Female cones have astringent properties, due to their tannic content, and are used internally in the form of aqueous extracts to treat diarrhea. They are used topically in the form of ointments or water baths in cases of uterine bleeding, hemorrhoids and varicose veins. The alcoholic extract of female cones also has an antiviral effect (HSV-1). The decoction of the cones is used popularly as an expectorant, to treat whooping cough, bronchitis, colds, and as a worm repellent. A soak of the cones is also useful in cleaning the feet and combating excessive sweating.

Other uses:

Giving them a distinctive smell. Wood is very Volatile oil is used in the manufacture of perfumes, soaps and detergents Solid, used in the manufacture of cabinets and wardrobes because it retains its scent and repels moths and is immune to woodworms, and for the manufacture of sieve frames and screens.

Use warnings:

Its use in high doses can cause kidney irritation.

Environment:

Cypress is found in several bioclimatic floors from the semi-humid to the semi-dry and upper dry floors. Cypress is a tree that can withstand cold and high temperatures, and has a high tolerance to winds, which makes it desirable for planting fences and windbreaks. It is a flexible species towards rainfall, and is widespread in the countries of the Eastern Mediterranean in areas with varying rainfall (1300-200 mm annually). It occurs on brown soils arising from the Marne, and on soils arising from Marnite limestone, which are calcareous clay soils, and it also occurs on sandy soils arising from rocks. Stony Sandy. It can live on poor surface soils, does not tolerate salinity and poorly drained, stagnant soils.

Cultivation and productivity:

Cypress is propagated by winged seeds that are planted in bags in the nursery in the fall, at a rate of 3 seeds per bag, After germination, they are separated and selected, and one seedling remains in the bag. Then it is transferred to the permanent land after a year, and planted at distances that vary according to the purpose of cultivation, and the required service operations are provided to it, including irrigation, fertilization, and control.

Juniperus communis L.

Juniperus borealis Salisb., Juniperus communis subsp. eucommunis Syme, Juniperus communis var. vulgaris Aiton, Juniperus vulgaris Bubani

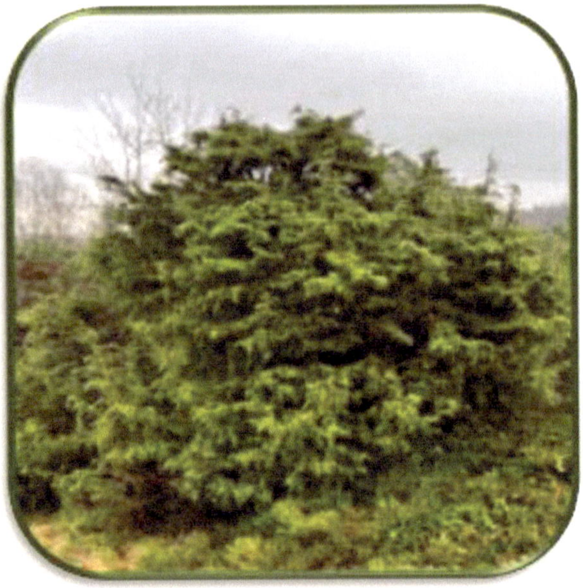

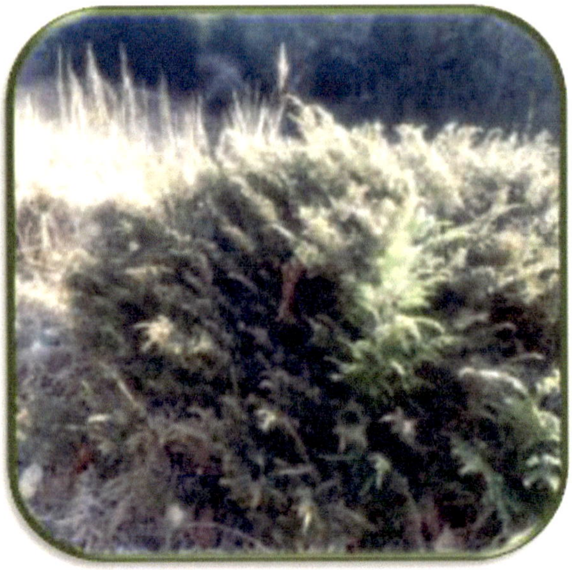

Family: *Cupressaceae*

Common names: *Common juniper.*

Foreign names:*Eng. Common juniper, Fr. genévrier commun, peferon*

Occurrences: 699,804Occurrences

Distribution in the world

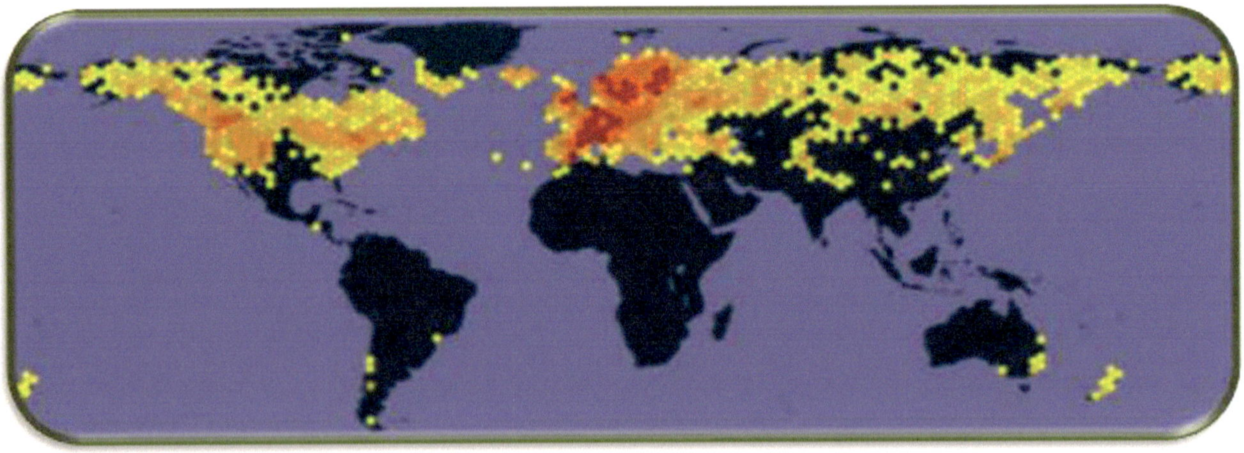

Botanical description:

Shrubs or small trees, dioecious, usually up to 4 m tall (or up to 10 m in some cases.) Stems numerous, extending on the ground to ascending (rarely erect.) Bark brown, fibrous, barking off in strips; young stem bark smooth. Twigs erect. Leaves are green (sometimes silvery), conical, flat, acute to rounded at the tip, and stalked. The female cones take two years to mature, and are of two distinct sizes, their holder is straight, spherical to ovate, 6-13 mm in diameter, bluish-black, resinous, and has 2-3 seeds. Blooms in spring.

Habitat and geographical distribution: Europe and North Africa In Algeria and Morocco.

History and Heritage:

The scientific name of the genus Juniperus is derived from the Latin language, which is the Latin name for the tree among the Latin peoples in Europe. Some references mention that the origin of the word is "astringent" in reference to the taste of its fruits. The species name communis means "common."

Part used:

Flowers, fruits, leaves, and stems.

Chemical components:

The plant contains 2% volatile oil, rich in monoterpene hydrocarbons, including alpha-beta pinene, camphine, para-cenole, myrcine, and sabinene, in addition to containing monoterpene and diterpene compounds. In addition to the volatile oil, the fruits contain catechine tannins, flavonoids, simple sugars, and proanthocyanidins.

Properties and medical uses:

Cyclooxygenase inhibitor, anti-inflammatory, antimicrobial, digestive, choleretic, antispasmodic, diuretic, expectorant. The essential oil is used internally to treat digestive disorders, and externally to treat rheumatism. The essential oil is popularly used as a diuretic, and to treat prostatitis, flatulence, and colon spasms. It is used topically as a reddening massage for the skin in cases of rheumatism, as a pain reliever for disc herniation, and to treat gout and peripheral blood flow deficiency. It is also used as a lotion in cases of eczema and acne. It is traditionally used to treat renal failure, acute and chronic cystitis, cystitis, albuminuria, hematuria and menopause. It has antimicrobial, antioxidant, anti-hypercholesterol, anti-hyperlipidemia properties, and has neuroprotective and Parkinson's disease treatment effects.

Other uses:

The essential oil is used in the preparation of many cosmetics.

Side effects, interactions and warnings:

The oil should not be used internally in cases of kidney inflammation, and prolonged use causes hypocalcem. Caution should be exercised when used by diabetics, and should not be used in cases of congestive heart disease. Topical use may cause irritation, skin injuries, damage and edema. It is not used on large and wide skin wounds and in acute skin diseases. It is not used in cases of pregnancy and lactation.

Environment:

The common juniper grows in multiple bioclimatic levels. And on different types of soil, stony and sandy, but it prefers well-drained lands. It is also found on sand in coastal areas, and may be found near fields and pastures. It grows at altitudes that may reach 3000 m above sea level. Tolerant of wind and sun. Prefers neutral soils, but tolerates a wide range of pH. Juniper is damaged by fires.

Cultivation and productivity:

Juniper is propagated by seeds (slow germination) in early fall or spring. The seeds are soaked in water for 24 hours before planting, then planted in bags at a rate of 2-3 seeds per bag, then they are separated after reaching the appropriate length. It is also propagated by cuttings that are planted in well-drained soil, and in a sunny to semi-shaded place. The plant is affected by some diseases, such as rust and red spider mites.

Juniperus phoenicea L.

Juniperus terminalis Salisb., Juniperus tetragona Moench, Sabina phoenicea)L.(Antoine, Sabinella phoenicea)L.(Nakai.

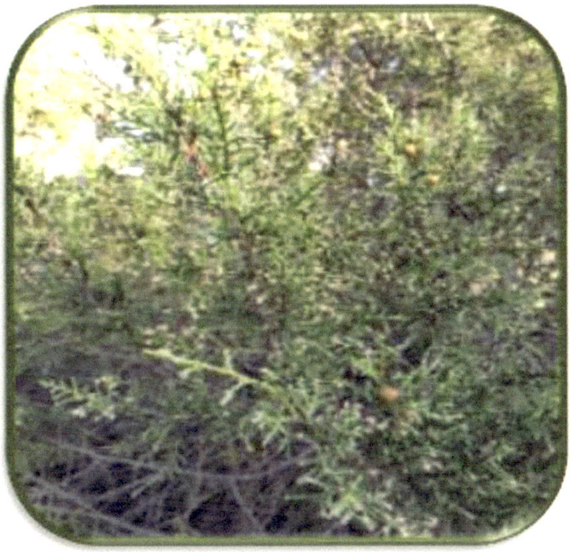

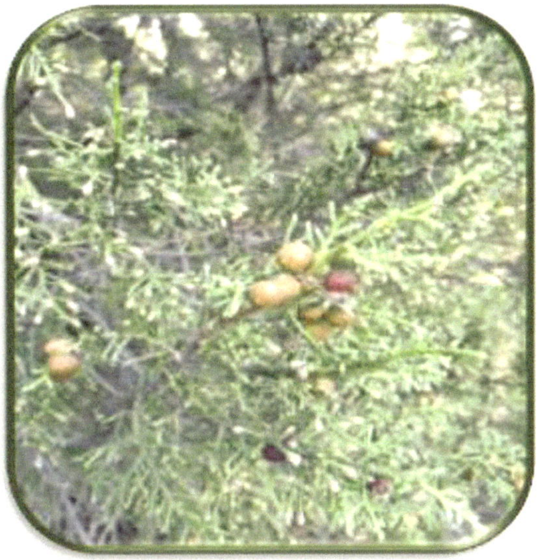

Family: *Cupressaceae*

Common names: *Phoenician juniper.*

Foreign names: *Phoenician juniper*

Occurrences: 82,277 Occurrences

Distribution in the world

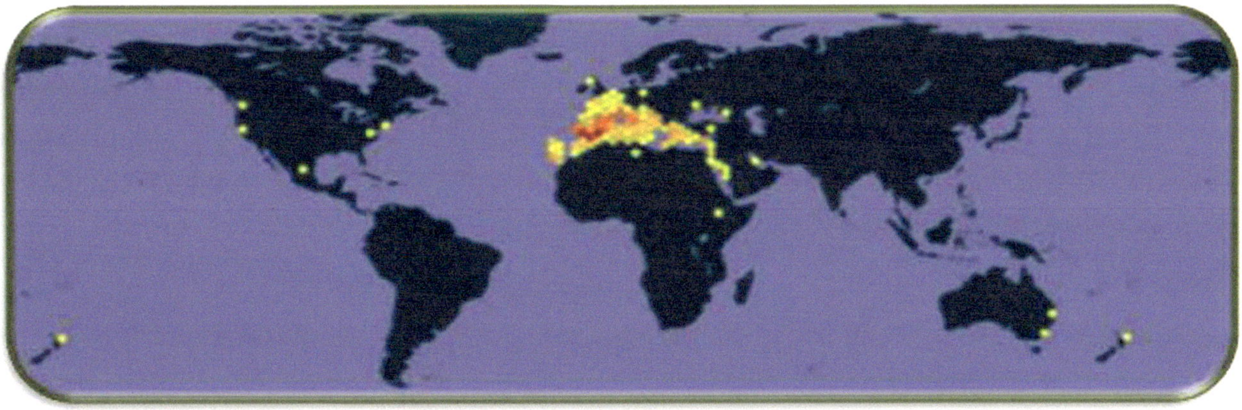

Botanical description:

Very long-lived trees or shrubs (may reach 1000 years), single-living, 6-8 m high. Branches erect or ascending, dense, cylindrical when young. Leaves 1-2 mm, semi-squamous, oblong, arranged in whorls, or opposite and overlapping, ovate-rhomboid, convex dorsally, marked by a linear resinous canal. Male cones terminal, sessile, ovate-oblong, scales rounded. Mature female cones are spherical to sub-spherical, 8-15 mm in diameter, semi-flattened, fleshy, reddish-brown to yellowish-brown, shiny, composed of 6-8 scales. Seeds 3-9 free, oblong, ripening in summer from the second year of formation. Flowering from March to April.

Habitat and geographical distribution:

Mediterranean, extending to southwestern Arabian Peninsula. It is distributed in Libya, Tunisia, Morocco, Algeria, and eastern Jordan.

History and Heritage:

The scientific name of the genus Juniperus is derived from the Latin language, the word describing the species phoenicia meaning "purple" in reference to the color of its fruits, or "Phoenician" in reference to the ancient Phoenicians who inhabited the Syrian coast and traded in purple, despite its non-existence naturally in that region. Phoenician juniper was mentioned in Pharaonic recipes in the "Hearst" and "Ebers" papyri as therapeutic recipes for pain relief, treating urinary tract infections, and relieving renal colic. The Greeks and Romans knew it and used it to treat their diseases. They also burned it to ward off bad thoughts and diseases. Dioscorides said about it: “There is a large and small amount of it, and both of them warm, soothe and increase urine flow. Ibn Sina also mentioned that juniper is good for chest pain, cough and stomach.”

Part used:

Leaves, fruits, and wood oil.

Chemical components:

The percentage of volatile oil in the plant parts ranges between 0.5 - 2%, depending on the geographical source of the plant and the method of drying and distillation. The wood contains 0.6% volatile oil, rich in mono- and semi-terpene compounds (sescoterpenes) 58%, the most important of which is cedrol 13%. The leaves contain 1.7-0.8% volatile oil, rich in mono- and semi-terpene compounds (sescoterpenes) 87%, while the monoterpenes include α-pinene 48%, α-thujene 36%, delta-cadinene δ 6%, and mono- and semi-terpene caryophyllene 5%, in addition to some Alcoholic compounds: Monoterpenes geraniol. The fruits contain 0.7% volatile oil rich in monoterpenes 60%, the most important of which are: alpha-pinene 13%, verbinone 6%, terpene alcohol: sapinol. Sabinol In addition to carbohydrates 30%, catechic tannins 3-5%, flavonoids, and anthocyanins such as leucanthocyanes.

Properties and medical uses:

Juniper oil has antibacterial and antifungal properties, and is used in the treatment of urinary tract infections. Some references mention the properties of lignins in the treatment of tumors. The oil is used topically in the treatment of wounds and skin diseases. Juniper leaves are popularly used in the form of an infusion or decoction to get rid of intestinal gases, treat pulmonary tuberculosis and asthma, treat diarrhea, increase urination, get rid of urinary tract stones, and treat renal colic.

It is used topically to treat rheumatism and skin diseases, such as eczema, pimples, and boils. Juniper wood is distilled to obtain black tar, which is filtered, and tar oil is taken from it, called "Safwa." It is used as an antiseptic and bacteria killer. Roasted juniper fruits are eaten as an appetite stimulant and digestive aid. The decoction is also used topically as a compress to treat skin ulcers and blisters, and as a gargle to get rid of bad breath. Alcoholic extracts of the aerial parts have shown antibacterial activity against both gram-positive and gram-negative bacteria.

Other uses:

Tar oil is used in veterinary medicine to get rid of ticks in the skins of farm animals. Juniper wood is used in carpentry in Algeria and Tunisia. In addition, it is used mainly in the production of charcoal and fuel in Africa.

Precautions for use:

It is not recommended to use the fruit oil internally, due to the presence of the irritating compound sabinol, which may cause digestive, nervous, cardiac, respiratory, hepatic and renal disorders. Bees visit it to collect the sap secreted by the plant.

Environment:

The Phoenician juniper grows in dry and semi-dry environments in various bioclimatic levels, from the fresh humid in the Canary Islands, to the upper dry and semi-dry lower levels in southern Jordan. It is resistant to cold, is light-loving, and is found on different types of soils, even calcareous, stony and sandy. It is suitable for moderate to slightly acidic soils, relatively tolerant of salinity and resistant to winds. It grows from sea level to an altitude of 2400 m in the Atlas Mountains and the Asir Mountains.

Cultivation and productivity:

The Phoenician juniper is propagated by seeds by treating them with sand to remove the gum layer to facilitate germination. The seeds can be treated with 30% sulfuric acid for 20 minutes. It is preferable to collect the seeds from ripe, soft fruits, i.e. not dry, from medium-aged trees. The fruits take two years to mature.

Juniperus oxycedrus L.

Juniperus glauca Salisb., Juniperus oxycedrus subsp. rufescens Debeaux, Juniperus oxycedrus var. rufescens Carrière, Juniperus rufescens Link.

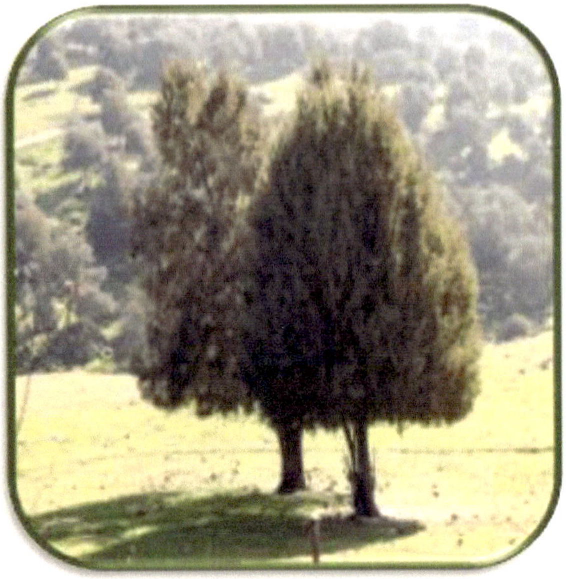

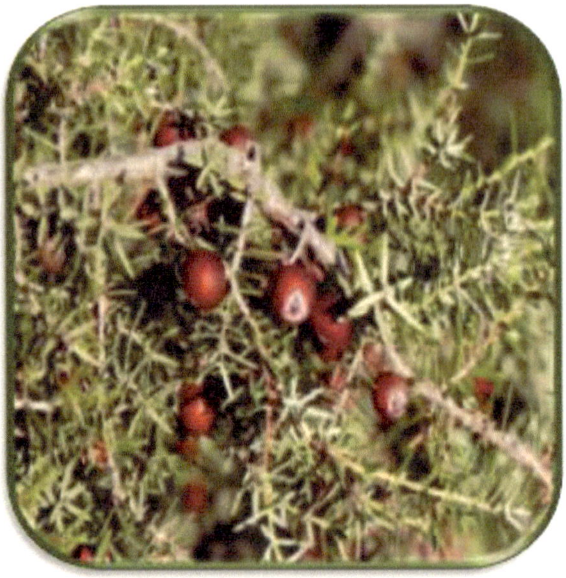

Family: *Cupressaceae*

Common names: *Kadi Juniper, Sherbini Juniper, Sherbeen, Thorny Juniper, Thorny Cedar.*

Foreign names*: Genievre Fr. juniper, Prickly Eng.*

Occurrences: 175,305 Occurences

Distribution in the world

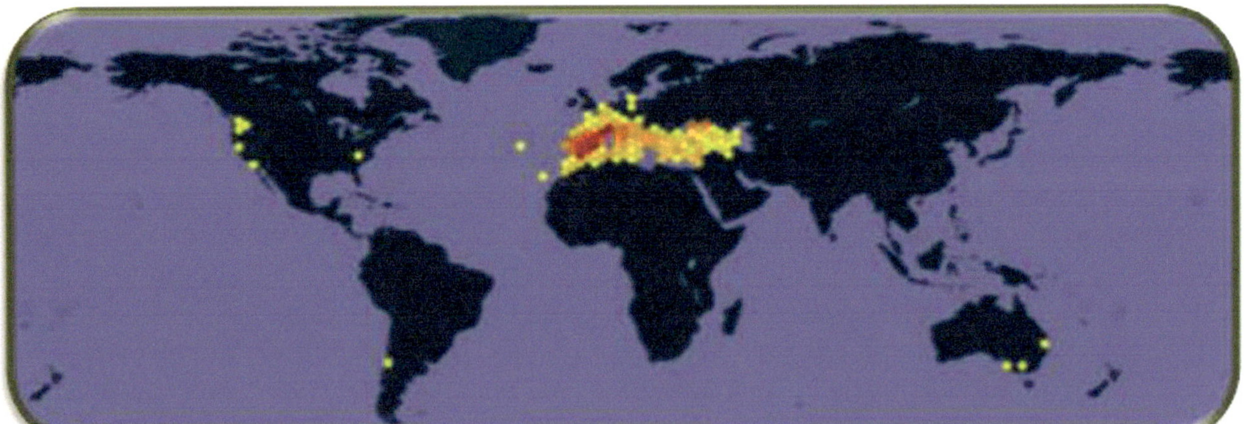

Botanical description:

Trees or shrubs, dioecious, can reach 10 m in height, young branches are not completely clear triangular in section, stem bark is rough, grey-brown in colour. Leaves are stinging, needle-like, linear-lanceolate, 15-20 mm long, 1-2 mm wide, bluish-green, hard, gathered every third together, and are characterised by the presence of two white lines on the upper surface. Male cones solitary, semi-spherical, semi-spherical or ovoid. Mature female cones spherical, 6-10 mm in diameter, reddish-brown to brown, consisting of several fused scales 3-6 (covering the fruit in a thin, bluish-coloured form.) Seeds 2-3 (rarely one), ripening the following year.

Flowering: March to April.

Habitat and geographical distribution:

Mediterranean, southeast Asia, and southern Europe, and is spread in the forests of the countries of the eastern Mediterranean basin as a mountainous element from Syria and Lebanon to northern Africa.

Part used:

Fruits, leaves, and cade oil. cade oil: a thick liquid with a dark brown color, a strong smell, and a pungent and bitter taste. cade oil is extracted by dry distillation of tree wood, and the remaining residue is neglected, which is asphalt in consistency and is called tar.

History and Heritage:

The descriptive name of the species oxycedrus is derived from the Greek: the syllable "oxy" means "sharp" in reference to its sharp leaves and the syllable cedrus means "cedar", i.e. prickly cedar. The plant was famous in ancient times, as it was burned to ward off the devil and evil thoughts, and to repel lice and fleas.

Chemical components:

The parts of the plant contain resins, volatile oils, flavonoid glycosides, tannins, organic acids, and terpenoid compounds. Cade oil: It is mainly composed of phenolic compounds -17-26%, the most important of which is guaiacol 12%, monoterpenes and semiterpenes (sesquiterpenes), the most important of which is delta-cadinene - δ 14.5%, cis-thujopsene 9%, alpha-muurolene 5% and alcoholic terpenes cardinol. Tar: It is mainly composed of cadinene, guaycol, and cresol. The fruits contain volatile oil, the most important components of which are α-pinene 27%, β-myrcene 19%, α-phellandrene 7%, limonene 7%, δ-cadinene 2.2%, and germacrene. The leaves contain volatile oil composed mainly of monoterpene compounds α-pinene 40-57% and manoyl oxide 5-10%, in addition to acid. Dahni Sabinic a. .sabinic

Properties and medical uses:

Cade oil has antioxidant, antiseptic, antimicrobial, antiparasitic, and wound-healing properties. Cade oil is included in the composition of preparations used topically to treat hemorrhoids, wounds, diseases, and skin inflammations der matitis, such as dermatitis, ulcers, chronic eczema, acne, and psoriasis. Research has shown the anti-inflammatory properties of the leaves (volatile oil).

Other uses:

Cad oil is used in the manufacture of perfumes, soaps and shampoos designed to care for the scalp, strengthen hair, prevent hair loss and get rid of dandruff. In some countries, the fruit is made into a powder that is drunk instead of coffee.

Side effects and warnings:

It is not recommended to use cad oil or its fruits internally for pregnant women, or for those suffering from intestinal infections or kidney problems, due to the fact that the oil and fruits contain compounds that irritate the kidneys and urinary tract if used in excessive doses for long periods.

Environment:

It is considered one of the species that loves light, tolerates cold, and is adapted to the high mountain environment. It lives on different types of soils, even dry and shallow, with a preference for non-calcareous soils.

Cultivation and productivity:

Common juniper is propagated by seeds that require alternating treatment with hot and cold water as the seeds have a hard coat. They can also be treated with boiling water for 3-6 seconds.

Cyperus rotundus L.

Chlorocyperus rotundus (L.) Palla, Pycreus rotundus (L.) Hayek.

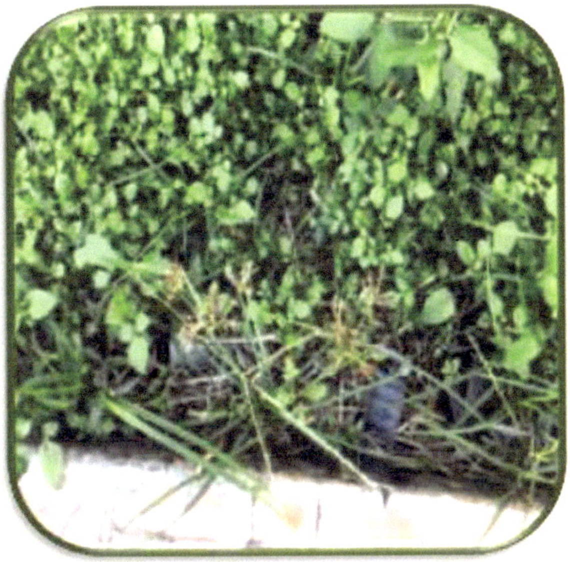

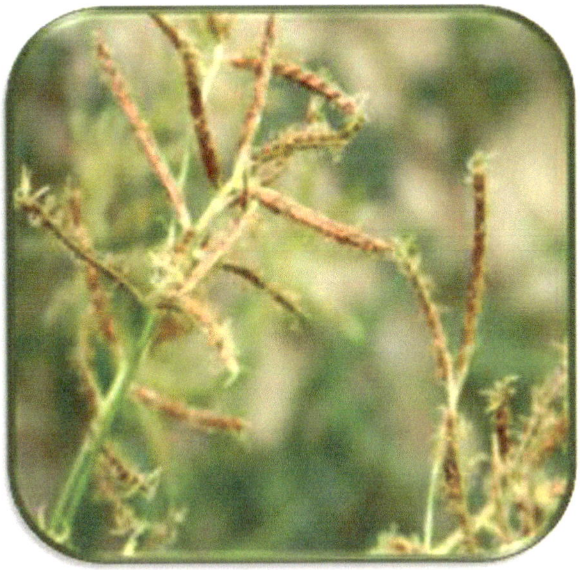

Family: Cyperaceae

Common names: Hab Al-Aziz, Hab Al-Zalm, Al-Saad, Saadi, Saadi Al-Himar, Saad Kouf (Damascus countryside).

Foreign names: Purple nutsedge, Nutgrass, Fr. herbe à oignon

Occurrences : 27,388 occurrences

Distribution in the world

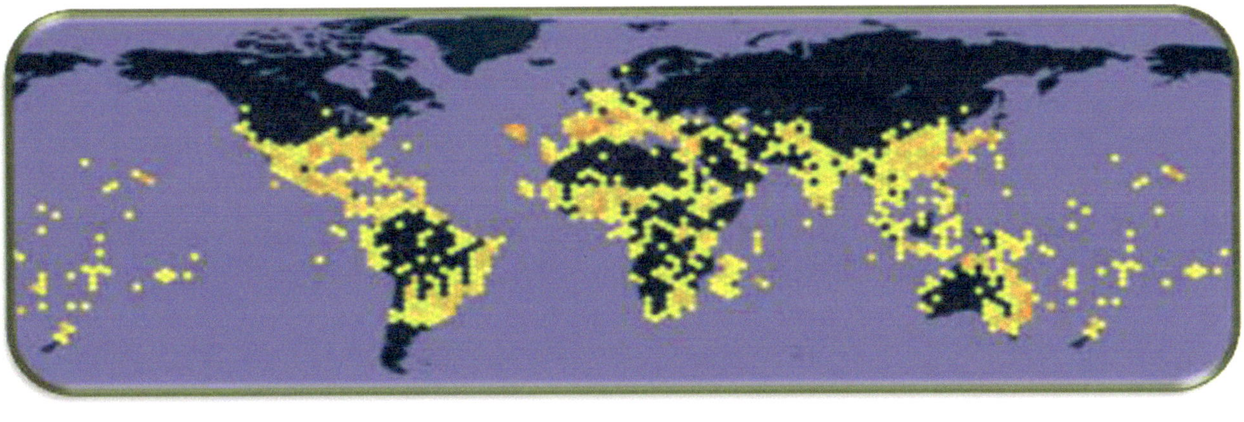

Botanical description:

A perennial herb, 15-60 cm tall, with a slender rhizome, bearing red to brown scales, and producing slender stems, ending in a dark brown semi-spherical tubercle. Stem Slender, three-sided, leafy in the lower part. Leaves up to 6 mm wide, flat, pointed at the apex, often shorter than the stem. Inflorescence simple or compound, rays (axes) 3-9, unequal, up to 10 cm long, each ending in a short spikelet or a group of spikelets. Bracts surrounding the inflorescence 2-4, flat, longer than the inflorescence. Spikelet 3-2×35-10 mm, many-flowered, linear, strongly compressed, winged axis. The two stamens are overlapping, ovate, scaphoid, reddish to dark brown, membranous on the edge, bearing 5-7 nerves 3. Stamens. 3. Pistils. Fruit: Acorn, oblong-ovate-inverted or ellipsoid, trilobate, glossy, rarely reaches maturity, propagation is mostly by peduncles.

Flowering: From February to December.

There is another type almond (Earth . L. esculentus (Cyperus), similar to the above type in its components and uses.

Habitat and geographical distribution:

Mediterranean, Iranian-Turanian and tropical. It is naturally distributed in large areas in Asia, Africa and Australia.

History and heritage:

The scientific name of the genus is derived from the Greek kypeiros, which is the name of one of its edible species, C. esculentus, meaning "edible" or "nutritious", as its sweet-tasting tubers are eaten, and it is known as the man's seed. Another species is the papyrus plant C. papyrus, from whose bark papyrus was made. The species called in the Levant is C. conglomeratus, meaning "clumped", and is a sand-loving plant, and is important in stabilizing sand dunes in the dry regions of the Maghreb and the Levant. It is believed that it was called Hab Al-Aziz because one of the kings of Egypt was fond of eating it, as he used to call the name of the king of Egypt "Aziz Misr." It was mentioned in the Pharaonic recipes to expel intestinal worms, treat eczema, and against skin itching and uterine infections. Some archaeologists found its fruits in one of the rooms of "Deir Abu al-Naja" where they found a cup filled with the fruits of the Aziz seed. The Aziz seed was also found around the neck of the mummy of Prince "Kent." The Arabs called the plant "Hab al-Zalm" and they used it as a type of fruit. Ibn Sina wrote about it that it is "very good tasting, and increases semen.

Part used: The aromatic root tubers, and the rhizomes.

Chemical components:

The tubers contain fixed oil, and volatile oil, which has a camphoraceous smell, and a bitter taste. The most important compounds of the volatile oil are cy-perene, rotundene, α-cyperone, cyperorotundene, α-corymbolol, α-pinene, caryophyllene oxide, D-germacrene, mustakone, Zierone, which give the plant extracts their medicinal properties. The rhizomes and tubers contain sugars such as glucose and fructose, in addition to a large amount of starch, alkaloids, tannins, bitter substances, and vitamin C.

Medical properties and uses:

The volatile oil of the tubers exhibits cytotoxic, antioxidant, and antitumor properties. The tubers and rhizomes of the plant are popularly used for their sedative, antiemetic, and carminative effects. The tubers are used as a headache reliever, to treat anxiety, stress, urinary tract infections, and menstrual disorders. Clinical studies have proven the properties of the plant's chemical components, as they are antioxidants, antimicrobials, anticancer, antineuritis, antidepressants, anti-inflammatory, anti-obesity, vasodilator, antispasmodic, bronchodilator, anti-allergic, anti-oomycete, anti-spasmodic, anti-diarrheal, anti-vomiting, anti-parasitic worms, anti-histamine, anti-hyperglycemia, anti-hypertension, anti-malarial, and have estrogenic biological functions. The flavonoid compounds present in the essential oil have analgesic and anti-inflammatory properties, and are a safe and effective treatment for the side effects of laser hair removal. The oil is used to treat trichomoniasis caused by the nematode Trichinella, especially when combined with albendazole.

Other uses:

The tubers are used as a type of fragrant incense, especially for fumigating baby clothes. The tubers and rhizomes are eaten after grinding them, despite their bitter taste.

Environment:

It grows on the edges of swamps and shallow muddy ponds, between rocks, and on the edges of roads, in tropical and temperate hot regions. It loves warm, humid environments. Its green group is affected by spring frost. It grows on different soils, provided that they are well-drained. Sedimentary soils that contain relatively large amounts of sulfur, magnesium, calcium, and boron are the most suitable soils for its growth. It is found in sandy loamy soils, whose pH ranges from Between -5.5 and 6.5 It is used in many countries such as China to stabilize river banks and earth dams.

Cultivation and productivity:

It is propagated by seeds that are scattered on fertile soil. The seeds germinate within 2-6 weeks at a temperature of 18°C. It is characterized by the rapid growth of its rhizomes and tubers underground, leading to the formation of large colonies that compete strongly with cultivated plants, causing many problems for farmers. It can be propagated by tubers collected from its colonies, especially those growing in agricultural land.

Dryopteris filix-mas (L.) Schott

Polypodium filix-mas L., Aspidium filix-mas (L.) Sw, Lastrea filix-mas (L.) C.Presl, The- lypteris filix-mas (L.) Nieuwl., Aspidium nemorale Gray

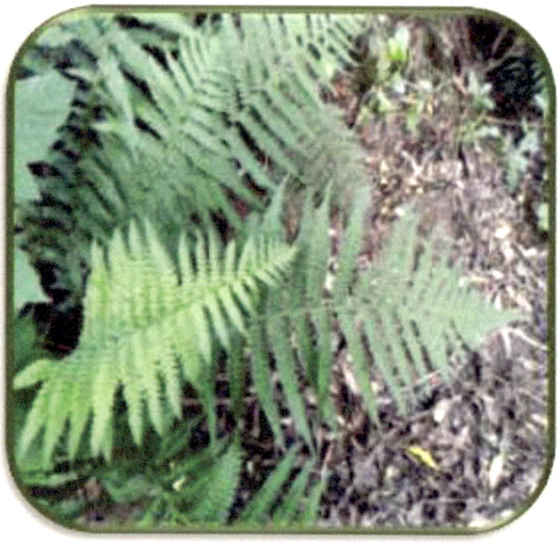

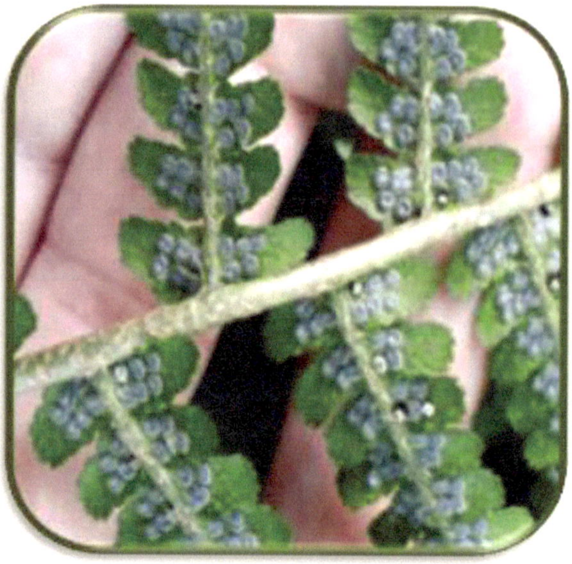

Family: Polypodiaceae (formerly Dryopteridaceae)

Common names: Male fern, dagger, shard.

Foreign names: mâle Fougère Fr. Fern, Male Eng.

Occurrences : 645,867 occurrences

Distribution in the world

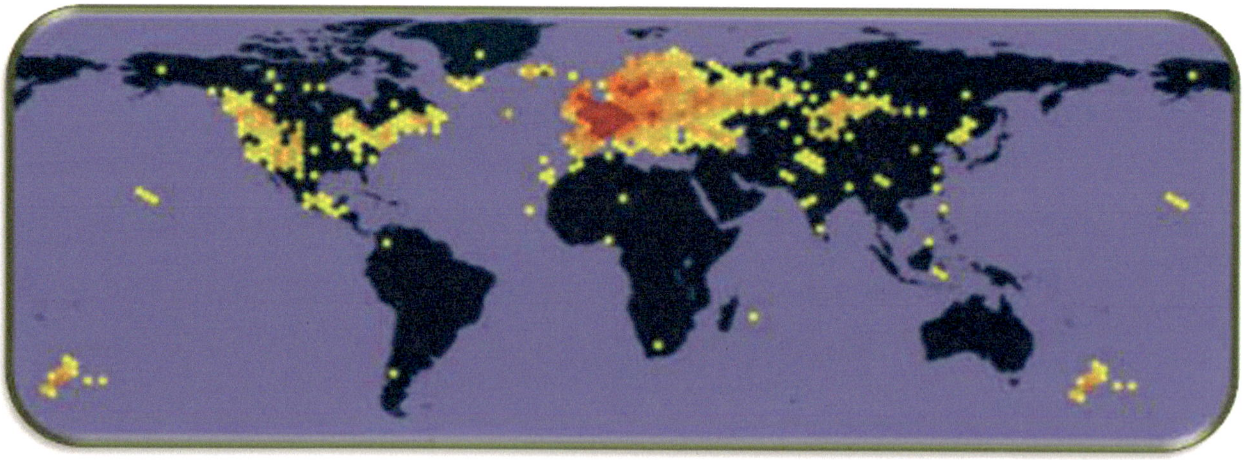

Botanical description:

A perennial herb with thick rhizomes. The leaves are uniform in shape, die in winter, their dimensions are 10-30 x 28-120 cm. The length of the leaf is less than a quarter of the length of the leaf, bearing scales at the base, the scales are scattered, brown, and have two patterns: the first is broad, and the second is hair-like (only this species has two distinct patterns of scales, without intermediate cases.)

The blade is dull green, solid, ovate-lanceolate, deeply divided twice into ovate-lanceolate parts, its edge is serrated to lobed. The spores are kidney-shaped, arranged in two rows in the middle of the distance between the median nerve and the leaf margin. The chemiscle is also spherical, glabrous and lacks glands. Spores are produced from June/July to September.

Habitat and geographical distribution: Europe,Siberian, Mediterranean.

History and heritage:

The scientific name of the genus Dryopteris is the Greek name for it, and the descriptive name for the species Filix-mas means "fern". The scientific name for the genus Dryopteris is the Greek name for it. It was used in ancient times as a repellent for various types of worms. Dioscorides, Al-Ghasani, Ibn Al-Baytar, and Al-Antaki mentioned it. Ibn Sina wrote about it: "It has bitterness and kills worms." The part used: The rhizome, dry or tender rhizomes, the basal leaves, and the apical bud. The rhizomes are usually collected in late summer and autumn.

Chemical components:

Rhizomes contain a mixture of phloroglucinoles derivatives 2%, called filicin crude, present in the form of mono, di, tri, and tetracyclic compounds, concentrated in the internal secretory hairs of the rhizomes and the leaf base parenchyma. The condensation of the cyclic compounds produces several compounds, the most important of which are: flavaspidic acid, filicinic acid, aspinidol, and albasidine. Tannins, saponins, mineral substances 4-5%, sugars, starchy substances, and fatty substances 4-6%. The leaves contain the same previous compounds in proportions of less than 0.2%, in addition to some flavonoid compounds, saponins, terpenoids, and reducing sugars. The compound quercetin-3-O-α-L-rhamnopyranoside

Properties and medical uses:

A poisonous plant, which has antiviral and anthelmintic properties due to its content of phaspidic acid and filicenic acid, such as liver flukes and band worms, but it does not affect roundworms and oxyuris (a type of snake worm). The extract of the male fern is popularly used to expel worms, and is used topically in the treatment of rheumatism and sweat. Women Muscle pain and treatment of hemorrhoids. It is also used to treat inflammation, arthritis, hemorrhoids, rheumatoid nerve pain, wounds and ulcers. Plant extracts are effective against foot edema, do not cause skin ulcers and have no side effects of stomach irritation. The plant is considered safe in treating acute cases of inflammation.

Warnings for use:

Poisonous plant, skin irritant, high doses of it can cause permanent disabilities such as paralysis, blindness and possibly death, which requires its use under medical supervision. The male fern or any of its preparations are not prescribed for patients with liver, kidney, heart and diabetes, and are not prescribed for the elderly and pregnant women. Environment: It grows in shady, humid places in forests. It tolerates low temperatures of up to -30°C. It likes moisture on its roots, but it tolerates drought in shady locations. It grows in places exposed to light, but it grows better in shady locations with 2-3 hours of sunlight per day. It likes moderate or acidic soils, it succeeds in fertile or poor soils, and does not like clay soils.

Cultivation and productivity:

It is rarely planted as a crop, it grows wild or is planted as an ornamental plant. It is propagated by spore-bearing blisters on the underside of the leaves, and by dividing the stem with part of the rhizomes. The blisters containing the spores are scattered in pots containing sterile compost, and kept moist by placing the pot in a black nylon bag. The spores germinate after 1-3 m. The seedlings are placed in a shady place until they grow, and are planted during the spring in the permanent ground. Months at 20 degrees Celsius. The plant can be propagated by division in the spring. Divided plants with their rhizomes can be planted directly into the permanent soil if they are large enough, and it is best to plant them in a nursery or greenhouse first in moist, humus-rich soil, in a shady location, by burying them shallowly in the soil, then watering them with a spray, taking care to drain excess irrigation water well, until they form strong rhizomes, then transferring them to the permanent soil in the following spring. The rhizomes are usually collected at the end of summer when they have reached their maximum growth.

Elaeagnus angustifolia L.

Elaeagnus angustifolia var. normalis Kuntze, Elaeagnus angustifolia var. biebersteiniana Kuntze, Elaeagnus angustifolia var. caspica Sosn., Elaeagnus angustifolia var. iliensis Musch., Elaeagnus angustifolia subsp. orientalis (L.) Soják, Elaeagnus angustifolia var. orientalis (L.) Kuntze

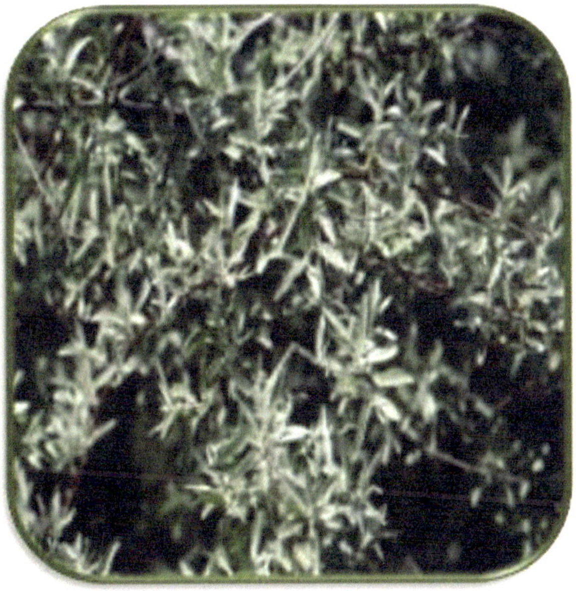

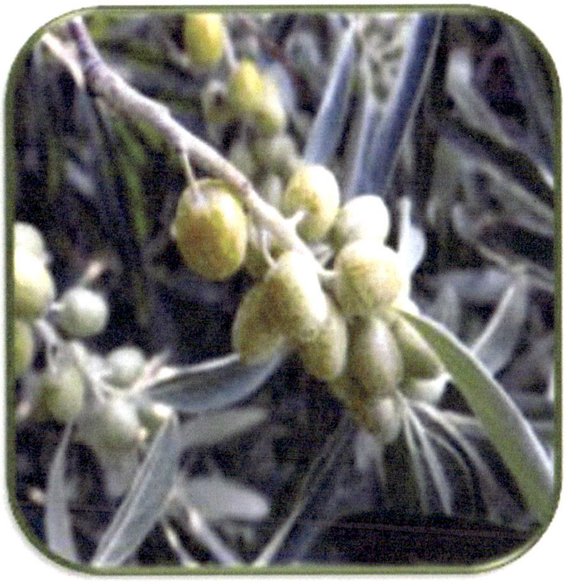

Family: Elaeagnaceae

Common names: Linden, fragrant olive, Bohemian olive, silver olive

Eng. Russian olive, Fr. L'olivier de Bohème Foreign names:

Occurrences : 41,484 occurrences

Distribution in the world

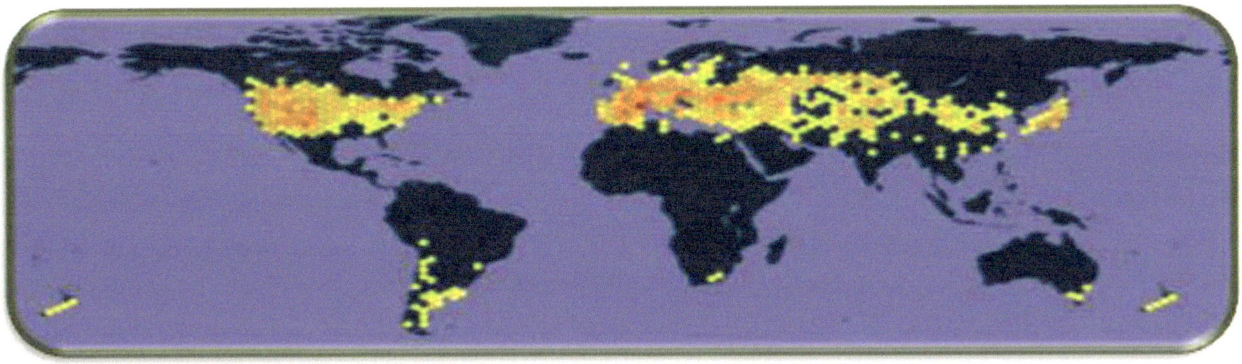

Botanical description:

A shrub or small tree, 3-8 m tall. The branches are often thorny. The leaves are deciduous, alternate, short-petiolate (5 - 8 mm), lanceolate or lanceolate-linear, light green on the upper surface, silvery on the lower surface, their dimensions are 1.6-0.6×2-5 cm. Flowers solitary or in groups of 2-3, 4-8 mm long, short panicle (2 mm), fragrant. Calyx tubular, about 5 mm long, sepals 4, short, triangular, silvery-white outside, yellow inside, corolla absent. Male 4 stamens, short filaments. The ovary is semi-spherical, the fruit is nuclear, elliptical, yellow or red, has a sweet taste, its dimensions are about 1.5 x 2 cm, ripens at the end of autumn (it blooms and bears fruit in Damascus and its countryside, with the exception of Jabal al-Sheikh.)

Flowering: from April to July.

History and Heritage: The scientific name of the genus Elaeagnus, comes from the ancient Greek: the syllable "elaia" means "olive tree", and the syllable gnusa means "leaf" Vitex is an aromatic plant, so the name aromatic olive becomes a reference to the scent of its fragrant flowers. The descriptive name of the species angustifolia means "sharp-leaved", a characteristic of the plant's leaves. The common name is linden, and it is also given to the genus Tilia, and it is also called "Bohemian olive", which is the literal translation of the plant in French, and it is also called "silver linden" due to its shiny silver leaves.

Part used: fruits, flowers and leaves.

Home and geographical distribution:

Southern Europe, western and central Asia, and Egypt, from where it spread to large areas of the world.

Chemical components:

Saccharides, the most important of which are fructose 27%, glucose 22%, proteins and amino acids 10%, The fruits contain the most important of which are glutamic acid and arginine, as well as fatty oil, the most important of which are linoleic acid 52%, linolenic acid a. linolenic acid 12%, and oleic acid. a oleic 5%, and also contains polyphenols, tannins and catechins, phenolic acids cafeic acid and tannic acid, rutin flavonoids, in addition to phospholipides, the most important of which are phosphatidylcholine 52%, phosphatidylethanolamine 16%, and many vitamins, the most important of which are A, C, E and minerals such as calcium Ca, potassium K, magnesium Mg. The flowers contain volatile oil, the most important component of which is trans-ethylcinnamate 79%. The leaves contain phenolic compounds Similar to those found in fruits.

Properties and medical uses:

The fruit extract has antibacterial activity against Staphylococcus aureus, Pseudomonas aeruginosa, and is analgesic and antioxidant due to its rutin content. The seeds have properties (flavonoid compounds) that reduce muscle tension, and the fruit extract has benefits in treating stomach ulcers. The fruits and flowers are popularly used to treat nausea, vomiting, insomnia, asthma, jaundice, tetanus, and flatulence. The decoction of the flowers (steam) is used, as it contains volatile oil, to improve heart function. The decoction of the leaves is used for its sedative properties in cases of anxiety and spasmodic cough. The decoction of the leaves and flowers is also used as a diuretic and to treat fever.

The fresh fruits are eaten as an appetizing fruit, and the fruit paste is used topically to treat rheumatism and arthritis. The plant is known for its therapeutic applications, and is added to food products as a vital ingredient to enhance antioxidants, polyphenols, fiber, flavonoids, sterols, carbohydrates and protein content. Other uses: Linden is a multi-purpose species that can be used as a windbreak and a beautiful ornamental shrub. Its fragrant flowers are desirable for bees and for producing good honey. The leaves have a high fodder value. The wood is porous, suitable for light uses, and excellent for fuel. The fruits are sugary and eaten by birds. They can also be used in jam making.

Environment:

A light-loving tree, resistant to drought and pollution, does not require special care. It can live on different types of soils, even moderately saline, provided they are well drained. There are fungal symbiotic nodes on the roots of the plant that help improve the growth of the tree and allow it to live on poor soils.

Cultivation and productivity:

The tree is fast-growing, leaves a lot of fruit after cutting, and can be easily propagated by cuttings and suckers, which gives it a great advantage in spreading and expansion. The plant can be planted in normal, well-irrigated soil in autumn or spring, and can be propagated by seed. The tree is pruned in winter to encourage branching, taking into account organic fertilization in spring. To obtain good growth and branching, it is preferable in the first years to prune about a third of the plant at the end of winter, noting that the plant tolerates pruning well, as it tolerates pests and diseases. Flowering begins in the sixth year of the plant's life, and the flowering period does not exceed one week. The flowers are harvested when two-thirds of them open.

***Ephedra alata* Decne.**

Ephedra alata var. *decaisnei* Stapf

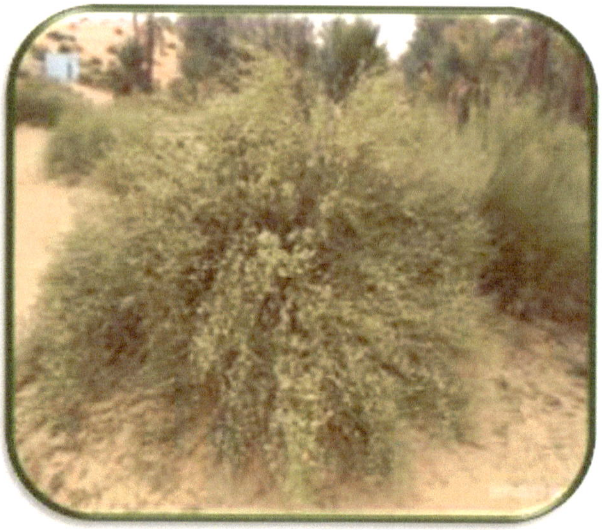

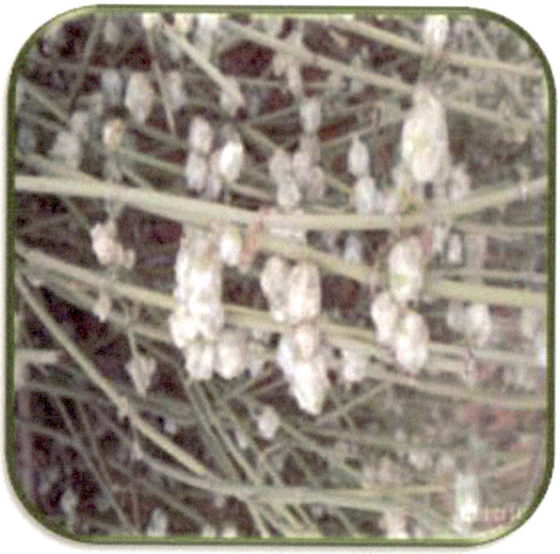

Family: Ephedraceae

Common names:winged ephedra

Foreign names: Ephedra Fr. pine, Joint Eng.

Occurrences : 1,285 occurrences

Distribution in the world

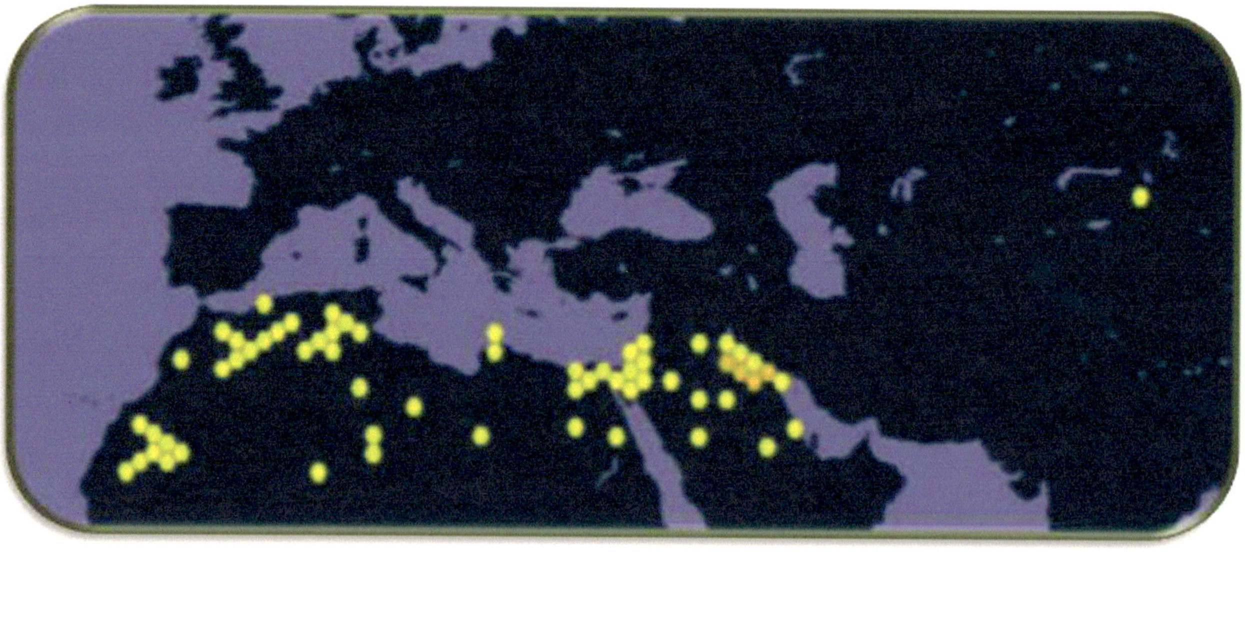

Botanical description:

A small shrub of coleoptiles, dioecious, gray-green in color, 25-75 cm high, sometimes more depending on environmental conditions. The stems are solid, rough, jointed-nodular. The leaves are reduced to a short simple sheath, 3-4 mm long, and 1-2 mm wide.

Flowers are unisexual, male flowers are sessile, gathered in spherical groups, emerge from the axils of the leaves at the top of small branches, about 3 cm long, reminiscent of conifer cones. There are 4 anthers at the top of branched filaments. Female cones are 5×7 mm, axillary or apical at the end of small branches, about 2 cm long. The bracts are fused to the middle to form 4-5 small cups, the interior of which becomes fleshy at the end of its development. The seeds are oblong, blunt at the apex, about 2.5 mm wide, and about 6 mm long. The pollen grains are released in mid-March, and the fruits appear in May.

Habitat and geographical distribution:

Arabian Peninsula, the Levant, and North Africa. It is widespread in Saudi Arabia, Kuwait, Iraq, Jordan, Syria, Egypt and Palestine, and has become rare in many Arab countries. The genus Ephedra includes about 70 species, the most important of which are: E. sinica Stapf, E. distachya L., E. maxima, E. vulgaris Rich, E. equisetina Bunge, E. intermedia Shrenk ex Meyer, E. geradiana Wallich ex Meyer, E. alte C.A. Mey, E. campy- lopoda C.A. Mey.

History and heritage:

The scientific name of the genus Ephedra is from the Greek, where epi means "on", and hedra means "chair" or "seat", i.e. "on a seat", which is a name given by the ancients in Europe to a climbing plant devoid of leaves. The word alata means "winged", and the name is derived from the shape of the plant and the wings sitting on the branches. As for the name of the alanda, it came from the tall and strong one, as well as the horse. The Chinese knew the effectiveness of al-Anda In Taj al-Arus by al-Zubaidi that it is the weak camel treatment for asthma 5000 years ago, and a Chinese chemist studied ephedrine in 1924, and it was synthesized industrially in 1929.

The part used:

The aerial parts, especially the spaces between the nodal branches. The soft branches and terminal tips of ephedra are collected in the fall, because the alkaloids contained in the aerial parts double from spring to fall, and the highest percentage of alkaloids is found in plants that are 4 years old.

Chemical components:

Ephedra species are generally similar in their compounds, with differences in the proportions of these compounds. Ephedra species contain alkaloids belonging to the group of non-traditional amino alkaloids, 0.2 - 0.5%, especially the easy ephedrine (L-Ephedrin 90-30%) and pseudoephedrine. It also contains a volatile oil that consists mainly of terpenoids (alpha-terpineol, limonene, tetramethylpyrazine, terpineol, linalool) in addition to many other compounds. Secondary: flavonoids (kaempferol), lacenin, tannins, glycans, and organic acids. 11 phenols have been identified, including gallic acid and quercetrin. Ephedra seeds are a valuable source of biologically active natural compounds and minerals that can be used for industrial and pharmaceutical purposes, as they contain significant amounts of sodium, potassium, calcium, magnesium, copper, zinc, and iron, with high levels of polyphenols, flavonoids, and concentrated tannins.

Properties and medical uses:

Ephedrine alkaloid has sympathmimetic activities, and antagonistic properties of alpha 1, alpha 2, and beta 2 receptors. It also causes vasoconstrictive activity, cardio-stimulation (tachycardia), a sharp increase in blood pressure, insomnia, dizziness, headache, and nervousness. Pseudoephedrine has beta-2 receptor-antagonist properties, including bronchodilation, and nasal capillary vasoconstriction. Ephedra generally has antiviral, hypotensive, male sexual stimulant, enzyme-inhibiting, anti-vertigo, bronchodilatory, alpha- and beta-adrenergic, and weight-reducing effects. Ephedrine is used to treat asthma, allergies, nasal congestion, upper respiratory symptoms, and nerve damage in diabetic patients. Ephedra is popularly used to treat asthma (oral sprays or nasal drops to dilate the bronchi), whooping cough, hay fever, colds, fever, urticaria, low blood pressure, rheumatism, joint diseases, edema, bone pain, and as a cardiovascular stimulant. The polysaccharides extracted from the plant have antihypertensive and antioxidant effects. It is a promising natural source of food additives.

Pharmaceutical forms:

It is available as a herbal or special substance or tincture, sold under names such as efadrin.

Side effects, interactions and warnings for use:

Irregular heartbeat and tachycardia, insomnia, anxiety, and nervousness. Tremors, dry mouth, circulatory disorders, high blood pressure, skin rash, eczema, and urinary retention may also be observed. Its hallucinogenic effect has also been observed in children. Ephedra should not be used in cases of coronary bleeding, diabetes, glaucoma, thyroid disease, enlarged prostate, melanoma, and renal dysfunction. Ephedra and its preparations should be avoided with monoamine oxidase inhibitors, and should not be given to patients who will be anesthetized with cyclopropane, halothane, or other volatile surgical anesthetics. Giving ephedra in combination with cardiac glucosides, quinidine, or tricyclic antidepressants can cause tachycardia, and the risk of vasoconstriction may increase in those taking ergot alkaloids (rye spur fungus). It should be avoided during pregnancy and lactation.

Environment:

Ephedra is a plant of dry, sunny, and very dry areas. It lives in critical environmental conditions. It occurs in the form of solitary groups, and sometimes accompanying other plant communities on gypsum soils and pale brown or structural soils, and is also widespread on fixed or mobile calcareous sand dunes. It grows on limestone rocks belonging to the Senonian and Turonian phases of the upper Cretaceous in mountainous areas of medium altitude.

Cultivation and productivity:

The plant is propagated by seeds.

Equisetum arvense L.

Allostelites arvensis (L.) Börner, Presla arvensis (L.) Dulac.

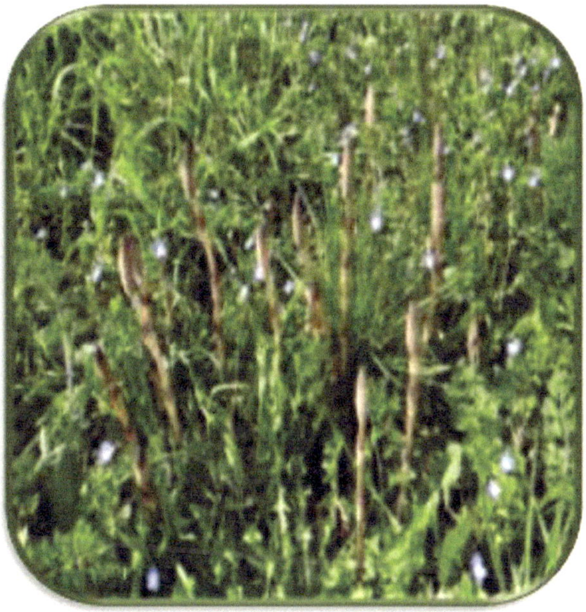

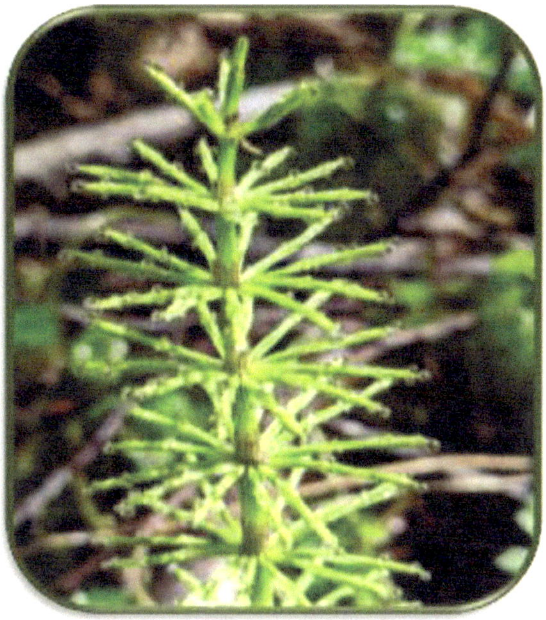

Family: Equisetaceae

Common names: Field horsetail, Field horsetail.

Foreign names: champs des Prele Fr. tail, Horse Eng.

Occurrences : 728,557 occurrences

Distribution in the world

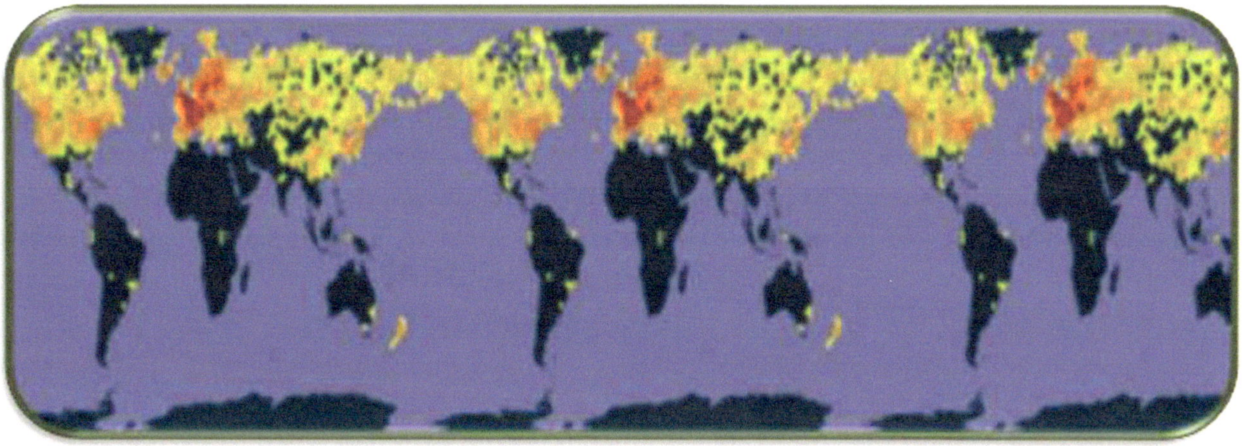

Botanical description:

A perennial plant with creeping rhizomes, dark brown to black, with two types of stems: In spring A fertile, erect, solid, short (35 cm), non-green, unbranched stem appears, ending in elongated spikes, bearing many brown sporangia. In summer, sterile branches grow, about 60 cm long, and are ribbed (with 6-19 prominent longitudinal ribs), 35-2 cm thick, branched, and their branches are whorled. The stem is hollow and thick, consisting of a succession of nodes and ribs. The ribs are 6-2 cm long. At the level of the nodes, there is a membranous sheath, edged with brown, triangular to lanceolate teeth, the number of which is consistent with the number of ribs, and they are equivalent to the leaves.

Flowering: February to October. The genus has several species, including the marsh horsetail E. maxima.

Habitat and geographical distribution:

The original habitat of the plant is Europe and Asia. History and heritage: The horsetail is a translation of the scientific name of the genus Equisetum, where equus means "horse" or "mare" and seta means "long hair", alluding to the resemblance to the horse's tail. This genus is considered a remnant of prehistoric times, as it is a very close relative of the trees that grew on the surface of the earth 270 million years ago, which are the source of the known layers of coal. The ancient Greeks used it to treat wounds. It was mentioned by Al-Antaki, Ibn al-Baytar, and Al-Ghasani. Ibn Sina mentioned that horsetail is astringent, especially its juice, and that it is very useful in stopping bleeding.

Part used: Flowering heads and herbaceous plant.

Chemical components:

Organic phenolic acids, including caffeic acid, gallic acid, and flavonoids: kaempferol, quercetol, and flavonoids isoquercitoside and luteoline glycosides, and saponins: equisetonine, and traces of alkaloids (nicotine, palustrine, methoxypyridine), silicic acid -60-80%, and mineral salts, including potassium chloride.

Properties and medical uses:

The plant has diuretic properties (potassium and flavones), antispasmodic, and also has Astringent and uric acid-lowering activities. It is used internally to treat edema, to wash the urinary tract in cases of infection, and to treat kidney and ureter stones. It is used externally to treat wounds and burns. It is popularly used to treat cancer, diarrhea, gout, rheumatism, mouth infections, and nosebleeds, and to treat hemorrhoids and fluid or urine retention in elderly people with enlarged prostate (edema). The decoction of the plant is used topically to treat Intractable skin lesions such as eczema and lupus (tuberculosis that affects the skin of the nose on both sides and ulcerates it), and is used as gargles in the treatment of tonsillitis, tooth decay and bad breath. The species has antibacterial effects against Gram-positive bacteria, and may be a new therapeutic approach for diseases associated with hypertension or oxidative stress and programmed cell death if given in low doses. It has an anti-inflammatory effect and has been added to toothpaste and mouthwashes to prevent gum disease. Combining horsetail extracts with licorice improves the development of new oral health products aimed at promoting gum health and may enhance anti-inflammatory effects. The nourishing properties of horsetail products for hair, bones, nails and connective tissue have not been confirmed.

Pharmaceutical forms: Horsetail is available in the form of liquid extracts.

Side effects, interactions and precautions for use:

Possible side effects of equine tail: allergic reaction, fever, irregular heartbeat, weakness, loss of coordination, and weight loss. Special care should be taken when mixing horsetail with diuretics and stimulants of the nervous system. It should be noted that the plant contains nicotine, and the use of large amounts of it may cause nicotine toxicity. This plant should be avoided by pregnant and breastfeeding women.

Other uses: Cleaner for vessels, furniture and floors.

Environment:

The plant grows on the banks of rivers, swamps, wet meadows, forest edges and shady, humid places. The plant is suitable for aquatic, semi-aquatic, humid, semi-humid and semi-humid environments, and it also grows in the appropriate soil temperature is 10-24C, and warm regions of the world. The suitable air temperature for the plant is 6-30. It can also tolerate relatively cold air. Horsetail is a shade-tolerant species, and prefers fertile soil rich in organic matter.

Cultivation and productivity:

It is propagated by rhizomes and spores (seeds) that germinate after 25-40 days, and vegetative growth continues for 40-90 days, and floral growth for 90-120 days. During its growth, the plant needs the necessary service operations of pruning (during the dormant period of the sap), fertilization, weeding and weeding. The plants mature in the summer, and are harvested in late summer and autumn, by cutting the stems and growths and placing them in bundles, then drying and storing them until use.

Arbutus unedo L.

Arbutus serratifolia Salisb., Arbutus unedo var. serratifolia Rouy.

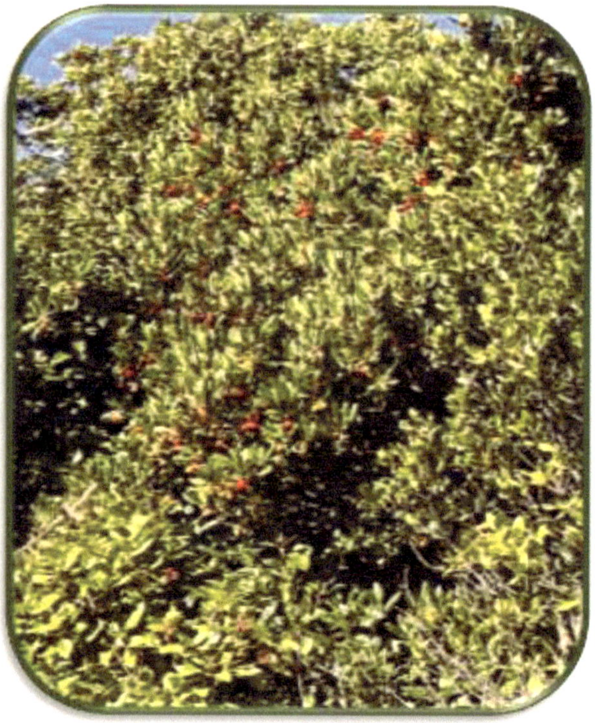

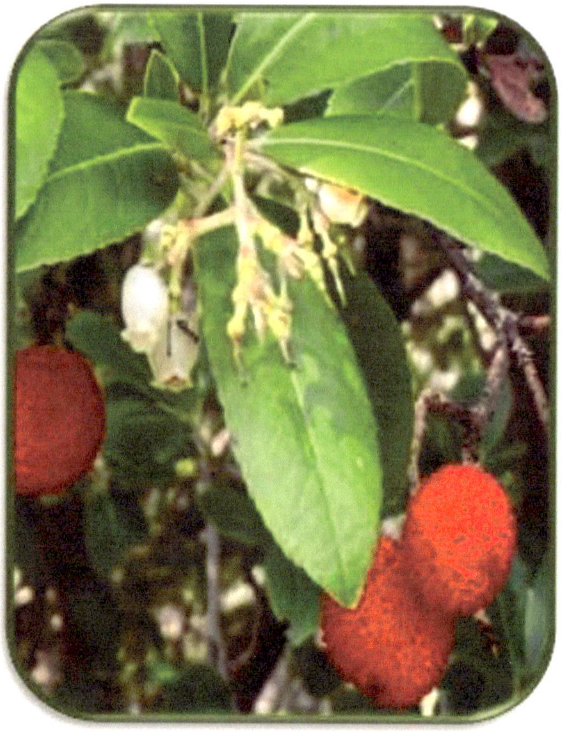

Family: Ericaceae

Common names: Qutlab, Qutlab Unida, Bear Juice, Red Henna, Father Killer, Sisno, Lang.

Foreign names: Arbousier Fr. arbutus, Common Eng.

Occurrences : 142,874 occurrences

Distribution in the world

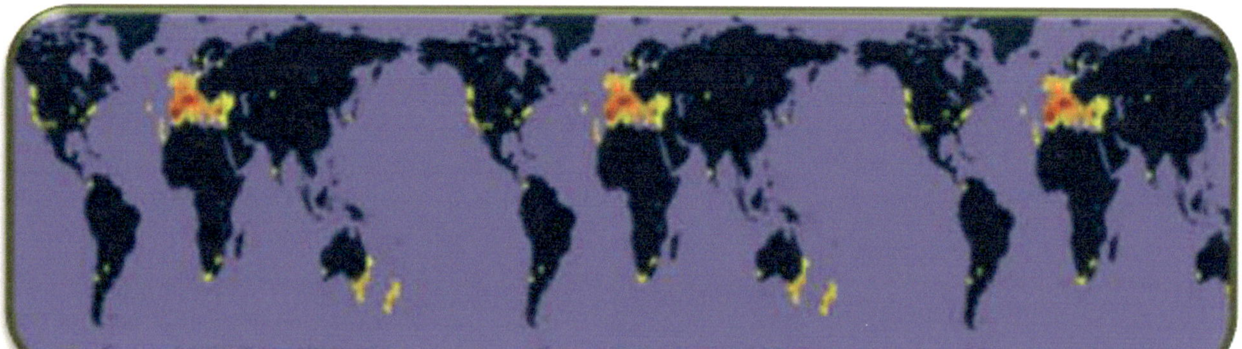

Botanical description:

Small trees or evergreen shrubs, 1-4 m tall. Branches erect, bark brown, rough-grained when young. Leaves simple, alternate, obtuse, leathery, ovate, serrated margin, short obtuse, 4-6 cm long. Flowers pentagonal, gathered in drooping terminal panicles, bracts very small, scaly. Calyx very small, disc-shaped, lobes triangular, deeply lobed. Corolla proximal, white, 5-7 mm long, narrow at the apex, lobes fringed, backwardly coiled. Male 10 stamens, filaments hairy, bases slightly widened. Ovary superior, pentagonal. The fruit is a grape, spherical in shape, bearing warts, red or purple in color, 1.5-2 cm in diameter, many-seeded, edible.

Flowering: December to March.

Habitat and geographical distribution:

warm and temperate regions of the Eastern Mediterranean countries. It is widespread in Greece, Europe, and also grows in the area extending from Albania to the Crimean Peninsula, passing through the coast of the Black Sea, Turkey and the west of the Black Sea to the north of Iraq, Syria and Lebanon, as well as in Morocco, Tunisia, Spain, Malta, Cyprus and the southern part of Italy.

History and Heritage:

The genus name Arbutus is the ancient Latin name for this tree, some believe it is of Phoenician origin, and means "red trunk" in reference to the distinctive trunk of the tree. The descriptive name for the species unedo is the ancient Latin name for this species in Europe Un-edo in reference to its single fruit. The word "Qatlab" is of unknown origin, but is commonly used in the Levant. Al-Antaki mentioned that the fruit of the cattail is useful for poisons, and for all types of diseases, and its leaves dissolve tumors.

Part used: Leaves

Chemical components:

The leaves contain tannin compounds, hydroquinone glycoside: arbutine 3-8%, methyl arbutine . The main volatile compounds in the plant are decenal, α-terpineol and palmitic acid. The species is an inhibitor of α-amylase, α-glucosidase and lipase enzymes.

Properties and medical uses:

Arbutin has diuretic and antiseptic properties for the urinary tract. A decoction of the leaves is popularly used to treat kidney and bladder inflammation, with attention paid to the irritating effect of the tannic compounds on the mucous membranes. The plant has antioxidant, antibacterial, anti-inflammatory, anti-acetylcholinesterase, and hypoglycemic properties. The plant extracts also have the ability to inhibit the growth of most microorganisms, and therefore the plant has been suggested as a promising source of natural medicines.

Precautions for use: It is not recommended to use it during pregnancy and breastfeeding. Its use may cause nausea and vomiting.

Environment:

The plant is widespread in forests, accompanying pine and oak, resistant to cold, lives on siliceous and calcareous soils, its roots contain mycorrhizae, which helps it live on poor rocky soils, relatively tolerant of lime in the soil. It is considered a fire-resistant species, and grows back strongly after a fire starting from the stem, but it does not give offshoots from the root system, and as a result of its resistance to fire, it occupies sites where fires recur.

Cultivation and productivity:

It reproduces naturally and in a limited way by seeds that are transmitted by birds that eat its fruits, or by seedlings that can be planted starting from autumn until the beginning of spring. It can be propagated by seeds in the nursery, but the seedlings are very susceptible to wilting.

Ricinus communis L.

Ricinus communis var. genuinus Müll.Arg., Ricinus communis var. typicus Fiori.

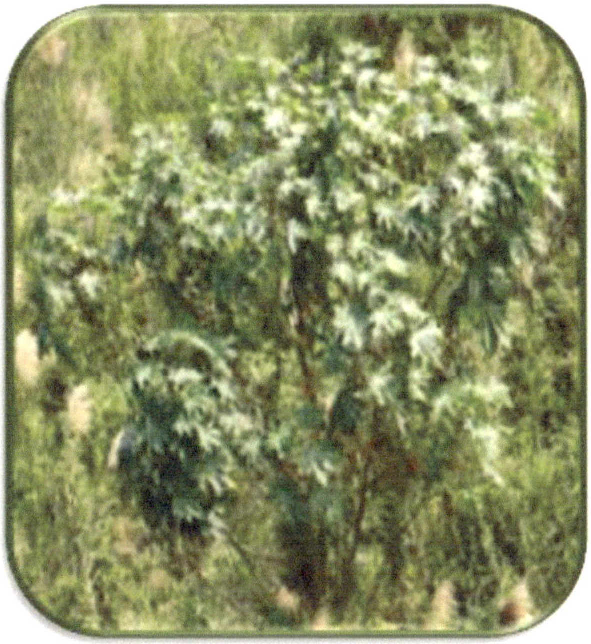

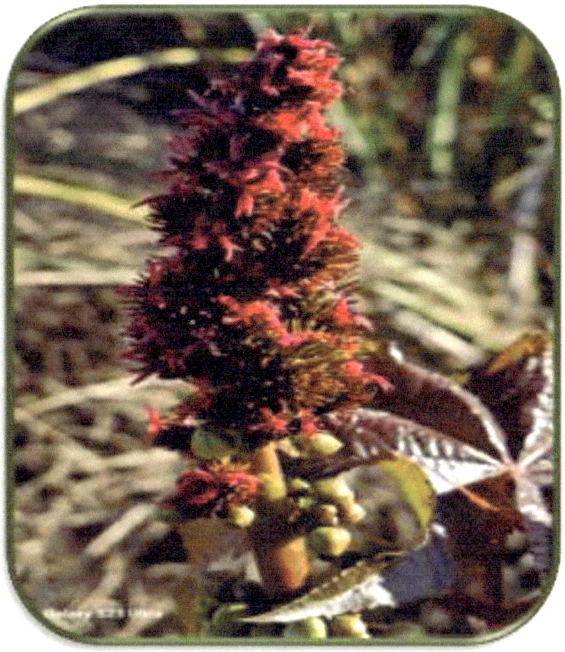

Family: Euphorbiaceae

Common names: Castor

Foreign names: ricin Fr. oil, castor Eng.

Occurrences : 73,116 occurrences

Distribution in the world

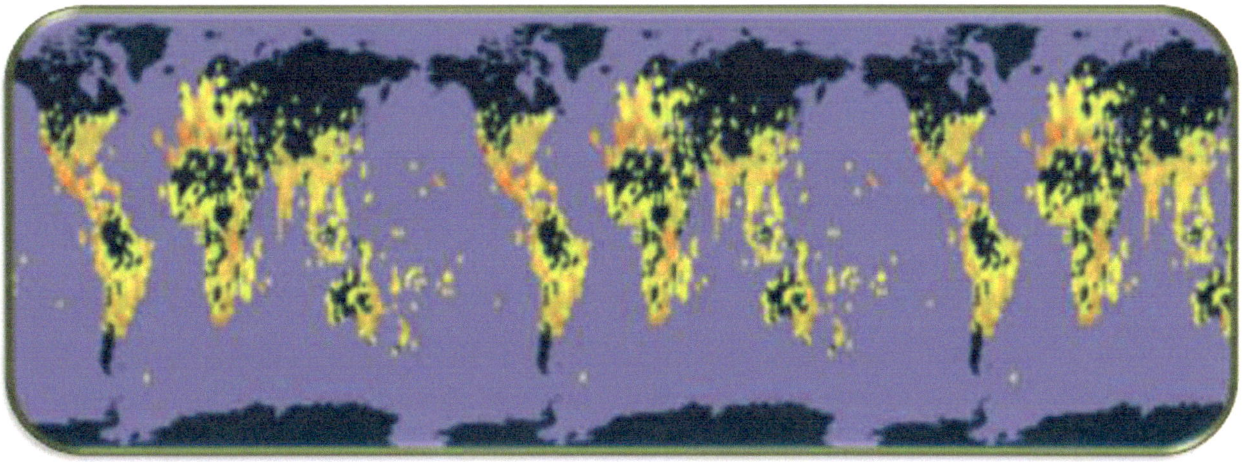

Botanical description:

A shrub or shrub, grayish green, bare, 1-4 m tall. Stem erect, heavily branched from above, thick, hollow. Leaves simple, alternate, 6-25 cm long (or more), obtuse. The blade is palmate, lobed, containing 7-11 lobes ovate-lanceolate, serrated edge. Ears fused. Flowers are unisexual and monoecious, gathered together in axillary or terminal racemes, with male flowers at the top of the raceme and female flowers at the bottom. Male flowers about 1 cm long, simple, composed of 3-5 lobes, stamens numerous and fused, branching several times into multiple anthers. Female flowers about 1 cm, simple panicle, 5-lobed, sessile, ovary tri-chambered, spherical or ovate, each chamber containing one ovule, stigma short, pistils 3, red, bi-lobed, fruit capsule, 1-3 cm, oblong-elliptic, covered with soft thorns, rarely smooth, each chamber opens in two valves. Seeds 1.5-1 cm, scaly, glabrous, variegated, bearing a very small bilobed papilla at the top.

Flowering: March to November.

Origin and Geographical Distribution:

India or tropical regions of Africa, has become globally widespread, and has adapted well to tropical and temperate regions of the world. It is widely cultivated in Brazil, North America, India, Sudan, Egypt and China.

History and Heritage:

The scientific name of the genus Ricinus is the Latin name for this plant, meaning "dog tick," referring to the shape of the seeds, and the species name communis means "common." Castor oil has long been known for its ivory properties, and archaeological evidence has shown the presence of its seeds in some graves of the ancient Egyptians, who believed that routinely softening the abdomen at least three times a month was necessary to ensure continued good health. The ancient Babylonian writings also recommended the use of its oil to treat stomach disorders, and it was used for the same purpose by the Greeks and Indians.

Part used: Seeds and the oil extracted from them (castor oil).

Chemical components:

The plant in all its parts contains alkaloids from pyridine derivatives, including ricinin, in addition to traces of cyanhydric acid. The leaves contain phenolic compounds, and the stems contain terpenoids, sterols and steroids. The seeds contain 42% (-55%) fatty oil, rich in ricinoleic acid esters (which account for the laxative effect), a. linoleic acid, and a. oleic acid. The seeds also contain the toxic alkaloid ricin, the non-toxic alkaloid ricinin, and vitamin E. Castor oil is prepared by cold pressing the seeds, after which the oil is exposed to sufficient heat to inhibit the lipase enzymes.

Properties and medical uses:

The oil has laxative and digestive system emptying properties. This property in castor oil is due to the presence of ricinoleic acid. Pure castor oil free of ricin is used to empty the digestive system before surgical operations and before childbirth. Castor oil is popularly used in cases of severe constipation, intestinal infections, and to get rid of worms. It is also used topically in cases of skin inflammation, boils, abscesses, otitis media and headaches (in the form of compresses.) The plant has strong effects on microbes, especially Escherichia coli, Staphylococcus aureus, Pseudo-monas aeruginosa and Klebsiella pneumonaie.

Other uses:

Castor oil is used in the manufacture of soap and shampoo to care for hair, increase its shine and prevent hair loss and breakage. The remains of the plant can be used as organic fertilizer after removing toxins.

Side effects, interactions and warnings:

Do not use in cases of intestinal obstruction, inflammatory bowel diseases, appendicitis, abdominal pain of unknown origin, during pregnancy and lactation, and do not give the drug to children under 12 years of age. Side effects may be observed in the form of allergic skin rash in rare cases. Overdose may lead to stomach irritation with nausea, vomiting, colic and severe diarrhea. Long-term use leads to loss of electrolytes, especially potassium, which may lead to hyperaldosteronism, inhibition of intestinal motility, and enhances the effect of cardiac steroids.

Pharmaceutical preparations:

Castor oil is available as a complete medicine in solid form, semi-solid form, and in pharmaceutical preparations for internal and external use.

Environment:

The plant grows in barren and neglected lands, on the sides of roads and valleys, in all tropical and temperate regions. It is successfully cultivated in light, sandy soil with good drainage and aeration.

Cultivation and productivity:

The plant is propagated by seeds that do not require any treatment, or may be soaked in normal water for 24 hours before planting. Seeds are planted during the months of February and March in temperate and hot areas, while in cold areas they are planted in April and May.

A dunum requires 10 kg of seeds, planted at a depth of 3 cm in the soil, in lines with a distance of 50 x 75 cm, and irrigated moderately during the summer. The fruits are harvested when they are ripe and light yellow in color, at a rate of once every four days. The harvesting process continues for a month, and the fruits are kept in a clean, dry place, where their valves open and the seeds fall easily.

Acacia arabica (Lam.) willd.

A. nilotica (L.) Del.□ A. adansonii Guill. & Perr, Vachellia nilotica subsp. tomentosa (Benth.) Kyal. & Boatwr.

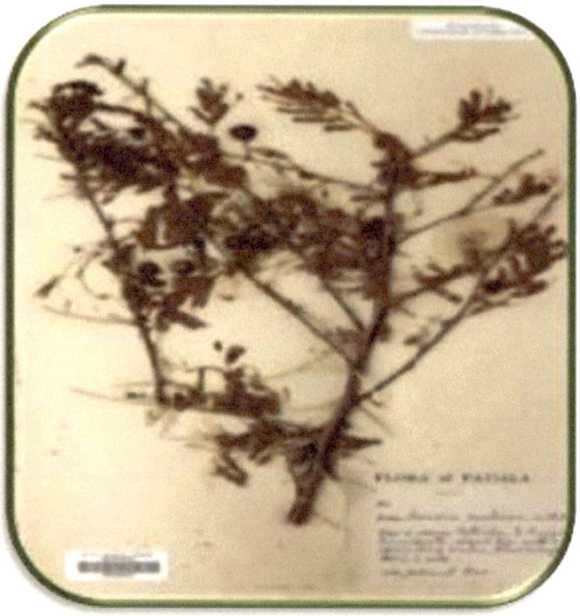

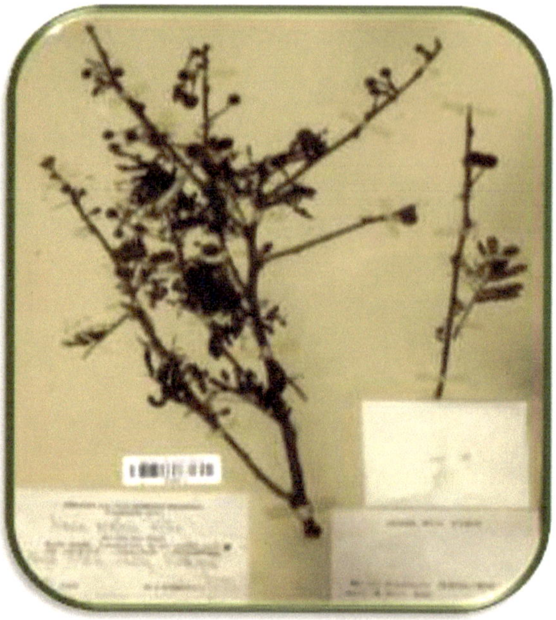

Family: Fabaceae (Mimosoideae)

Common names: Nile acacia, Arabian acacia, Nile acacia, Arabian acacia, acacia gum

Foreign names: Eng. Acacia gum, Egyptian thorn, Black thorn, Prickly acacia, Fr. babul, arabe.palmier

Occurrences : 340 occurrences

Distribution in the world

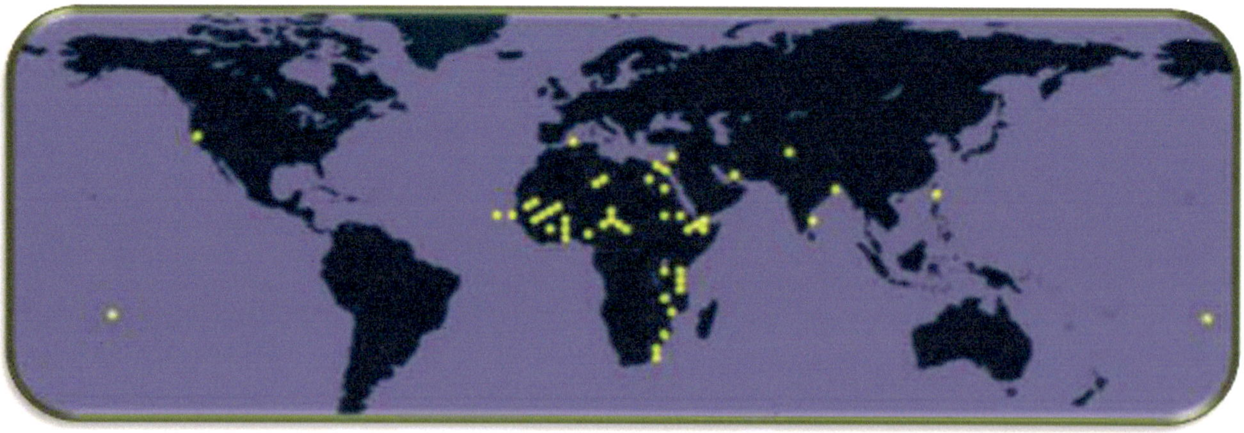

Botanical description:

A small tree, 2.5-14 m high, old branches are bare, while young branches are red to dark brown in color, the thorns are slightly curved, up to 3 cm long. The bark is thin, rough and cracked The leaves are compound Double pinnate, with one or two glands at the base of the peduncle, and other glands at the base of all secondary axes, or only the upper ones. Secondary axes are 2-12 pairs. Each secondary axle bears 7-25 pairs of leaflets. Leaflet is elongated, blunt-apical, 1.5-7 mm long, 0.5-1.5 mm wide, glabrous or hairy. Inflorescence is capitate, 6-15 mm in diameter, axillary, clustered on young branches, The bract is at the base of the inflorescence or in its lower half. Flowers are bright yellow. Calyx 1-2 mm, glabrous to hairy. Corolla 2.5-3.5 mm, fused at the ends, glabrous to hairy on the outside. Pod linear, indehiscent, 8-20 cm long and 13-22 mm wide, straight or arched, glabrous or velvety, swollen, narrowing between the seeds, blackish in colour, containing about 12 seeds. Seeds are smooth, semi-spherical, 6-7 mm in diameter, compressed.

Flowering: October to December.

Habitat and geographical distribution:

The range of the Nile acacia extends from South Africa to Iraq in the north and India in the east. It grows in Egypt, Sudan, Libya, Mauritania, the Sultanate of Oman and the Kingdom of Saudi Arabia.

History and heritage:

The word acacia is derived from the Greek akakia, meaning "gentle" or "non-aggressive", and the species name arabica means "Arabian", and it may be called nilotica meaning "Nile", i.e. Nile acacia. The main importance of the fruits (pods) lies in their use in tanning leather, as adding the ground pods to any other tanning material gives the leather a reddish-brown color. The trees also produce a gum called gum arabic, which is of lower quality than the gum arabic produced by the Acacia senegal tree.

Part used: Stem bark, fruits (pods), and gum.

Chemical components:

The fruits and bark contain tannins, quercetin, and campherol.

Properties and medical uses:

A decoction of the stem bark (tannins) is used in folk medicine to treat gum diseases, inflammation of the mucous membranes of the mouth and throat, to reduce diarrhea, and to treat vaginal infections. It is also used in the form of an enema to treat hemorrhoids. The plant is traditionally used to treat a variety of diseases, including type 2 diabetes, or as a nutritional supplement or source of antidiabetic agents. The use of hot water extract increases insulin secretion, and isolated plant components, including quercetin and kaempferol, have been shown to increase insulin secretion and glucose tolerance in vitro. All plant extracts have also shown antiviral activity, especially against avian influenza virus H9N2.

Environment:

The plant is widespread in hot desert valleys. In areas with rainfall ranging from 250-750 mm/year, sedimentary and loamy soils. It tolerates high temperatures up to 50 on C, and high salinity up to 5000-6000 ppm.

Cultivation and productivity:

The plant is propagated by seeds, which are planted after soaking them in hot water at 80 C and left for a period of 24 hours.

Acacia senegal (L.) Willd.

Mimosa senegal L., Senegalia senegal (L.) Britton.

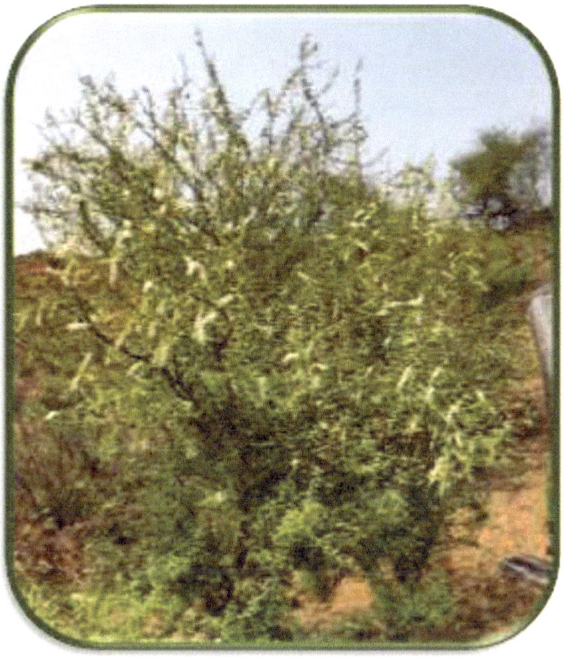

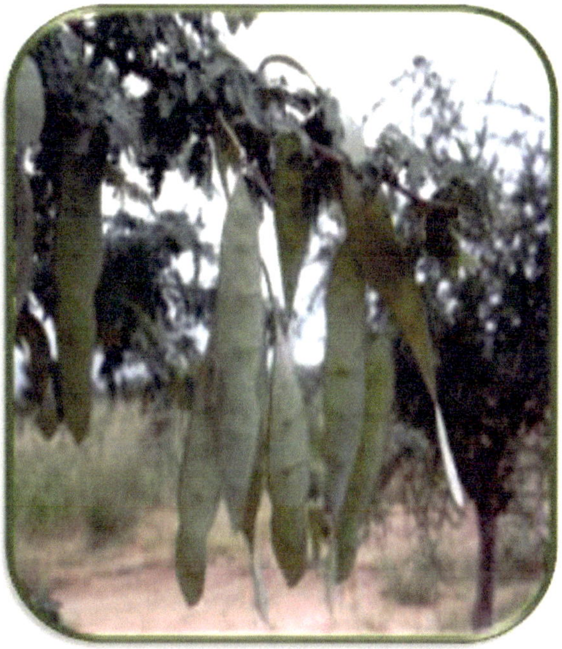

Family: Fabaceae (Mimosoideae)

Common names: Hashab, Gum Arabic

Foreign names: Eng. Gum Arabic Tree, Fr. Gomme arabique

Occurrences: 3,509 occurrences

Distribution in the world

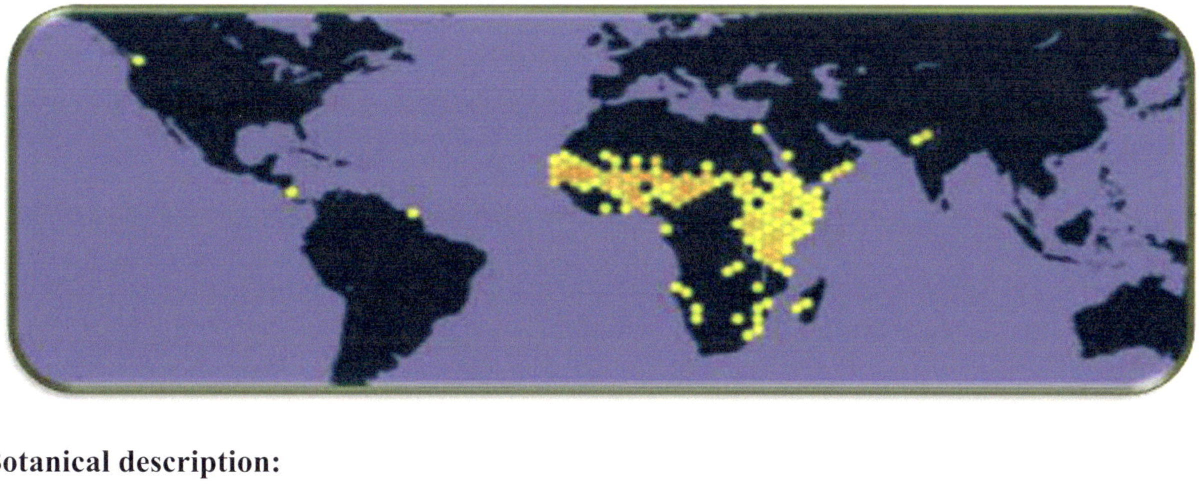

Botanical description:

A small tree, 3-6 m high, young branches. A fluffy, old branches are bluish-green to gray, barking. The bark in the old stem is in the form of dark-colored flakes. The thorns are found in triads at the base of the leaf stalk, two lateral thorns are straight or slightly curved upwards, and the thorn The third is curved, its length is about 5 mm. The axis of the compound leaf is 2.5-5 cm long, there are glands between the lowest and highest pair of secondary axes. The main axis carries 3-5 pairs of secondary axes opposite each other (sometimes alternate), their length is 1-2.5 cm. The leaflets carried by the secondary axes are 8-15 pairs, their length is 2-5 mm and their width is 1-1.5 mm, linear, semi-substrate. The inflorescence is a spikelet, its length is 5-10 cm. The flowers are substrate. The calyx About 2 cm, bell-shaped, glabrous. Corolla about 4 mm long. Stamens numerous, filaments 6-7 mm long. Horn 5-8 cm long, 1.7-2.5 cm wide, thin, flattened, almost straight, tipped with slightly curved beak. Seeds 5-6, disc-shaped, rounded to oval.

Flower: August to December.

Habitat and geographical distribution:

Tropical savanna regions from Sudan (Kordofan region) and Senegal to Zambia and northern Nigeria, forming across central Sudan the gum arabic belt in the region between latitudes 10° - 14° N

History and Heritage:

The use of gum arabic dates back about 3,500 years, as it was transported from the Gulf of Aden to ancient Egypt. The ancient Egyptians used it for adhesives and pain relief. Theophrastus mentioned that it was produced in Upper Egypt. Arab doctors used it to treat a wide range of diseases, which earned it its current name (gum arabic). The Europeans, especially the Portuguese, knew the commercial importance of gum arabic and imported it from Africa. They used it in the silk industry, and many naval wars broke out between them in the nineteenth century in order to monopolize this commercially profitable gum product.

Part used: Gum.

Chemical components:

The chemical composition of gum arabic is not fully known yet. The gum consists mainly of branched polysaccharides composed of galactose units, and carries side chains of arabinose, rhamnose, and linked uronic acids, and contains protein, oxidase enzyme, and water (14%). Phenolic, flavonoid, and astringent compounds were obtained in the aqueous ethanolic extract of the leaves. Six new triterpene saponins, called 6(1-A-F) senegalosides were isolated from the seeds and roots of the plant.

Properties and medical uses:

Gum Arabic maintains the stability of suspensions and emulsions, which made it Excellent stabilizer, thickener, binder and adhesive. Resists organic decomposition caused by bacteria in the mouth that leads to tooth decay. Gum Arabic is used in the manufacture of pharmaceutical capsules, medical tablets prepared for sucking, and is used for its emollient properties in various preparations, such as cough syrup, throat medications, runny nose and diarrhea. Research has shown the positive properties of gum in reducing kidney problems by reducing uric acid in the blood, which leads to To reduce the risk of kidney failure. It is used in the preparation of facial cosmetics, hair fixatives, and to maintain the freshness and clarity of the skin. Recent studies have shown that gum arabic is commonly used as a natural product and a home remedy for various diseases in sub-Saharan Africa. The plant has been successfully used to treat sickle cell anemia, rheumatoid arthritis, metabolic disorders, gingivitis, digestive system diseases, and kidney diseases. It is used against multidrug-resistant bacteria. It has the effects of chloramphenicol and florfenicol against E. coli strains. The plant has a toxic effect on rat hepatoma cells (H4IIE).

In Gum Arabic (a water-soluble dietary fiber rich in calcium ($Ca2+$), $Mg2+$, and $K2+$) is used to treat chronic kidney disease. The plant resists the development of tumors after chemotherapy for cancer. The plant has a positive effect on the treatment of Maria mice. It is useful in cases of chronic kidney failure and diabetic nephropathy. It may be Useful in the prevention and treatment of obesity and diabetes, and for the prevention of colon cancer, and in the treatment of inflammatory diseases and malaria. It is used for the prevention or treatment of diseases of the urinary system and in the treatment of cancer and osteoporosis.

Food and industrial uses:

Gum Arabic receives great attention due to its distinction from other types of natural gums by maintaining its natural properties for a long period without change, and its ease of dissolving in water, and its low degree of viscosity, which qualifies it to be one of Materials that are globally permitted to be added to food, beverages and medicine. It is used in food processing and manufacturing, and is considered one of the best materials that maintain flavor and taste, as it reduces the crystallization of sugar (candy), and prevents the crystallization of water in ice cream (ice cream and milk). It is used in the manufacture of some types of beverages, and is the basic component of all solutions that require stability even in difficult conditions imposed by the acidic medium. The soft drink and confectionery industry consumes about 70% of the global gum arabic trade, and its high fiber content has recently added many new uses to it in healthy diet foods.

In addition to the above, gum arabic is used in other industries, the most important of which are:

1. The manufacture of dyes, glass coatings and high-tech ceramic works.

2. Purification and refining of some metal ores and materials that prevent metal corrosion.

3. Stationery (glue, adhesive tapes, printing ink, wrapping paper, etc.)

Habitat:

A widespread species due to its drought tolerance. It is generally found in areas with an altitude of 100-1700 m, and an annual rainfall rate of 300-400 mm, but it can grow in areas with annual rainfall as low as 100 mm, and a dry period of 8-11 months. It tolerates high temperatures, but is sensitive to frost. Prefers light sandy and sandy loamy soils with good drainage and a pH of 5.8-

Cultivation and productivity:

This species is important in fixing creeping sand and fixing atmospheric nitrogen in the soil. Also, the leaves and fruits that fall on the ground represent rich feed for animals with nutrients. It is propagated by newly collected seeds, and they germinate well without any treatment, while the seeds collected in the previous season need to be treated by soaking in cold water for 12-24 hours. Gum Arabic productivity varies greatly from one region to another depending on the age of the trees, climatic conditions, and insect infestation. Productivity ranges between 200-240 kg/ha, and may decrease in other regions to 30-40 kg/ha. The Hashab trees start producing gum at the age of 5 years.

Some of the gum oozes freely from the trees as a result of the cracking of the bark, but the most valuable gum is obtained from the trees through a process called "stripping" (stripping the gum), which is done by scratching the bark of the tree trunk and branches between September and January, and another stripping is done in March or April. Each tree produces between 200-500 gum per year. Gum Arabic is a sticky, viscous substance, its types and shapes vary according to its origins, its color tends to be orange-brown (the gum of the Kordofan origin is yellowish in color), it has no smell, does not dissolve in alcohol, and dissolves in hot water, forming sticky threads, its taste is sour. The world consumes between 50,000 and 60,000 tons of gum arabic annually, and Sudan (Kordofan State) is the world's largest producer of gum arabic, producing 75% of the world's need.

Alhagi maurorum Medik.

Hedysarum alhagi L., Alhagi alhagi (L.) Huth.

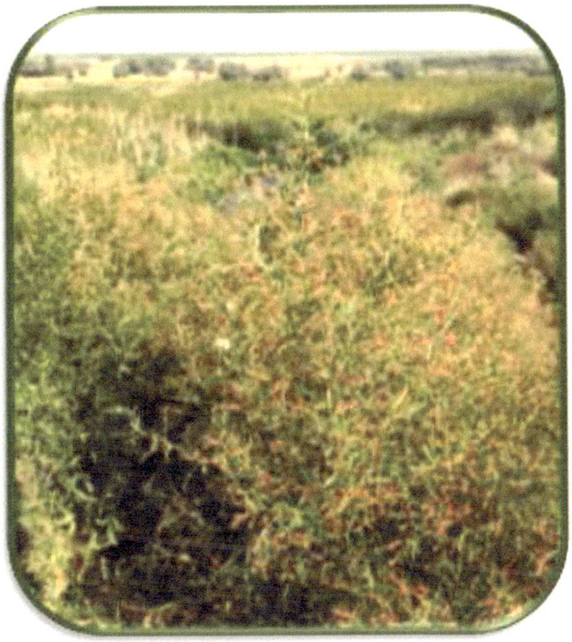

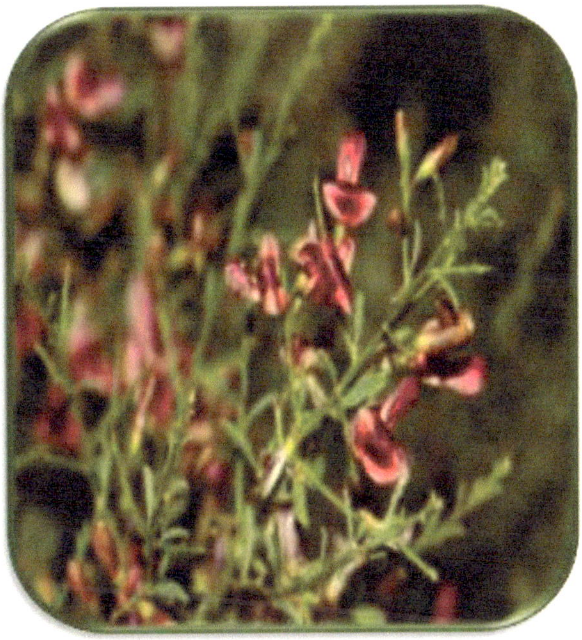

Family: Fabaceae

Common names: Moroccan Aakoul, Aakoul.

Foreign names: Manna tree, camelthorn, Fr. Alhagi des maures

Occurrences : 2,375 occurrences

Distribution in the world

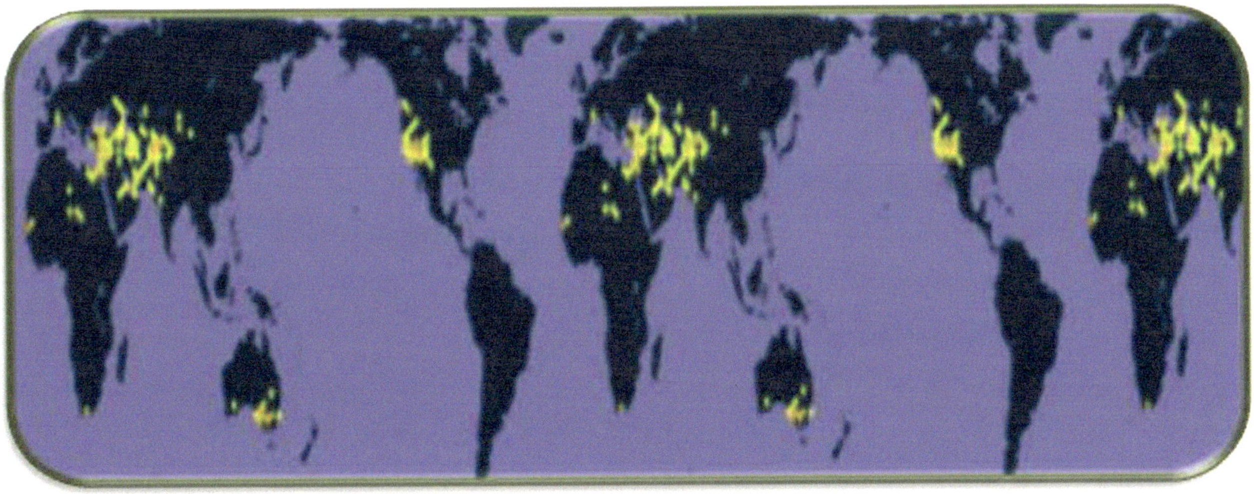

Botanical description:

A small shrub, bare or semi-bare, 40-100 cm high. Stems are erect to ascending, highly branched, notched, bearing short, flat branches, the end of which forms a stinging thorn. Leaves are simple, 1-

2 cm long, oblong to obovate-ovate, blunt or acute at the apex, with entire margins. Ears are small, bead-shaped. The short-flowered peduncle. Flowers hermaphrodite, solitary, axillary, on short, spiny branches, their panicles as long as the calyx or slightly longer. The calyx is 3-4 mm, consisting of a tube ending in five short, triangular to ovate teeth. The corolla is 5-petaled, pink to crimson, about three times longer than the calyx. The flag is inverted-ovate, its apex is notched, and turns upwards. Male 10 stamens, biconcave (1+9). Female monocarpal, ovary superior, silky hairy, containing many seeds. Carpel 30-12 x 4-3 mm, containing 8-2 seeds, linear to cylindrical, narrowing between seeds, glabrous or almost glabrous. Seeds about 2 mm, kidney-shaped, brown, smooth.

Flowering: April to September.

Habitat and geographical distribution:

Iranian-Turanian extending to the Mediterranean and Sudanese regions, It is spread in most countries of the Arab world and the Arabian Desert.

History and Heritage:

The scientific name of the genus Alhagi is derived from the Arabic word meaning "pilgrim", and the species name maurorum means "Moroccan."

The Sumerians used it to improve the soil, and it has long been used as a medicinal plant. David of Antioch wrote in Al-Aqoul: "It is the camel's thorn, and it is a plant with many thorns. It has white and yellow flowers, and its seeds are round. All other parts of the plant cure hemorrhoids by drinking, incense, and rubbing, even with its ashes."

Part used: All parts of the plant, including the roots.

Chemical components:

The plant contains: kae-, isorhamnetin, chrysoeriol-7-O-xylosoid, chrysoeriol, kaempferol, the most important of which are flavonoids,.mpferol-3-galactorhamnoside anthraquinone and saponin glycosides, tannins and resinous substances, coumarin, organic acids, unsaturated sterols, reducing sugar, vitamins and volatile oil, noting that the roots do not contain volatile oil. The plant also contains a wide range of pharmacologically active secondary metabolites such as flavonoids, alkaloids (alhacidin and alhacin), stimulants, pseudalhagin, and phospholipids. During the flowering period (summer), the leaves and branches secrete a honey-like liquid called manna in the form of small, light brown grains with a sweet taste (mannitol). The pods secrete another type of manna with laxative properties.

Properties and medical uses:

Flavonoids are effective in treating gastric ulcers, and research indicates the effectiveness of the plant as an antifungal skin agent. The fresh juice of the plant or its decoction is used popularly as a cough suppressant, digestive system disinfectant, sugar lowering,and diuretic, and helps get rid of kidney and bladder stones. The plant powder, especially its flowers, is used topically to prepare a paste or ointment used to stop bleeding, dry and disinfect wounds (anti-inflammatory) and treat hemorrhoids. The oil extracted from the leaves is used in the form of compresses to treat rheumatism, arthritis, and eye inflammation, especially in children. Manna is also used to increase the body's vitality and sexual activity, and it works to increase the strength of the heart and improve digestion. The manna secreted by the pods is used by mixing it with milk or hot water as a laxative or as a light dab. It is noteworthy that scientific research on the plant is limited, and studies are currently being conducted on its effect on the kidneys. Recent studies have proven that the plant has antioxidant uses and nutritional value with various medical properties, and is a rich source of digestible proteins and rare minerals. The plant is used to treat heart and blood vessel diseases, as a fever reducer, anti-ulcer, liver diseases, anti-spasm, diarrhea, pain, rheumatism, bacteria and fungi.

Environment:

A deep-rooted plant, spreads on hills, steppes, valleys, and on the edges of fields and roads in semi-arid and dry environments. Suitable for heavy and loamy soils with high groundwater level, tolerant of salinity, and occurs in saline soils (sabkhas).

Cultivation and productivity:

It is considered an invasive species for pastures around sabkhas and valleys, and is rarely cultivated. It is propagated by seeds that must be soaked in lukewarm water for 12 hours, then planted in plastic bags in the nursery, and transferred to permanent land after at least a year. It can also be propagated by young cuttings. It blooms in the summer, bears fruit in the middle and end of the summer, and enters a winter dormancy during the winter.

Astragalus gummifer Labill.

Astracantha gummifera (Labill.) Podlech, Tragacantha gummifera (Labill.) Kuntze

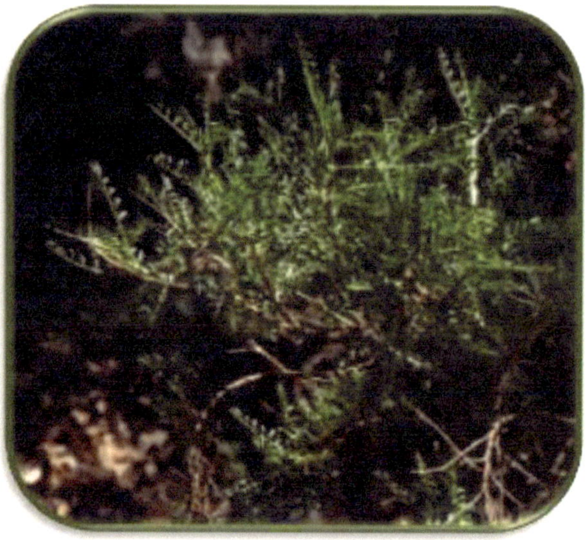

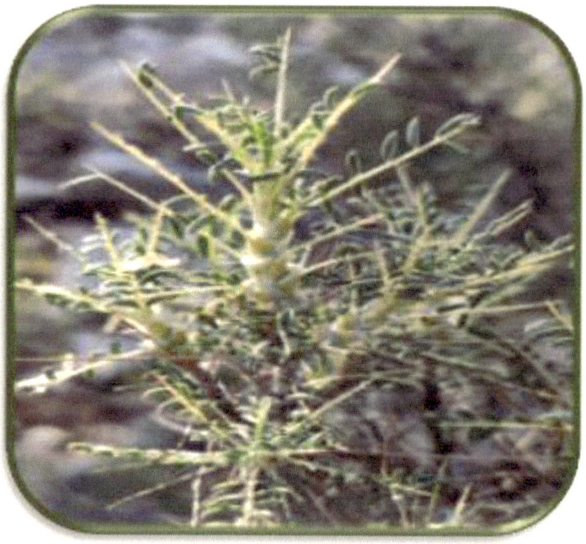

Family: Fabaceae

Common names: Gum Tragacanth, Gum Gomme adragant

Foreign names:

Occurrences : 281 occurrences

Distribution in the world

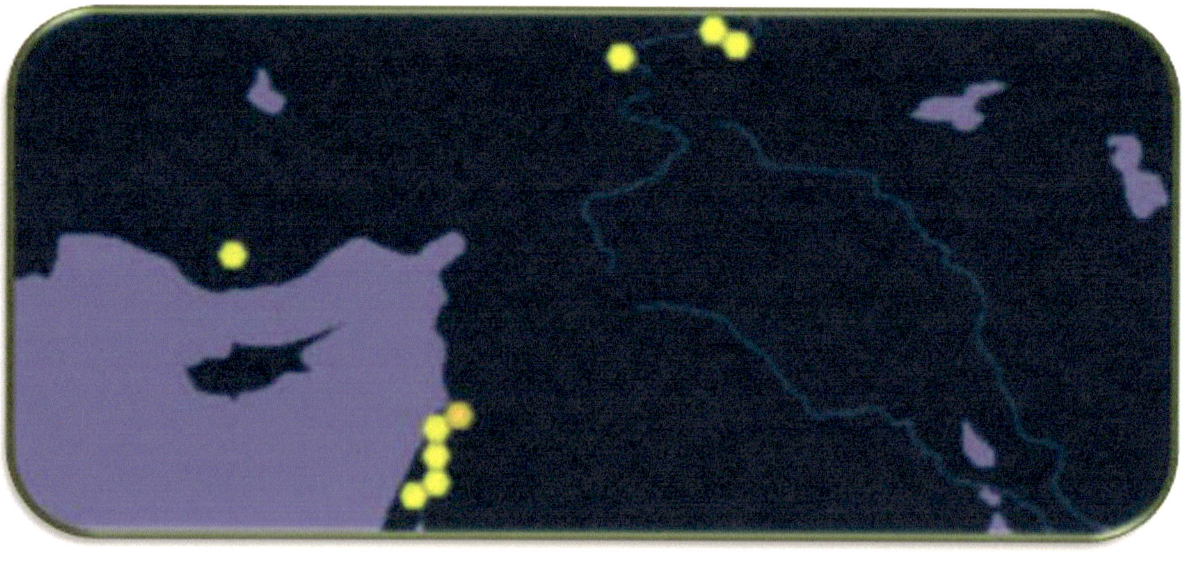

Botanical description:

A small shrub, 20-60 cm long, branched from the base, bare, its bark is brown. The bases of the stems and branches are surrounded by whitish leaf stalks. Leaves are compound, pinnate, composed of 4-7 pairs of glabrous leaflets, 5-8 mm long, the leaf stalk is glabrous, 2-3 cm long, and has a stinging spine at the end. Ears are glabrous, 7-9 mm long. Flowers are paniculate, gathered in a main racemose inflorescence, composed of 2-3 flowers, emerging from the axils of the leaves, and surrounded by the ears of the adjacent leaves. The bracts are ovate, their apex is oblique, membranous, and longer than the calyx. The calyx is densely hairy, its teeth are shorter than the tube. The corolla is white to yellow, the flag is notched. The fruits are legumes, round to oval, about 4 mm long, hairy, and single-seeded. This species produces gum only when the plant is healthy.

Flowering: From May to August.

Habitat and geographical distribution:

It grows naturally in southern and eastern Europe, the highlands of Syria, Lebanon, Palestine, Jordan, Turkey and Iran. Turkey is one of the most productive countries.

History and Heritage:

The genus Astragalus is derived from the Greek word meaning "small bone" in the wrist, and the name of the species is gum. The scientific name mifer from gum, meaning "gum", referring to the gummy substance (worm gum) secreted by the bark of the woody part of the stem and taproot when the plant is injured. Tragacanth gum is one of the oldest known drugs, used by Arab doctors to treat coughs.

Part used:

Tragacanth gum. Tragacanth gum is very valuable and is considered one of the best types of gums that help in giving a stable gelatinous texture for a long period of time, even in acidic media or when exposed to heat. The gum is extracted from the layer directly under the bark of the plant's stem and branches during the period between May and September, by making an incision in the bottom of the trunk. The gum liquefies immediately after the wound, and hardens when exposed to air, turning into strips or ribbon pieces, fragile in structure, ivory white in color. The ribbon pieces (2.5 cm) are collected manually. The best types are the white or very light yellow, transparent and horny strips. Odorless, mild taste, pure from impurities.

Chemical components:

Tragacanth gum consists of a complex of several sugars, the most important of which are: Tragacanthin 40% tragacanthin, polysaccharides (soluble in water) Basorin 60% (basorin =) tragacanthic acid, polysaccharides (insoluble in water), and both components. Insoluble in alcohol, and when tragacanth gum is placed in water, tragacanthin dissolves in water to form a solution Glue, and the insoluble bassorin swells to form gatin.

Properties and medical uses:

Gum tragacanth has laxative properties, and is used as a laxative and astringent, increasing the spiral movement of the intestines. Studies indicate that gum tragacanth stimulates the production of red blood cells. It is used as an adhesive for pills and tablets, and in the manufacture of medical suspensions.

Cosmetic, food and industrial uses:

Gum tragacanth is used in the manufacture of many cosmetics (adhesive agent for powders), coatings (lotions), creams and toothpastes. It is used in the manufacture of many food industry products (jelly), vinegar, regular or flavored drinks, creams, mayonnaise, candies and ice cream. Gum lava is also used in drawing on marble, where the gum is soaked in distilled water for three days to dissolve, then filtered to produce a thick liquid, which is used in drawing on marble. Precautions for use: There are no health problems or side effects associated with its use. Using large quantities of it without drinking plenty of fluids leads to intestinal obstruction and esophageal congestion.

Environment:

A mountain plant, lives on light, well-drained sandy and clayey soils, and is also found on neutral and alkaline soils, and also grows on highly acidic soils.

Cultivation and productivity:

The plant is propagated by seeds that are collected in the summer and planted in the spring. Cold stratification can increase the germination of stored seeds. Stored (and sometimes fresh) seeds need to be soaked in warm water for 24 hours before planting. Germination may be slow or irregular, but usually occurs in 4-9 weeks or more at 13°C if the seed is treated or sown soft.

Cassia italica *(Mill)*

Cassia italica (Mill.) Spreng., Cassia obovata Collad., Senna obovata Link.

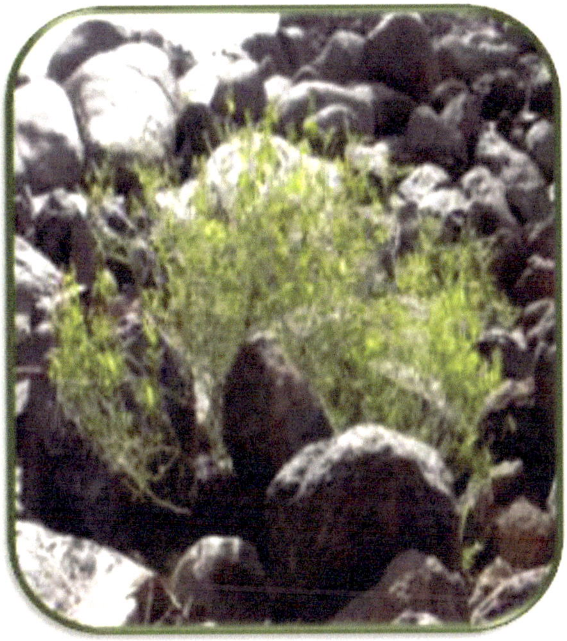

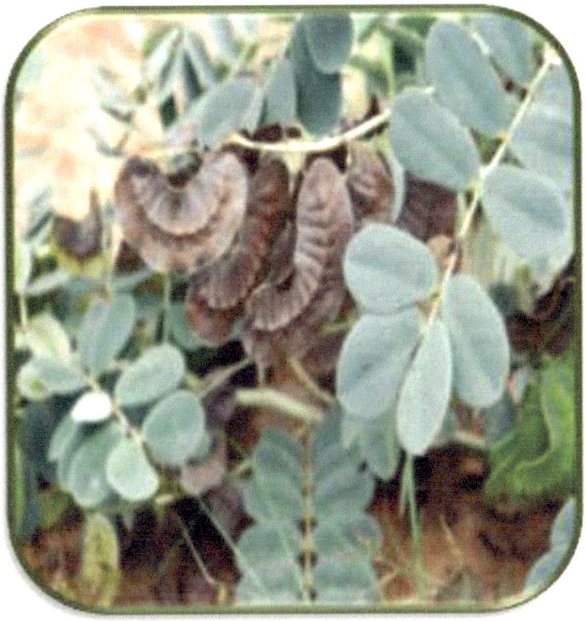

Family: Fabaceae (Caesalpinoideae)

Common names: Asharq

Foreign names: Séné Fr. senna, Italian Eng.

Occurrences : 717 occurrences

Distribution in the world

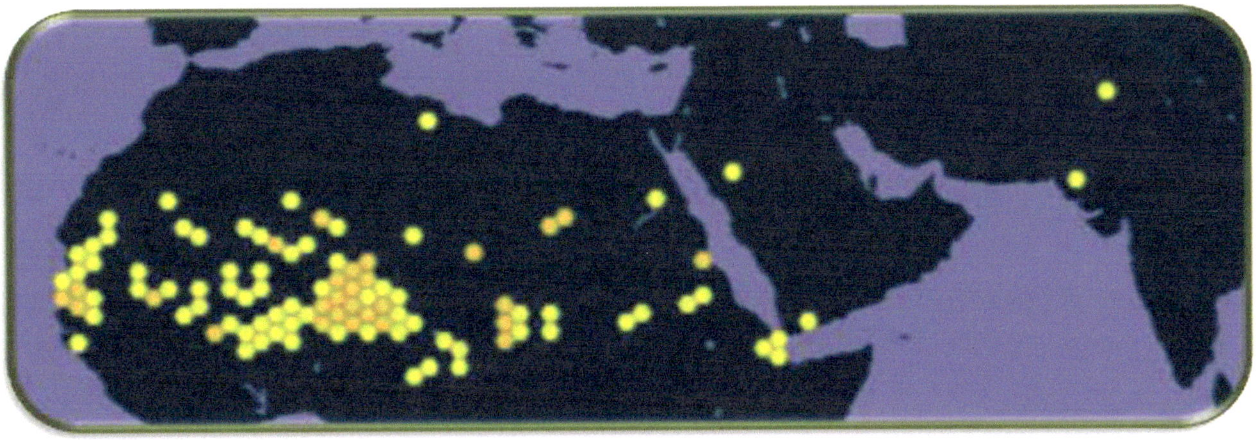

Botanical description:

Perennial herb, woody base, 50-70 cm tall. Stems branched from the base, bluish-green, almost glabrous. Leaves are compound pinnate, composed of 4-7 pairs, alternate, about 10 cm long or more. Ears 3-5 mm, lanceolate Shape. Leaflets 0.7-2×1-3 cm, obliquely inverted ovate, rarely oblong, blunt-topped (sometimes peduncles). Inflorescences are clustered, axillary, erect, not compact. Flowers are longer than the leaves Supporting, bracts Deciduous, rounded to ovate. Inflorescences short. Calyx 5 sepals, free, overlapping in bud. Corolla 5 petals, overlapping, yellow streaked with violet veins, posterior smaller. Male 10 stamens free, anthers unequal, the anterior two larger, about 1 cm long, the others gradually smaller, one about 7 mm long, four 5 mm long, three 2 mm long. The ovary is downy. The horns are 2-1.5×6-3 cm, Carried on a short, arched, flattened, rounded-ended stalk, divided transversely by a membranous septum, the two valves are leathery to the touch, protecting a network of dark-coloured veins, and a wavy crest along the median rib. The seeds are small, 4×6 mm in size, compressed, inverted oval, and truncated at the apex.

Flowering: September to April.

Habitat and geographical distribution:

Sudanese, extending to the eastern part of Africa, distributed in Egypt, Libya, Algeria, Nigeria and Somalia.

History and heritage:

The genus Cassia has no known linguistic origin. Nahal (2009) states that the name may have come from the local Indian name, while the species name italica means "Italian."

Part used: Leaves.

Chemical components:

The leaves contain anthraquinone compounds and their derivatives, including senoside glycosides A.B.C and amodin.

Medical uses: Laxative and purgative.

Environment:

Senna species are widespread in valleys in desert and semi-desert areas, and grow in dry sandy environments Generally. The soil is Light sandy soil is the most suitable for it.

Cultivation and productivity:

Senna is planted at the beginning of spring, when the temperature begins to rise, and it is preferable not to delay after April. It is propagated by seeds, and the hectare needs 8-10 kg of healthy seeds, and may increase to 13-16 kg. The seeds can be soaked in water for 12 hours before planting, and this increases the germination rate. It is preferable to irrigate every 5 days after the plants begin to grow and become established in the soil. Soil, with the necessity of reducing irrigation after flowering. Excessive irrigation water causes yellowing of plants, and this appears clearly on the leaves. It is recommended to fertilize the plant with basic elements and fertilization by spraying can be used. The date of harvest depends on the drug used, either leaves or pods, or both, and in the case of a desire to obtain leaves, the harvest is two or three times, and this depends on the irrigation and fertilization process. In case of adding small amounts of fertilizers, the number of harvests is reduced to two instead of three during the growing season. In case of collecting the pods, this begins in July on a regular basis. The hectare produces 1.5-2.5 tons of fruits.

Ceratonia siliqua L.

Ceratonia coriacea Salisb., Ceratonia inermis Stokes, Ceratonia siliqua var. latissima Risso, Ceratonia siliqua var. siccata Risso, Ceratonia siliqua var. sterilis Risso , Ceratonia siliqua var. vulgaris Risso.

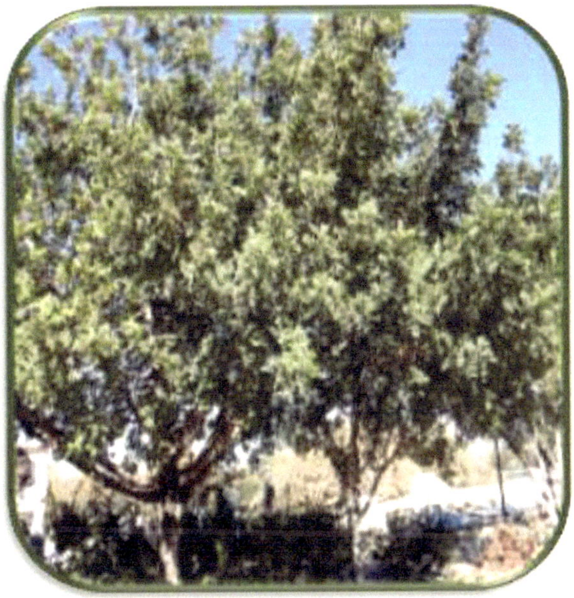

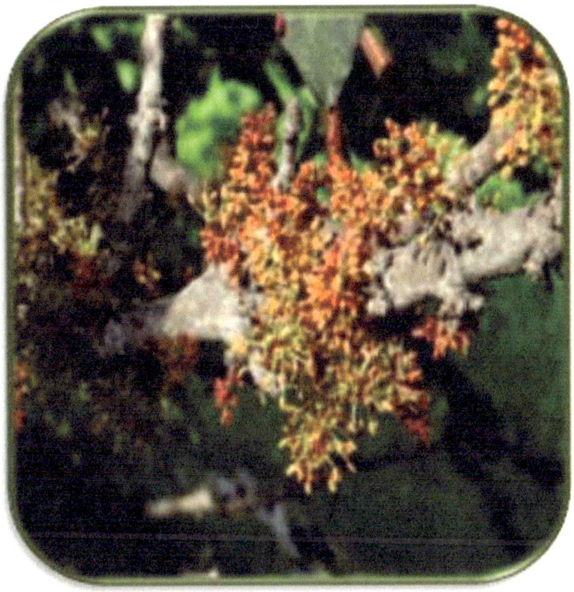

Family: Fabaceae (subfamily Caesalpinoidaceae)

Common names: Carob, Carob.

Foreign names: Caroubier Fr. Carob, Eng.

Occurrences : 67,668 occurrences

Distribution in the world

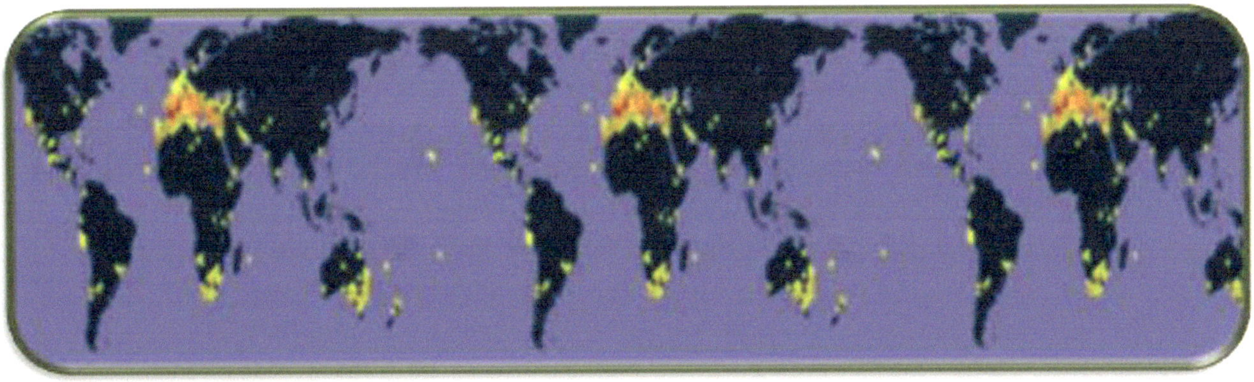

Botanical description:

Evergreen tree, dioecious, 4-10 m high. Branches are curved, sinuous, crown is spherical. Leaves are compound, pinnate, with 2-5 pairs, short-petiolate, 10-25 cm long. Leaflets are oblong-ovate, blunt or notched at the apex, leathery in texture, glossy on the upper surface, and hairy on the lower surface, 3-7 cm long cm, and its width is 3-4 cm. The inflorescence is racemose, axillary, cylindrical, erect, solitary or in groups. The flowers are unisexual, small, reddish-yellow to green in colour. The calyx is pentagonal. The corolla is absent. The male in male flowers is composed of 5 stamens. The female in female flowers is composed of one carpel, the ovary is superior, thick and oblique. The horn is linear, straight or slightly curved, its length is 10-30 cm, and its width is 2-3 cm. Thickness about 4 mm, many seeds, brown to purple-brown in color and dark when ripe. Seeds are flat and convex on both sides, separated by barriers from the fruit pulp, sweet in taste. Pods are formed in late summer and early autumn.

Flowering: August to November.

Homeland and geographical distribution:

Mediterranean Basin. It is found naturally in the countries of the Eastern Mediterranean: Syria, Lebanon, Palestine, Cyprus, Jordan, Egypt, and Turkey, southern Europe, and northern Africa.

There are a number of cultivated varieties, highly productive, spread in many regions of the world (America, Australia, southern Africa, and the Mediterranean Basin.)

History and heritage:

The name of the genus Ceratonia is derived from the Greek Kerâtonia from Kèras, meaning "horn", in reference to its horny fruits. The descriptive name for the species siliqua also means "thorny" and is the Latin name for the carob horn.

It was cultivated in the Mediterranean region 4000 years ago, and the Greeks were aware of its benefits and uses. Its seeds were among the reference units of weight for the ancients (it is said to be the origin of the carat weight used in weighing precious stones), and Ibn Sina mentioned it as drying and astringent.

Part used: pods or fruits (fruit pulp) and seeds that give a white powder called "carob gum"

Chemical components:

The fruit contains 70% sugars (sucrose, fructose, xylose and ceratose), 2-3% salivary substances, pectins. flavonoids: isoschaftoside, neoschaftoside, schaftoside, proteins and butter-like acid (responsible for the distinctive flavor of the fruit pulp.) The seed flour contains 40-45% of its weight salivary substances, which are hydrolyzed and give carobin (a polysaccharide compound) Gum Rich in galactomannanes in particular. The plant contains phenolic compounds, tannins, anthocyanins, alkaloids, and glycosides. Carob pods contain high amounts of carbohydrates (40-60%), polyphenol compounds, especially tannin (18-20%), dietary fiber (27-50%), minerals (potassium, sodium, iron, copper, manganese, zinc) and small amounts of protein (3-4%) and fats (0.4-0.8%). These trees are famous for their richness in sugars, which are mainly composed of sucrose (32-38%), fructose (5-7%) and glucose (5-6%).

Properties and uses Medical:

The pulp of the fruit is used for its laxative properties and to reduce coughing. It is also used to treat colitis, acetonemic hyperacetonemia, and diarrhea caused by salmonella bacteria or viruses, especially in infants and children. It makes the stool semi-dry and reduces the loss of water associated with diarrhea, which leads to the loss of body salts. Studies have proven the effect of carob gum in regulating blood sugar and lowering blood fats through Activating digestive enzymes and increasing the viscosity of digestive juice. Carob gum is used to reduce blood clotting, and is included in diets to treat obesity. It is also used in many food industries and medical preparations due to its antiviral and intestinal disinfectant properties. Carob seeds are used to make flour, which is used to make bread that is beneficial in treating cases of vomiting in pregnant women and infants, and in producing gluten-free gluten, which is used in treating cases of malabsorption resulting from the gluten found in regular bread. The extracts of this plant have an antioxidant effect against sugar bacteria, fungi, inflammation and diabetes. It is used as a natural alternative to treat neurodegenerative diseases. It is used in traditional Tunisian medicine to treat digestive system disorders The plant has multiple pharmacological activities in the digestive system, especially including antioxidants, ulcers and inflammation.

Other uses:

The pulp of the fruit is used for its sweet and nutritious taste, mixed with nuts, and a type of chocolate has been made from it.

Environment:

Carob is a tree that is sensitive to cold, especially in the young seedling stage, where it can hardly tolerate low temperatures of less than -7°C, and its fruits fall at -4°C to -5°C. Cold weather harms the growth of young trees, making them soft and succulent, but they can tolerate low temperatures as they age. Carob needs sunny places, resistant to hot summer winds, high temperatures, dry air and desert weather, tolerant of thirst, but grows better when water is available. Carob tolerates calcareous and poor soils, and it is recommended to use it in afforestation of these soils in moderate temperature areas, but an excess of lime beyond the necessary limit causes yellowing of the leaves due to lime fixing the iron element. It can also live in relatively saline soils, but it fears saturated, poorly drained soils. Carob cultivation does not succeed in poorly aerated soils, and this plant responds to nitrogen fertilization, because its roots are unable to fix atmospheric nitrogen.

Cultivation and productivity:

Carob is propagated by seeds. It can also be propagated by budding, and it is difficult to propagate it by cuttings. The seedlings are transferred from the nursery to the permanent ground after being grafted with buds taken from hermaphrodite trees, at the age of one year, and their height is between 90-120 cm. The trees are raised in the first years of their life on 4-5 branches distributed regularly around the main axis, followed in the following years by thinning the dense and crowded branches and cutting the diseased and dry branches, and this throughout the life of the tree, and good training is beneficial in the regularity of the yield. The tree bears fruit starting from the age of 15-20 years, and the female trees bear their crop every two years (reciprocally), and here it is necessary to take into account the presence of the male trees close to the female ones for the purpose of pollination and fertilization.

Glycyrrhiza glabra L.

G. glandulifera Waldst. et Kit., G. hirsute Pall., alalensis X.Y.Li. alaschanica Grankina, brachycarpa Boiss., .echinata Lepech.

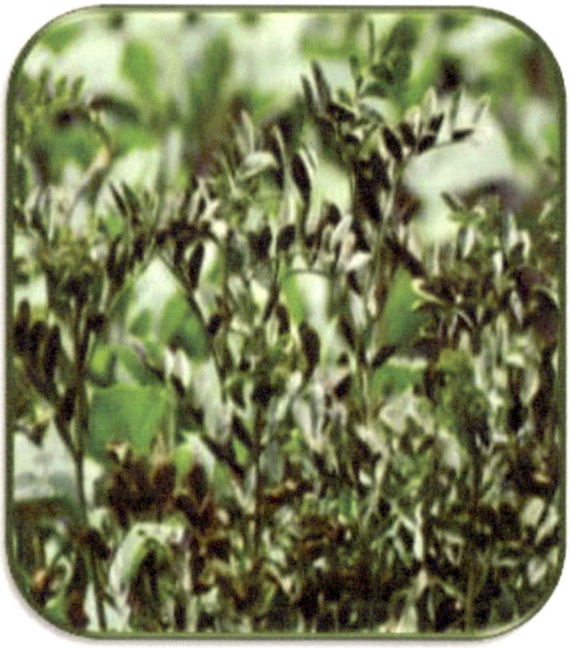 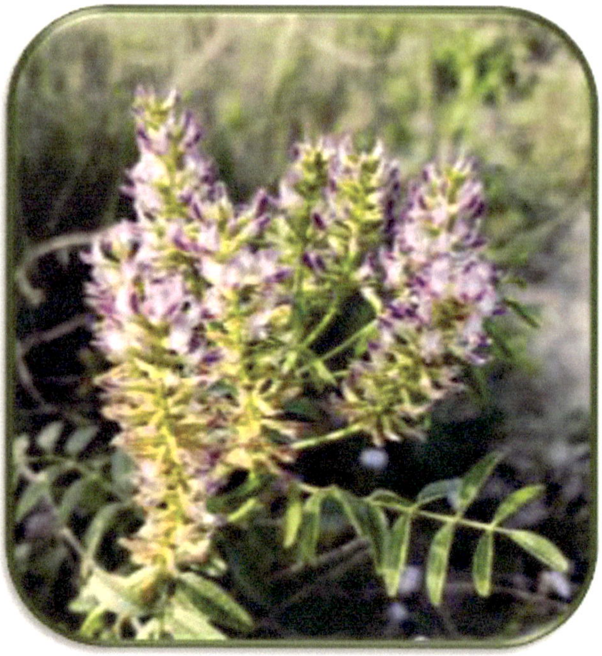

Family: Fabaceae (Leguminosae)

Common names: Licorice, Licorice

Foreign names: Réglisse Fr. Licorice, Eng.

Occurrences : 5,154 occurrences

Distribution in the world

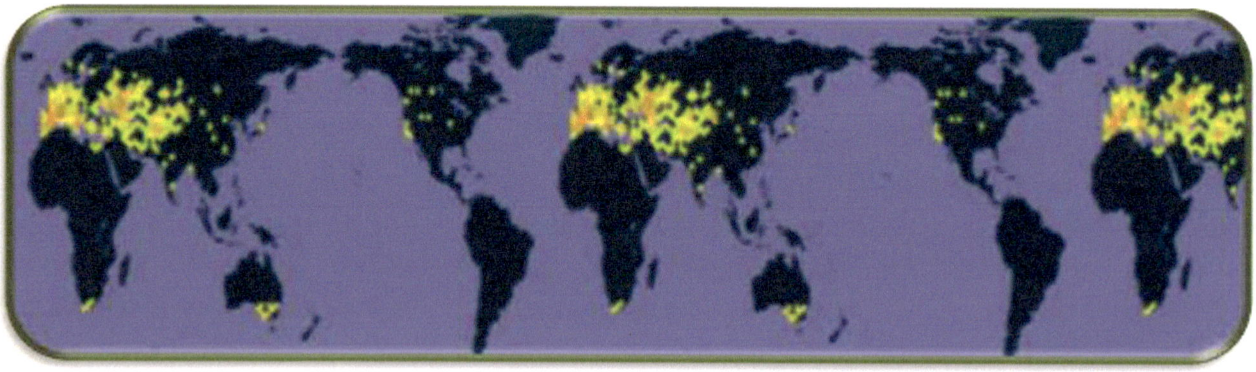

Botanical description:

Erectile perennial herb, sticky, 50-100 cm tall, thick, long roots, sweet-tasting. Stems numerous, few stringy, 5-15 cm long, composed of 4-8 pairs of leaflets. Ears oblong Branching. Leaves compound pinnate Shape, hairy, may be absent. Leaflets 2-1×5-3 cm, oblong to elliptic, acute or blunt at the apex, glabrous on the lower surface. Inflorescence racemose or spike-like, axillary, shorter than or as long as the supporting leaves, not clustered, cylindrical. Flowers hermaphrodite, bisymmetrical, about 1 cm long. Calyx 5 sepals, united in a tube, ending in 5 equal teeth, longer than the tube. Corolla 5-petalled, blue or violet. Flag whitish Colour. Male 10 stamens, bi-segmented. Female uni-carpel. Ovary superior, Graw or covered with glandular hairs, stigma arched, ending with terminal stigma. Fruit pod, 0.7-0.4×3-2 cm, flat, oblong to linear in shape, fruiting pericarp leathery in texture, graw or covered with glandular hairs in varying degrees, opens late, contains one to several seeds, renal to spherical in shape.

Flowering: From May to October.

There are two varieties of the species:glabra var. G.g., pod bare, containing 7-1 seeds.glandulifera var. G.g., pod covered with glandular hairs, containing 3-2 seeds.

Homeland and geographical distribution:

Mediterranean, European-Siberian, and Iranian-Turanian. It is widely cultivated in the United States, Russia, Spain, Turkey, Greece, India, Italy, Iraq, and Syria.

History and heritage:

The scientific name of the genus is derived from the Greek Kglykys, meaning "sweet" or "sugary" and rhiza means "root", alluding to its sugary roots, while glabra means "naked." Licorice syrup is used in many Arab countries, especially during the summer and the month of fasting.

Part used: dried, unbarked roots.

Chemical components:

triterpene saponins 3-15% (glycyrrizin), flavonoids, such as liquiritin and isoliquiritin (chalcone), isolicoflavo- nol (compounds responsible for the yellow color of the roots), isovflavones such as glabren, glabridin, glabrol, cumestan derivatives, such as glycyrol, liqcoumarin, hydroxycoumarins, herniarin, umbelliferone, glycocoumarin, licopyranocoumarin, and steroids, such as beta-sitosterol, and stigmasterol. The drug also contains a small percentage of volatile oil, the most important components of which are anethole, estragole, eugenol, and hexanoic acid. Many organic acids, liquirtin, rhamnoliquirilin, liquiritigenin, prenyllicoflavone A, apio-glucoliquiritin side, 1-metho-xyphaseolin, shinpterocarpin, shinflavanone, licopyranocoumarin, glisoflavone, B semilicoisoflavone, licoriphenone, 1-methoxyficifolinol, R kanzonol and many volatile components. The highest concentration of biologically active substances were found: 3,4-dihydroxybenzoic acid, n-coumaric acid, luteolin-7-glucoside, acacetin, apigenin-7-O-glucoside, chicoric acid, and hesperetin. The alcoholic extract contains rosmarinic acid and large amounts of catechin.

Properties and medical uses:

Licorice has anti-ulcer properties (inhibits Helicobacter pylori bacteria that cause ulcers), affects the reception of steroid hormones, has immunomodulatory, anti-mutagenic, anti-tumor, anti-edema (free radical suppressant), and hemolytic, affects blood electrolytes, has anti-lipid and anti-anemia effects. It also has effects on enzyme activity, estrogenic effects, and anti-allergic effects. Licorice also has antiviral effects. Studies have shown its effect in treating chronic viral hepatitis, as the glycyrrhizin compound affects the hepatitis B virus, as well as the herpes simplex virus that causes ulcers in the genital areas. It enhances the body's resistance to the Candida albicans fungus. It is used in treating respiratory tract infections (cough, sinusitis accompanied by abundant, yellowish, foul-smelling mucus secretions, and nasopharyngitis and bronchitis). Licorice, which contains glycyrrhizinic acid, is especially used in treating chronic stomach infections, as it increases the mucus that protects the stomach wall, reduces acid secretion, and helps On ulcer healing. Coumarin compounds Thin the blood, prevent clotting and reduce blood clots and brain clots. Phenolic compounds BHP were isolated from liquorice roots, which showed the ability to stop the development of breast cancer in women and prostate cancer in men, by disrupting the activity of the protein responsible for the proliferation of cancer cells. Liquorice is popularly used as a refreshing, moisturizing and expectorant drink. Digestive, and treatment of cold sores, common cold, cough, stomach pain, constipation, increased milk secretion, and treatment of epilepsy and headache. It is used externally in cases of dermatitis, eczema, mouth ulcers, wound healing, and eye diseases.

Pharmaceutical forms: It is available in the form of capsules, especially liquid, infusion, tobacco products, candies, chewing gum, and sugary phlegm. It is sold under different names.

Other uses:

The sweetening power of licorice is 50 times greater than sugar, and is currently widely used as a flavoring and sweetener for bitter medicines, candy, drinks, foods, chewing gum, tobacco manufacturing, toothpastes, and soaps.

Side effects, interactions, and warnings for use:

Possible side effects include headache, water retention, and high doses can cause heart failure and rhabdomyosarcoma. Licorice should not be combined in particular with carotene, procaine, quinidine, steroids such as prednisone and nicotinic steroids, dactone, diuretics, antihypertensive drugs, and anoxin. Licorice should not be consumed by people with heart disease, high blood pressure, liver and kidney diseases, and should also be avoided by pregnant or breastfeeding women. Glycyrrhetinic acid (prepared from licorice) enhances the effect of steroids applied to the skin. Scientists have discovered the possibility of removing 97% of glycyrrhetinic acid, and the result is called lico-deglycyrrhizinated (DGL) rice, and pharmaceutical companies are currently resorting to removing glycyrrhetinic acid from the plant to reduce its negative effects.

Environment:

It grows naturally near swamps, river banks, and flooded lands in winter. Licorice adapts well to different environmental conditions in areas between 35-45° north latitude. The plant tolerates high temperatures, but it does not tolerate cold, especially at a young age. It tolerates relative salinity.

Cultivation and productivity:

It is propagated by seeds or by cuttings that result from cutting the ground stem cuttings (rhizomes) into small pieces. The planting date varies according to the propagation method. In sexual propagation, the seeds are planted in the spring in the nursery soil, and the seedlings are transferred to the permanent soil after a year. In the case of vegetative propagation, which is the best method, the rhizomes are planted in the permanent place before the sap flows in them at the end of winter and the beginning of spring. After preparing the land, lines are drawn at 110-120 cm intervals, then the seedlings are planted in the line at a distance of 40-50 cm between each seedling. As for planting by cuttings, it is done in holes at distances of 60 cm, and at least three cuttings are placed in the hole horizontally at a depth of 5-8 cm, then they are irrigated directly. Licorice needs close irrigation in the first months of planting in order to help the cuttings form roots and grow, then the soil is irrigated once every month, and this varies according to the type of soil, the degree of its water retention and the weather conditions. Fertilization improves production clearly. It is recommended to start collecting the roots 2-3 years after planting, and the best time to cut the roots is during the fall when the plant begins to turn yellow, i.e. two months after the flowering stage. The collection begins by cutting the green growths aerially at a height of 5 cm from the ground, then the lines are plowed to loosen the soil, and then the stems and rhizomes are cut with special sharp knives, then pulled out of the ground. The cutting process helps the remaining parts in the soil to grow quickly and fill the void. After the cutting process, the roots and stems are cleaned, then cut into small parts, 5-10 cm long. The cut parts are dried under the sun for a week, and turned daily to prevent fermentation and fungal rot and to speed up drying. One hectare yields about 5 tons of dry roots.

Lupinus albus L.

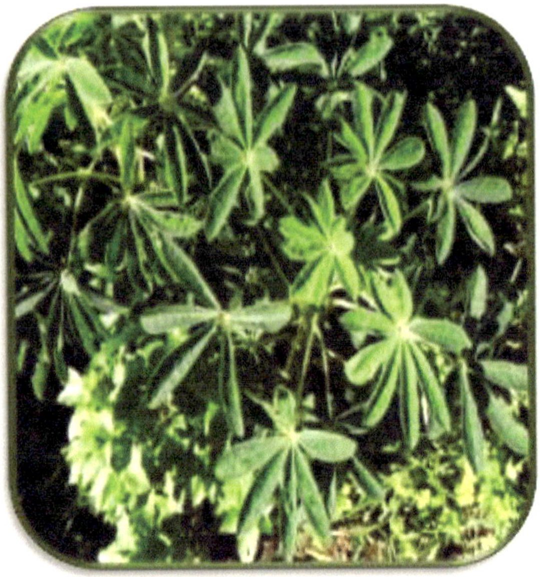

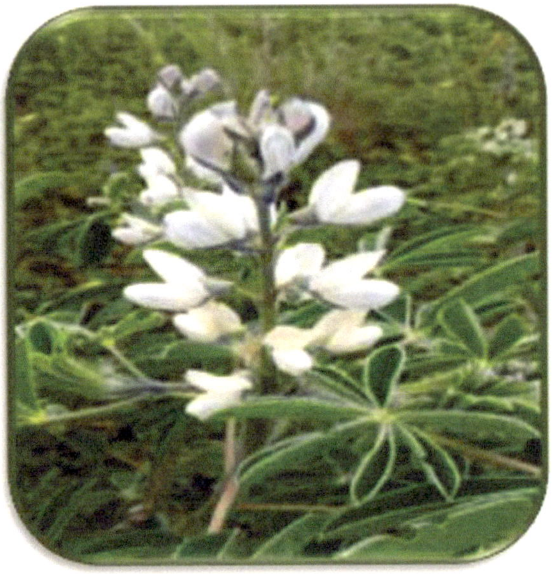

Family: Fabaceae

Common names: Lupin

Foreign names: blanc Lupin Fr. Lupin, Eng. Kafiya,

Occurrences : 170,122 occurrences

Distribution in the world

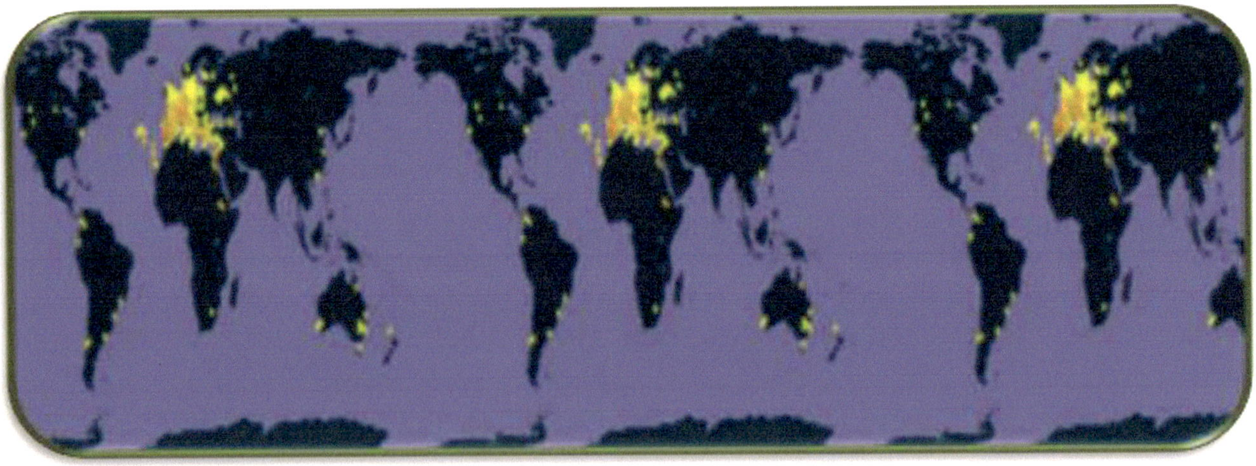

Botanical description:

An annual herb, covered with silky hairs, 20-60 cm long. Stems erect, branched. Leaves compound 5-20 cm long. Ears usually exceed 2 cm, fused to the base of the petiole, conical to obovate, hairy. Petiole Longer than the leaf blade. Leaflets 6-9, oblong-lanceolate to lanceolate, base scalloped, apex pointed, glabrous above, hairy below. Inflorescence racemose, many-flowered, erect, oblong-lanceolate, exceeding leaves. Bracts rapidly falling. Flower spikes shorter than calyx. Flowers about 1.5 cm long, usually alternate, or clustered in widely spaced whorls. Calyx persistent, green to bluish, hairy below, bilipped. Corolla twicc as long as calyx, flag white to lilac, bluish around margin, as long as wings. Pod 5 x 1.3 cm, 2-4 seeds, flattened, linear, ending in short beak. Seeds compressed, lenticular, white to pale brown, smooth.

Flowering: February to April.

Homeland and geographical distribution:

Eastern Mediterranean basin, as well as many countries in the northern hemisphere. Its cultivation is concentrated in Australia, Europe, Russia, Poland and South Africa. The countries of the Soviet Union used to produce more than 50% of the world's production.

Cultivated varieties include: white lupine, yellow lupine, and sweet lupine.

History and heritage:

Al-Shahabi (1978) mentioned, on the authority of Meyerhof, that the word “lupine” came from the Greek “thermos,” and that it was transferred to Coptic, Hebrew, and Aramaic, and from there to Arabic and Persian. Nahal (2009) believes that the scientific name of the genus is likely from the Greek “lupus,” meaning “wolf,” meaning “wolf bean,” referring to the bitterness of its seeds. Lupin seeds have been used since ancient times as an appetite stimulant and diuretic. The Arabs considered it a sexual tonic, and Ibn Sina mentioned it.

Part used: seeds and leaves.

Chemical components:

The leaves contain quinolizidine alkaloids at a rate of 1.6%, and this rate in the seeds reaches 3.3%, including sparteine, lupinine, and gramine, and 6% fatty substances, and carbohydrates, including stachyose 6%, in addition to 48% proteins. The percentage of alkaloids in the seeds of cultivated species (sweet lupine) decreases to less than 0.1%.

The plant contains a high percentage of protein, dietary fiber, and low Fats make lupine a suitable substitute not only for animal protein, but also for processed flour, which is less balanced from a nutritional point of view. It is also used in the preparation of bread, cakes, biscuits, etc.

Properties and medical uses:

Lupin seeds have anthelmintic properties. It is popularly used as a nerve tonic, heart stimulant, diuretic, anthelmintic, and to treat some skin diseases, such as eczema and psoriasis. It helps lower blood sugar in patients, especially since fiber slows the body’s absorption of glucose (simple sugar) resulting from the breakdown of starches and sugars, which limits the occurrence of high blood sugar levels. It has been found that these fibers, which are generally found in grains, resist high cholesterol levels and limit Constipation, and protects against colon cancer. Boiled lupine seeds are used as an enema to eliminate worms, or massaged into the hands and body to get rid of scabies and eczema. Lupine seeds are used in cardiovascular diseases, high blood pressure, and glucose and insulin reception.

Lupins contain inhibitors of metalloproteinases (MMP-9) and (MMP-2) that cause diseases in the digestive system, and therefore the inhibitor is of great importance in reducing inflammatory diseases and tumors, and in stopping the growth of colon cancer cells.

Side effects and warnings for use:

Increased salivation, difficulty swallowing, with vomiting, diarrhea, headache and difficulty seeing, and in case of using large quantities, paralysis is observed, and perhaps death due to respiratory arrest.

Environment:

It can be found naturally in sandy soils, lupins grow in many types Soils, it is successfully cultivated in red or calcareous clay soils, prefers sunny locations.

Cultivation and productivity:

It is propagated by seeds, the seeds are planted at a distance of 25 cm between each seed after the soil has been opened and prepared for planting. The plants are harvested in the summer, dried and threshed to extract the seeds. It fixes nitrogen thanks to the bacteria that live in symbiosis with its roots, so it is preferable to cut the plant after harvesting and not to uproot it.

Medicago sativa L.

Medica sativa (L.) Mill., Medicago sativa var. vulgaris Alef., Medicago sativa subsp. vulgaris (Alef.) Arcang., Medicago vera Kirschl.

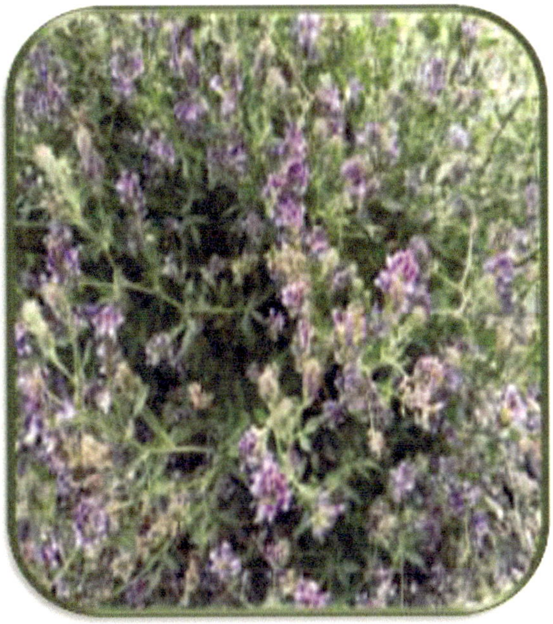

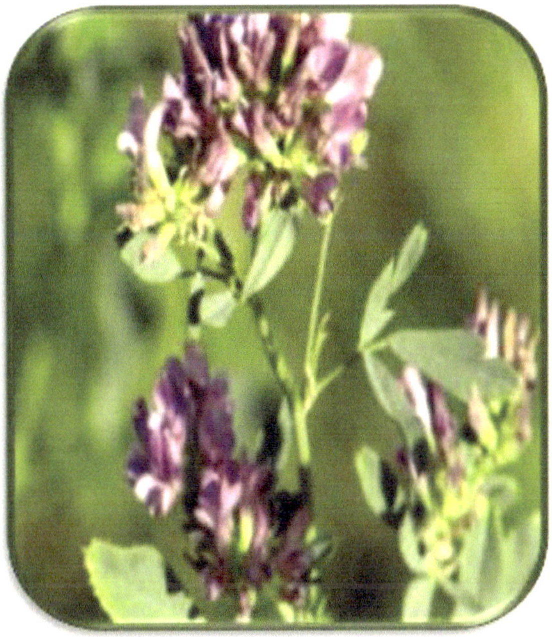

Family: Fabaceae

Common names: cultivated alfalfa, Hijazi clover, wet rod

Foreign names: Luzeme: Fr. Alfalfa, Eng.

Occurrences : 273,200 occurrences

Distribution in the world

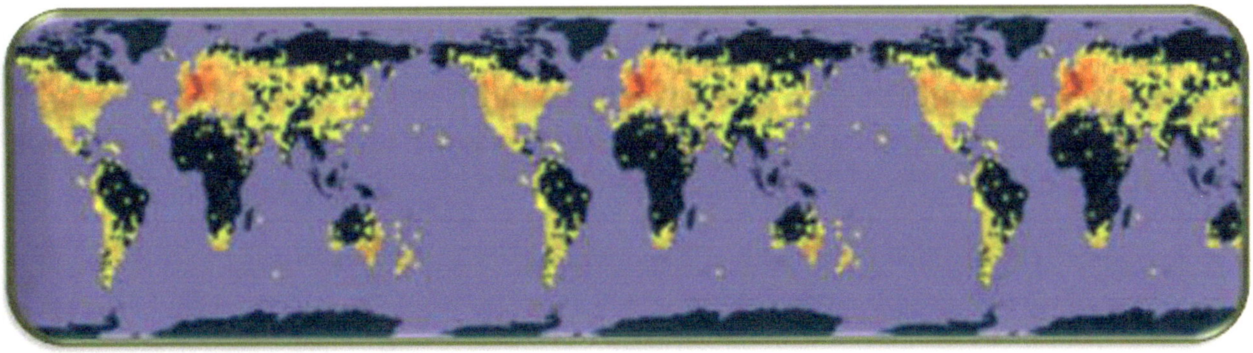

Botanical description:

Perennial herb, woody base, glabrous or bearing dense hairs, 10-50 cm long or sometimes more. Stems numerous, supine to ascending, branched, leafy. Leaf Trifoliate. Ears ovate-lanceolate, apexed, complete. Leaflets 1-1.5 cm × 3-6 mm, in the lower leaves they are inverted ovate to oblong, in the upper leaves they are lanceolate, rounded or truncated and lanceolate at the apex, serrated at the upper part only. Inflorescence: Clustered, containing 8-20 flowers, their spikes are longer than the supporting leaves. Flowers 6-10 mm, the length of their spike is equal to the length of the calyx tube or twice its length. Calyx about 5 mm, hairy, the length of the tube is equal to the length of the teeth. Corolla Blue or yellow in color. The horn is spiral, consisting of 2-3 spaced coils, linear or sickle-shaped, hairy, not thorny. The seeds are straight or slightly curved.

Flowering: April to May.

Habitat and geographical distribution:

Mediterranean, European-Siberian, western Iranian-Turanian region. It is cultivated in many countries of the world.

History and heritage:

The scientific name of the genus is derived from the Latin name of the plant Medica, meaning "herb of Medica", and the name of the species sativa means "cultivated."

Part used: Leaves, seeds.

Chemical components:

The leaves contain carotenoids, including lutein and others. Triterpene saponins: sojasapogenols A-E, aglycones hederagenin and medicaginic acid. Isovavonoids including: glycosides formononetin, gentistein, daidzein. Coumestans, the most important of which are: coumestrol, lucernol, sativol, trifoliol, and steroids including spinasterol, stigmasterol, and other compounds. Cyanogenic glycosides. Vitamins, especially vitamin K. The seeds contain L-canavaine, betaine, homostachydrine, stachydrine, trigonelline, and fatty oil. It also contains the following components: proteins, carbohydrates, saponins, lignins, phenolic compounds, tannins, alkaloids, carotenoids, sterols, phytoestrogens, favones, and isovavonoids. Alkaloids: Asparagine, Trigonelline, Staccidrine, L-Homostacdrine. Amino acids: Medicanin, Lysine, Arginine, Histidine, Tyrosine, Phenyl Alanine, Methionine, Aspartic Acid, Glutamic Acid, Serine, Alanine, Coumarin, Myrceiminol, Scopoletin, Esculetin, Digestive enzymes, Other enzymes such as: Isovavon reductase, Festetone reductase, Iminopeptidase, and Aminopeptidase. Flavonoids: Quercetin, Myristin, Luteolin, Apigenin, Cresceriol, Tricin, Medicarpine, Coumestrol, Sativane, Festetol, and Formonetin. Phenolic compounds: Hydroxybenzoic acid, vanillic acid, coumaric acid, ferulic acids, salicylic acid, sinapic acids, caffeic acid, hespertin, chlorogenic acid, tannic acid and heterosides. Phytoestrogens: coumestrol, genistein, formometin, diadzein, biochanin, beta-sitosterol, stigmasterol. Polyamines: norspermidine, norspermin. , esculetin, scopoletin, myrsellinol, stigmasterol, β-sitosterol, α-spinasterol, dihydrospinasterol Protein: ferritin, protein phosphatase 2A, beta amylase. Saponins: soy sapogenol, hydragenin, medicagenin acid, pyogenin. Minerals: Ca, K, P, Mg, Fe, Zn, Cu, Al, B, Cr, Co, Mn, Mo, Se, Si, Na Amino acids: non-protein such as L-canaverin, organic acids: citrate, malate, malonate, succinate, fumarate, lactate, Benzoate. Vitamins A, B1, B6, B12, C, D, E, K, niacin, pantothenic acid, biotin, folic acid. Volatile components: terpenes, limonene, linalool, trans-ocymine, furanoids, benzaldehyde, ethyl benzaldehyde, butanol.

Properties and medical uses:

Saponin contents affect the cardiovascular system, nervous system and digestive system. The drug is popularly used to treat diabetes, thyroid dysfunction, kidney, bladder and prostate problems, and to increase urine flow. It is also useful in treating menstrual disorders and menopause, due to the estrogenic effect of the lozenge. The seeds are used to reduce high cholesterol levels, treat rheumatoid arthritis, and are a source of vitamins A, E, and K, and some minerals. The leaves and young branches are used as salads, and the powder of the leaves or seeds is used in the form of capsules and tablets as nutritional supplements (vitamins A, E, K, and C). Eating alfalfa reduces the absorption of cholesterol and hardening of the arteries in animals. Saponins contribute to reducing the concentration of cholesterol in plasma without changing the concentration of high-density lipoprotein cholesterol, reduce the absorption of cholesterol by the intestine, cause an increase in the secretion of bile acids, prevent hardening of the arteries, and contribute to the regression of hardening of the arteries. Cholestaid™, a product available in the USA, contains 900 mg of alfalfa extract with 100 mg of citric acid, facilitating the elimination of cholesterol from the body without any side effects. The plant is important in reducing blood sugar levels caused by streptozotocin. The manganese content is an important factor in alfalfa plant for controlling diabetes. The methanol extract of alfalfa showed estrogenic activity on breast cancer cells, where the pure antiestrogen ICI 780,182 suppressed cell proliferation. The alfalfa leaf extract is used in the treatment of symptoms of nervous menopause. Hot flashes and night sweats completely disappeared with the treatment, and the plant product caused a significant increase in the response of prolactin and thyroid hormones. Purified polysaccharide components of alfalfa have been shown to inhibit the reverse transcriptase activities of the human immunodeficiency virus (HIV). Beverages prepared from alfalfa are beneficial in maintaining normal digestive function, balancing nutrition in the human body, and preventing osteoporosis, atherosclerosis, and aging.

Precautions for use:

No health incidents or side effects have been reported with the proper administration of the specified ivory dose. It is preferable to avoid it during pregnancy, due to what is believed to affect the level of estrogen. It is warned against feeding young and growing alfalfa shoots to ruminants, especially sheep, as this leads to bloating of the stomachs of these animals. Environment: Alfalfa grows wild on the edges of fields and neglected lands. Its germination is fast, from long-day plants that love light, especially in the early stages of growth. The seeds can germinate at a temperature of 2-3 ° C. Alfalfa tolerates High temperatures that reach 40 C, and also tolerates low temperatures in the basal branching area even -15 ° C. Alfalfa needs large amounts of water, but it is resistant to drought thanks to the depth of its roots in the soil. Alfalfa is a crop that tolerates soil salinity.

Cultivation and productivity:

Alfalfa is propagated by seeds, and is planted in autumn or spring. Alfalfa cultivation requires deep plowing of the land, followed by several shallow plowings to soften the soil, then rectangular basins or basins are prepared with dimensions of 10 - 20 X 2 - 3 m if the irrigation process will be done by irrigation or without basins if the irrigation process will be done by spraying. Then the seeds are scattered in two stages and in opposite directions, then the soil surface is stirred with a comb or plant branches (pomegranate for example) or burlap to cover the seeds in the soil, then it is irrigated by spraying or by resting with low-flowing water. Alfalfa responds to phosphorous and potassium fertilization, and to a lesser extent nitrogen. Alfalfa grows in various types of agricultural lands, and prefers deep, loose, well-ventilated lands. The most important service operations are eliminating weeds and regular irrigation, especially in the early stages. The production of seeds per hectare reaches up to 360 kg.

Melilotus officinalis (L.) Lam.

Trifolium melilotus oficinalis L,.Brachylobus oficinalis (L.) Dulac, Medicago oficinalis (L.) E.H.L.Krause, Sertula maior Lunell, Sertula oficinalis (L.) Kuntze, Trifolium ofici- nale L., Trigonella oficinalis (L.) Coulot & Rabaute.

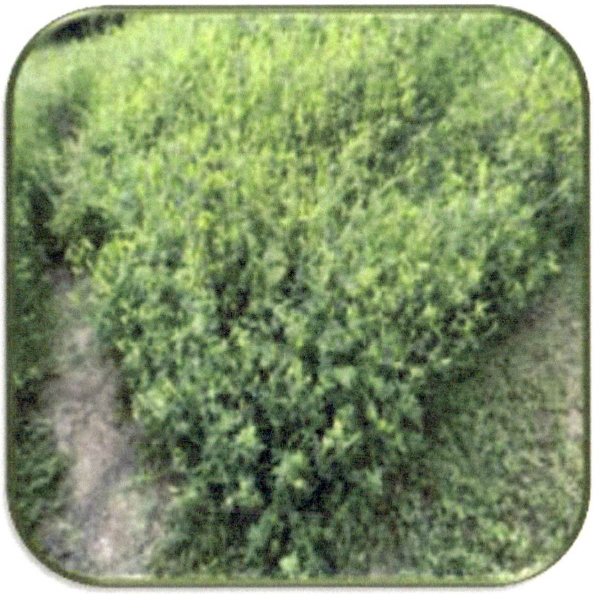

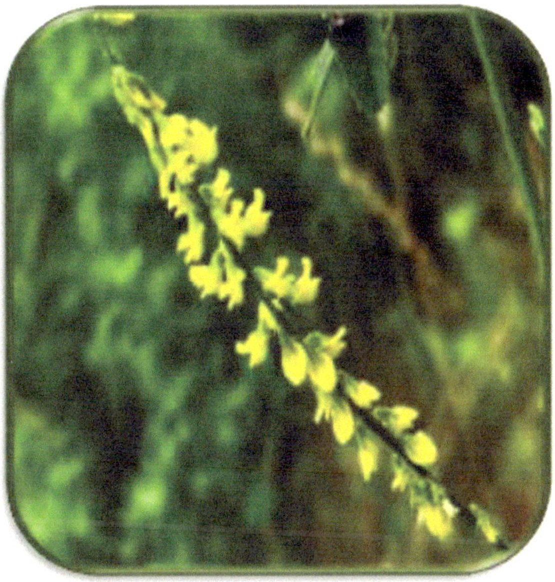

Family: Fabaceae

Common names: Handoq, King's wreath, Melilot

Foreign names: Sweet clover, Sweet melilot, Fr. Melilot

Occurrences : 127,649 occurrences

Distribution in the world

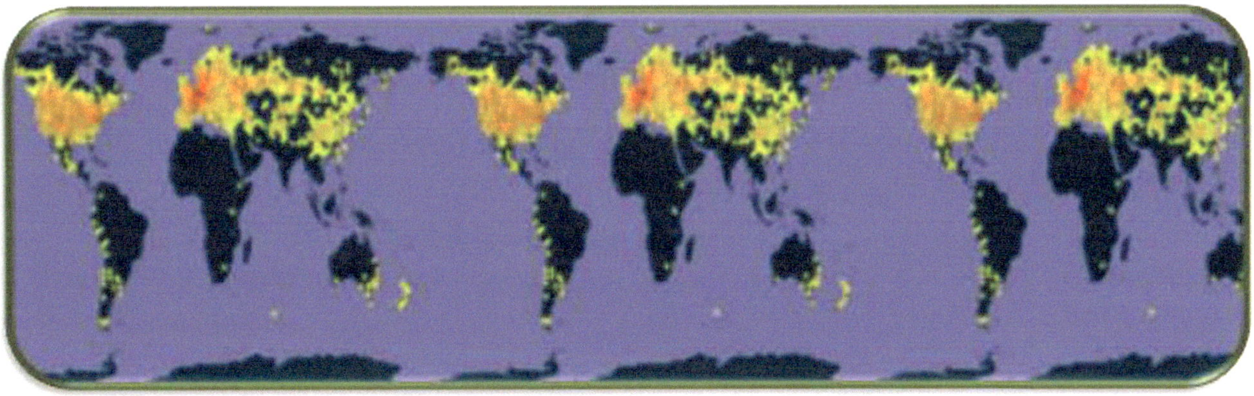

Botanical description:

A biennial herb, 50-100 cm tall. Stem erect, branched. Leaves alternate, trifoliate, long-petioled. The lateral leaflets are ovate and inverted, the central leaflet is oblong, with serrated margins, the ears are fused to the petiole. The inflorescence is densely clustered, axillary, much longer than the leaves.

Flowers are small, about 6 mm long, short-stalked. The calyx is short, ending with five teeth of equal length. The corolla has 5 petals, yellow in color. The stamens are biconcave. The pod is not open, single-seeded, oval in shape, its apex ends in a stigma, its length is about 3 mm, its surface bears irregular transverse wrinkles.

Flowering: From March to May.

Habitat and geographical distribution:

Europe, Asia, northern Turkey, Syria, and Lebanon. The genus includes several species that are similar to each other. Their distinction depends on a set of characteristics, the most important of which are:

1) The color of the flowers (white in M. albus and yellow in the rest of the species.)

2) The dimensions of the horn and the shape of the decorations on its surface.

History and Heritage:

The scientific name of the genus is derived from the Greek melilôtos, the name of the plant, from meli meaning "honey", and lotus meaning "lotus." The descriptive name of the species oficinalis means constitutional (medical). This herb was used in ancient times to treat a number of conditions as a carminative and expectorant, an anticoagulant, and an antibiotic.

Handsome syrup aids digestion, and its flowers attract bees and repel moths. The fennel was used as a powder, and its leaves could be eaten, but they are somewhat bitter. Prospero mentions that the fennel is a warming herb, and is used among other ingredients in making compresses to treat fevers. Its seeds are also added to a basic drink, which relieves pain. In a "Coptic Medical" papyrus, the fennel was mentioned as an ingredient in one of the medicines used to treat diseased testicles.

Part used:

Fresh or dried flowering tops. (The dried herb has an aromatic smell.)

Chemical components:

Free coumarins (0.4-0.9%), formed from coumarinic acids during the drying process.

Coumarin derivatives:

Some of them are in the form of glycosides, or in the form of hydroxycoumarins, including: herniarin, coumarin, melilotol, melilotin, umbelliferone, scopoletin, fraxidin. Phenolic acids, including: melilotic acid, a. cafeic, a. ferulic, a. salicyc, chlorogenic acid and rosmarinic acid. Favonoids, the most important of which are: glycosides quercetin, kampferol-, rutin and isoquercitrin.

Terpene saponins, including: Melilotigenin, aglycones soya sapogenols B, E, azuki saponin II, azuki saponin-V-carboxylate.The seeds also contain the alkaloids trigonelline and canavanin.

Properties and medical uses:

Handhuq is used to treat disorders related to chronic venous insufficiency, edema, and as a complementary treatment for hemorrhoids and lymphatic congestion. The drug is used in folk medicine to treat bronchial diseases and wash the eyes. It is used topically in the form of compresses to accelerate wound healing, treat bruises, contusions, and joint sprains. Plant extracts rich in polyphenols have inhibitory activity on α-amylase and alpha-glucosidase enzymes.Sugar and inflammation.It is a promising plant for developing natural nutritional supplements against diabetes. Studies have revealed its effectiveness in treating multiple sclerosis.

Pharmaceutical forms:

Infusion (tea), liquid used as injections, ointments, suppositories, patches, or compresses.

Other uses:

The compound dicoumarol is extracted from the plant on an industrial scale to produce rodenticides. The leaves are used in salad preparation, and the seeds are used for their flavoring properties. Raised by livestock.

Drug effects, interactions and precautions for use:

There are no health risks or side effects if the prescribed dose is adhered to. However, when taken in high doses, this leads to headaches and confusion, and may cause temporary damage to the liver. The dried leaves can be toxic if they rot, because the coumarins in the plant turn into dicoumarol, an anticoagulant, when they rot. Therefore, the plant should be taken with caution and should not be given to people who suffer from slow blood clotting, or who are taking warfarin. The drug should be kept away from light in sealed containers, so that the coumarins do not spoil. Environment: The plant grows in fields, meadows, fallow lands, on roadsides, and in steppes. Acidic soils are not suitable for it, and it prefers moderate or basic soils, well drained. It prefers sunny locations and does not like shade. Mature plants tolerate drought. Its seeds spread with the manure of animals that graze it during the fruiting stage, so it is considered a harmful weed in agricultural lands.

Cultivation and productivity:

It is propagated by seeds, which are scattered directly in the permanent soil in the spring and until early summer. Seeds are soaked in lukewarm water for 12 hours before planting. Germination takes approximately two weeks. The plant is collected during the flowering period, then dried in the shade. Some types of nitrogen-fixing bacteria in the soil coexist with the plant roots.

Prosopis farcta (Banks & Sol.) J.F.Macbr.,

Mimosa farcta Banks et Sol., Lagonychium farctum (Banks et Sol.) Bobr., Prosopis stephaniana (M.B.) Kunth ex Spreng., Mimosa stephaniana M.B., Acacia stephaniana (M.B.) Wilid., Lagonychium stephanianum (M.B.) M.B.

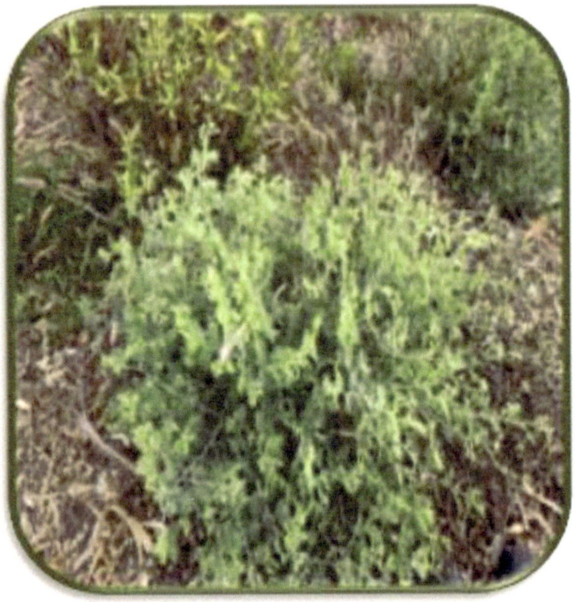

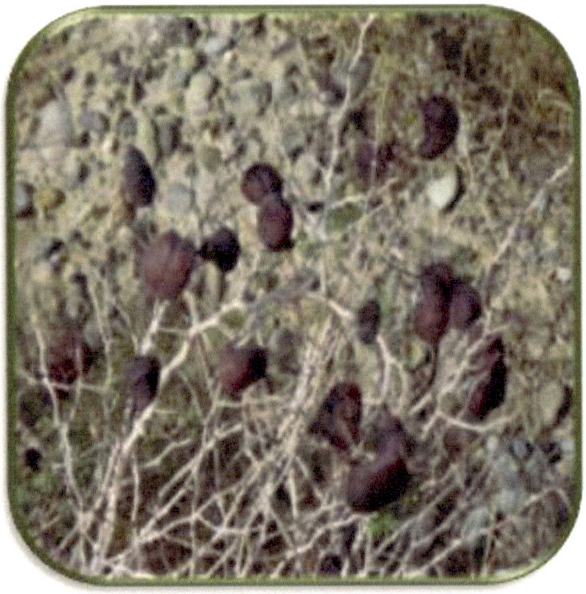

Family: Fabaceae (Mimosoideae)

Common names: Kharniba, goat's carob, Yanbut, Arak, Sheshan

Foreign names: Mesquite mesquite, Syrian Eng.

Occurrences : 2,560 occurrences

Distribution in the world

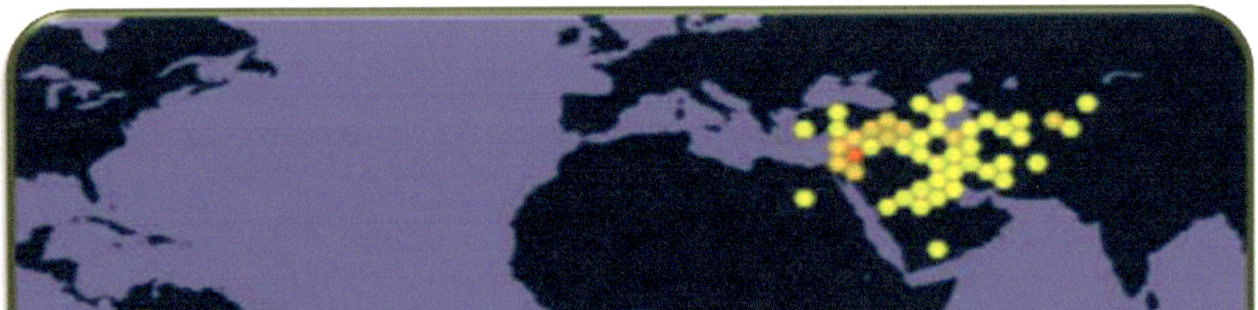

Botanical description:

A small shrub, 40-100 cm tall and more, branches from the base, and reproduces through adventitious roots that arise below the stem,and through rhizomes. The roots and rhizomes extend deep into the soil for a distance of 15 meters or more. The branches are slender, thorny, and the young ones are hairy. The leaves are compound, double pinnate, and up to 5 cm long. cm, ovate in general shape, the main axis of the leaf bears 3-7 pairs of secondary axes each bearing 10-15 pairs of leaflets. The leaf is semi-palmate, oblong, acute at the apex, covered with short hairs, its dimensions are 2-3 x 3-7 mm. The ears fall quickly. The flowers are gathered in spike-shaped inflorescences, axillary, about 7 cm long. The flower is short-branched, hermaphrodite. The calyx is pentamerous. The corolla is 4-5 mm, Pentameric, pale yellow. Male 10 stamens, free, slightly protruding from corolla. Female unicarpal, ovary superior. Fruit indehiscent pod, 3-1×5-2 cm, oval, ellipsoid, dark brown when ripe, medium fruiting pericarp spongy. Seeds compressed, few in number, dark brown.

Flowering: April to August.

Homeland and geographical distribution: Iranian-Turanian, extending to the Mediterranean and Arabian desert regions.

History and heritage:

The Arabic name is Khreiniba, a diminutive of carob, referring to the similarity of the fruits to it.

Part used: Leaves, fruits, and seeds.

Chemical components:

Phenolic compounds, volatile compounds, sugars (glucose, fructose, sucrose.) Favone glycosides: 7-O-glucoside, luteolin vitexin, isovitexin, rutin, myricetin Lactate (salivary substances), especially in seeds 19%. And organic acids including: oxalic, malic, citric, tartaric. The seeds contain tannins, fatty oil, composed of unsaturated fatty acids (oleic, linoleic, linolenic) and saturated fatty acids (palmitic), phenolic acids, flavonoids and glycosidic derivatives, flavonoids O, C, phenolic acid derivatives. The extracts contained gallic acid, vanillic acid, luteolin, apigenin, phloridzin, and vicinin. Fatty acids, organic acids, steroids, terpenoids, and hydrocarbons.

Properties and medical uses:

Research has shown moderate to weak effectiveness of the aqueous extract of the aerial parts against some types of bacteria and fungi that cause some skin diseases. The decoction of the leaves is popularly used to treat kidney stones and reduce sugar. The decoction of the leaves, flowers and fruit is also used as an expectorant, and in the treatment of rheumatism and insect stings. The pods and seeds have astringent properties (tannins) and are used to treat diarrhea. The aqueous and alcoholic extract of the leaves and fruits is used against cutaneous leishmaniasis caused by Leishmania major compared to current reference drugs (Glucanthem).

Other uses:

The tannins extracted from the plant are used in tanning leather.

Environment:

The plant grows on loamy, salty, warm, sunny soils, in neglected places, valleys, depressions, and the walls of neglected fields, whether in the interior or near the coasts.

Cultivation and productivity:

An invasive plant, it can be transformed into A pest that is difficult to get rid of in agricultural lands. It reproduces through adventitious roots that arise at the bottom of the stem and through rhizomes.

Retama raetam (Forssk.) Webb & Berthel.

Lygos raetam (Forskal) Heywood Genista raetam Forssk., Lygos raetam (Forssk.) Hey- wood, Spartium raetam (Forssk.) Spach

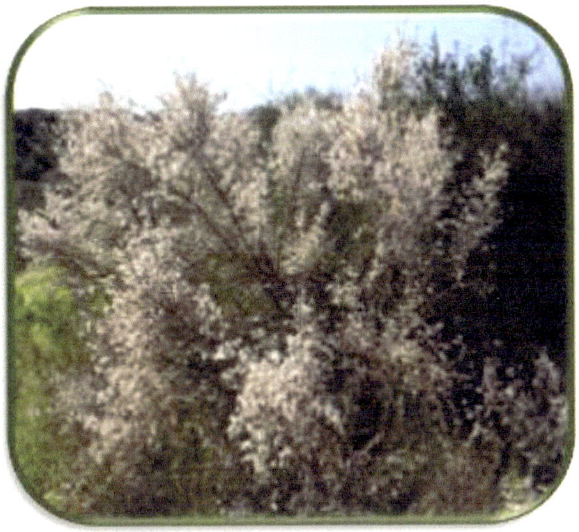

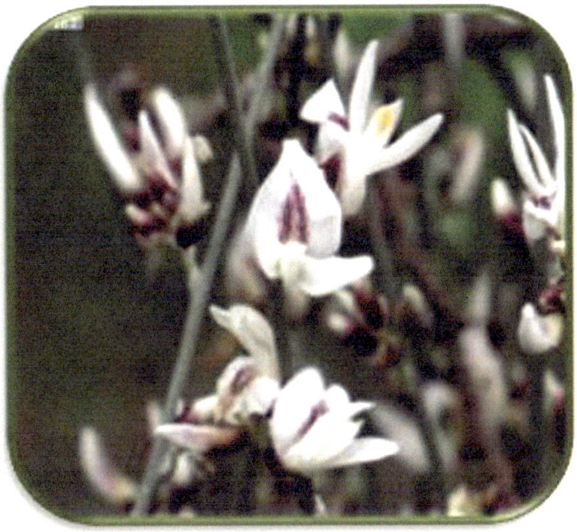

Family: Fabaceae

Common names: Rattam

Foreign names: désert du Genêt Fr. broom, White Eng.

Occurrences : 5,101 occurrences

Distribution in the world

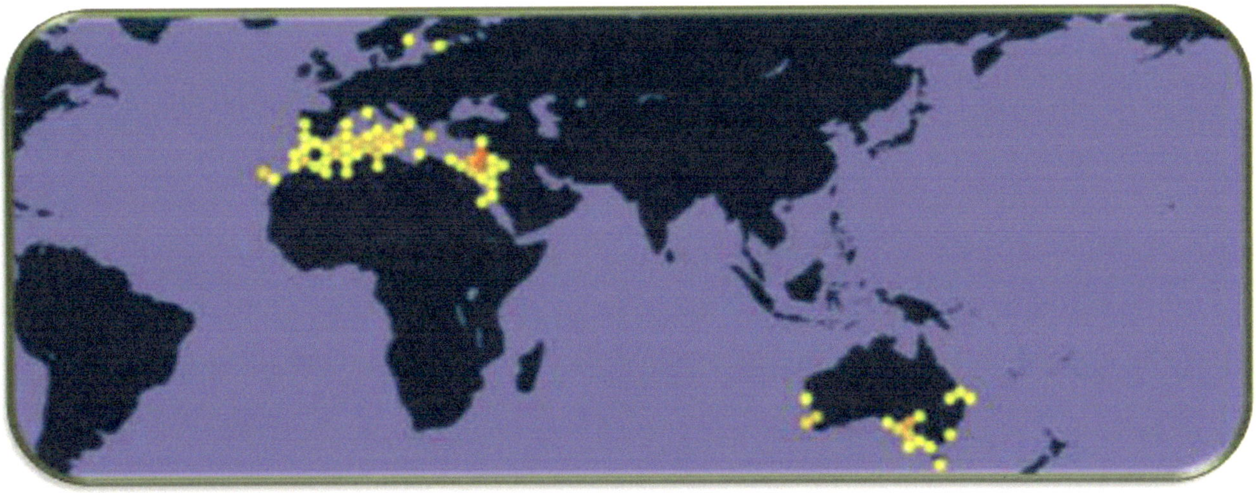

Botanical description:

A shrub resembling a sedge, 1-3 m long. The roots are thick, sparsely branched, spreading vertically penetrating the soil reaching a depth of 20 m. The stems are thick, notched, the branches are erect or flat, the young ones may be drooping. The leaves are simple, live for a very short period, linear to oblong in shape, their dimensions are 3-8×5-20 mm. Inflorescences are racemose, containing 1-5 flowers, distributed along the branches. Flowers are hermaphrodite, bisymmetrical, 10-15 mm long. Calyx is crimson, bilipped, the upper lip consists of two broad triangular teeth, and the lower lip consists of three short teeth. Corolla white, petals pentagonal, descending butterfly-shaped, crimson at the top, flag streaked with violet, ovate to round, navicular shorter than wings. Fruit small pod, 9-5×20-7 mm, unopened or late-opening, ovate to oblong, or ellipsoid, apex terminated in a stigma with a small beak, erect or arched, pericarp leathery or fleshy, smooth or wrinkled. Seeds yellow or brown.

Flowering: February to April.

Habitat and geographical distribution:

Arabian-Sindhi, and is naturally distributed in the Canary Islands, North Africa, Egypt, the Arabian Peninsula, Palestine, and Syria.

History and heritage:

Ratam is an Arabic name, and it is the origin of the scientific name of the genus and species, i.e. "Ratam al-Ratmi." Part used: The stem, leaves, and flowers that are collected in the spring.

Chemical components:

The fruits contain the alkaloid cytisine, the glycosidegenistein, phenolic compounds, proteins, and fats. The flowers contain an alkaloid anagyrine. Organic components: spartanine, benzenepropanoic acid, phthalic acid, 1-octadecanol, squalene, and argentamine. Inorganic components: aluminum, chlorine, calcium, bromine, magnesium, phosphorus, and chromium. The essential oil contains 50 components, including: nonanal, alpha-humulene, acetaldehyde, linalool, myrcene, tridacanal, beta-caryophyllene, alpha-terpenyl acetate, terpineol, and methyl anthranate.

Properties and medical uses:

Genistein glycoside is an antitumor and an enzyme inhibitor (kinase). Research on mice indicates the effectiveness of the aqueous extract of the aerial parts in limiting the growth of some fungi, reducing blood sugar, and increasing urine production. The decoction of the leaves is used popularly as a diuretic, reducing blood sugar, and in treating stomach cramps and liver disorders, especially in patients with fever, high temperature accompanied by diarrhea and jaundice.

A mixture of powdered branches and honey is popularly used as an emetic, astringent, anthelmintic, and abortifacient. The decoction of the leaves and flowers is used topically as a compress to treat back pain, disinfect wounds, skin rashes and itching, and wash inflamed eyes. The plant is used in veterinary medicine to treat scabies. The essential oil has antibacterial and antifungal activity, and has antioxidant properties, and is therefore used as a natural ingredient in preserving food and pharmaceutical preparations.

Precautions for use:

The fruits of the wormwood are poisonous, and are believed to cause hallucinations. Eating large quantities of flowers leads to urinary tract disorders. Not to be used by pregnant women.

Environment:

Xerophyte species, widespread in hot regions. Found in the moderately dry Mediterranean bioclimatic zone. Grows on sandy, calcareous, inland or coastal soils, and on moving sand dunes. The plant resists burial by sand, as well as sand erosion. Cultivation and productivity: It reproduces naturally by seeds that can remain in the soil for a long period of time, up to 20 years. Young plants give deep taproots, which makes it difficult to pull them out. It can also reproduce vegetatively by offshoots. The plant begins to flower at the age of two years. It can also spread widely sometimes, making it difficult to get rid of.

Senna alexandrina Garsault

Senna alexandrina var. alexandrina

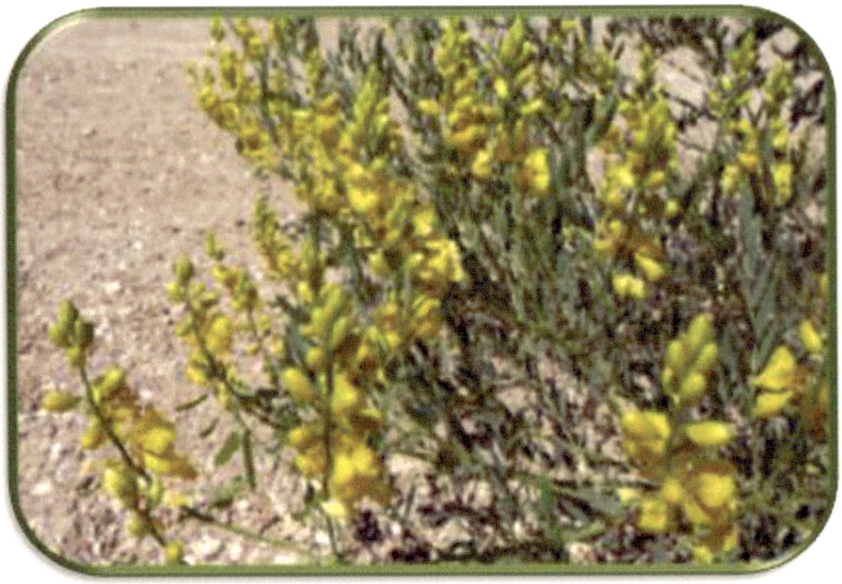

Family: Fabaceae (subfamily Caesalpinoideae)

Local names: Senna, Senna, Senna, Senna Hegazi or Alexandrian, Ashreq

Foreign names: séné Le, Fr. senna Alexandrian Eng.

Occurrences : 3 occurrences

Distribution in the world

No occurrences with coordinates

Description of the plant

A shrub, up to 1 m tall, covered with some short, ascending hairs, herbaceous. The leaves are compound, pinnate, pinnate, composed of 3-7 leaflets, 8-10 cm long, the leaflet is semi-palmated, lanceolate to oblong, sharp-pointed, the ears Perennial, conical. Inflorescence axillary, erect, longer than supporting leaves. Bracts Drop, membranous, ovate or inverted ovate. Inflorescence 4-6 mm, elongated in fruit. Flowers 1-1.5 cm. Calyx 5 sepals, united in a very short tube, then its segments overlap. Corolla yellow, composed of 5 stamens. Male 10 stamens, unequal, the upper (posterior) of which is shorter and without anthers. Horn 2.5-2×6-3 Poison, carried on a short stalk, flat, oblong to elliptical in shape, ending in a short stalk, straight or slightly curved, bearingndown. The seeds are compressed, inverted oval to pedicel in shape.Narrow, bare, or winged on both sides of the seam

Flowering: Between March and June.

Habitat and geographical distribution:

It is spread in the Arabian Peninsula, Egypt, Sudan, India, Pakistan, and Iran, which is considered one of the most important countries exporting Senna.

History and Heritage:

The name Senna is the Arabic name for the leaves of the plant. The plant was known to Arab and Indian doctors, and the leaves, flowers, fruits and branches were used in herbal mixtures. The inhabitants of North Africa and Southwest Asia have also been accustomed to using Senna as a laxative for centuries. It is said that the first to introduce Senna into medicine were the two Arab doctors Serbion and Ibn al-Musawi.

Part used: Dried leaves and ripe fruits.

Chemical components:

Senna leaves and fruits contain: 2.5-4% anthraquinone derivatives, some of which are free and reduced anthrone di-, and some of which are linked in the form of anthraquinone glycosides: sennosides a, b, and there is a third glycoside (C) emodin. Senna fruits contain a smaller amount of anthraquinone compounds compared to the leaves. And important substances, flavonoids, and volatile oil.

Senna glycosides interact with immune cells in the colon,

Properties and medical uses:

Senna leaves and fruits are currently considered among the best Laxatives and herbal tinctures registered in European, American, Indian and Chinese pharmacopoeias. Research on senna leaves and fruits has proven that it is a mild laxative if taken in small, moderate doses, and turns into a laxative if taken in large doses. The action of anthraquinone compounds begins in the colon (large intestine) specifically, where anthraquinone glycosides are decomposed by intestinal bacteria into sen-A,B nidin, which in turn are split into the two compounds renin Rhein and anthrone, which stimulate the colon to move, Senna is characterized by its lack of effect on the stomach and small intestine. In practice, the laxative effect of Senna begins when it reaches the colon, and this requires 6 to 12 hours or more. Senna is used internally in the form of a cooked form (ten leaves are enough to soften the stomach), or soaked, or in the form of granules or manufactured tablets, available in pharmacies. Senna leaf infusion can also be used topically in the form of enema for children with constipation, using an infusion of 1 g for each year of age, while for adults the enema ratio is 10-15 g for every 500 ml of water. Senna is popularly used to treat kidneys, jaundice, enlarged spleen, anemia, and typhoid.

Pharmaceutical forms: Pharmaceutical companies have produced many senna preparations, including: puresenid, sennakot.

Precautions for use:

It is not recommended to use dry powdered leaves, and the use of senna compounds infrequently (once a week) and in a small dose does not usually lead to significant side effects, especially in the elderly, but continuing to use it for more than ten days causes colon problems. Senna is not used in cases of inflammation or obstruction of the intestines, in cases of appendicitis, or liver problems. Pregnant and breastfeeding women should not use Senna. If it is accidentally swallowed by infants, it can cause side effects such as severe rashes on the bottom.

Environment:

The plant is widespread in desert and semi-desert areas, and generally grows in dry, sandy environments. Light, sandy soil is the most suitable soil type for its growth. It is not preferable to plant it in heavy soils. It is also recommended to add organic fertilizer or other fertilizers to improve productivity.

Cultivation and productivity:

The plant is propagated by seeds, which are planted at the beginning of spring. It is preferable to soak them in water for 12 hours before planting, which increases germination. The hectare produces about one ton of fruits.

Spartium junceum L.

Cytisus junceus (L.) Vuk., Genista juncea (L.) Scop.

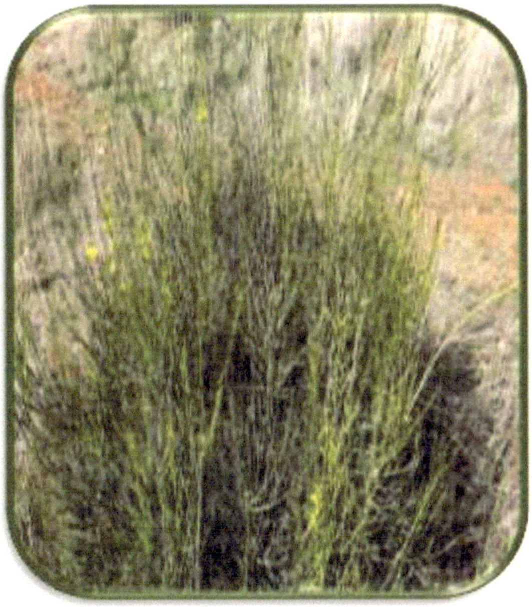

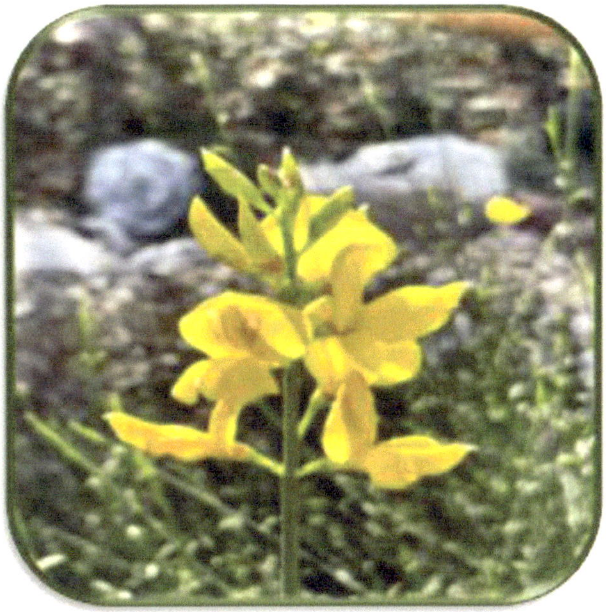

Family: Fabaceae

Common names: Wazzal, Wazzal A

Foreign names: d'Espagne Gene't Fr. broom, Rush Eng.

Occurrences : 51,508 occurrences

Distribution in the world

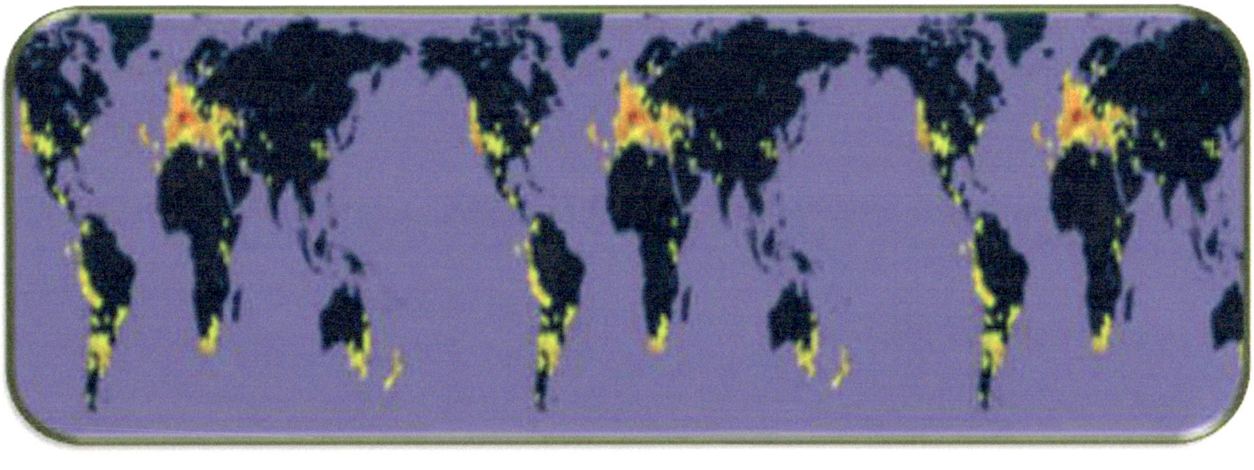

Botanical description:

A shrub, bare, 1-3 m high. The stem is gray, the branches are green, notched. The leaves are simple, auricular, fall early, lanceolate to linear in shape, gradually tapering towards the base, bare or semi-bare, its dimensions are 0.5-1.7×1-4 cm, The petiole is slightly widened at the base, and resembles a sheath. Flowers about 2 cm long, pleasantly scented, short-stalked, gathered in terminal panicles, flowers not compact. The calyx is membranous, sheath-like, bilipped, the upper lip ends in two teeth, and the lower lip in three very small teeth. The corolla is yellow, the flag is inverted oval, broad to semi-rounded, shorter than the scaphoid. Stamens 10, their filaments all fused in a stamen tube. The ovary is superior, flat. Pod 6 - 0.8-0.6×9 cm, 6 or more seeds, linear, glabrous or hairy, dark brown when ripe, The valves are open when opened. Seeds linear, compressed, reddish-brown, shiny.

Flowering: April to June.

Habitat and geographical distribution: Mediterranean, grows wild in Syria, Lebanon, and Jordan, and is also found in northern Asia, southern and central Europe

History and heritage:

The scientific name of the genus is derived from the Greek "spartos" or "spartion", which are two ancient names for species of the genus Genista, in reference to the province of Sparta in Greece, where this plant is found in its natural state. The species description junceum is derived from Juncus, meaning "root."

Part used: Herbaceous plant, and flowers.

Chemical components:

All parts of the plant contain chinolizidin alkaloids, including: cytisin and its derivatives, rhombifolin, in addition to the following compounds:

Ethyl benzene, dimethyl-benzene, Mesitylene, Decane, Phenylethyl Alcohol, Benzothiazole, Propenoic acid, phenyl, methyl ester, Pentadecane, trimethyl-Naphthalene, Dodecanoic acid, ethyl ester, Hexadecane, Pentadecane, tetramethyl, Heptadecane, tetramethyl-Penta-decane, Phenol, Tetradecanoic acid, Phenanthrene, Octadecan, Nonadecane Chemical study of the plant showed the presence of a large amount of cytisin, which is an antagonist of nicotinic acetylcholine receptors.

Properties and medical uses:

The drug has sympathicomimitic, vasoconstrictive, and blood pressure-raising properties. It is used medically in the treatment of circulatory disorders.

The plant is used in folk medicine to treat constipation, stomach ulcers, relieve fluid retention, treat vomiting, and treat liver diseases, gout, and rheumatism. The aromatic water of the plant is toxic to cancer cells (RPMI 7932 melanoma, K562 leukemia, CF7-ICLC cells, SW480), while it did not change the viability of normal keratinocyte cells, indicating the possibility of using the plant as an antitumor and cancer prevention agent.

The plant has a toxic effect on animals when mixed with feed, and causes nervous disorders, and tension spasms, followed by dilated pupils, tremors, irregular heartbeat, rapid breathing, and diarrhea. Muscle paralysis

Side effects, interactions and warnings:

Large doses cause nausea, vomiting, tinnitus, drooling, pain in the mouth, throat and throat, sweating, headache, and severe vomiting, colon spasms, and then paralysis, and death may occur. It is not given to pregnant women, breastfeeding women or children under 12 years of age. It is also not given in case of high blood pressure, and it is not given with drugs that are anti-monoamine oxidase.

Environment:

An environmentally flexible plant that grows in rocky and high mountainous areas, dry and degraded forests, and on the sides of roads. It tolerates different temperature conditions, and does not tolerate frost for long periods, as it tolerates drought. It grows on different types of soil, especially calcareous soils, and is considered a type indicative of deterioration. Cultivation and productivity: The large, mature seeds are planted directly after they ripen in winter in warm, sunny locations. It can also be propagated by cuttings. Flowers, new shoots and seeds are collected in spring and summer. The plant is also grown for ornamental purposes.

Trigonella foenum-graecum L.

Buceras foenum-graecum (L.) All., *Fenugraecum oficinale* Czechov, *Foenum-graecum oficinale* Moench, *Foenum-graecum oficinale* var. *cultum* Alef., *Foenum-graecum sativum* Medik., *Medicago foenugraeca* (L.) E.H.L.Krause, *Telis foenum-graecum* (L.) Kuntze, *Xiphostylis erectus* Gasp.

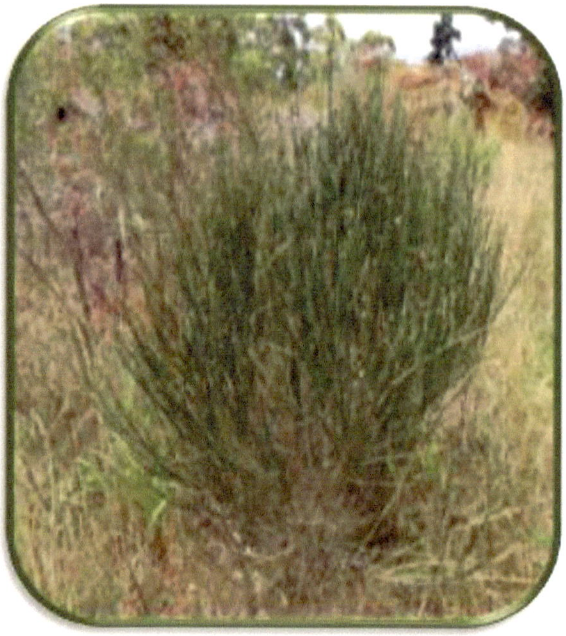
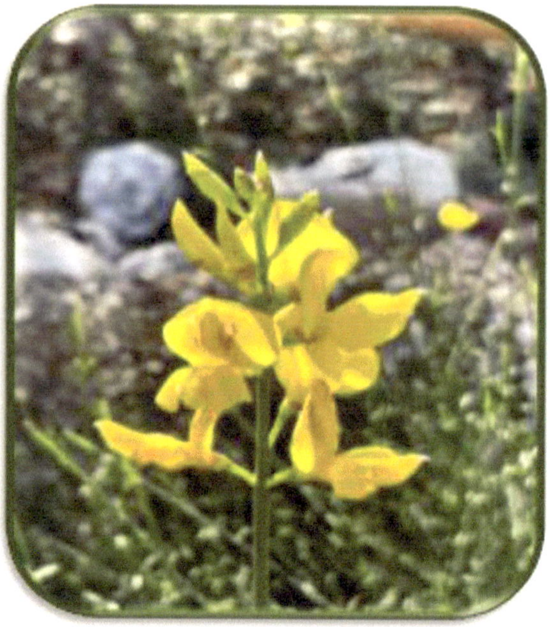

Family: Fabaceae

Common names: Fenugreek

Foreign names: Trigonelle Fr. Fenugreek, Eng.

Occurrences : 51,508 occurrences

Distribution in the world

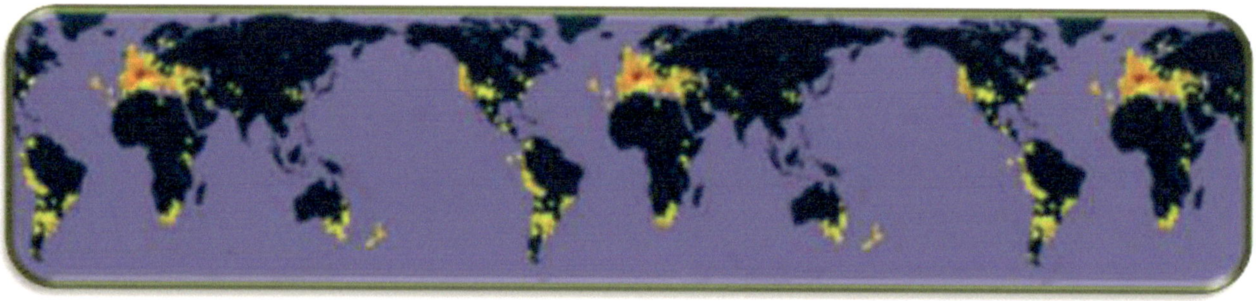

Botanical description:

Annual herb, hairy or glabrous, 15-50 cm tall. Stem simple or slightly branched, erect. Leaves composed of three leaflets, auricular, alternate, obtuse. Ears triangular to lanceolate, acuminate, entire. Leaflets 1.5-0.8×3-1 cm, oblong to inverted ovate, blunt at the apex, serrated at the upper part, glabrous. Inflorescence racemose, racemose or semi-raceous, few-flowered (usually 2 flowers). Flowers 13-18 mm. Calyx tubular, teeth equal and shorter than tube, hairy. Corolla white to creamy, twice as long as calyx. Flag inverted ovate, notched at apex, longer than wings. Horn 6-15 cm x 4-5 mm, flat, linear, straight or arched, hairless or hairy, the scutellum bears a network of longitudinal nerves, gradually tapering to form a beak 2-4 cm long. Seeds numerous, 3-5 mm long, 2-3 mm wide, light brown or reddish-grey to yellowish, many-lobed, rhombic, irregularly rounded, wrinkled and leathery. Hard, with a distinctive aromatic smell. Flowering: March to April. Its wild species include: T. arabica, which is the most widespread species of fenugreek in the dry and semi-dry regions of the Arab region, T. filipes, T. stellata, and T. caerulescens.

Homeland and geographical distribution:

North Africa (Nile Valley), and the countries of the Eastern Mediterranean Basin. Its cultivation has spread to tropical and subtropical countries. The most important countries producing fenugreek are Pakistan, India, China, and Egypt. Syria and the Arab Maghreb countries

History and heritage:

The scientific name of the genus is derived from the Latin trigonus, meaning "triangular-shaped", referring to the shape of the corolla of the species foenum-grae- T. cum in particular, while the species name foenum-grae-cum means "fodder-Greek", as foenum means "fodder" in Latin and graecum means "Greek." Its Arabic name, fenugreek, comes from the name "Halba", which is originally hieroglyphic. Fenugreek has been cultivated and its seeds used since ancient times in food and folk medicine in India and the Nile Valley. The ancient Egyptians used it to facilitate childbirth, and the Egyptian Ebers Papyrus recorded a recipe for treating burns with fenugreek. The Greek physician Hippocrates mentioned it as one of the most important and beneficial plants, and Dioscorides recommended fenugreek as a medicine for women's diseases, including inflammation of the uterus and vagina. The ancient Arabs used it as medicine and food.

Part used: Seeds.

Chemical components:

Fenugreek seeds contain important compounds mucilage -25-45%, mannogalactans, proteins -25-30%, and fatty substances 10-6%, in addition to steroid saponins steroid compounds 1 - 1.5%, the most important of which are: tri-gofoennosides, and aglycones, including diosgenin, tigogenin yamogenin, gitogenin, smilagenin. Saponoid peptide steroid ester: foenugraenin. isovitexin, orientin, saponaretin, vicenin. Favonoids Alkaloids: choline 1.3%, trigonelline 0.4% Volatile oil consisting of monoterpenes and sesquterpenes and ketones. Sugars, including: galactose and mannose. And minerals (phosphorus, iron, sulfur, calcium, magnesium), and vitamins A, C and B1. All parts of the plant contain Chinolizidin alkaloids, including rhombifolin in addition to spartein and ammodanderin and lupinin.

Properties and medical uses:

Fenugreek seeds have properties that lower cholesterol and triglycerides, and contribute to the prevention of factors that help in The emergence of vascular and heart diseases. It also has properties that lower blood sugar and protect against liver diseases, especially cirrhosis. It seems that the antioxidants found in fenugreek can contribute to the prevention of liver, colon, and breast cancers.

Steroidal saponins, especially diosgenin, are the main source in the semi-synthesis of sex hormones, and research has shown the benefits of fenugreek seeds in facilitating the process of childbirth. It also stimulates milk production in breastfeeding mothers. (tigogenin, diosgenin)

Saliva substances help in soothing sore throats and treating asthma. The seeds are popularly used as an appetite stimulant, for people with anemia, to lower blood sugar, as a stomach and digestive tonic, to treat stomach and duodenal ulcers, chest diseases and coughs, to expel intestinal worms, to treat hemorrhoids, dysuria, menstruation and diarrhea. Fenugreek is used topically for its laxative and antiseptic effect in treating burns, skin diseases, cracked skin, eczema, boils, foot ulcers and anal abscesses.

Drug interactions and precautions:

Due to the effect of fenugreek in lowering blood sugar, its use with blood sugar-lowering medications leads to severe hypoglycemia. It is recommended to avoid using fenugreek at the beginning of pregnancy, as it helps in abortion in the first three months of pregnancy.

Food uses:

Fenugreek is widely used all over the world as both food and medicine. Fenugreek seeds are characterized by their high nutritional value, and it is recommended to be consumed by people who do strenuous work, as it helps to endure fatigue and stress, and it seems that it preserves the muscles of the elderly and strengthens their immune system and helps them resist diseases. Fenugreek seeds are used in the countries of North Africa and the Middle East in preparing appetizing spicy mixtures. Many popular dishes of these countries. Consuming fenugreek seeds gives urine a distinctive smell. The green tops and leaves of the plant are eaten due to their high nutritional value (Alzheimer's disease). Other uses: Fenugreek is an inexpensive raw material in the preparation of sex hormones (contraceptive pills) and cortical steroids. The fruits are used to dye tissues a beautiful crimson red color.

Environment:

Fenugreek grows under different climatic conditions. It tolerates drought, high temperatures and cold, but it grows well in temperate regions. Although Fenugreek is a winter crop with a short photoperiod. The long photoperiod and the intensity of sunlight accelerate vegetative growth, early flowering, and rapid fruit ripening. Fenugreek grows in all types of soil except for rich and alkaline soils. It is successfully cultivated in soils containing a high amount of calcium carbonate and absorbable phosphorus and light soils.

Cultivation and productivity:

The plant is propagated by seeds and planted in early fall. Fertilization with essential elements improves the amount of production.

The pods are collected at Drying of the basal part of the plant, yellowing of most of the leaves, and when the pods become almost dry and light brown in color and their seeds are fully ripe and hard in texture. The plants are packed on the surface of the soil in the early morning so that the pods do not open and the seeds are scattered. The hectare gives 1.2-2 tons of seeds.

Quercus infectoria G.Olivier

Quercus infectoria subsp. euinfectoria A.Camus, Quercus lusitanica subsp. Infectoria (G.Olivier) Mouill., Quercus lusitanica var. infectoria (G.Olivier) A.DC.

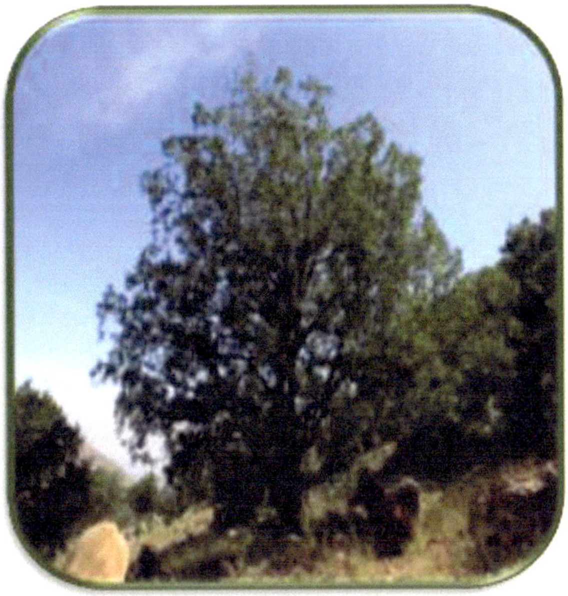

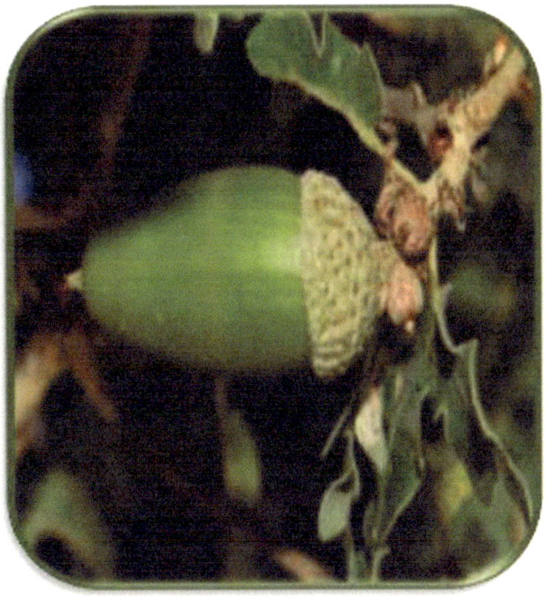

Family: Fagaceae

Common names: Mulul, Oak, Oak, Gall oak

Foreign names: chêne Fr. oak, Gall Eng.

Occurrences : 2,169 occurrences

Distribution in the world

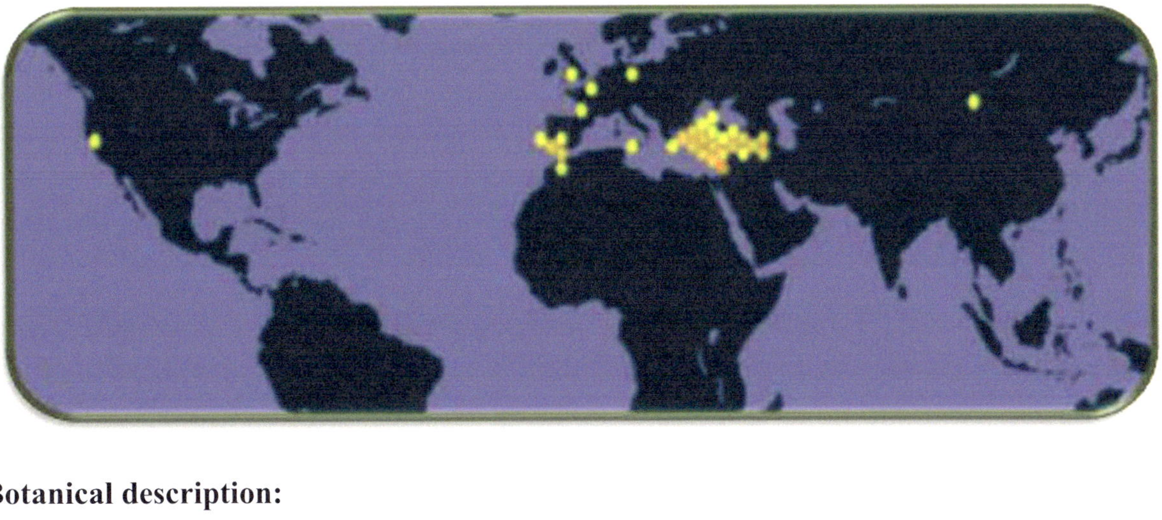

Botanical description:

A deciduous tree, 4-15 m high, the bark is grey, scaly, not corky; the crown is ovate. The branches are ascending and horizontal. The buds are ovate, their scales are ovate, with hairy or bare edges. Leaves simple, alternate, 4-2×7-4 cm, ovate-oblong to oblong-lanceolate, blunt at the apex, base rounded or gradually tapering, wavy to sinuous at the margin, glossy on the upper surface, hairy on the lower surface when young, later glabrous or almost glabrous, bearing 7-9 lateral nerves. The obstructed 0.5-2 cm, glabrous or almost glabrous, ears hairy, falling off quickly. Flowers unisexual. Male flowers are gathered in loose racemes, 4-6 cm long, with a hairy axis, simple bract, composed of 4-6 hairy segments, stamens 4-12. Female flowers are less numerous. Female 3 carpels. Ovary inferior, three-chambered. Stamens 3, in which only one ovule develops as a result of abortion of other ovules. The fruit is a nut (or acorn), 2-1×5-3 cm, single or in pairs, short-stalked or sessile, cylindrical in shape, surrounded at its base by a semi-spherical calyx. The scales of the calyx are compact, not protruding, triangular to oval in shape, the length of the acorn exceeds the length of the calyx by 3-5 times.

Flowering: From March to April, fruits in October.

Habitat and geographical distribution:

Eastern Mediterranean and western Iran Turanian. It is widely distributed in the forests of the eastern Mediterranean in Syria, Lebanon, Palestine, Jordan, Iraq, Iran, Turkey, Cyprus, and other countries in western Asia, as well as in southern Europe and northern Africa. It is cultivated in Europe, the Maghreb countries, and Egypt.

History and Heritage:

The scientific name of the genus Quercus is the Latin name used by the ancient Romans in Western Europe, and some trace the name back to the ancient Celtic origin Kaër quez, meaning "beautiful tree." The descriptive name for the species, infectoria, means that the tree is infected with an insect (a type of tumor-making wasp) Oliv-gallae tinctoriae Cynips. It lays its eggs on the branches and leaves, causing the formation of tumors (gallon) rich in tannin. The name oak is of Persian origin, and the name oak is of Aramaic origin. Ancient legends mention that the oak tree is rarely struck by lightning and has been attributed to the god Zeus, the god of thunder in Greek mythology, and to the god Donar, the god of lightning among the ancient Germans. It is also considered the tree of Jupiter in Roman mythology, and was a symbol of courage and strength among the Celts. It was mentioned by Ibn Manzur in the dictionary "Lisan al-Arab", Ibn al-Baytar, al-Antaki, and Ibn Sina. Oak was used in ancient times to treat diarrhea, digestive system infections, involuntary urination, skin rashes, and hemorrhoids. The wood of the tree was used for heating, building houses, and making food stores, and the fruits were collected and used as food, such as nuts such as walnuts, pistachios, almonds, and dried figs. Part used: Leaves, and galls (globular tumor).

Chemical components:

Leaves contain cyclitol, including quercitol, expensive tannins (gallo), including ellagitannin. Gallic acid contains expensive tannins at a rate of up to 70%, in addition to expensive acids (galic acid), sugars, starch, gum, resin, and traces of volatile oil. The main components of the tubers (gallics) include: tannins, phenolic acids, flavonoids, and triterpenes.

Properties and medical uses:

Oak has astringent, sedative and analgesic properties, and lowers blood sugar. It is used in the supportive treatment of skin inflammations. It is popularly used to treat intestinal bleeding, coughing up blood, and bronchitis. The decoction of the leaves is used topically as a gargle to treat gingivitis, ulcerative stomatitis, and tonsillitis. The leaf and tannin preparations are also used as ointments to treat skin infections, eczema, impetigo, syphilis, heavy menstruation, and hemorrhoids. It has a long history of use in traditional Chinese medicine to treat diarrhea, bleeding, skin diseases, and many other human diseases. Its medical applications are becoming increasingly popular in Greece, Asia Minor, Syria and Iran. Studies have shown its potential against a wide range of enzymes, such as cholinesterase, monoamine oxidase, tumors, hypertension, microbes, insecticide, parasiticide and antioxidant. The extracts can be used as an effective and natural disinfectant to clean eggshells of pathogenic microorganisms. Its effectiveness against microbes such as Staphylococcus aureus, Escherichia coli, Candida albicans, Salmonella typhimurium, Pseudomonas aeruginosa, and others has been proven.

Other uses:

It is used in industry to obtain tannins used in tanning leather and ink manufacturing.

Side effects and warnings:

It is not recommended to use it internally for long periods, as it may cause liver damage. Prolonged and concentrated topical use may cause the appearance of some skin tumors.

Environment:

A type that is friendly to light, relatively tolerant of cold and dryness. Grows well in calcareous soils, preferring red soils, although it can live in poor rocky soils.

Cultivation and productivity:

Oaks are propagated by acorns after they are stacked at 5°C for 45 days. The acorns are planted by placing them on their sides in plastic bags in the nursery, and watered moderately. Germination occurs about 15 days after planting.

Centaurium erythraea Rafn.

Centaurium centaurium (L.) W.Wight ex Piper, Centaurium minus Moench, Chironia centaurium (L.) F.W.Schmidt, Erythraea centaurium (L.) Pers., Erythraea vulgaris Gray, Gentiana centaurium L., Gonipia linearis Raf.

Occurrences : 180,670 occurrences

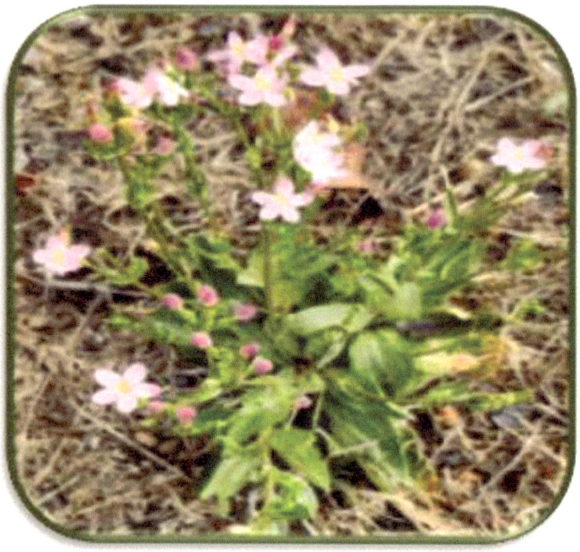

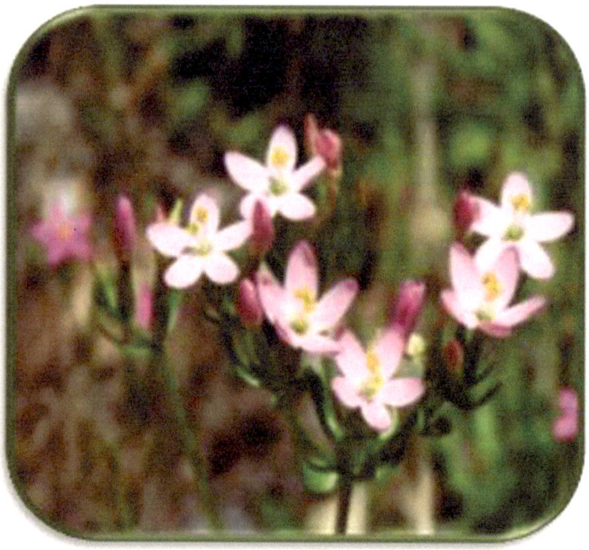

Family: Gentianaceae

Common names: Centaury, small Centaury, snake gall, snake's horn.

Foreign names: Centaurée Petite Fr. Centaury, Eng.

Distribution in the world

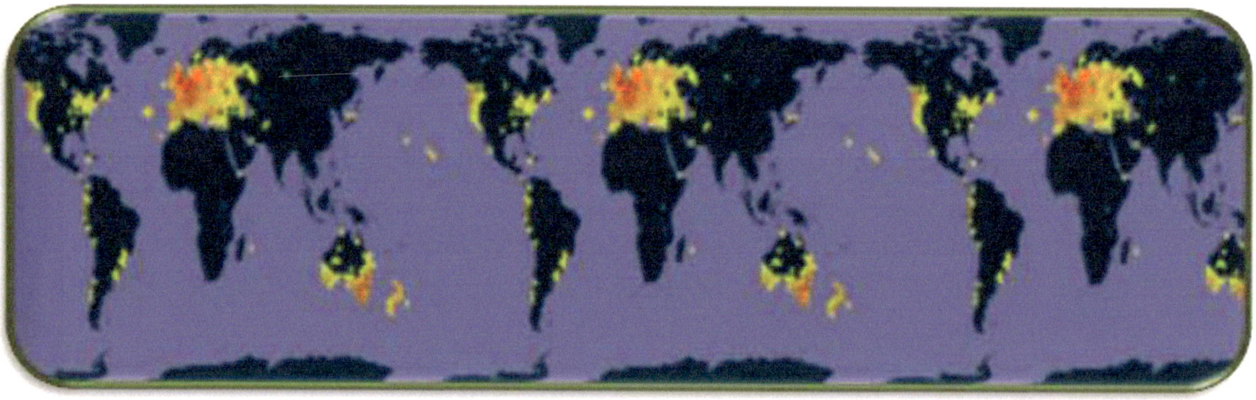

Botanical description:

An annual or biennial herb (sometimes perennial), 20-40 cm tall. Stems erect, quadrilateral, ending in a comb-shaped inflorescence composed of a group of dichotomous, closely-spaced inflorescences. Leaves simple, opposite, petiolate, entire, auricular, elliptic, rounded to sub-acute, basal leaves emerge above the soil surface in the form of a rosette, stem leaves are spaced. Flowers pentagonal, with short peduncle. Calyx 5-7 mm, its length is approximately equal to the length of the corolla tube. Corolla funnel-shaped, pink, 17-20 mm long, tube cylindrical, membranous after flowering. Stamens are located on the upper part of the corolla tube, the anthers are prominent, and spirally twisted after opening. The ovary is superior, bicarpal, the style is threadlike, perennial, the pistils 2.

Flowering: May to August.

Habitat and geographical distribution: Mediterranean, Iranian-Turanian.

History and heritage:

It was mentioned by Ibn al-Baytar, al-Antaki, Ibn Sina, and al-Ghassani. Ibn Sina wrote that the centaury is called in Arabic the small loofa. Centaury is a plant praised since ancient times by ancient doctors until today. It is the herb of a thousand medicines, and it is the herb of fever. It is also beneficial for the stomach, as it eliminates bloating and expels intestinal worms.

Part used: The herbaceous plant (the aerial part of the plant.)

Chemical components:

Secoiridide compounds, including: sweroside, swertiamarin, gentiopikrin. Alkaloids such as gentianine, gentianidine. xantones, such as bellidifoline. terpenoids, flavonoids, phenolic acids, fatty acids.

Properties and medical uses:

An important medicinal plant in many countries (Morocco and Algeria). It is used in medicine. Popular for treating various diseases, anti-inflammatory, anticoagulant, pneumonia, blood purifier, blood pressure lowering, and other diseases such as diabetes, fever, rhinitis, stomach diseases, urinary tract infections, indigestion, loss of appetite, hemorrhoids, diuretic, and for many heart and blood vessel disorders, such as high blood pressure.

The drug is used to increase saliva and digestive secretions, as a fever reducer, and to treat indigestion and digestive disorders

The plant is popularly used as a bitter tonic, and in the treatment of kidney stones. The decoction of the plant is used topically for wound healing.

The essential oils and extracts of the plant have shown many biological properties, antibacterial, anti-oxidant, anti-fungal, anti-leishmanial, anti-cancer, anti-diabetic, anti-inflammatory, insecticide, diuretic, hepatoprotective, skin-protective, neuroprotective, and larval growth inhibitory. For the digestive system The plant extracts stimulate endothelium-dependent vasodilation and inhibit angiotensin II-induced fibroblast proliferation, which may explain the hypotensive effects. The plant is recommended for the treatment of gastrointestinal disorders and to reduce hypercholesterolemia. The plant has the ability to inhibit the enzyme acetylcholinesterase (AChE) and -3-hydroxy-3-methylglutaryl Co-enzyme (HMGR(A). Reduces free radicals: 2,-2-diphenyl-1-picrylhydrazyl (DPPH)

Other uses:

It is included in the composition of cosmetic skin tightening products, hair coloring and dyeing.

Side effects and warnings for use:

The plant should be avoided by pregnant and breastfeeding women, and patients with gastric and intestinal ulcers, and its prolonged use should be avoided.

Environment:

The plant grows wild on the sides of roads, water channels, and neglected places, on hard and stony soils, Tolerant of alkaline soil, and does not prefer shady places.

Cultivation Productivity:

Centaureas are propagated by seeds, which are scattered in early spring. In warm areas, they can be planted in the fall, where the plant blooms early.

Pelargonium odoratissimum (L.) L'Hér.

Cortusina odoratissima (L.) Eckl. & Zeyh., Geraniospermum odoratissimum (L.) Kuntze, Geranium odoratissimum L.

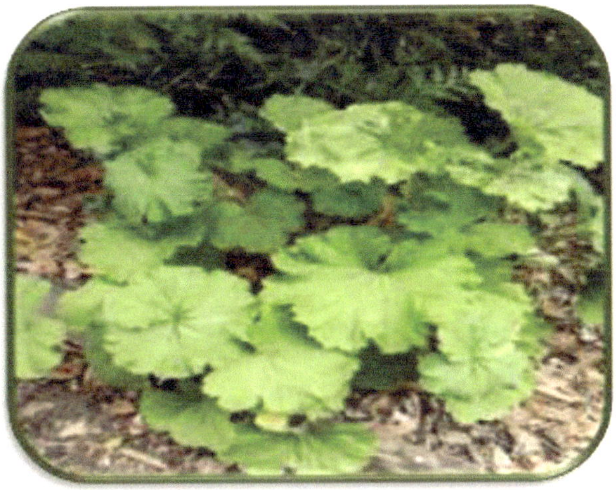

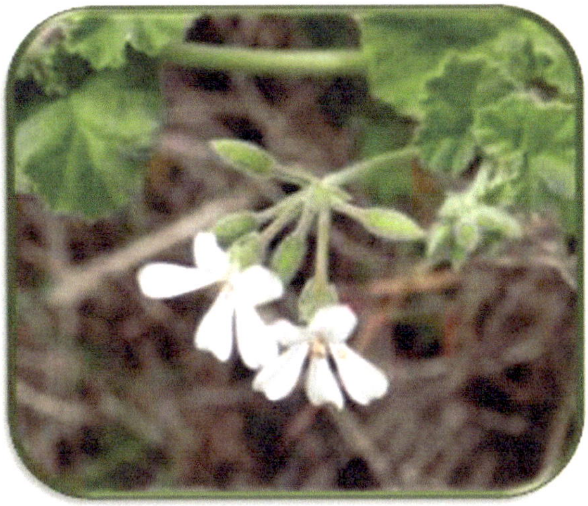

Family: Geraniaceae

Common names: fragrant, atrah, geranuq Perfume, aromatic, stork

Foreign names: Eng. Apple Geranium, Fr. Pélargonium odorante

Occurrences : 248 occurrences

Distribution in the world

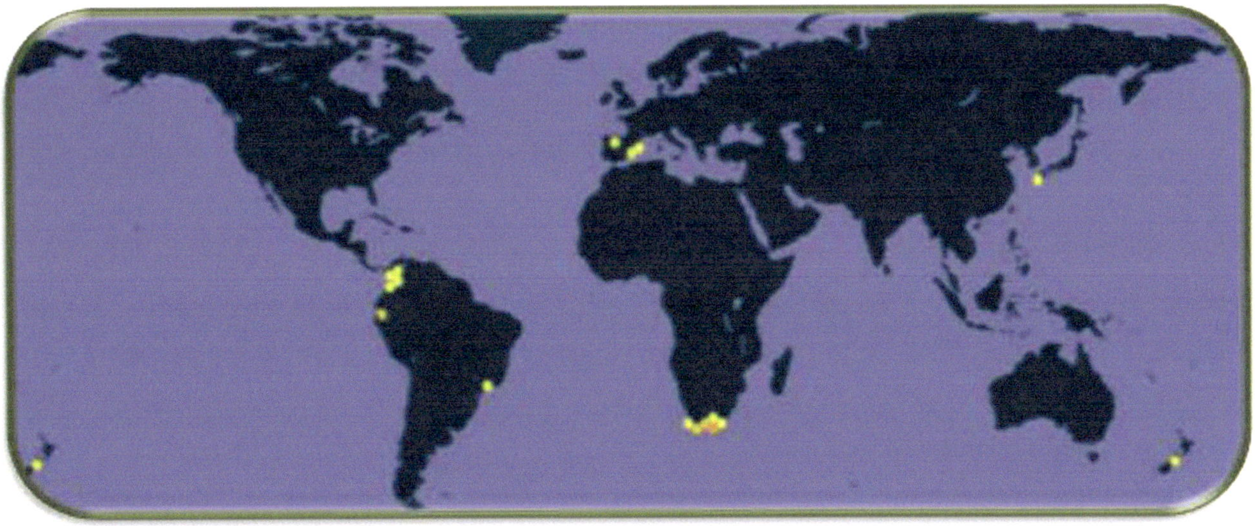

Botanical description:

Evergreen shrub, much branched, 20-80 cm long. Leaves alternate, thick, light green, palmately lobed, with a distinctive aromatic scent, auricles. Flowers hermaphrodite, tending to be symmetrical, gathered in semitic inflorescences. Calyx 5 sepals, free, hairy, perennial. Corolla 5-petaled, free, pink. Male 10 stamens arranged in two whorls. Female 5 carpels, their ends extend to form a central column, which separates from it when ripe, forming a long beak for the fruit. Ovary superior, ending in five free linear stigmas. Fruit lobate, composed of 5 fruit sections, single-seeded, separate from the bottom towards the top.

Flowering: April to June.

Homeland and geographical distribution:

South Africa, and its cultivation has spread to many countries of the world (ornamental houseplant.)

History and heritage:

The scientific name of the genus is from the Greek word pelargos meaning "stork", alluding to the shape of the fruit, which is similar to a stork. Species name odoratissimum means "fragrant." The plant is grown in home gardens for decoration and for its aromatic scent.

Part used: Flowering plant.

Chemical components:

The plant, especially its leaves, contains 2-3% volatile oil, the most important components of which are geraniol 60-70%, citronellol and linalool. Some flavonoid compounds, gallic acid and its derivatives have been identified.

Medical properties and uses:

The plant is used in the treatment of viral infections. The fragrant plant is available in the form of Potpourri, aromatic oil, tea flavoring, and a mixture of its dried leaves with some spices. The methanolic extract of the plant inhibited the growth of methicillin-resistant Staphylococcus aureus (MRSA) bacteria, as it caused partial inhibition of biofilm formation. The results showed that the plant extract has antioxidant, antibacterial and anti-inflammatory activity by improving the stability of the lysosomal cell membrane. The plant leaf extract is suitable for the manufacture of zinc oxide NPs (ZnO) as a general reducer. Zinc oxide can be used as a safe alternative to synthetic materials, and as an antioxidant, antibacterial and anti-inflammatory agent in the medical and pharmaceutical industries.

Other uses:

Insecticide (can be used as a natural insecticide in gardens), the volatile oil is used in the manufacture of perfumes and cosmetics (to prepare compresses and creams.) Its fresh leaves are added in the Damascene kitchen (Syria) when preparing (rice with milk) with starch to give it a fragrant flavor.

Side effects and warnings for use:

Researchers do not have information about whether this plant is safe and effective for use in humans. A doctor should be consulted if any possible side effects appear, such as allergic reactions, dermatitis from touching the plant. Pregnant or breastfeeding women should avoid using the plant. Environment: The plant thrives in semi-arid, semi-humid and humid bioclimatic floors with moderate, warm and even fresh climates if protected from frost. It grows in various types of soils including sandy and clayey soils with high calcium carbonate content, but it does not tolerate flooding or salinity.

Cultivation and productivity:

The plant is propagated by terminal cuttings without hormonal treatment during the spring and until mid-summer. The soft parts of the plant are collected after 50% of the flowers open, and the crop can be collected three times a year. One hectare produces more than 70 kg of oil.

Hypericum perforatum L.

Hypericum oficinale Gaterau, *Hypericum oficinarum* Crantz , *Hypericum perforatum* var. *Vulgare* Spenn., *Hypericum perforatum* subsp. *vulgare* (Spenn.) A.Fröhl., *Hypericum vulgare* Lam.

Occurrences : 694,092 occurrences

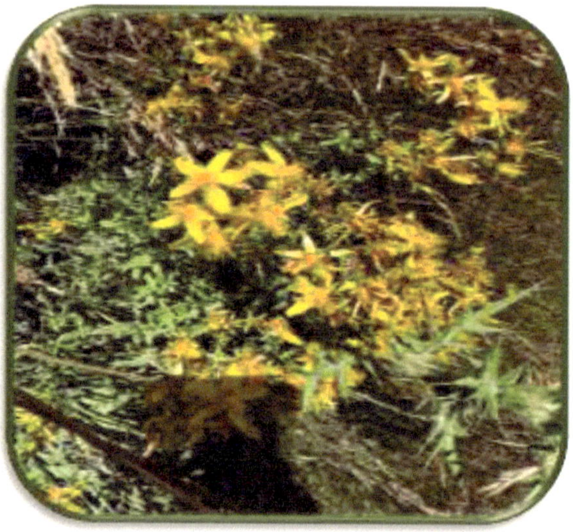

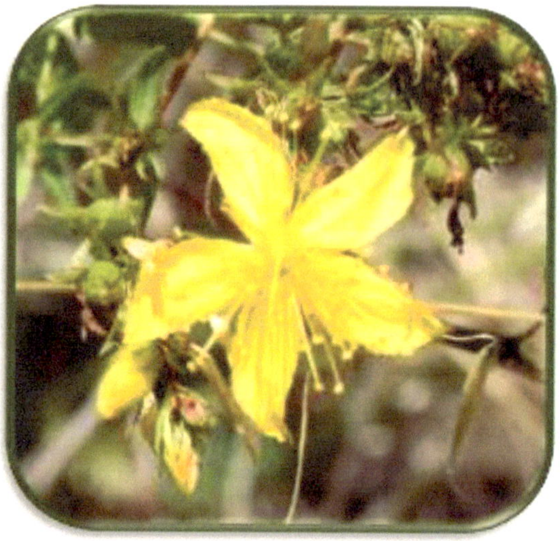

Family: Hypericaceae (Guttiferae)

Common names: Perforated-leafed arn, St. John's wort, Sidi Yahya, Dadi Rumi, `Usbat-sab,The heart, Mansia, Perforated St. John's wort, Common St. John's wort.

Foreign names: Eng. Saint – Johns wort, Fr. Millepertuis

Distribution in the world

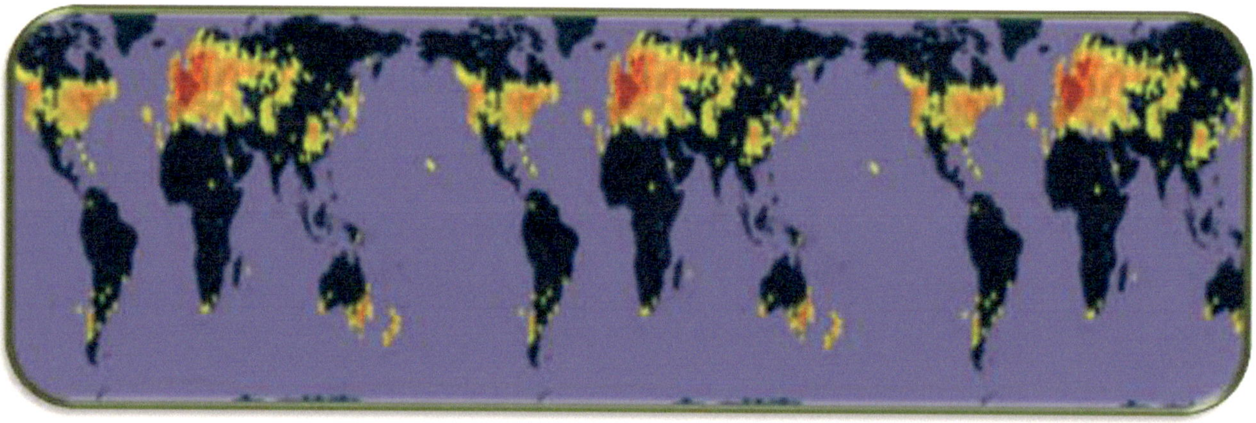

Botanical description:

A perennial herb, bare, 50-100 cm tall, the stem is erect or ascending, bearing leafy lateral branches, and has two prominent longitudinal ribs. The leaves are opposite, petiolate, elliptic, bearing dots representing transparent glands, so the leaf appears as if it is perforated, and on its edge are black dots (glands), spaced apart, the edge is curled downward to varying degrees. The flowers are gathered in primary, semi-pinnate inflorescences, which in turn are gathered in wide, terminal, comb-like paniculate inflorescences. The calyx is twice shorter than the corolla. The sepals are complete, sharp-pointed, neither glandular nor dotted. 5-petals, yellow, bearing black hairs, especially on the margin. The male has many stamens that are united in 3 groups. The female has three carpels, topped with long red stigmas. The fruit is an inverted oval to conical capsule, characterized by the presence of parallel vesicular bundles, three-chambered. The seeds are numerous, their surface bears minute pits.

Flowering: From May to July.

Habitat and geographical distribution: Europe and western Asia.

History and Heritage:

The genus name Hypericum is derived from the Greek hypo meaning "close" or "similar", and ereike, meaning "heather", i.e. a plant similar to heather. The species name perforatum is derived from the perforated leaf. It is said that the plant took its English name John's St. St. John's Wort (St. John's Wort) was used by the Knights of St. John of Jerusalem to treat wounds on the battlefield. The ancient Egyptians used it to treat many diseases, and called it "the balm of wounds." The Greeks and Romans also used it. It was popularly believed that the plant was useful for repelling evil spirits, so it was common to hang a bouquet of the plant on the doors of homes. It was used as a diuretic, to treat menstrual disorders, and as a treatment for intestinal worms and snake bites. To relieve pain, treat anxiety, depression, water retention, and gastritis. Plant extracts are used to treat ulcers, wounds, and minor burns, especially those involving nerve damage.

Part used: Aerial parts, especially flowering tops.

Chemical components:

The flowers and leaves of the plant contain a volatile oil rich in hydrocarbons called (red hyphae). It also contains dianthrone naphtone compounds, the most important of which are hypericin, pseudohypericin, and phloroglucinol derivatives such as the compound Hyperforin (naphtodianthrones hyperforin Red pigment. Flavonoids 2-4%, including: quercitrin. rutin, amentoflavone, (hyperin), hyperoside. Catechin tannins 15-7%. Organic acid derivatives, such as caffeic acid, and chlorogenic acid a. The flowering tops contain a fixed oil, the most important fatty acids of which are palmitic acid 30%, and linoleic acid a. 15-7%. The oil is prepared by soaking a quantity of flowers in olive oil in a closed, opaque bottle, under sunlight for several weeks until the oil turns blood-colored. The plant contains flavonoid compounds: favonol (kaempferol, quercetin), favon (luteulin), glycosides (isoquercitrin, rutin), pivafon (piabigenin), mentovafon, myricetin, hyperan, proanthocyanidin, oligomeric proanthocyanidin.

Additional compounds: include tannins, xanthones, phenolic compounds (caffeic acid, chlorogenic acid, and p-coumaric acid), hyperfolin. acids (nicotinic, myristic, and palmitic), carotenoids, choline, pectin, hydrocarbons, and long-chain alcohols. Several amino acids that have been isolated from the herb include cysteine, glutamine, leucine, lysine, and aminobutyric acid.

Properties and medical uses:

The drug has neuroleptic, antidepressant, anti-inflammatory, antibacterial, antitumor, antioxidant, steroid hormone secretion stimulant, blood sugar lowering, and wound healing properties. The plant is used to treat depression, psychological disorders, anxiety (tension), fear and lack of concentration.

It is also used topically to treat dermatitis, suppurating wounds and burns, to treat HIV viruses and in phototherapy for psoriasis (raised and scaly spots) and warts. The drug is popularly used to treat insomnia, depression (mild to moderate), bronchitis, asthma, jaundice, gastritis and ulcers, kidney disease, gout, rheumatism, nocturnal enuresis, burns and wounds, bleeding, insect bites, scabies, and hypothyroidism. The main antibacterial component is hyperforin, which inhibits the growth of all types of gram-positive bacteria, but does not inhibit the growth of gram-negative bacteria. Experiments have shown that methicillin-resistant Staphylococcus aureus (MRSA) and penicillin-resistant Staphylococcus aureus (PRSA) are highly sensitive to hyperforin, which has been resistant to several types of penicillin, ofloxacin, clindamycin, erythromycin, cephalosporins and gentamicin. Studies have also indicated that the flavonoid and catechin-containing parts are effective against influenza virus. The plant has anti-cancer properties: Hyperforin inhibits the growth of cancer cells in the laboratory. The mechanism involves induction of programmed cell death through activation of caspases, which are cysteine protease enzymes. Hyperforin also causes the release of cytochrome C from isolated mitochondria. Inhibits the growth of tumor cells, including glioma, neuroblastoma, benign tumor, epithelioma, carcinoma, sarcoma, leukemia, and melanoma. Recent research shows that plant extracts reduce oxidative stress, thus preventing neurotoxicity, inflammation, and digestive system problems. Flavonoid-rich extracts are effective against hydrogen peroxide-induced apoptosis in PC12 cells, a cell line derived from rat adrenal melanoma. The extracts can prevent DNA fragmentation and cell shrinkage due to hydrogen peroxide activity. Flavonoid-rich extracts effectively treat oxidative stress-related neurodegenerative disorders such as Parkinson's disease and Alzheimer's disease. The plant has promising results as an antidepressant. Anti-inflammatory. Rats given doses of plant extracts showed:

There was a decrease in the levels of blood and intestinal enzymes associated with colitis, and the incidence of gastric ulcers was lower. Lipophilic extracts were found to have greater anti-inflammatory activity than ethyl or hydroalcoholic extracts. Quercetin and the dimeric apigenin I3,II8-biapigenin showed anti-inflammatory and protective activity for the digestive system.

Pharmaceutical forms:

St. John's wort is available in the form of oral suppositories, creams, and liquid tinctures, and its products are sold under the names: Hypericalm, Hypericum, Kira, Mood support, St. John's wort

Side effects, interactions and precautions for use:

Use of the drug may cause allergic reactions, constipation, dizziness, dry mouth, anxiety, sensitivity to sunlight, stomach upset, and sleep problems. The drug should be avoided with alcohol or other medications that slow down the nervous system such as cold medications, allergy medications, flu medications, decongestants, narcotic or hypnotic pain medications, amphetamine compounds, antidepressants called selective serotonin reuptake inhibitors and tricyclic antidepressants. The drug should be avoided in case of an allergic reaction, and should be avoided in pregnant and breastfeeding women. When using the plant, you should avoid foods and drinks that contain tyramine, such as wine, beer, aged cheese, chicken liver, chocolate, bananas, and meat tenderizers, and avoid exposure to the sun. You should check the source before purchasing this plant, because its quality varies between producers. High doses may lead to phototoxicity in susceptible individuals.

Environment:

The plant grows on the edges of forests, forest steppes, river banks, roadsides, and shady slopes in areas with cold winters. It prefers moist, well-drained, acidic soils.

Cultivation and productivity:

The plant is propagated by seeds and division. Seeds are planted at a rate of 3-4 kg / hectare in basins, and germinate within 1-3 months at a temperature of 10 °C. The resulting seedlings are planted in the permanent soil at a distance of 40 cm between them, and irrigated in the summer. The plant is harvested at a height of 15-25 cm from the ground surface. Productivity is estimated at 3-5 tons/ha of dry matter, and seed productivity is estimated at 400-950 kg/ha.

Crocus sativus L.

Crocus sativus var. *oficinalis* L. *Crocus oficinalis* (L.) Honck., *Safran oficinarum* Medik., *Crocus setifolius* Stokes., *Geanthus autumnalis* Raf.

Occurrences : 1,427 occurrences

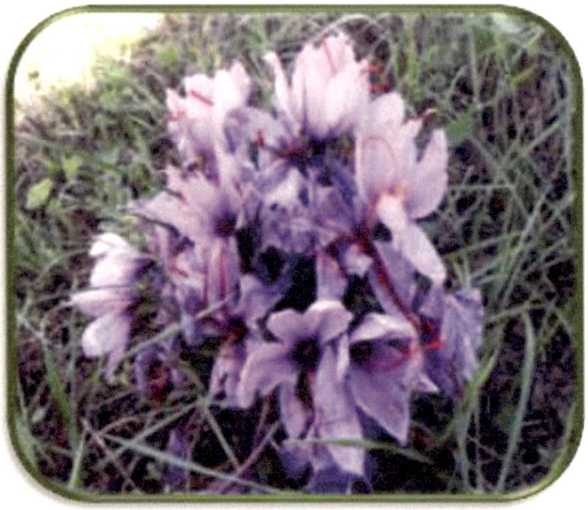

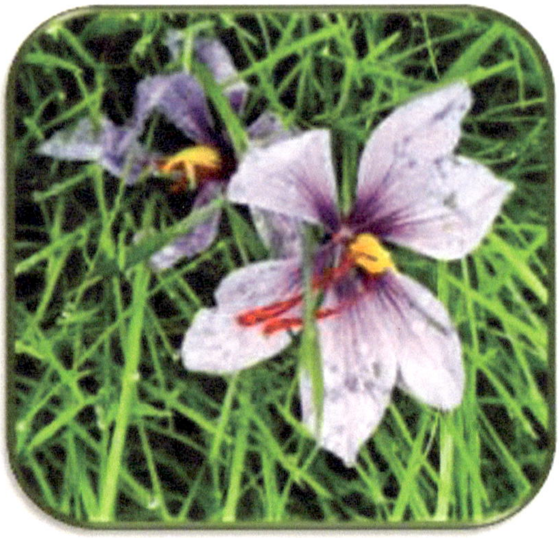

Family: Iridaceae

Common names: Saffron, saffron hair, saffron head, Jadi.

Foreign names: cultivé Safran Fr. Saffron, Eng.

Distribution in the world

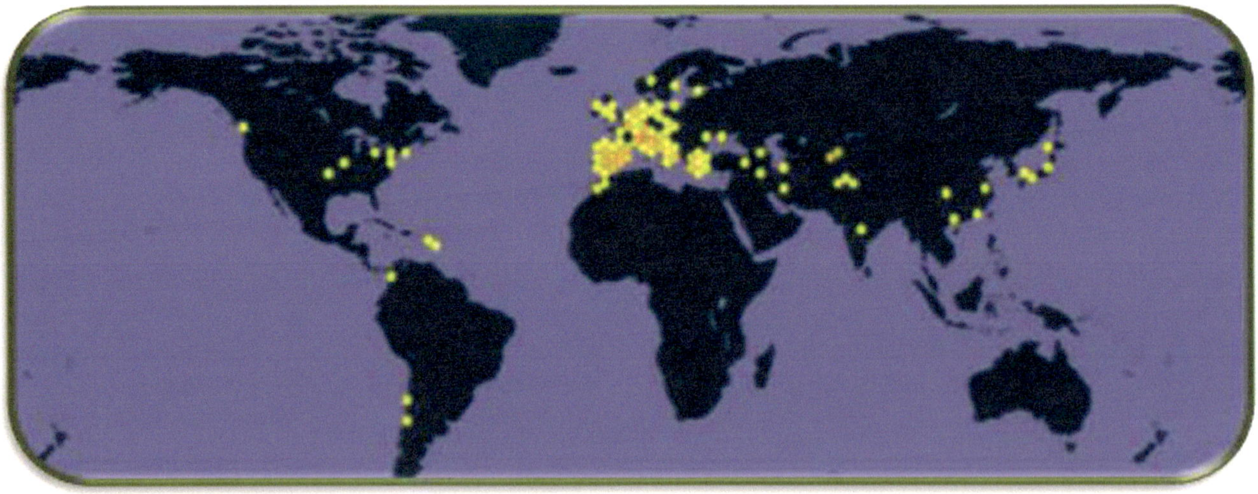

Botanical description:

A small, perennial herb with a fleshy corm, 1-4 cm in diameter, covered with silky, brown scaly leaves, their surface consists of a network of fine fibers, extending above the corm neck for a distance of 2-5 cm. Leaves basal, erect, long, narrow, parallel-veined, 5-10 mm wide, appear at the end of flowering or with it. Flowers single or double. The bract is hexagonal, lilac-veined with violet, its segments are fused at their bases, lobes 10-12×25-40 mm. Male 3 stamens, filaments white-yellowish, short. Anthers -12-17 mm, yellow. The ovary is tri-chambered, the style is long and pink, divided into three long, lobed, reddish-orange branches. This type of saffron is genetically sterile, while other wild types have a pomegranate fruit, spindle-shaped, about 2 cm long.

Flowering: October to November.

Types of saffron:

yellowish green, reticulated, and Damascene, which is called in Damascus and its countryside "Harsanin and Hasranin" and "Hallouz" in Jabal al-Sheikh in Syria, where its ground clusters (corms) are eaten and are the size of a hazelnut or chickpea. Homeland and geographical distribution: Its original homeland is southwest Asia, and its cultivation has spread to Iran, Greece, France, Italy, and Spain, and it has recently entered Syria.

History and Heritage:

The scientific name of the genus is derived from the Greek krokos, which is the name of saffron, and the descriptive name of the species, sativus, means "cultivated." The plant is famous for its purple flowers, its large, fragrant stigmas, and its orange color, which is the part used, called saffron. It has been used to color foods and drinks, and is believed to have been known for more than 4,000 years. Saffron was planted in the tenth century AD in Iran. It was and still is planted in the Kashmir region. With the Mongol attack on Iran, saffron found its way to China. In the tenth century AD, the Arabs brought it to Andalusia.

Part used: Stigma, and the tip of the style. It has an aromatic scent and is orange-red or red in color.

Chemical components:

The pistils contain carotenoid glycosides, especially the compound α-crocin, which results from an esterification reaction between crocetin and gentiobiose sugar (β-D-gentiobiose). Crocin is a water-soluble carotenoid pigment, and is responsible for giving saffron its orange-yellow color. Crocin constitutes 2% of the pistils' weight. It also contains a bitter glucoside, picrocrocin, which constitutes 4% of the pistils' weight, and results from the union of Picrocrocin is responsible for the distinctive flavour of saffron. Heat and enzymatic activity affect picrocrocin, causing it to split into glucose and the free safranal molecule. In addition to 1.3-0.4% volatile oil, its most important components are safranal aldehyde and saffron, which are compounds sensitive to changes in pH, and decompose quickly in light and oxidizing agents, which requires keeping them away from light and oxygen. Picrocrocin, safranal aldehyde, and saffron are compounds responsible for the smell of saffron. Carotenoid compounds: lycopene, beta-carotene (which are cancer prevention and treatment factors.) In addition to fatty oils and starch.

Properties and medical uses:

Saffron has digestive properties, stimulates the secretion of digestive juices, expels intestinal worms, is used to treat depression and psychological disorders, improve physical energy, improve hearing and memory, and is a cardiac stimulant and a stimulant for the central nervous system. Studies have shown the possibility of using saffron as a preventive and therapeutic agent for cancer. It has been shown that saffron not only prevents the formation of cancerous tumors, but also contributes to the shrinkage and contraction of existing tumors.

Partly due to its content of carotenoid compounds, which include lycopene and beta-carotene. Lycopene is believed to help reduce damage caused by harmful free radical molecules that lead to diseases of aging. Research has shown the benefits of saffron in reducing vision loss in the aging stage, and the possibility of its help in improving vision in some people who suffer from eye diseases that cause blindness. A clinical trial of treating patients with age-related macular degeneration using saffron supplements showed early indications of the possibility of healing and restoring damaged eye cells. The active components of the plant have many beneficial pharmacological effects, such as anticonvulsants, antidepressants, anti-inflammatory, and antitumor, and are beneficial in learning and improving memory. Clinical trials have shown that saffron is more effective than a placebo in Alzheimer's disease, comparable to the effectiveness of the drug Donepezil. Trials have confirmed the anti-itching effect of saffron. The plant is used in cases of desire to lose weight, as it can reduce the frequency of snacking. It can reduce the symptoms of suffering from premenstrual syndrome. The plant has effects on erectile dysfunction, allergies, the heart, blood vessels, and the immune system. The results indicated that saffron significantly reduced blood glucose, waist circumference, diastolic blood pressure, total cholesterol, and low-density lipoprotein cholesterol concentrations, and alleviated symptoms of depression, cognitive function, and sexual dysfunction. Crocin was shown to be able to regulate glutamate levels, reduce oxidative stress, and modulate Aβ and tau protein accumulation. Saffron powder decoction is popularly used for chest tightness, colds, asthma, cough, bronchitis, soothing intestinal colic, and indigestion. It is also known for its stimulating effect on the circulatory system, spleen, liver, and heart, and for lowering blood pressure. Moderate use is useful in relieving menstrual pain and uterine bleeding. Saffron oil or tincture is used topically in the case of arthritis, and to relieve gum pain in children when teeth begin to appear. Its powder is used in the composition of some types of alcohol that help remove cataracts from the eye. Food and industrial uses: It is mentioned that one gram of saffron stigmas is enough to color one hundred liters of water yellow, and stigma powder is used to give food and beverages an amber yellow color, and a distinctive aromatic flavor and taste. Its hot drink is used in cold countries. Saffron is used in industry to color carpets, furniture, clothing, etc., and in the perfume industry.

Warnings for use:

It is not given to pregnant women, because it causes abortion in doses of 10 g, while larger doses (12-20 g) may cause death. The manifestations and symptoms of saffron poisoning are dizziness, vomiting, uterine bleeding, intestinal cramps, diarrhea, bloody urine, bleeding of the lips, nose and eyelids, numbness and paralysis, and yellowing of the skin. Environment: Saffron prefers areas with cold winters and warm summers, with rain in the fall, winter and spring. It grows well in most soils, especially light, well-drained and aerated soils with a pH of 6 - 7. Cultivation and productivity: Saffron is propagated vegetatively. New corms are planted during the months of September and October in temperate regions and the Mediterranean basin, and in March and April in cold regions to produce flowers. Early planting is done during the month of August to produce large, well-specified corms, with a diameter of no less than 3.5 cm. And at a distance of 25 cm between one corm and another. And it is irrigated immediately after planting, it needs organic fertilization when preparing the soil for planting, and small amounts of potassium in particular. Saffron cultivation is expensive financially.

Economic value of saffron:

Saffron is one of the most valuable spices in the world, and is usually bought by the gram, and therefore it is called red gold. The global production of saffron is about 300 tons annually, and it requires obtaining 100 grams of dry pistils -15,000 20,000 flowers, i.e. 150-200 flowers to obtain one gram of dry pistils. The most important countries producing saffron currently are Kashmir, Iran, Spain, and Morocco.

Iris germanica L.

Iris spectabilis Salisb., *Iris alba* Savi., *Iris australis* Tod., *Iris cypriana* Baker & Foster., *Iris amoena* DC., *Iris atroviolacea* Lange, *Iris glauca* Salisb. , *Iris humei* G.Don.

Occurrences : 16,766 occurrences

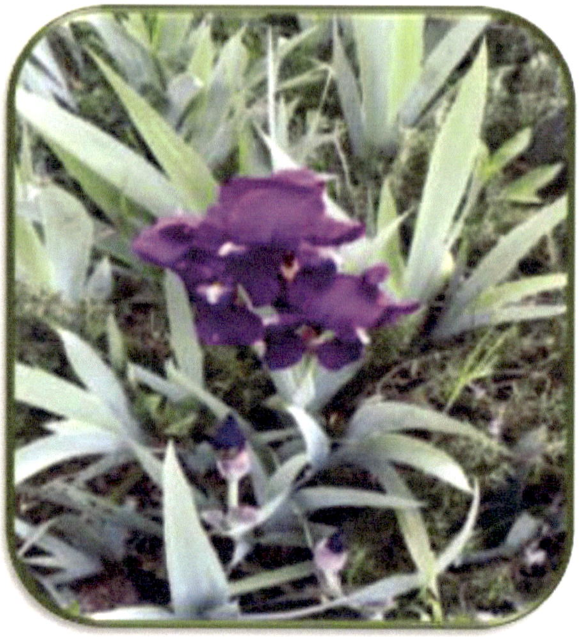

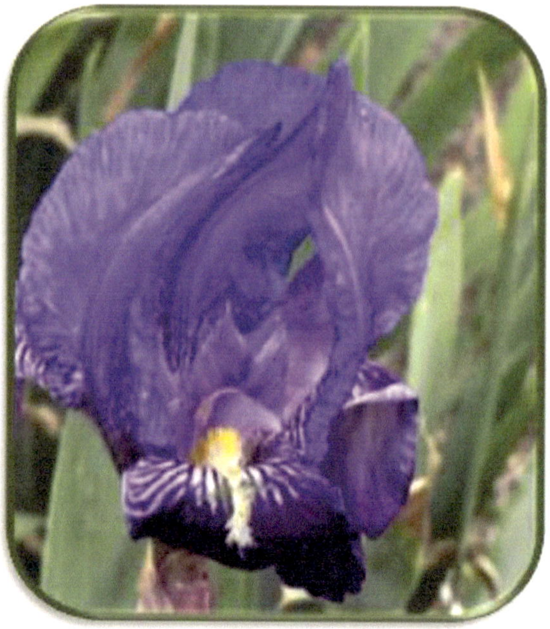

Family: Iridaceae

Common names: German Iris, Iris odorata.

Foreign names: Iris Allmagnd Fr. Iris, German Eng.

Distribution in the world

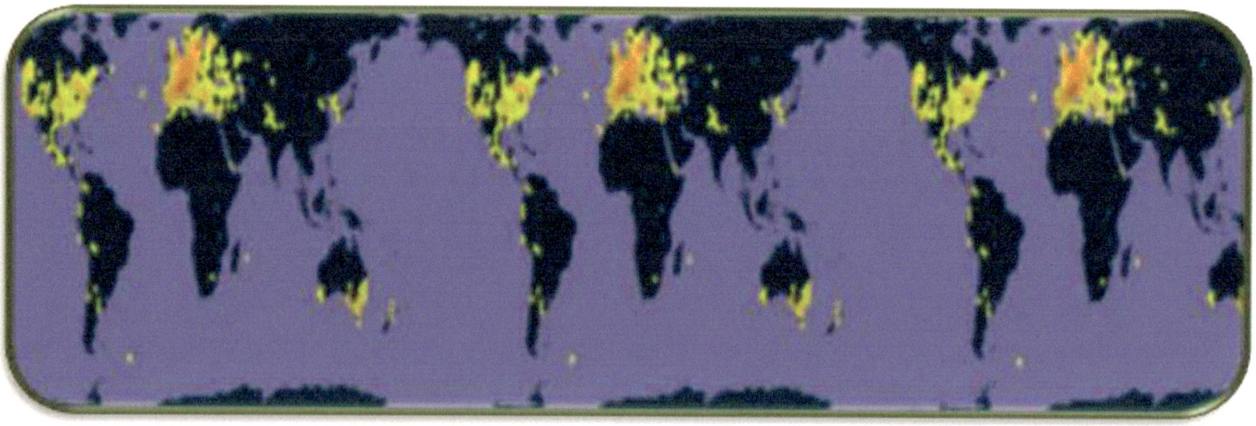

Botanical description:

A perennial herb with a thick rhizome, flower stalk length 30-100 cm. Leaves are basal, bluish-green, sword-shaped, 30-40 cm long, and 2-4 cm wide.Flower stalk is simple, or branches into several branches, bearing 4-5 flowers. Flowers are large and fragrant, their color varies from one type to another (often blue, yellow, purple, white).., each surrounded by two membranous bracts. The bract has 6 sepals, arranged in two whorls, the outer sepals are flat or curved downwards, often bearing a multi-colored line of cilia (often yellow), the inner sepals are erect, lacking cilia. Male 3 free stamens. Female: 3 fused carpels, ovary tri-chambered, inferior, topped by a style ending in three stamens, their appearance resembling petals.

Fruit: ovoid capsule.

Flowering: March to May.

Habitat and geographical distribution:

Southern Europe, Mediterranean countries, and northern Africa, its species are grown in most parts of the world.

History and heritage:

The scientific name of the genus comes from Greek mythology, where it is said that "Iris" is the winged messenger chosen by the gods, whose seven-colored handkerchief was likened to a rainbow, alluding to the variety and strength of flower colors in the species of this genus. The descriptive name of the species germanica means "German." Iris has been considered a symbol of power and magic since ancient times. It was dedicated to Juno, the king of heaven, by the Romans. The ancient Egyptians placed it on the scepters of their kings, and the three leaves of its flowers were considered to represent faith, wisdom, and courage. The Arabs used its roots for medicinal purposes.

Part used: Rhizome.

Chemical components:

Volatile oil, yellow in color, its percentage ranges between 0.3-0.1%, the main compound is irone (with an aromatic smell, resembling the smell of violets.) Fixed oil (9%) known as iris oil, its most important components are myristic acid Flavonoids, including iridale, irilon, irisolone and their glycosides. Xanthones, such as iris xanthone, magniferin. Starch 20-50%.

Biologically active compounds: flavonoids, triterpenes, sterols, phenols, ceramides, and benzoquinone.

Medical properties and uses:

Iris rhizome has expectorant properties and is used in the treatment of bronchitis, asthma, and whooping cough.

Flavones have an inhibitory effect on the enzyme phosphodiesterase c-AMP. Studies have shown that oral use of irisolidone stimulates the formation of T-cells and cytokine Th1 cells. Irisolidone is an immunosuppressive compound. The plant has many biological and therapeutic effects, including neuroprotective, hypoglycemic, and hypolipidemic effects, antimicrobial, antioxidative, anti-inflammatory, anti-intestinal spasm, and antifungal effects, in addition to its immunomodulatory and cytotoxic effects.

The rhizome is popularly used to treat ulcers and spasms. It has an anti-serotonin effect, detoxifies the body, increases urination and bile production, and has a mild laxative effect. This combination of effects makes it useful for treating chronic skin diseases such as acne and eczema.

Other uses:

Aromatic dried rhizome powder (Ironate) is used in the manufacture of cosmetics, perfumes, toothpastes, and scented and antiseptic soaps.

Precautions for use:

There are no known risks if the required therapeutic dose is adhered to. High internal doses cause vomiting, abdominal pain, bloody diarrhea, and severe inflammation of the mucous membranes. It is not used during pregnancy.

Environment:

Iris grows in varying environmental conditions, as it tolerates high and low temperatures during its growth and flowering. It is suitable for most soils, especially light, yellow, fertile, well-drained and ventilated soils. It tolerates slightly high acidity, and prefers neutral or alkaline soils.

Cultivation and productivity:

Iris is propagated vegetatively by dividing the rhizomes taken from the second-year plants two to three days before the planting date so that their length is 5 cm, and their roots are well developed. The rhizomes are placed on lines with a distance between them of 65-70 cm, and the distance between one plant and another is 25-30 cm, at a depth of 10-12 cm. A hectare needs about 50 thousand rhizomes.

Juglans regia L.

Juglans duclouxiana Dode, Juglans fallax Dode, Juglans fertilis short. ex Dippel, juglans frutescens short. ex Dippel, juglans fruticosa short. ex Dippel, Juglans kamaonia Dode, Juglans orientis Dode, Juglans quercifolia N.Pierce, Juglans regia subsp. fallax Popov, Juglans regia subsp. sinensis (C.DC.) Ohle, Juglans regia var. kamaonia C. DC.

Occurrences : 221,109 occurrences

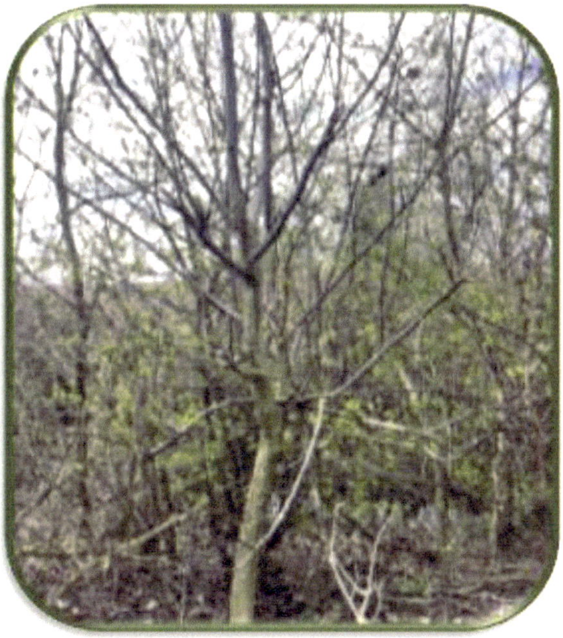

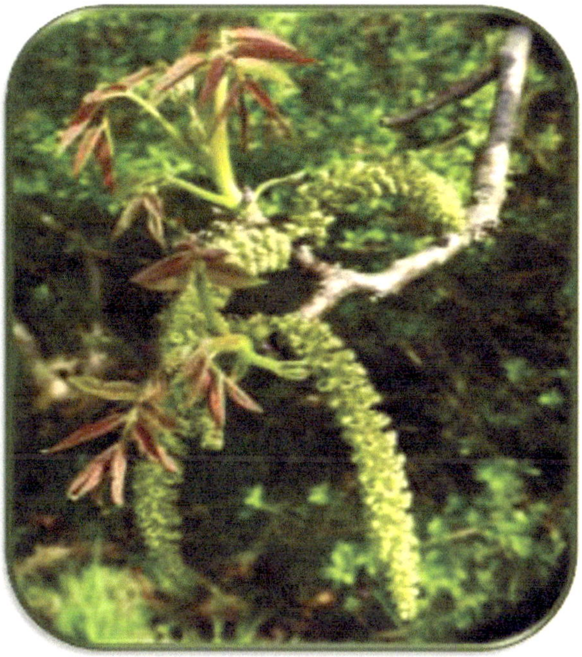

Family: Juglandaceae

Common names: Walnut, Persian Walnut, English Walnut, Royal Walnut, Common Walnut.

Foreign names: Noyer Fr. Walnut, Eng.

Distribution in the world

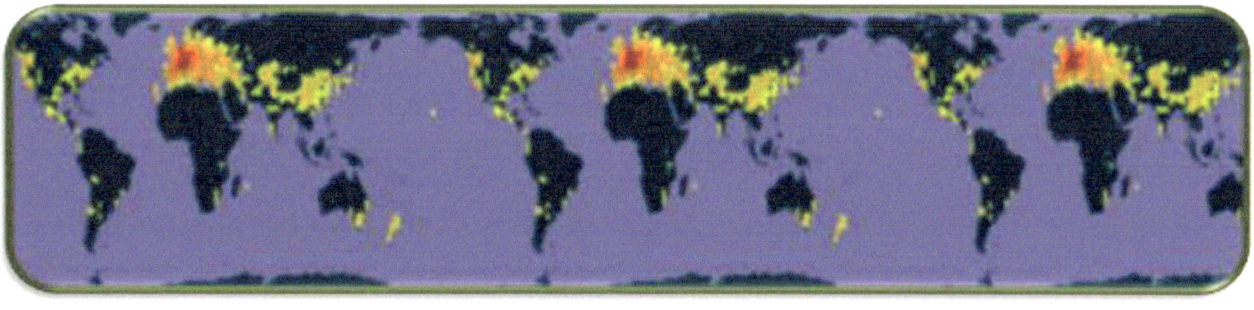

Botanical description:

A tree 10-25 m tall, its bark is smooth in the early stages of life, then cracks with age, gray stringy, initially reddish then becomes green, its length is about 25 cm light. Leaves are compound, pinnate or more, and consist of 5 to 9 leaflets, entire, elliptic in shape, somewhat leathery in texture. Male flowers are gathered in green, elongated, terminal or lateral, about 10 cm long, their bases bear a number of bud scales, and appear on the branches of the previous year. Female inflorescences are shorter, consist of 1-3 flowers, and appear on the young of the current year. The fruit is nuclear, its outer pericarp is transparent, the middle is fleshy and green in color, then turns brown, and the inner is woody and hard, it opens through two valves. The seed is divided into four lobes, the cotyledons are large, fleshy, and wrinkled.

Flowering: From April to May.

Homeland and geographical distribution:

Iran, South Caucasus and the Middle East, and is now cultivated in many areas, especially in southeastern Europe, Asia Minor, Syria, northern India, China, and northern Africa.

History and heritage:

The scientific name of the genus Juglans is derived from the Latin "Glans" Jovis, meaning "Jupiter's fruit", while the descriptive name of the species regia means "royal", in reference to the distinctive shape of the tree, and it is also called Persian walnut in reference to its origin. The name walnut is derived from Persian, and some associate it with the nature of the tree's bearing, as the walnut fruit is usually borne in pairs or three on the tree.

Part used: Leaves, fleshy fruiting cover, seeds, stem bark.

Chemical components:

The leaves and fruit pericarp contain 10% tannins, including galloylglucose and ellagitannins. Naphtoquinone derivatives decompose to give hydrojuglone, which soon turns into juglone when the leaves or fruits are exposed to bruises or drying, and polymerizes easily into yellow or brown components (causing skin staining), and therefore juglone is almost never found in the drug. Flavonoids 3.4%, the most important of which are: quercitrin and hyperoside, a volatile oil rich in monoterpene compounds, and phenolic acids. The leaves also contain significant amounts of vitamin C (0.85-1%). The seeds contain 40-60% fatty substances (walnut oil), and many amino acids.

Properties and medical uses:

Walnut leaves and bark have astringent (astringent) and antifungal (juglone and essential oil) properties. Research has shown that both the stem bark and leaves have shown high effectiveness against tuberculosis germs. A study conducted on mice showed that the alcoholic extract of walnut leaves significantly reduces blood sugar levels and returns them to values close to the normal level. It also raises blood insulin levels and reduces glycosylated hemoglobin values. Research indicates that consuming the fruit improves the functions of the lining of blood vessels in patients suffering from high cholesterol and restores the vessels to their natural elasticity. In the event of hardening, it reduces the risk of heart and blood vessel diseases, and coronary heart diseases.

Cultivation and productivity:

Walnuts are propagated using mature and healthy walnuts, where seedlings are produced and later grafted. The seeds are germinated for 30-35 days at a temperature of -2-3°C with sprinkler irrigation. The seedlings grow within a year, and are grafted in spring and summer to obtain seedlings of known variety and specifications, then they are transferred to permanent land and planted at distances of 10-12 m between trees. Walnut trees need special care in the first five years of growth. Before the tree starts bearing fruit, it is pruned to give it the appropriate structure. When fruiting begins, pruning is limited to removing tangles and replacing some main branches if necessary. Continuous fertilization and weeding are carried out in walnut orchards, along with uprooting the growing cankers near the root collar area. It is necessary to irrigate trees in summer during dry periods, taking care not to let the irrigation water touch the tree trunk, as this leads to crown rot. The number, quantity and timing of irrigations vary according to the climate, soil and age of the trees. Drip irrigation of walnuts using a suitable irrigation network is one of the best economical methods. Walnut trees begin to bear fruit at the age of 5-8 years after planting in the orchards. The productivity of a single tree varies according to environmental conditions, services and age. The fruits are harvested only when fully ripe. The productivity of a medium-aged tree from seeds can range from 10-25 kg per year.

Ajuga chamaepitys (L.) Schreber

Teucrium chamaepitys L., Chamaepitys trifida Dumort., Bugula chamaepitys (L.) Scop., Chamaepitys vulgaris Link, Bulga chamaepitys (L.) Kuntze., Ajuga chamaepitys subsp. Chamaepitys.

Occurrences : 47,400 occurrences

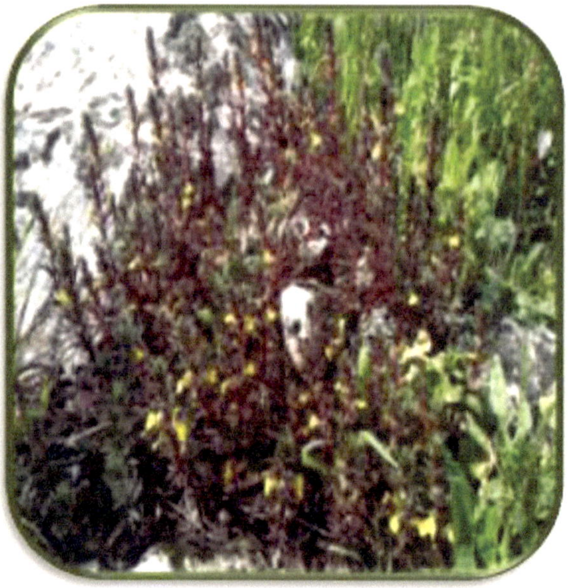

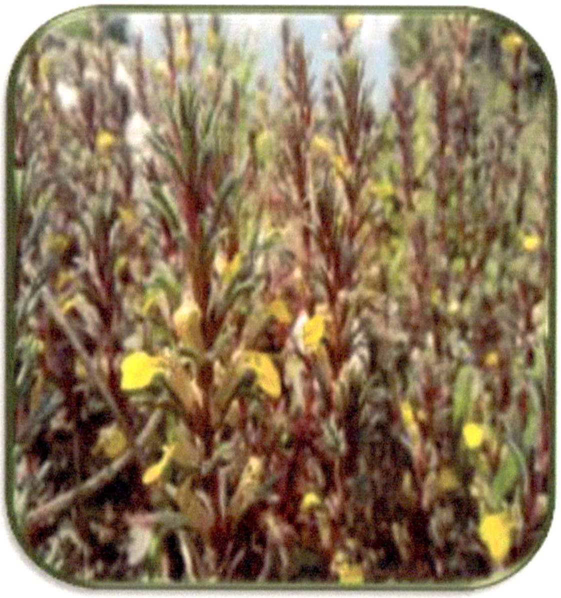

Family: Lamiaceae

Common names: Shanqoura, Musk al-Kabour, Ground Oak.

Foreign names: Jaune Bugle Fr. bugle, Yellow Eng.

Distribution in the world

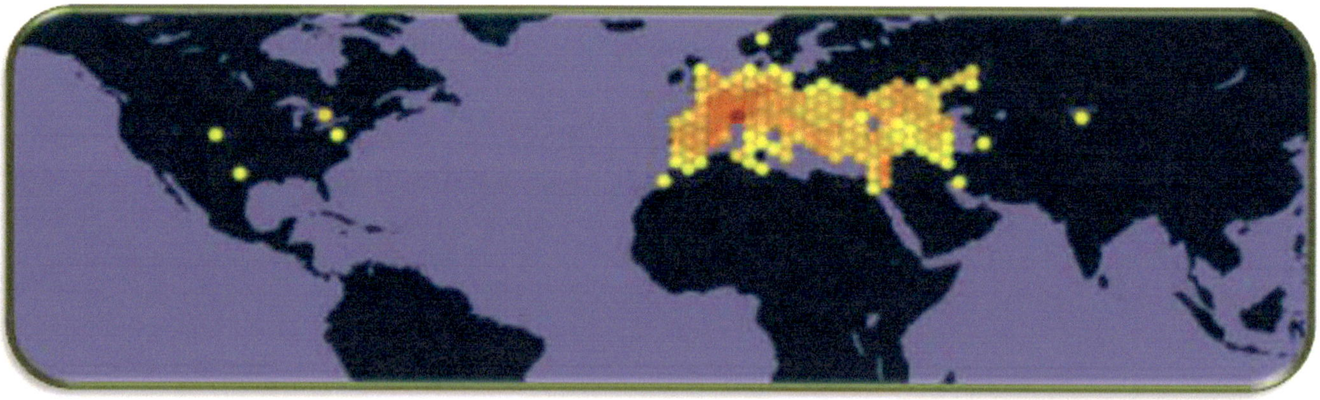

Botanical description:

A perennial herb, its base is semi-woody, branched from below, covered with long, white, flat and dense hairs, its length is 10-25 cm. The stems are lying, then ascending or erect. The leaves taper at their base to form spoons. The stem leaves are generally spoon-shaped, their apex is divided into three complete lobes. The floral leaves are usually shorter than the flowers. Flowers are arranged in sparsely flowered whorls (usually two flowers per whorl), axillary, forming a semi-clustered inflorescence. Flowers are hermaphrodite, bisymmetrical, sessile. Calyx about 5 mm, tubular, white-haired, terminating in five sharp-pointed lanceolate teeth shorter than the length of the tube. Corolla 12-15 mm, hairy white, streaked yellow and spotted with violet, its five petals united in a tube longer than the calyx, then split into two lips of unequal size, so that it appears unilipped. Upper lip very small, straight and notched at the apex. Lower lip composed of three flat lobes, the middle lobe larger, notched at the apex, appears to be composed of two lobes. Stamens 4, bipotent, prominent. Female bicarpal, ovary superior, divided into four chambers. Fruit tetracarpal, 1.5×3 mm, brown, transversely rough.

Flowering: January–May.

History and Heritage:

Researcher Edward Ghaleb called it in his encyclopedia the Ja'dah. According to Ibn al-Attar, the Ja'dah is the Camaphytus, and according to Dioscorides, it is the Teucrium polium, which some called Ajuchamaepitys ga. This agrees with what was mentioned by al-Antaki, who mentions that the Ja'dah in Greek is Polium and in Berber it is Artalas. As for Ibn al-Baytar, he describes the Ja'dah as a small, white, thin plant, about a span long, and it is a seed. According to Ibn Sina, "Ja'dah is a type of wormwood, with a slight heat and sharpness. The small one is sharper and more bitter, has stems and white or yellowish downy flowers, filled with seeds, and its head is like a ball, with a heavy scent like white hair with the slightest fragrance. The largest one is weaker and is also bitter, and has a pungency, and the mountain one is the smallest." The student of the term "ja'dah" in the works of Al-Antaki, Ibn al-Baytar and Ibn Sina finds that it applies to what is known as the herb Teucrium polium, i.e. wind grass or jinn musk, while the "shanqura" is a type of Ajuga, including creeping and hairy ones.

Homeland and geographical distribution:

Eastern Mediterranean and western Iranian Turanian.

Part used: Flowering plant

Chemical components:

Volatile oil, its most important compounds: muurolene 40%, limonene, 20%, B.germacrene 8%, and bitter diterpene compounds, tannins, mineral salts, glycosides, saponins and caf- derivatives. Feic acid. Chemical analysis of the essential oil by GC-FID and GC-MS showed the following compounds: ethyl linoleate, corin, beta-pinene, and phytol. The plant contains mainly polyphenols and iridoids, ajugoside, asperulosidic acid, and diacetylspiruloside a. .deacetyl-asperulosidic , 5-O-β-d-glucopyranosyl-harpagide, harpagide, 8-O-acetylharpagide, reptoside , and 5-O-β-d-glucopyranosyl-8-O-acetylharpagide

Properties and medical uses:

The plant has a sharp, pungent taste. It was previously known to be used in the treatment of nervous tremors, rheumatism, wounds, jaundice and dropsy. The decoction of the leaves is popularly used as a diuretic and emmenagogue, and to treat diseases of the urinary system, gout and rheumatism.

The aerial parts are used in folk medicine to treat diarrhea, for their diuretic and anti-inflammatory properties, and for wound pain. The plant has anti-inflammatory and anti-ulcerative effects on the intestines and colitis. The effect of plant extracts to inhibit cells in the inflammatory response, through the modulating effects of oxidative stress, was studied in both colon cancer in mice and skin cancer cells, where the plant showed antitumor activity, and represents an important source of biologically active compounds, and is an additional form of treatment alongside traditional anticancer drugs, where tests revealed that the essential oil and ethanolic extracts are toxic For cancer cells.

Environment:

The plant is spread in semi-arid and humid environments on sunny hills and slopes with calcareous soils and prefers acidic soils. The plant can be considered one of the species suitable for decorating gardens.

Cultivation and productivity:

The plant is propagated by seeds that are scattered in the spring.

Ajuga iva (L.) Schreb

Ajuga humilis Porta*, A. pseudoiva* Robill & Castagne *ex DC.*, *Bulga iva*)L.(Kuntze, *Cha- maepitys iva*)L.(Fourr., *Teucrium iva* L.

Occurrences : 12,558 occurrences

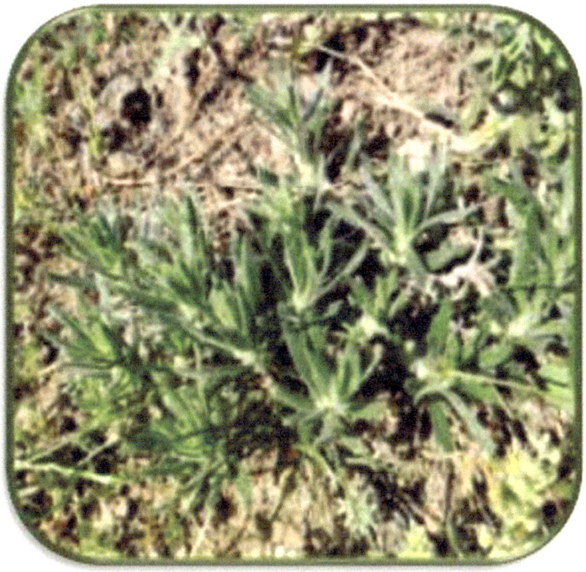

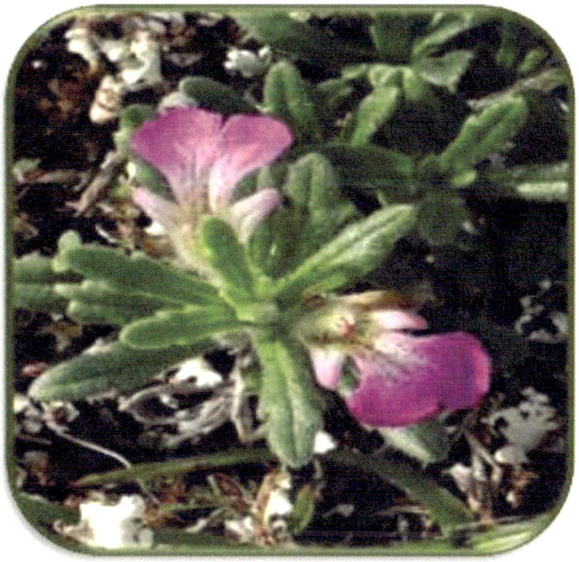

Family: Lamiaceae

Common names: Chandkoura, Aromatic Ajouqa

Foreign names: Jaune Bugle Fr. bugle, Yellow Eng.

Distribution in the world

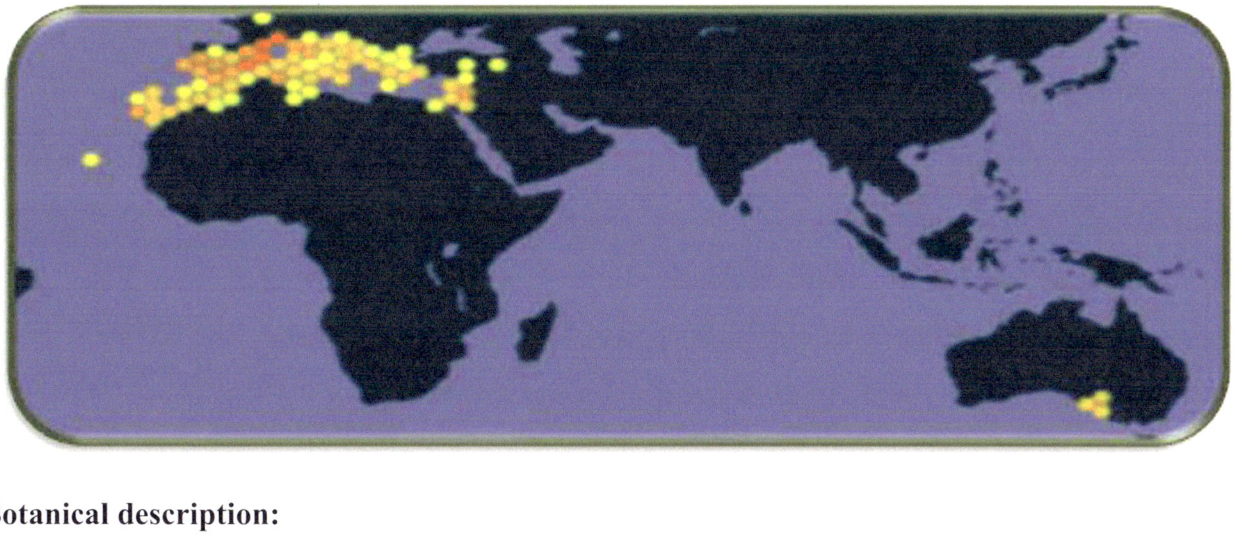

Botanical description:

Perennial herb, semi-woody base, branched from below, hairy, gray in color, 20-30 cm long. Stems are supine or ascending, densely leafed. Leaves are linear to oblong in shape, their edge is curled downward, entire or bear 1-3 teeth on each side. Floral leaves are usually longer than flowers. Flowers are gathered in few-flowered whorls (2-4 flowers in each whorl), axillary, forming a semi-clustered inflorescence. Flowers are hermaphrodite, bisymmetrical, sessile. Calyx about 5 mm, tubular, white-haired, ending in five ovate to lanceolate teeth, equal in length to the length of the tube or shorter. Corolla about 15 mm long, purple, pink or yellow, its five petals fused into a tube longer than the calyx, then split into two unequal lips so that it appears uni-lipped. The upper lip is very small, straight and notched at the apex. The lower lip is composed of three flat lobes, the middle one is the largest, its apex is notched, it appears to be composed of two lobes. Stamens 4, bipotent, prominent. Female bicarpal, ovary superior and quadripartite. Fruit quadripartite, about 1.5×3 mm, black, pitted.

Flowering: February to June.

Habitat and geographical distribution: Mediterranean.

Part used: Aerial parts (collected during the flowering season)

Chemical components:

Tanins, volatile oil, polyhydroxylated-sterols, steroids phytoecdy makisterone, cyasterone, polypodine. The plant mainly contains potassium and magnesium, and the leaves contain linoleic and linoleic acids. The essential oil is mainly composed of thymol, 4-phenylguaiacol, and linalool. The plant contains many chemical compounds such as 20-hydroxyecdysone, cyasterone, ajugas-palmitic acid, ecdysterone, carvacrol, apigenin, apigenin dihexoside, and terone.

Properties and medical uses:

Research conducted on laboratory mice has shown the antioxidant properties of the aqueous extract of the plant. The research has also shown the presence of antibacterial and antiulcer properties. And lowers blood sugar.

The decoction of the plant is used popularly for its purifying, anthelmintic properties, and to treat digestive disorders, enteritis, asthma, sinusitis, and diarrhea. It is used topically to treat mouth ulcers, wounds, hemorrhoids, and rheumatism.

The extracts and compounds isolated from the plant have shown pharmacological, anti-hypercholesterolemia, insecticide, and kidney stone dissolving effects. The results confirmed the possibility of using the plant as a treatment to lower blood pressure, and the decrease in systolic blood pressure can be attributed to glycosylated phenolic compounds (polar phenolic compounds) such as flavonoids and/or their metabolites.

Other uses: The plant is very suitable as fodder for ruminant animals in pastures.

Environment: It is widespread in rocky areas within the Mediterranean basin.

Cultivation and productivity: The plant is not cultivated, grows wild.

Ballota nigra L.

Ballota foetida Lam., *Ballota sordida* Salisb., *Marrubium nigrum*)L.(Garsault, Stachys *ballota* Kuntze.

Occurrences : 137,038 occurrences

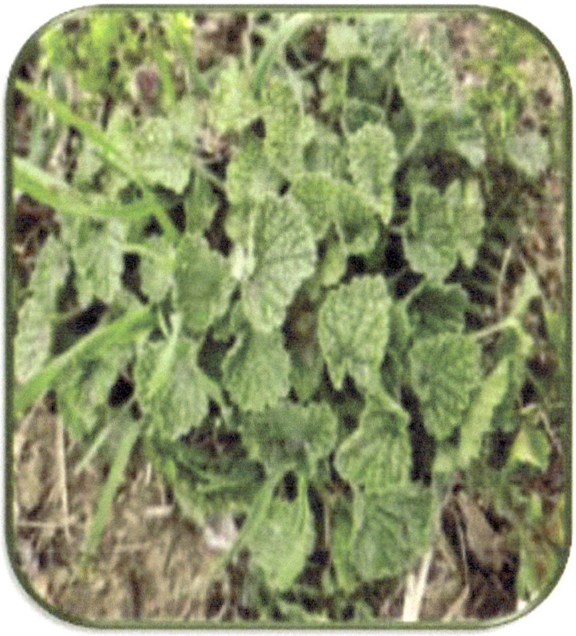 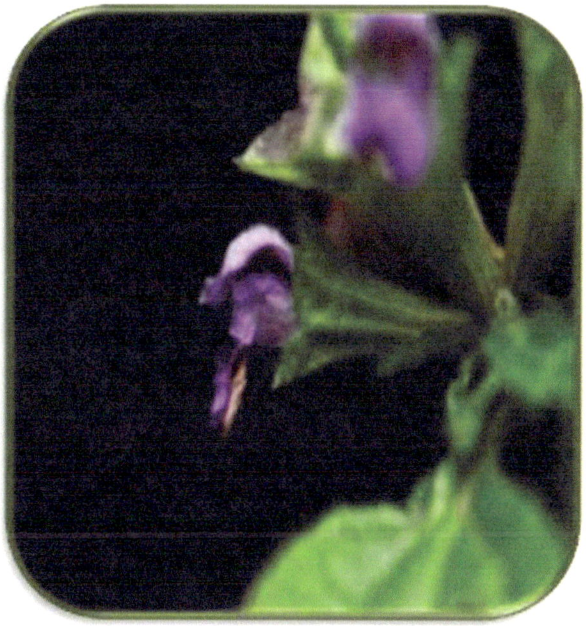

Family: Lamiaceae

Common names: Black phlox, ground oak, ketila, sharmaa. Black danah or black ghassa

Foreign names: noire Ballote Fr. orehound, Eng.

Distribution in the world

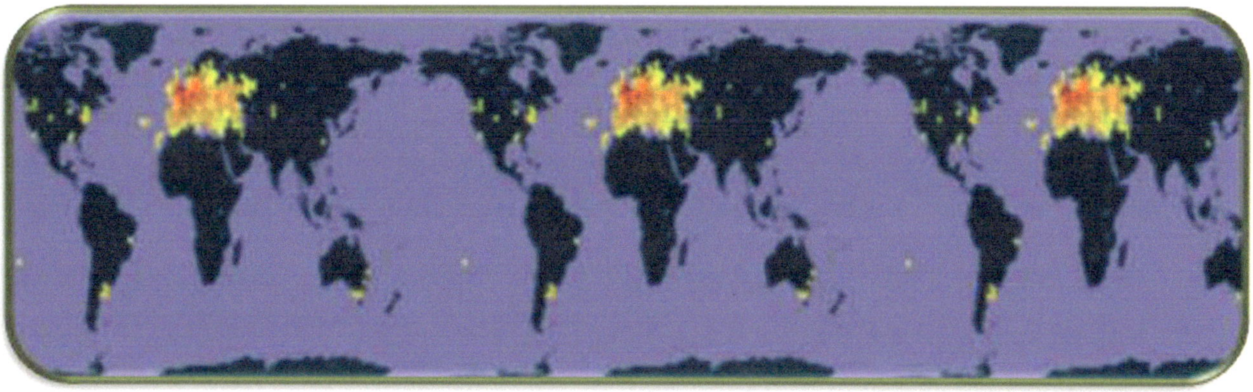

Botanical description:

A perennial plant, 30-80 cm high, with a rhizomatous stem that produces a strong, erect, angular stem. The entire plant is downy and green, turning brown to purple in autumn. The leaves are opposite, ovate, the lower ones are larger, oval to round in shape, their margins are serrated to serrated, and both sides are downy at first, then the upper side becomes bare and shiny. Flowers are 10-15 mm long, gathered in widely spaced racemes, 4-10 in number in the axils of the leaves, bracts are bead-shaped and solid, 4-8 mm long. The calyx is grooved, pentamerous, and the teeth end in barbs. The corolla is violet in color, bilipped. Stamens 4 with two different lengths. The fruit is an oval-shaped nut, 12 mm long and smooth.

Flowering: From June to July.

Habitat and geographical distribution: It is mainly distributed in the western Mediterranean basin.

History and heritage:

The scientific name of the genus Ballota is derived from the Greek ballôté, which is the name given to this plant in Greece, and its origin is unknown. The descriptive name of the species, nigra, means "black." The plant was used in ancient times primarily to treat respiratory disorders and vomiting. Dioscorides mentioned that a paste of the leaves of the plant with salt was used to treat dog bites, and a paste of the dried leaves with honey was used to treat wound infections.

Part used: Flowering tops.

Chemical components:

diterpenes lactone compounds (bitter principles) marrubiin, ballotenol, ballotinon, ballonigrin, 7-alpha-acetoxymarrubiin

Phenolic acids: caffeic acids, ferulic acid, chlorogenic acid and their derivatives. Tannins. A volatile oil with an unpleasant odor, rich in mono- and semi-terpene compounds (sesquiterpenes), the most important of which is germacrene-D. 33 components were found in the essential oils isolated from fresh aerial parts, and the most abundant components in the oil were: phytol, germacrene-D and caryophyllene. A phenylpropanoid glycoside, ballotetroside, was isolated from the aerial parts.

Properties and medical uses:

It is rarely used in modern herbal medicine due to its unpleasant taste. The plant has stimulating properties, is antispasmodic and digestive, and stimulates the secretion of bile. It is a sedative and analgesic, and is used to treat vomiting of nervous origin, anxiety, tension, depression, insomnia, and tachycardia. It is also used to treat whooping cough in children. The plant extract is used in the form of suppositories and enema to expel worms and parasites from the body. The plant is used internally or externally in the form of a decoction, extract, alcoholic tincture, or suppositories.

The use of plant extracts leads to a significant decrease in blood glucose, total cholesterol levels in the blood and serum creatine kinase CK levels. The results indicated that plant extracts have effects in reducing blood sugar, insulin release and cholesterol in mice.

Environment:

It grows in neglected lands, on roadsides and in shady places. It is suitable for moist, well-drained soils rich in nitrogen. It prefers sunny or semi-shaded locations. Rarely found on acidic soils.

Cultivation and productivity:

The plant is propagated by seeds that are scattered in spring or autumn in the nursery or in a greenhouse. The seeds germinate within 3-6 weeks at a temperature of 15°C. The seedlings are transferred to the permanent soil the following autumn. The plant can also be propagated by division, where the divided plants are planted directly in the permanent soil if they are large, or they are planted in plastic bags and left in the nursery for a year.

Ballota undulata)Sieb. ex Fresen.(Benth.

Pseudodictamnus undulatus)Sieber ex Fresen.(Salmaki & Siadati.

Occurrences : 1,824 occurrences

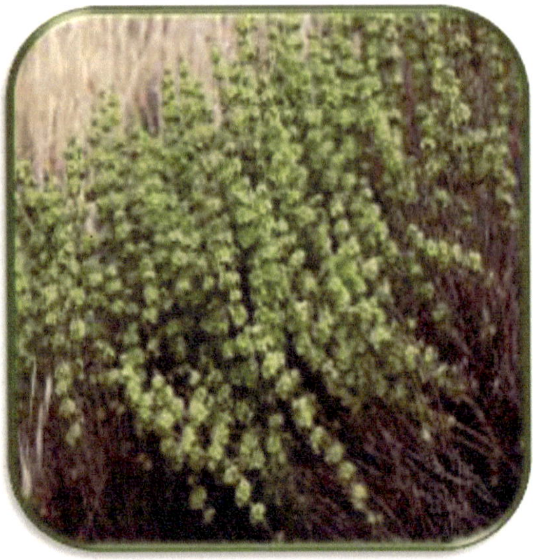

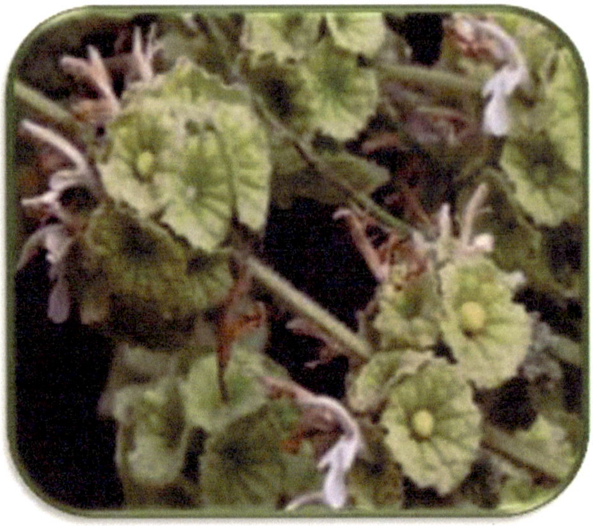

Family: Lamiaceae

Common names: Katila, Sharmaa

Foreign names: Eng. Common ballota, Fr. Ballote ondulée

Distribution in the world

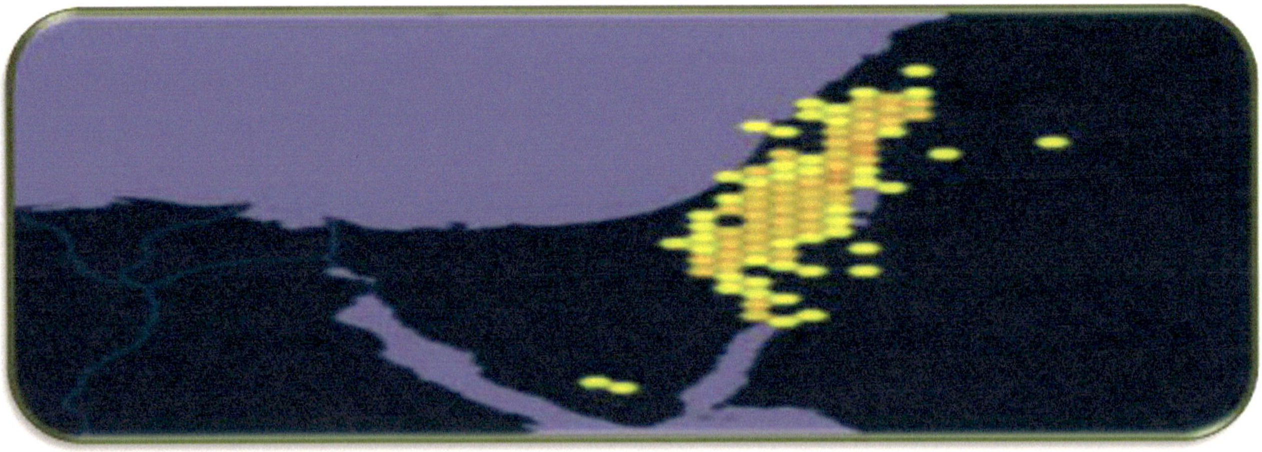

Botanical description:

Perennial herb, 30-80 cm tall, many stems, yellow-green in color, covered with glandular hairs and simple or star-shaped flat hairs. Stems erect or ascending, quadrilateral and notched. Lower leaves disappear quickly, middle stem leaves are spiculate, rounded or kidney-shaped, 25 x 35 mm, cordate or truncated at the base, crinoline to wavy at the edge, sunken-veined (curly). Floral leaves are shorter than whorls except the lower ones. Flowers are gathered in numerous whorls, the lower ones are widely spaced, the upper ones are compact. Bracts are short (3-4 mm), linear-spoon-shaped or conical, hard and hairy. The calyx is 9-12 mm, consisting of a tube with about 10 ribs, initially narrow and then widening from the middle to form blades 12-15 mm wide, with reticulate veins, its edge is cristaled and irregularly serrated. The teeth are cut or terminate in short barbs. The corolla is 15-18 mm, white, its three petals are fused into a tube that is included in the calyx, which soon splits into two lips. Stamens 4, of different lengths, located below the upper lip. Fruit: oblong-ovate, smooth.

Flowering: April to October. Habitat and geographical distribution: Eastern Mediterranean, extending to the western Iranian-Turanian and eastern Arabian desert regions.

History and heritage: The genus name Ballota was mentioned in the previous type, and the species name undulate means "wavy."

Part used: Flowering plant

Chemical components:

Volatile oil rich in mono- and semi-terpenes (sesquiterpenes), germacrene D-, ketone terpenes (bitter compounds) principles maruben and ballonigrinon .ballotinon, ballonigrin, flavonoid compounds, including: myricetin, kaempferol, rutin, and quercetin, and phenolic acids ( )acids, including: ferulic acid, a. chlorogenic, a. .coumaric acids, glycosidic compounds, including: forsythoside, verbascoside, and betonyoside.

Properties and medical uses:

The plant has antibacterial properties including Pseudomonas coli, Escherichia aureus, Staphylococcus .aeruginosa The glycosidic compounds have antioxidant properties. The decoction of the plant is popularly used to treat skin allergies.

The effect of plant extracts against two human cancer cells, the Hepg2 liver cell line and the MCF-7 breast cancer cell line, as well as the antioxidant effect, was studied. The oil was found to have an anti-proliferation effect on HepG2 liver cancer cells. The plant has antioxidant effects by scavenging free radicals in the body. In a study of the effect of the plant on body fat, the use of the plant extract led to a clear reduction in the level of cholesterol, phospholipid levels and triglycerides in the blood of rabbits.

Environment:

Grows on sunny hills with stony, semi-dry calcareous soils, indicating soil degradation and erosion. The plant prefers medium-acidic, neutral, moist, well-drained sandy and clayey soils. It tolerates low temperatures up to -10°C.

Cultivation and productivity: Grows wild.

Lamium album L.

Lamium vulgatum Benth., *Lamium vulgatum* var. *album* (L.) Benth.

Occurrences : 368,508 occurrences

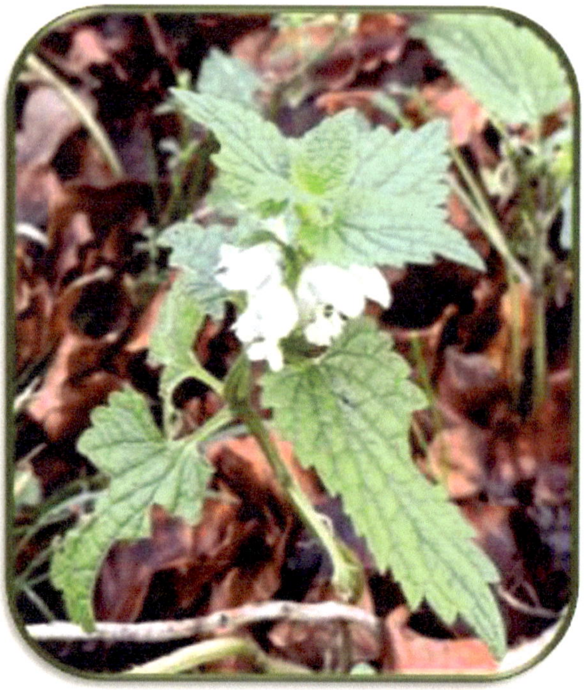

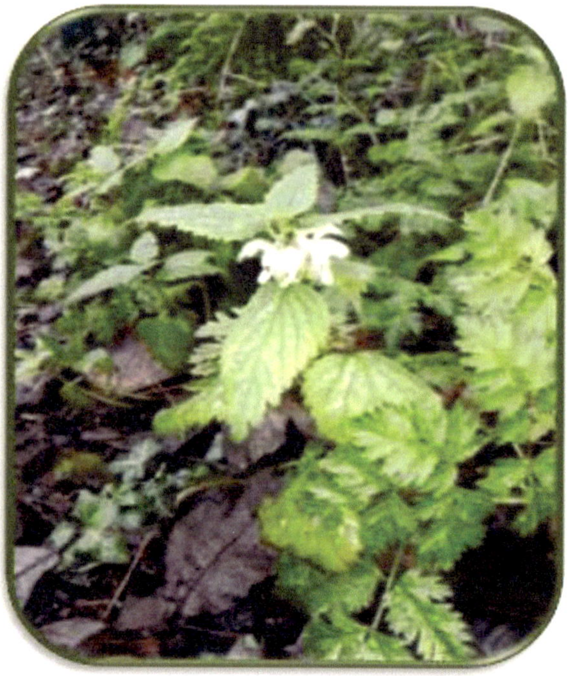

Family: Lamiaceae

Common names: White dead nettle, Fr. Lamier blanc

Foreign names:

Distribution in the world

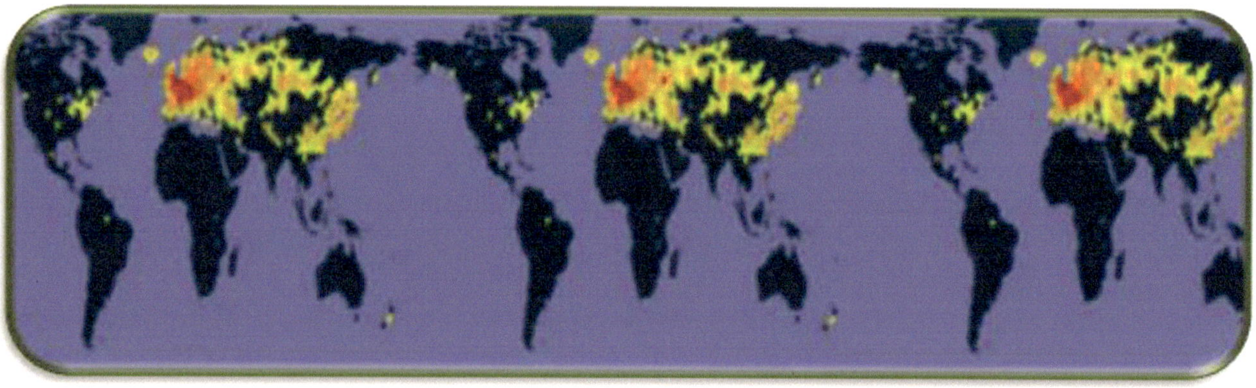

Botanical description:

A downy herb, 30-60 cm tall, perennial with a creeping rhizome, from which erect, square-sectioned aerial stems branch. Leaves are simple, opposite, ovate, ovate to heart-shaped, serrated on the margin, pointed at the apex. Flowers are white, about 2 cm long, gathered in whorls around the stem, each containing 6-16 flowers, forming clusters of flowers. The calyx is bell-shaped, ending in five equal teeth, perennial with the fruit. The corolla tube is prominent, curved in the shape of the letter S, the upper lip is arched, like a helmet, with a fringed edge, the lower lip is flattened, three-lobed, but the lateral lobes are greatly reduced. Male 4 stamens (long pair and short pair) located within the upper lip. The branches of the stem are equal. The fruit 4 triangular seeds.

Flowering: From April to May.

The shape of the plant before flowering resembles the stinging nettle, and therefore it is called the white or false nettle.

Habitat and geographical distribution: Europe and western Asia, and was introduced to North America.

History and heritage:

The scientific name of the genus is derived from the Greek and Latin lamia, which is derived from laïmos, meaning "throat", referring to the shape of the flower's crown, which resembles an open throat. The descriptive name of the species album means "white."

Part used: Flowering plant

Chemical components:

Iridoid monoterpenes, including: lamalbide, caryoptoside, alboside lamiridosins A, B, A, B . Triterpene saponins. Flavonoids, including: kaempferol Coffee acid and its derivatives, including: rosmaric acid, a. .chlorogenic tannins (gum) hydroxycinnamic acid, secoiridoids, anthocyanins, phenylpropanoids, phytoecdysteroids, benzoxazinoids, and betaine

Properties and medical uses:

The plant has expectorant (saponins and gum) and astringent properties due to its richness in tannins. It is used in the treatment of cough, bronchitis, stomatitis, laryngitis, and dermatitis. Research indicates that the aqueous extract of the flowering tops of the plant contains antiviral isomers iridoid B, A lamiridosins, which inhibit infection with hepatitis C virus. It is used in the treatment of cytotoxicity and cell protective activity. It prevents menstrual and skeletal muscle disorders, and improves fat metabolism. The plant is popularly used to treat upper respiratory tract infections, and digestive disorders such as gastritis and flatulence. It is used topically to treat moderate inflammation of the mucous membrane of the mouth and throat and superficial inflammation of the skin. It is also used in cases of menopausal and urinary tract disorders, and is used in the treatment of fractures, high blood pressure, blood flow, paralysis, sepsis, shocks, and some women's diseases such as heavy menstruation, uterine bleeding, vaginitis and cervicitis, and bleeding after childbirth.

Other uses:

The fresh leaves are used as a salad or cooked as a vegetable. The plant is nectarous and is sometimes called bee stinger.

Environment:

A plant that lives in diverse environments such as open meadows and forests. It likes sunny places, but it can grow in partially shaded places. It tolerates low temperatures up to -25°C, and tolerates most types of soil and environmental conditions, but it likes humidity, and grows well in heavy, fertile clay soils.

Cultivation and productivity:

It is propagated by seeds. The plant scatters its seeds automatically and rarely needs human help after planting it for the first time. It is also propagated by division in the spring, and can be successful at any time during the growing season. The divided plants are planted directly in the permanent ground or wait until the following spring, until they have formed strong roots, otherwise the plant can turn into a weed.

Lavandula angustifolia Mill.

Occurrences : 48,867 occurrences

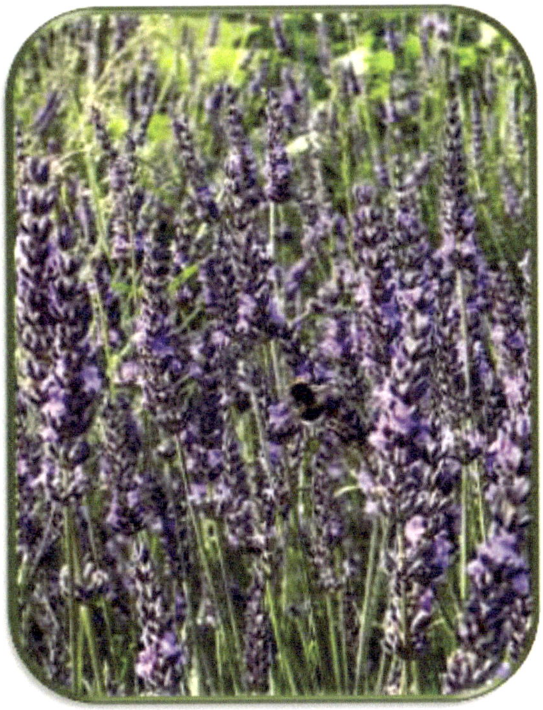

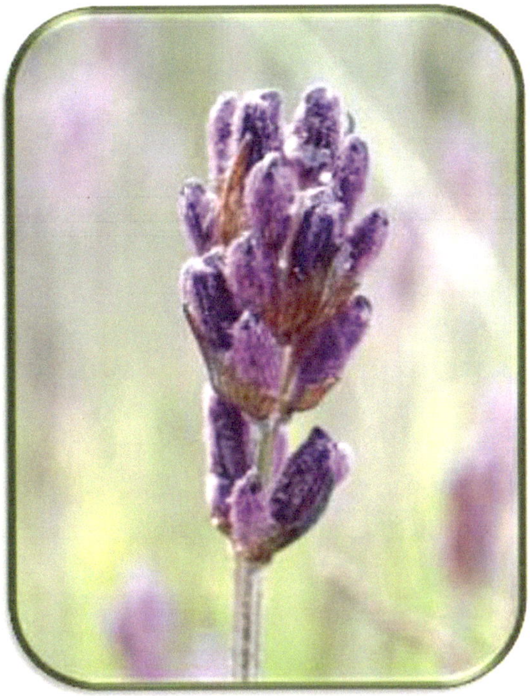

Family: Lamiaceae

Common names: Lavender

Foreign names: Lavande Fr. Lavender, Eng.

Distribution in the world

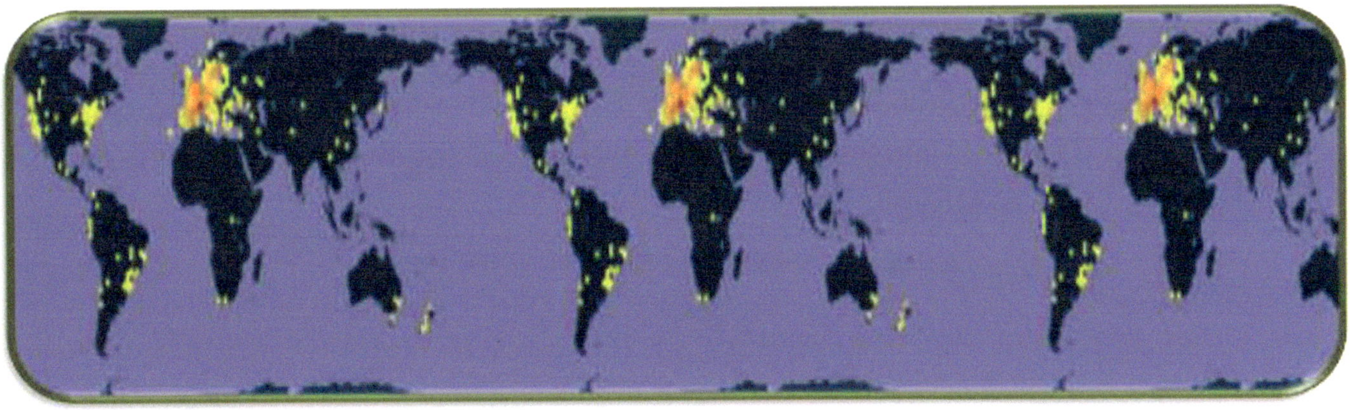

Botanical description:

A fragrant shrub, with many branches, 30-80 cm long, branches are erect and gray in color, the flowering ones are clearly longer. Folded to linear-lanceolate in shape, dimensions 2-5 cm x 3-5 than the leafy ones. Leaves are simple, opposite, short-spikelet, hairy, then bare, grey-green, with a strong aromatic scent, with an entire margin. mm, at first leaves of flowering branches are spaced apart, while leaves of non-flowering branches are in groups. flowers are blue, gathered in whorls of 6-10 flowers, forming long spikes. bracts are small, rhombic-ovate or acuminate-bead-shaped. The calyx is tubular, 4-5 mm long, ending in 5 teeth (4 short teeth and the fifth forming a small oval or heart-shaped lip), bearing 13 nerves, growing slightly with the formation of the fruit. The petals are blue in colour, wrinkled in texture, fused in a tube that protrudes from the calyx and then splits into two lips. The male has 4 stamens of different lengths, contained in the corolla tube. Ovary bi-chambered, each chamber divided into two by a pseudo-septum, each containing a single ovule. Fruit 4 smooth seeds.

Flowering: Late summer. Other species widespread and used in North Africa are multifida L.

Habitat and geographical distribution:

Sunny Mediterranean coasts and mountains up to 1800 m.

History and Heritage:

The scientific name of the genus is derived from the Latin lavare, which means "to wash", indicating that these plants were used to perfume laundry and bath water. They are also one of the most popular medicinal herbs since ancient times, as Tabernaemontanus (one of the famous ancient doctors) recommended using the flowers to restore speech to the tongue after suffering from cerebral palsy. Lavender species were used in Arab medicine as an expectorant, antispasmodic, and astringent. It is a heart and brain tonic, a chest purifier, and nothing compares to it in purifying the kidneys, spleen, stomach, and liver.

Part used: Flowers, leaves, and the volatile oil extracted from them.

Chemical components:

The flowers and leaves contain 3% volatile oil, the most important components of which are linalool, ac-linalyl acetate, lavanulyl acetate, and ocimene. Hydroxycoumarins, including: herniarin, umbelliferone, tannins, caffeic acid, and rosmaric acid. Sterol compounds and triterpenes in the flowers, in addition to tannic substances and phenolic acids. The plant is rich in polyphenols, sugars and biologically active polar compounds such as polyphenols and coumarins. HPLC analysis showed the presence of rosmarinic acid (10.82-2.52 mg/g), ferulic acid, caffeic acid (1.70 - 3.10 mg/g), morin (1.02 - 13.63 mg/g), coumarin (5.97-1.01 mg/g) and herniarin (8.02-1.05 mg/g).

Properties and uses Medical:

The drug has anti-inflammatory, lipid and cholesterol-lowering, antimicrobial, antitumor, central sedative, and carminative properties. It is used in cases of loss of appetite, digestive disorders, nervous conditions, insomnia, and circulatory disorders. The volatile oil is used in cases of nervous tension and sleep disorders. The flowers have cholagogue and cholagogue properties, and are used internally to treat functional upper digestive disorders, anxiety and restlessness, and sleep disorders. The flowers are popularly used in cases of spasms, migraines, bronchial asthma, for massage in cases of rheumatism, for relaxation, and in cases of poorly healed wounds.

Volatile oil is popularly used to treat bronchitis, rheumatism, migraine, and menstrual disorders. It is used topically in the form of water baths to relieve tension and relaxation, and to treat difficult-to-heal wounds and closure. It is also used to treat chronic anal and perineal eczema, to prevent colds, and to stimulate the circulatory system.

Side effects, interactions, and warnings:

The use of drug forms may cause digestive disorders, skin irritation, and a decrease in estrogenic activity. Do not take more than two drops of the volatile oil, high doses can cause central nervous system depression, constipation, respiratory depression, headache, vomiting, and effects similar to those of narcotic. Do not take it when taking alcohol or sedatives such as: valium halcyon, dalmane, and narcotic painkillers. Pregnant and breastfeeding women should avoid its use.

Other uses:

Volatile oil is used in the manufacture of perfumes, cosmetics, ointments, soaps, shampoos, and deodorants. It is also used in the food industry, especially beverages, to give them an acceptable smell and taste.

The essential oil is used in cosmetics, medicines, food, environmental and agricultural applications.

Environment:

The plant grows wild in neglected fields and in semi-forested areas that have a Mediterranean climate. It tolerates drought and heat, and can tolerate frost for a short period of time and is found in conditions of moderate temperature and humidity. Grows in various types of soils and lands, but prefers yellow soils, and is tolerant of salinity.

Cultivation and productivity:

The plant is propagated by seeds, stem cuttings (terminal or intermediate), or division, noting that vegetative propagation is the best. Seeds are planted in beds or in rows in the nursery at the beginning of spring, and seedlings are transferred to permanent soil during the fall and early winter. Old plants can be divided with their roots in the form of seedlings and replanted. It is preferable to plant the stem cuttings in the nursery in the fall in narrow lines, 50 cm wide, and at a distance of 10 cm between the cuttings within one line, then transferred to the permanent ground after 4-5 months. Service operations are provided by fertilization and moderate irrigation. The plant blooms in the summer. The plants are cut at the end of summer after harvesting the flowers at a height of 10 cm above the soil surface in order to strengthen the plants and increase their branching to resist the winter cold. Lavender production varies according to the type, environmental conditions and plant part. 1 ton of green herb of medicinal lavender gives 5-6 kg of volatile oil.

Lavandula stoechas L.

Stoechas oficinarum Mill.

Occurrences : 223,619 occurrences

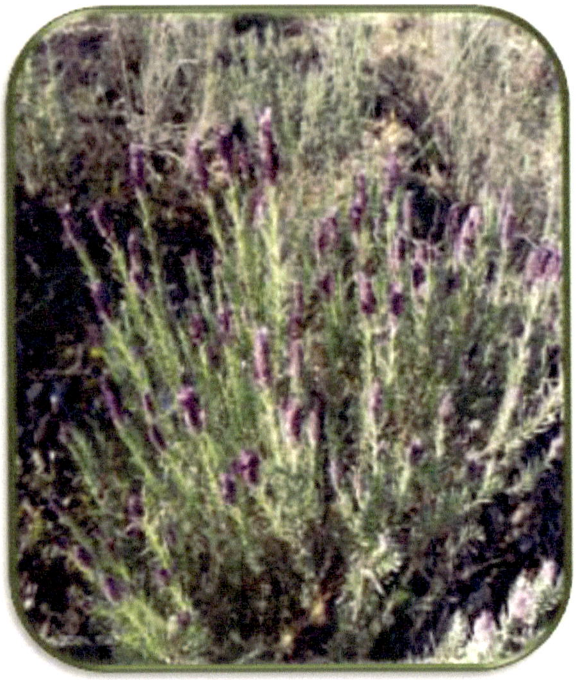

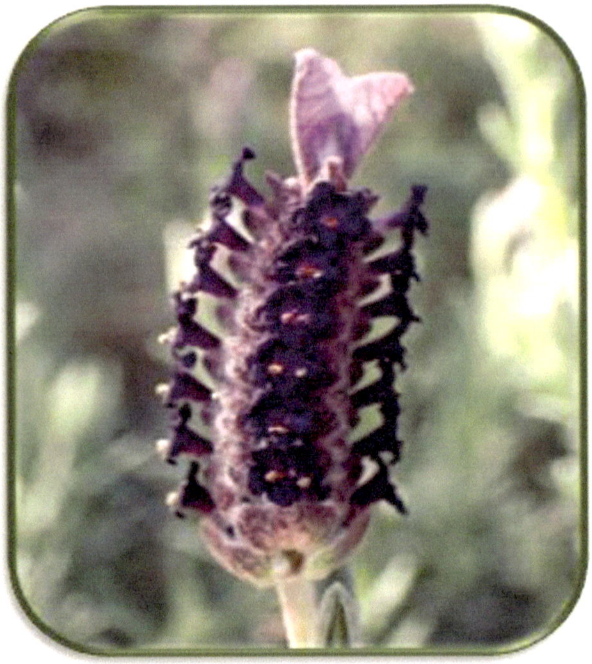

Family: Lamiaceae

Common names: Lamiaceae, Ascidian

Foreign names: Lavande Fr. Lavender, Arabian Eng.

Distribution in the world

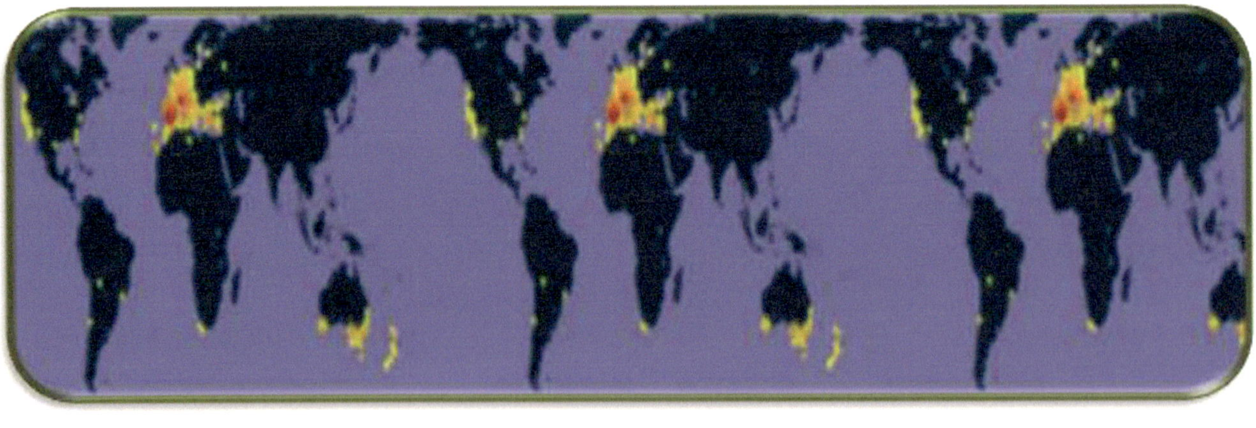

Botanical description:

A small shrub, 30-50 cm tall, highly branched, covered with dense grey hairs. Stem erect, many leaves. Leaves simple, linear to oblong, entire, blunt at the apex, their margins curling downwards, grey on both surfaces, and tufts of leaves are noted on very short branches in the axils of large leaves.

The flowers are gathered in close whorls, each containing 6-10 flowers, and their group forms oblong to oval spikes, their dimensions are 2-3 × 1 cm. The fertile bracts (which have flowers in their axils) are overlapping, have an inverted triangular shape with rounded corners, and carry a network of nerves. As for the sterile bracts (which do not have flowers in their axils), they are inverted oval in shape, their color is purple to violet, and they form dark-colored strands in Top of spikelet. The calyx is about 5 mm, grey Villiform, composed of a tube ending in five triangular teeth, the upper one ending in a heart-shaped sepal. Corolla dark purple, the tube slightly longer than the calyx.

Flowering: February to May.

Habitat and geographical distribution: Mediterranean basin and Black Sea.

History and heritage:

The genus name was mentioned in the previous type. Some say that the type description is attributed to islands located south of France, and was known as the islands of Khors, which means "arrayed in a straight line", while others see it as a reference to the spike-shaped flowers. Part used: Flowering tops

Chemical components:

The flowering parts contain 0.7 - 1.2% volatile oil rich in compounds such as camphor 17%, linalool 37%, and cineole 1-8 25%. They give the plant its distinctive smell. Phenolic compounds have been identified, such as caffeic acid, quercetin-O-glucoside, luteolin-O-glucuronide and rosmarinic acid.

Properties and medical uses:

The flowering tops have blood sugar-lowering properties and are popularly used in cases of lung pain, asthma, chest and stomach flu. Lavender oil is characterized by its ability to reduce the incidence of foot edema and acute ear edema in mice, as well as inhibiting the inflammatory response of the skin.

It also has anti-tumor activity against various cancers, such as stomach cancer and breast cancer. The aqueous extract of the plant has a high phenol content, and has antioxidant activity.

Side effects, interactions and warnings for use: Using high doses of the oil causes symptoms Toxicity.

Environment: The plant spreads on sunny slopes, and prefers siliceous soils. The plant cannot grow in the shade and tolerates relative drought.

Cultivation and productivity: The plant is propagated by seeds that germinate within 1-3 months at a temperature of 15°C, or by stem cuttings at any time of the year.

Marrubium vulgare L.

M. apulum Ten., *M. ballotoides* Boiss. & Balansa, *M. hamatum* Humb. Kunth., *Prasium marrubium* E.H.L.Krause

Occurrences : 83,783 occurrences

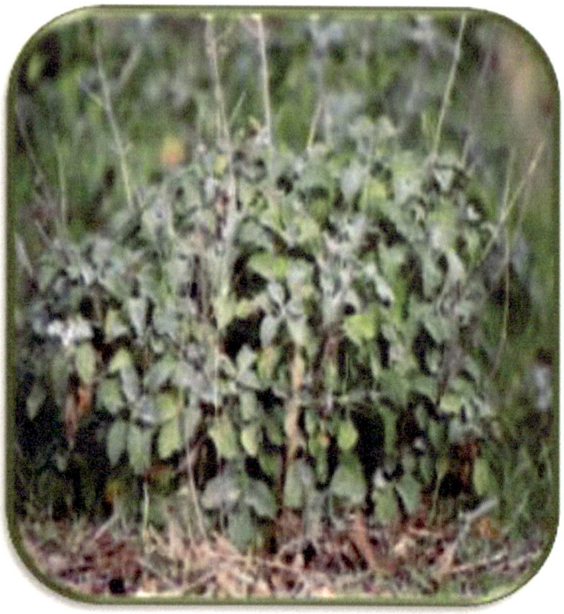

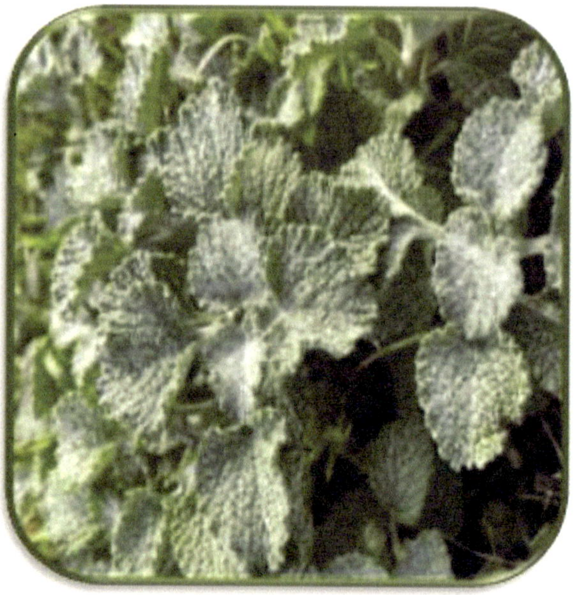

Family: Lamiaceae

Common names: Frasyon, Common Goddess

Foreign names:Eng. White horehound, Fr. Marrube blanc

Distribution in the world

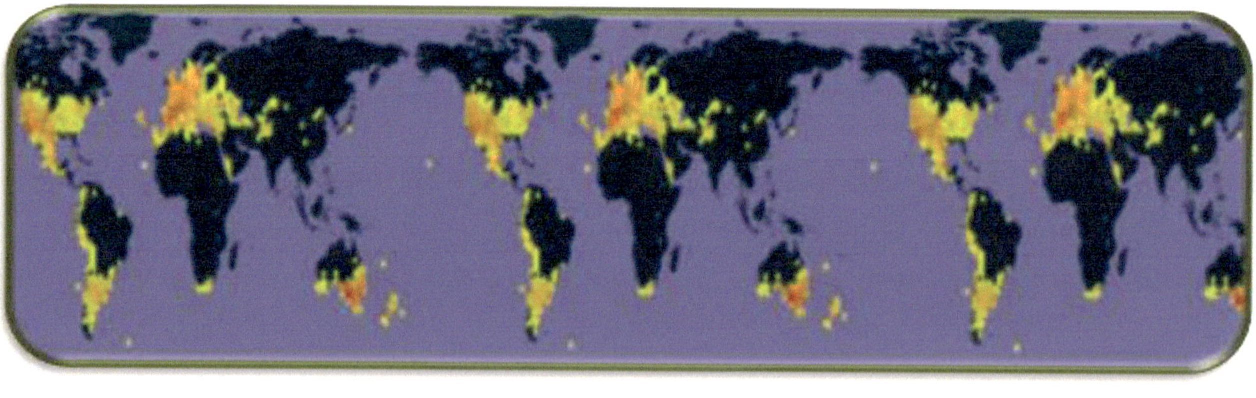

Botanical description:

Perennial herb, 30-60 cm tall, many-stemmed, woolly, especially in the lower part. Stem strong, ascending, square-sectioned. Leaves are simple, sessile, rough, covered with soft woolly hairs, grey or whitish on the underside, ovate to rounded, heart-shaped at the base, crest-shaped to serrated at the margin, 1-4 cm long. The floral leaves are short-spined, pedunculate to oblong, drooping downwards, longer than the whorls. The flowers are gathered in semi-pinnate inflorescences, forming numerous, spaced-out, spherical whorls. Bracts acuminate, acuminate, shorter than calyx. Calyx covered with stellate to woolly hairs, bearing 10 nerves; terminating in equal, flattened teeth, shorter than tube, each tooth terminating in a bare, hooked spine, calyx tube 4-7 mm, aperture blocked by woolly hairs. Corolla white, labial, upper lip erect, bilobed, lower lip flat. Stamens 4, embedded in corolla tube. The style is also included in the corolla tube. The fruit is a nut, oval, rounded at the top, smooth, black.

Flowering: April to June.

Homeland and geographical distribution: Mediterranean and Iranian-Turanian.

History and heritage:

The scientific name comes from Hebrew, the word mar means "bitter", and rob means juice, meaning "bitter juice plant", and vulgare means "common." As for the word phrasyon, its origin is Greek. The ancients used the phrasyon herb to treat chest diseases such as cough, asthma, and lung ulcers, and also in liver blockage and jaundice. It was mentioned by Ibn al-Baytar.

Part used: Flowering plant, (when rubbed, the leaves emit a strong smell and have a bitter and hot taste)

Chemical components:

Bitter), the most important of which is marrubiin (0.1-)%Diterpene lactone (compounds. marrubenol, 0.1% premarrubiin, Traces of volatile oil, the most important of which are: camphene, para-cymene, fenchone, caryophyl- lene, D germacrene, α-humulene and α-copaene from monoterpene hydrocarbons and semi- sesquiterpene hydrocarbons Contains marrubiin, which is a diterpene labdane, which is characteristic of this genus, In addition to a complex mixture of phenolic compounds. Phenolic acids (derivatives of caffeic acid), the most important of which are a.: a.caffeic, chlorogenic and a.apigenin, luteolin, vicenin, chrysoeriol, flavonoids, Tanins, traces of soap compounds, choline, mineral salts, especially potassium salts.

Properties and medical uses:

The plant has the properties of bitter compounds marrubinic acid, volatile oil, tannins and flavonoids, which stimulate the appetite, stimulate the liver, and stimulate the secretion of digestive juices. Digestive and gas expelling. Research indicates the antioxidant properties of the aqueous extract of the plant marrubiin, marrubenol, as well as its properties in relaxing and expanding blood vessels, in addition to its effect in reducing cholesterol levels, which makes it a reducer of high blood pressure. The plant has analgesic properties due to its marrubiin content, in addition to its anti-edema and blood sugar-lowering properties. The decoction of the plant is used popularly as an expectorant, and to treat respiratory tract infections (bronchitis, laryngitis, colds, coughs, and asthma), diarrhea, jaundice, and menstrual pain.

The decoction of the plant is used topically to treat wounds, skin ulcers, and as a gargle for inflamed throats. The fresh juice of the plant has antiseptic, diaphoretic, and diuretic properties, and helps in healing wounds and repels worms. The drug is an antioxidant, and a treatment for cancer, diabetes, and liver diseases. The drug is also an anti-inflammatory, antihypertensive, anti-lipid, and sedative.

It also has antimicrobial activity, especially against bacteria, fungi, herpes simplex virus, and parasites such as Toxoplasma gondii, Trichomonas vaginalis, and Plasmodium berghei-berghei. It can be used as a chicken lice repellent, herbicide, natural insecticide against mosquito larvae, and natural molluscicide. In veterinary medicine, the drug can be used as an anti-eggs and larvae of bovine parasites, and as an antibiotic for bacterial mastitis in bovines.

Other uses:

The leaves or the resulting volatile oil are used as a flavoring for some drinks (beer, tea). Warnings for use: It has been noted that consuming large quantities of the plant causes diarrhea and vomiting. It is not used by pregnant women and people with stomach ulcers, as the increase in digestive juices increases the pain of the ulcer in them.

Environment:

It grows on the edges of roads, on slopes and in steppes with gravelly-sandy soils. It is suitable for dry, calcareous, well-drained soils. It prefers moderate or alkaline soils. Its presence indicates overgrazing.

Cultivation and productivity:

It is propagated by seeds. The seeds are planted in the nursery either in early spring or early autumn, and germination is irregular. The seedlings are transferred individually to bags or pots after reaching a suitable size. The plants are transferred to the permanent ground in the following spring. The plant can also be propagated by division in late spring, by cutting the branches with parts of the stem below the ground when they reach a length of 8-10 cm. The plants are placed in bags or pots and left in a shaded place until they are well rooted, then transferred to the permanent ground.

Melissa officinalis L.

Faucibarba oficinalis)L.(Dulac, *Mutelia oficinalis*)L.(Gren. ex Mutel, *Thymus melissa* E.H.L.Krause

Occurrences :114,209 occurrences

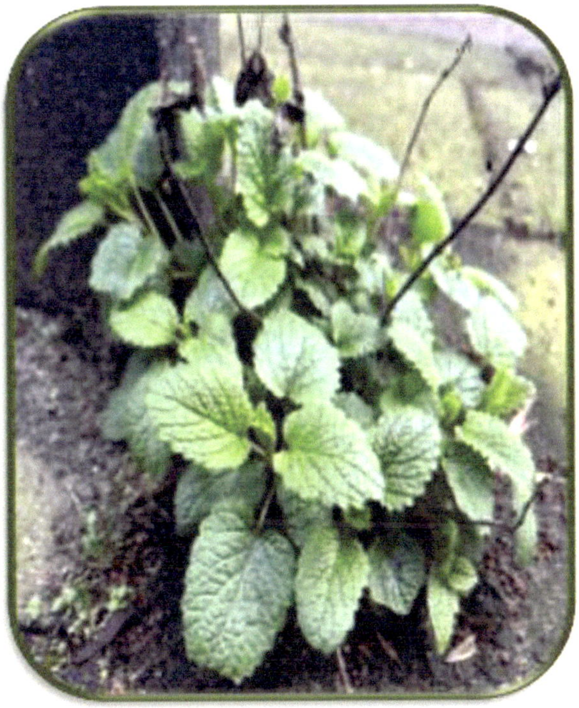

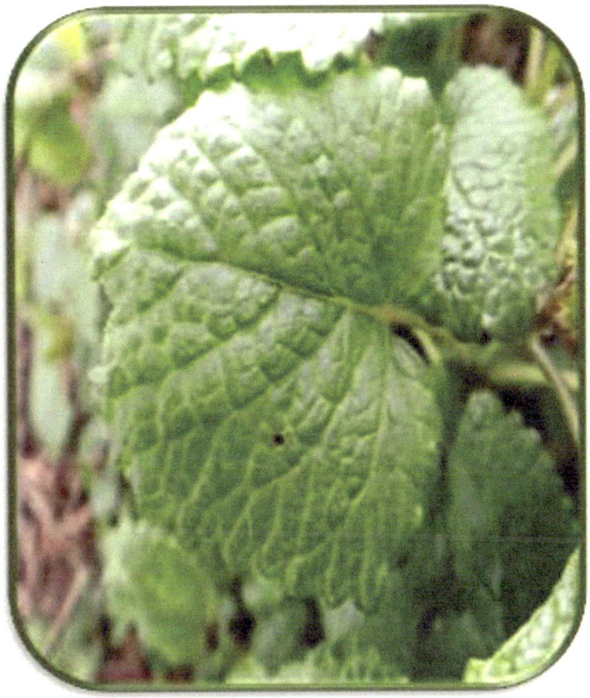

Family: Lamiaceae

Common names: Constitutional lemon balm, tarragon, bee weed, tangerine basil

Foreign names: Melisse Fr. balm, Lemon Eng.

Distribution in the world

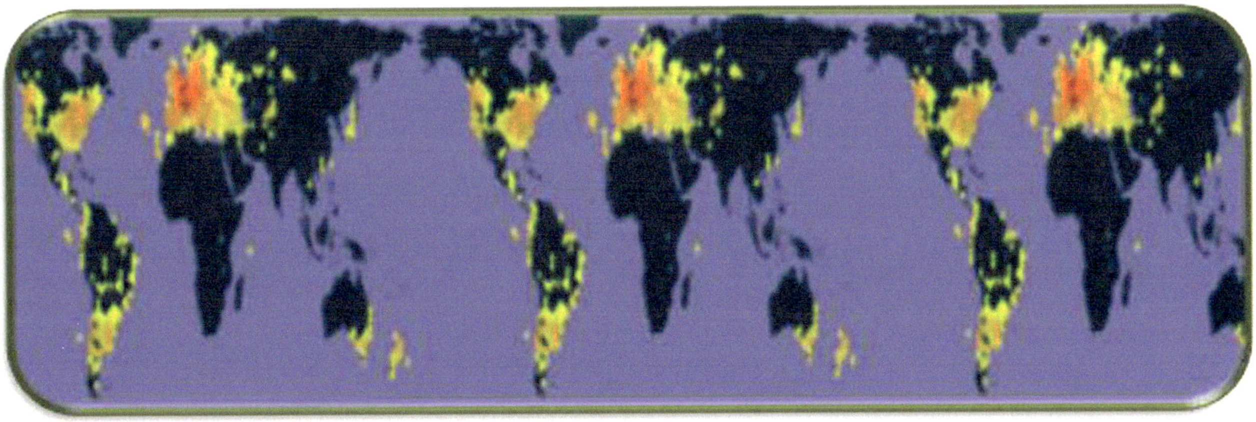

Botanical description:

A perennial herb, 60-100 cm tall, covered with hairs or down, with a lemon scent. The stem is square in section, erect, branched in the form of strong, solid bundles. The leaves are opposite, ovate, ovate in shape, blunt at the apex, cordate at the base, serrated to crescent at the edge, 2-6 cm long. The floral leaves usually exceed the whorls. The whorl contains 6-10 flowers, forming a spike or semi-clustered inflorescence. The bracts are elliptic to ovate. The flower stalk is rather long. The calyx is covered with hairs, bearing a network of nerves, drooping at maturity, bilipped. The corolla is 15-18 mm, white to pale violet (yellowish in bud), twice as long as the calyx, the tube is prominent. Stamens 4, including under the upper lip. Fruit 4, oval, smooth.

Flowering: May to September.

Habitat and geographical distribution: Mediterranean and Iranian Turanian. Cultivated in many countries.

History and heritage:

The scientific name of the genus Melissa is derived from the Greek, meaning "honey bee", and the descriptive name of the species oficinalis means "constitutional" or "medicinal." People have associated lemon balm with bees since ancient times. Lemon balm has properties Therapeutic and tonic properties similar to those of honey. The plant has been known for more than 2000 years, and was known to the Greeks, Romans and Arabs. Lemon balm was one of the favorite herbs in the Middle Ages to prepare what was called the "elixir of youth", and until the eighteenth century it was believed that lemon balm "rejuvenates" and that it "consoles the heart and drives away sorrows." Part used: stems and leaves (they have a lemony aromatic smell, collected before flowering.)

Chemical components:

Volatile oil -0.02 0.8%, its most important compounds: geranial aldahyd 30-35%, neral (citral = 25-20%), citronellal 3%, these compounds constitute between 40-75% of the components of the oil, and to them the distinctive flavor of the plant is attributed. In addition to monoterpene phenols linalol, geraniol gera-niol, citronnellol, eugenol, germacren, caryophyl-lene 13 %, beta-ocimene, geranylacetate, citro-methyl nellale, caryophyllene oxide. Glycosides of alcoholic or phenolic compounds found in volatile oil, such as eugenol glucoside. Derivatives of caffeic acid 4.7%, the most important of which are rosmaric acida.))=labiatic, and caffeic acid a. and others. The phenoids include: cynaroside, cosmosil, rhamnocitrin, and quercitrin. Tri- acids terpenes, including ursolic acid and a. oleanolic, and others. Catechin tannins (polyphenols) 4%, contribute with terpenic compounds to the plant's antibacterial and antiviral effectiveness.

Properties and medical uses:

The leaves of lemon balm and its volatile oil are among the best drugs that calm the nervous system and fight spasms associated with anxiety and insomnia. It also has antioxidant properties. The volatile oil is used to treat inflammation of the mucous membranes lining the respiratory system, with antibacterial, antiviral and anti-intestinal worm properties. The decoction of the plant's leaves is popularly used in cases of general weakness, chronic asthma, nervous weakness, high blood pressure, digestive disorders of nervous origin, to expel gases, stimulate the secretion of digestive juices, and menstrual disorders. Lemon balm oil is used topically in the form of compresses to treat rheumatism and nerve pain.

Environment:

Lemon balm grows in semi-arid and dry environments with moderate temperatures of 20-25°C. It is very sensitive to cold and loves light. Its growth is weak and the percentage of the active ingredient in it decreases in shady places. The plant needs moderate humidity, as its deficiency leads to weak growth, yellowing of the leaves and their falling, while its high humidity combined with low temperatures leads to the death of the plant. It grows well in soils rich in organic matter. It can be grown in various types of soil except saline, and it tolerates acidity (pH) up to 4.5.

Cultivation and productivity:

The plant is propagated by seeds that are planted in the nursery at the beginning of spring, and germinate after 20-25 days at a temperature of 10-12°C, Then the seedlings are transferred to the permanent ground and planted. The plant can also be propagated by suckers that are planted in the fall.The plant responds to fertilization with essential elements.

Mentha piperita L.

Mentha aquatica var. piperita)L.(Alef., Mentha aquatica f. piperita (L.) G.Mey., Mentha glomerata var. piperita (L.) Gray

Occurrences : 9,963 occurrences

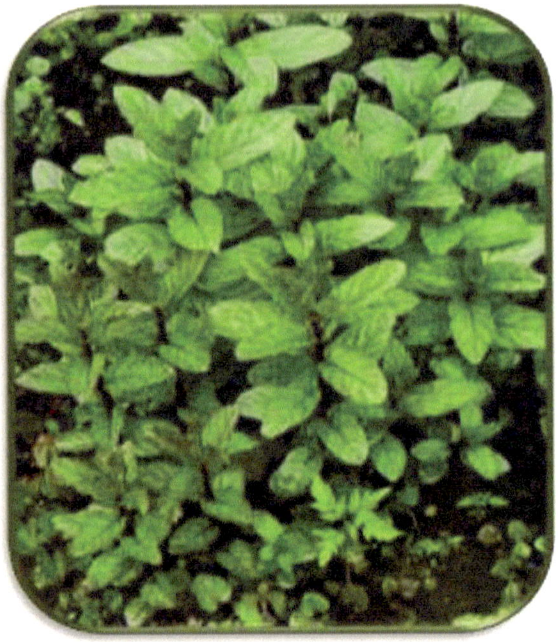

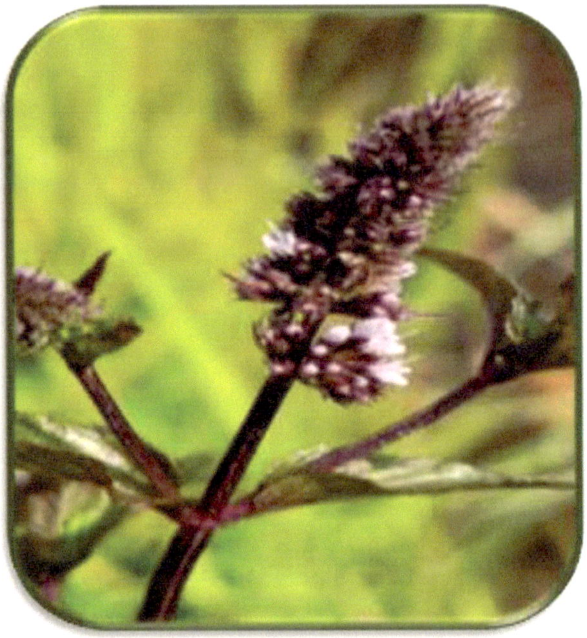

Family: Lamiaceae

Common names: Peppermint, Garden mint

Foreign names: poivrée Menthe Fr. Peppermint, Eng.

Distribution in the world

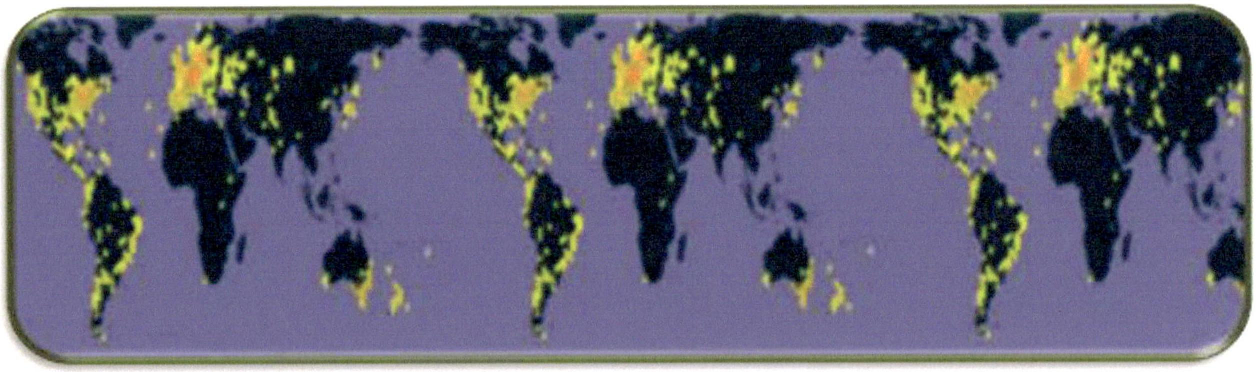

Botanical description:

Perennial herb with strong peduncles. Stem erect, branched, square-sectioned, reddish-purple in color, about 70 cm long. Leaves simple, opposite, ovate, lobate, serrated on the margin, bearing glandular glands filled with aromatic oil with a distinctive smell, 3-9 cm long, 1-3 cm wide. The flowers are blue-violet in colour, gathered in densely flowered panicles, which in turn gather in terminal spikes.

The calyx is tubular and five-toothed. The corolla is funnel-shaped, four-lobed and equal or nearly equal. The stamens are four-lobed, nearly equal in length, protruding from the tube and widely spaced. The plant produces fruits only exceptionally and they are sterile. The species is a hybrid between a number of mint species. There are a number of commercial varieties, including the brown or black Mentha vulgaris var. peperita and the white Mentha peperita var. oficinalis.

Habitat and geographical distribution:

European-Siberian, Mediterranean, and western Iranian Turanian. Native to the Americas, and cultivated in various parts of the world.

History and heritage:

The scientific name of the genus is derived from the Greek word Minthê, which is the name of the water nymph in Greek mythology, and the species name peperita means "peppery" and is cultivated and used as a spice. Dioscorides and others used it to refer to many types of mint, and Wilfrid Strabo wrote in the twelfth century: "If a man could name all the properties of mint, he would certainly know the number of fish that swim in the Indian Ocean." Part used: The flowering plant and the oil extracted from it. Chemical components: Volatile oil, its most important components are menthol 45-35%, menthone 20-15%, menthyl acetate 5-3%, neomenthol -2.5-3.5%, pulegone, alpha- and beta-pinene, carvone and other compounds. It also contains alcohols, alkanes, aldehyde, halocompounds, 1,2-benzene dicarboxylic acid, and 3-ethyl-5-dimethyl-6-phenyl-6-phenyl-dimethyl l-5-ethy linked to NS3 protease, which play a role in preventing health risks and combating mosquitoes. The plant is a source of chemical compounds used in the synthesis of insecticides. Coffee acid derivatives, including rosmaric acid

Flavonoids: apigenine, diosmetin, and others. .xanthomicrol, gardenine D: Flavones

Properties and medical uses:

The volatile oil has antispasmodic, antibacterial and antiviral properties. It is used for its sedative properties, and in the treatment of liver and gallbladder diseases, digestive disorders and spasms affecting the upper digestive system, biliary tract and irritable bowel syndrome. Antimicrobial, and effective antibacterial, especially gram-positive bacteria. It is used to treat inflammation of the mucous membranes in the mouth and throat, bronchitis and respiratory system. The volatile oil has a cooling effect on the skin. Antioxidant. Anticancer, especially colon and rectal cancer. The ethanolic extract of the plant is useful in combating mosquito larvae due to the presence of active components such as alkaloids, carbohydrates and flavonoids in the extract.

Warnings for use:

Peppermint is not recommended for gallstones and kidney stones, and is not recommended for bile duct obstruction and cholecystitis. It may cause colic for those with gallstones due to its cholestatic effect. Do not use the essential oil on the faces of infants and children, especially near the nose and mouth.

Environment:

Mint grows in all highly fertile, well-drained and aerated soils, preferring sandy soils. It also tolerates soil acidity pH up to 5.2.

Cultivation and productivity:

Mint is propagated vegetatively by creeping stems and rhizomes, which are divided into lengths of 5-8 cm, with each part bearing two nodes. Organic and mineral fertilizers are added, the land is plowed twice, then the seedlings are planted at a distance of 20-25 cm in the presence of water.

Mentha pulegium L.

Melissa pulegium (L.) Griseb., *Mentha aromatica* Salisb., *Mentha pulegium* subsp. *Vulgaris*) Mill.(Briq., *Mentha pulegium* var. *vulgaris*)Mill.(Briq., *Minthe pulegia* (L.) St.-Lag., *Pulegium vulgare* Mill.

Occurrences : 80,496 occurrences

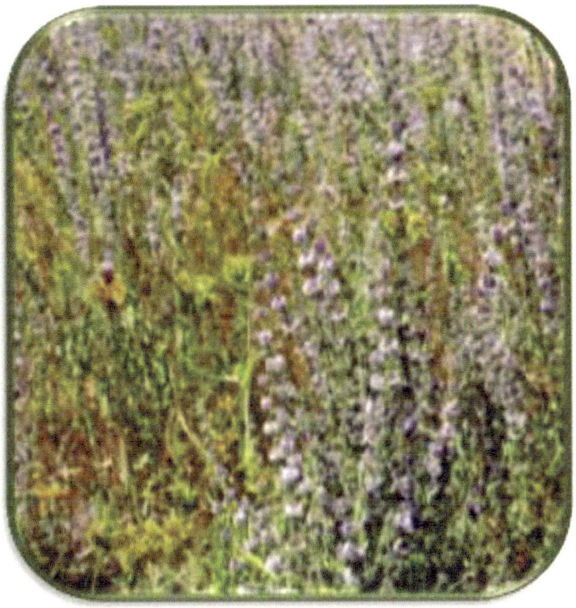

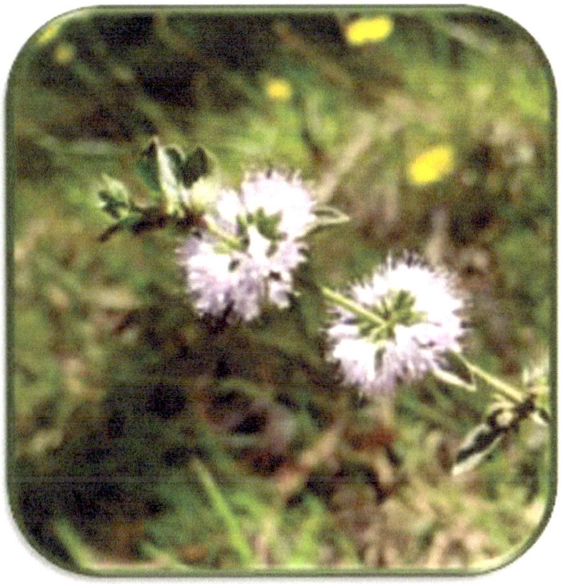

Family: Lamiaceae

Common names: Wild mint,Poulio mint, Wild mint, Wild pouilot

Foreign names: pouilot Menthe Fr. Pennyroyal, Eng.

Distribution in the world

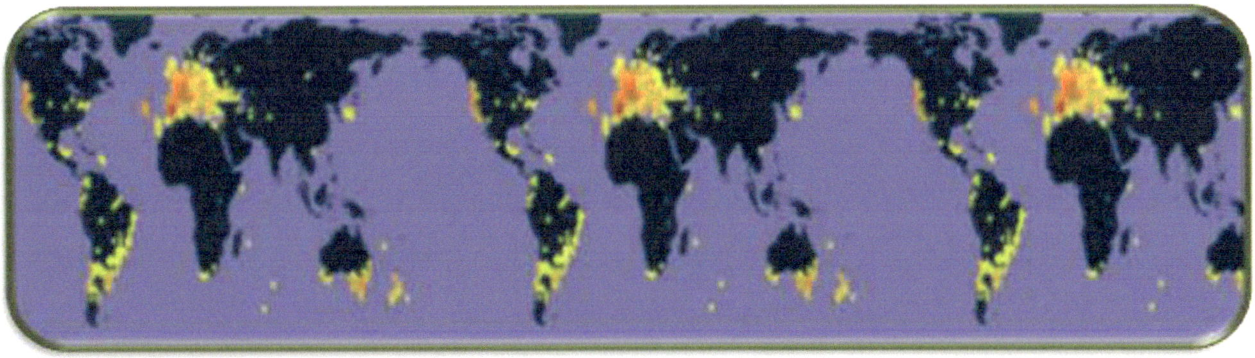

Botanical description:

A perennial herb, bearing glandular glands, with a strong aromatic scent, 20-50 cm tall, hairy to varying degrees. Stems reclining or ascending, mostly purple in color. Leaves short-spooned, ovate to oblong to elliptic, finely and faintly toothed, floral leaves similar in shape to stem leaves and usually exceed whorls. Flowers hermaphrodite, gathered in semi-spherical racemes, 1.5-1 cm in diameter, bracts absent. Calyx about 3 mm long, tubular, grooved, hairy, aperture hairy, 5 nearly equal teeth. Corolla funnel-shaped, ending in four almost equal lobes, pinkish-purple or pale purple. Male 4 stamens almost equal in length, protruding from the corolla and spaced apart. Fruit composed of 4 ovate, smooth or warty.

Flowering: From June to September.

Habitat and geographical distribution: European-Siberian, Mediterranean, and western Iranian-Turanian. Cultivated in various parts of the world.

History and heritage: Mentioned in the previous species.

Part used: Flowering tops, volatile oil extracted from the young plant.

Chemical components:

Volatile oil -1-2%, its most important compounds are pulegone 90-60%, menthone -10-20%, isomenthone -2-10%, piperitone, neoisomenthylacetate, limonene. Tannic compounds including rosmaric acid. Flavonoid compounds including: diosmin, hesperidin, in addition to some bitter compounds. Twenty-one mineral elements have been identified in mint: Ba, Br, Ca, Cl, Co, Cr, Cs, Eu, Fe, K, Mg, Mn, Mo, Na, Rb, Sb, Sc, Sr, Th, U, and Zn. HPLC analysis revealed flavonoid compounds, ferulic, cinnamic, caffeic, pyrogalol, coumaric acid, and salicylic acid. Properties and medical uses: The volatile oil, which contains the compound pulegone, has antimicrobial and anti-insect properties. Mint oil is used topically as a skin antiseptic. It is popularly used to treat digestive disorders (it stimulates the secretion of digestive juices). It is sometimes used to treat intestinal worms and menopause by strongly stimulating the uterine muscles and urging them to menstruate. The plant is an antioxidant and antibacterial against Staphylococcus aureus, Bacillus subtilis, Pseudomonas, Candida albicans, fungi, Escherichia coli and aeruginosa.

Warnings for use:

Excessive doses cause vomiting, high blood pressure, coma and then death due to respiratory collapse. Its use has been banned in many countries. Extreme caution should be exercised when using the oil internally, due to its high toxicity, especially to the liver, due to its polygon content. It should not be used by pregnant women, as it causes abortion.

Environment:

The plant lives in moist soils, and is severely affected by drought. It prefers slightly acidic soils. Its production of essential oil increases in sunny locations, and it can tolerate shady locations.

Cultivation and productivity:

The plant is propagated by seeds that are planted in the spring in the nursery or greenhouse, germination occurs quickly. The seedlings are transferred to pots when they reach a suitable length, then transferred to the permanent soil in the summer. The plants resulting from the seeds do not resemble the mother plants in the proportion of essential oil, so it is preferable to propagate them by division, which can be easily carried out at any time of the year, preferably in spring or autumn. Any part of the root will sprout into a new plant, so it is recommended to divide the roots into parts no longer than 3 cm, and place them in shade in a greenhouse to grow quickly, then transfer them to the permanent ground in the summer. The grass is cut just before the flowering period at a height of 8-10 cm above the soil surface and dried in the shade.

Micromeria nervosa (Desf.) Benth.

Satureja nervosa Desf., *Clinopodium nervosum*)Desf.(Kuntze, *Satureja graeca* subsp. *ner- vosa*) Desf.(O.Bolòs & Vigo.

Occurrences : 1,994 occurrences

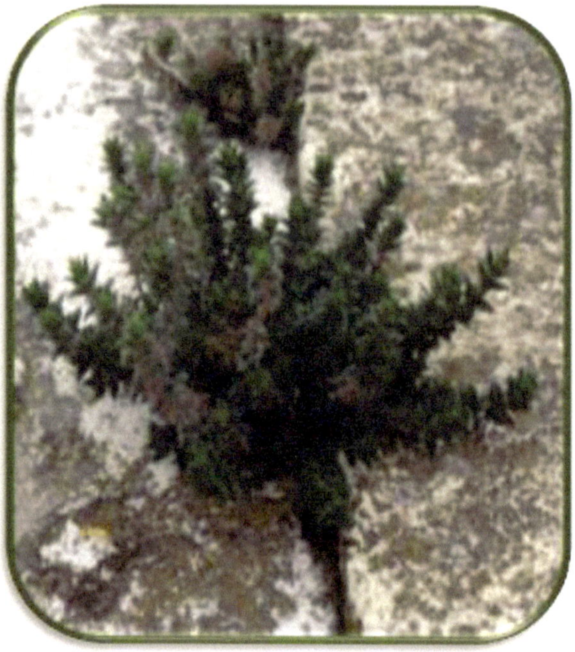

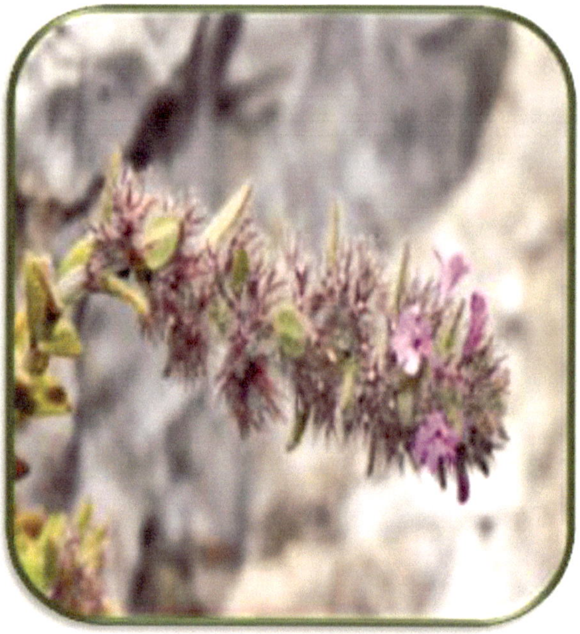

Family: Lamiaceae

Common names: Hyssop, Tea herb.

Foreign names: Micromerie Fr. Micromerie, Eng.

Distribution in the world

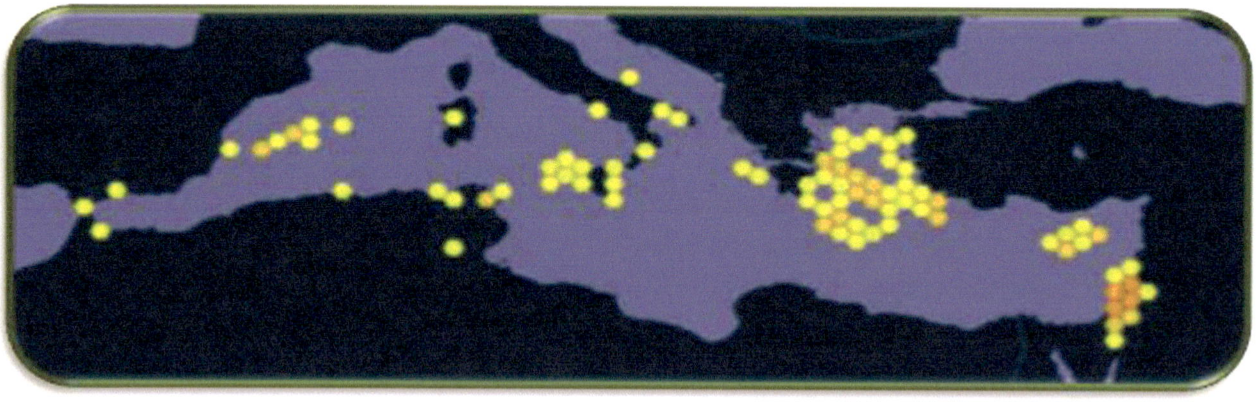

Botanical description:

Perennial herb, branching from the base, 15-40 cm tall, slightly hairy except for the upper part which is covered with flat hairs. Stems are solid, ascending, simple (single) or slightly branched, their color tends to purple, generated from a semi-woody rhizome. Leaves short to semi-spinate, edges slightly curled downwards, nerves prominent on the lower surface, semi-heart-shaped at the base, ovate-shaped, semi-acute at the apex. Floral leaves are equal to or slightly longer than flowers. Primary inflorescence semi-spiked, covered with abundant, hard hairs, many-flowered, gathered in secondary inflorescences resembling short spikelets, the lower whorls of which are spaced apart and the upper ones closely packed. Bracts are bead-shaped. Flowers short-stalked. Calyx tubular, grooved, violet-purple, about 3 mm long, covered with long hairs, teeth erect-flattened, shorter than the tube. Corolla violet, about 5 mm long, slightly hairy, corolla tube almost included in calyx. Fruit composed of 4 small oval seeds.

Flowering: February to May.

Other species include: Myrtifolia M., Fruticosa M. It is widespread in the countries of the Eastern Mediterranean.

Home and geographical distribution: Eastern Mediterranean.

History and heritage:

Hyssop has been used for a long time to treat coughs in the Eastern Mediterranean. There is hardly a house without it in that region, as the decoction of the plant is used as a hot drink as a preventive and therapeutic measure in winter. Hippocrates described hyssop to treat pleurisy and Dioscorides recommended it with agricultural rue for cases of asthma and colds. Al-Antaki mentioned it: "Nothing is equal to hyssop in diseases of the chest, lungs, asthma, cough, and shortness of breath, especially if it is mixed with figs, rue, and honey," as Ibn Sina and Ibn al-Baytar mentioned it.

Part used: The flowering plant.

Chemical components:

Hyssop species contain volatile oil, the proportions and main components of which vary according to the species. In the species myrtifolia M., the oil percentage reaches 0.5%, the most important of which is β-caryophyllen 44%, while the oil percentage reaches 4% in the species fruticosa M., the most important of which is pulegone 81%. One of the main active components of the plant, carvacrol, was isolated, and its antimicrobial effectiveness was shown to be The most sensitive organisms to this compound are the bacteria Proteus vulgaris. The plant also contains polyphenol compounds and flavonoid glycosides. Chromatographic analysis of the acetone extract of the plant revealed the identification of furanosquiterpene (a new natural alcohol), beta-sitosterol, a new natural type of 5-b-cholestane, nervosin, oleanolic acid and ursolic acid.

Properties and medical uses:

Hyssop species have expectorant and anti-inflammatory effects, and are included in the composition of preparations used in the treatment of respiratory diseases. They also have digestive and diuretic effects, are carminative and emmenagogues, and help in wound healing. The antibacterial and antifungal effects of the volatile oil have also been noted. Hyssop species are popularly used as a medicinal tea to treat coughs, asthma, and digestive system diseases. Its decoction or oil is also used topically to treat some skin diseases.

Precautions for use:

The presence of polygon in the volatile oil causes miscarriage in pregnant women, so it is not given during pregnancy.

Environment:

Hyssop species grow wild in poor and degraded rocky lands on the slopes of mountains and mountains, and their cultivation is successful in semi-humid and semi-arid environments with moderate temperatures, and their cultivation is very good in fertile lands.

Cultivation and productivity:

Seeds are planted in the fall by scattering in small areas. One hectare needs 4-5 kg of seeds. The basic mineral fertilizers are added in the fall before planting, and another amount of nitrogen is added after mowing. The plants are mowed in the flowering stage by cutting their stems at a height of 5-10 cm. The amount of green grass production in the first year is estimated at 2.3-2 tons/ha, and in the following years it reaches 8-9 tons/ha. The plants remain in the ground for 5-6 years.

Origanum syriacum L.

Majona srayriaca (L.) Rafin., *Schizocalyx syriacus*)L.(Scheele.

Occurrences : 2,546 occurrences

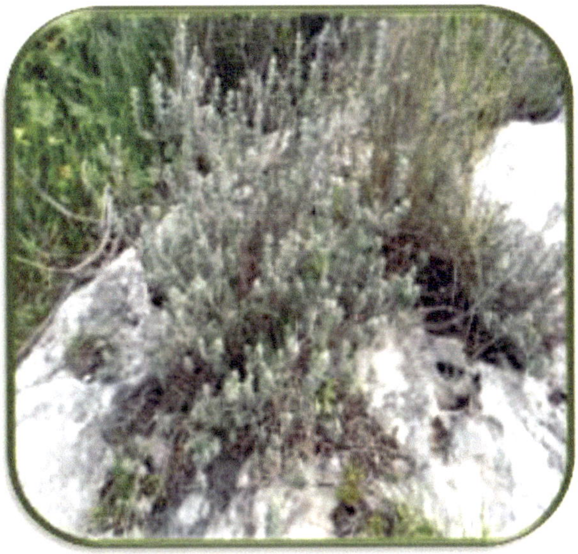

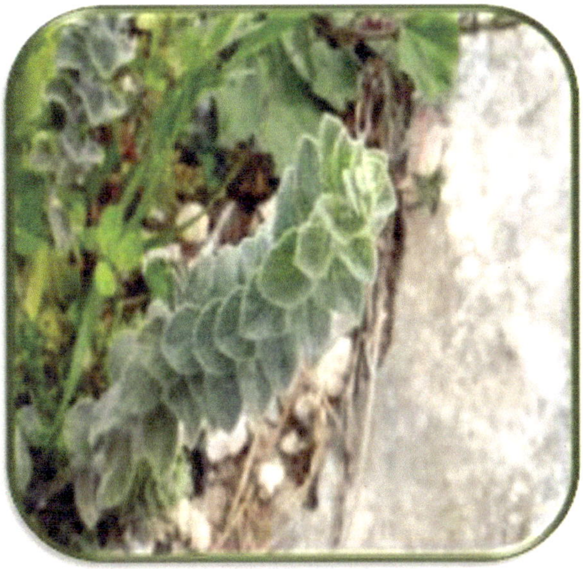

Family: Lamiaceae

Common names: Marjoram, Thyme Khalili, Whirlpool, Basil of the elders, Marroz

Foreign names: Eng. Syrian Marjoran, Fr. Marjolaine de la Syrie

Distribution in the world

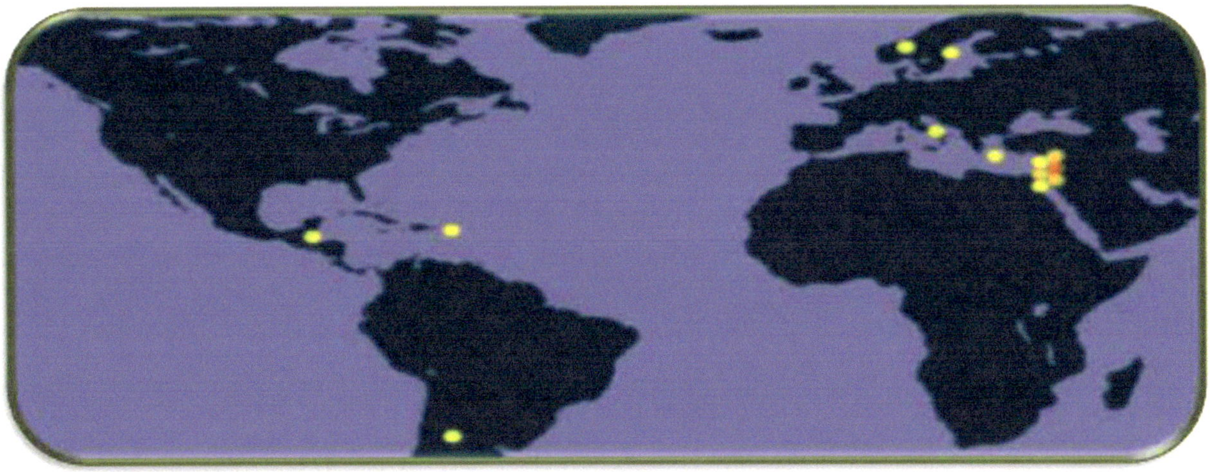

Botanical description:

A small shrub, 30-50 cm tall, covered with woolly to gray hair in addition to glandular hairs. The stem is erect, solid, and branches in a cluster. The leaves are simple, short-spiked to short-spiked, entire-edged, ovate-shaped, blunt-topped, slightly thick, and the nerves of the lower face are prominent. The flowers are accompanied by leaves that are inverted oval to round, overlapping, and their length is equal to the length of the calyx. The inflorescence is semi-ovate, short-branched, and gathered in an oblong spike in its general shape. The calyx is 2.5-2 mm long, its sepals are united in a very short tube, which soon splits from the outside to form a serrated plate. The corolla is white, about 4 mm long, double-lipped, the tube protrudes from the calyx. Stamens 4, prominent, diverging from the base. Ovary bicarpelic, containing 4 ovules. Fruit composed of 4 seeds, smooth, about 1 mm long.

Flowering: April to September.

Homeland and geographical distribution:

Eastern Mediterranean countries. It grows wild in southern Turkey, Syria, Lebanon, Palestine, and rarely in Egypt. It is cultivated in many countries around the world. History and heritage: The scientific name of the genus is derived from the Greek origanos and origanon, which are two names derived from oros meaning "mountain" and gano meaning "shine" or "sparkle" to indicate that it is a beautiful plant that embodies the beauty of mountains. The descriptive name of the species syriacum means "Syrian." Part used: flowering plant, volatile oil extracted from flowering plant.

Chemical components: Volatile oil 2%, phenolic in nature, contains carvacrol 44%, thymol 16%, monoterpene compounds, paracymene 30%, gamma terpinene 4%, monoterpene and a half (sesquiterpene), beta-caryophyllene 2%, in addition to tannins 8%, phenolic acids, including rosmarinic acid, flavonoids, including quercetin.

Properties and medical uses:

Volatile oil of marjoram (components of marjoram) has Phenolic) with antibacterial, antifungal and antiviral properties. Marjoram extract, which contains phenolic compounds and flavonoids, has antioxidant and immunostimulating properties. The drug is rich in essential oils that show antimicrobial, anti-inflammatory, antioxidant and antitumor activity. It can be useful in treating various diseases such as cancer, neurodegenerative disorders and peptic ulcers, which gives it great importance for pharmaceutical and medical purposes. The decoction of the aerial parts is used popularly for its expectorant, carminative, digestive and antispasmodic properties, and to treat inflammation of the mucous membranes of the digestive and respiratory systems (spastic cough, bronchitis, sinusitis and laryngitis), and urinary tract infections. Volatile oil is used topically to treat skin infections, wounds, burns, arthritis, and rheumatic pain.

Food uses:

Khalil thyme is in great demand in the countries of the Eastern Mediterranean, where people are keen to secure their needs of it by collecting it or buying it for food and medical purposes. Thyme leaves are considered a spice that adds taste and flavor, and are used in the preparation of many foods, pastries and sweets. The leaves are the main ingredient in the famous thyme mixture in the Levant.

Other uses:

Research has shown the effectiveness of marjoram oil as an alternative to chemical substances used to combat nematodes such as nematodes, as it has been shown that the compounds carvacrol, thymol and linalool present in the oil have a clear effect in preventing the hatching of nematode eggs.

Experiments have shown the effectiveness of the oil in treating varroa disease that affects honey-producing bees.

Environment:

Hebron thyme grows on mountain slopes In semi-humid and semi-arid environments within the maki and on stony hills. It is considered a long-day plant, and requires high temperatures during its growth period in the summer. It tolerates low temperatures in the winter, and does not tolerate frost for a long period. It grows well in various lands, and prefers yellow, moderately acidic, and calcareous lands, and tolerates drought.

Cultivation and productivity:

It is propagated by seeds, and the seeds are planted in special nurseries At a rate of 100-150 g to obtain seedlings sufficient to plant one hectare, then the seedlings are transferred to the permanent land when they reach the fourth or fifth true leaf stage in early spring. It can also be propagated vegetatively by dividing the mother plant and planting it directly in the permanent land. After that, various service operations are carried out. The plant is encouraged to branch in the first year and prevented from reaching the flowering stage by removing the flower buds before they appear. The first harvest yields 1-1.25 tons of dried leaves, which yields 20-25 kg of aromatic oil.

Origanum vulgare L.

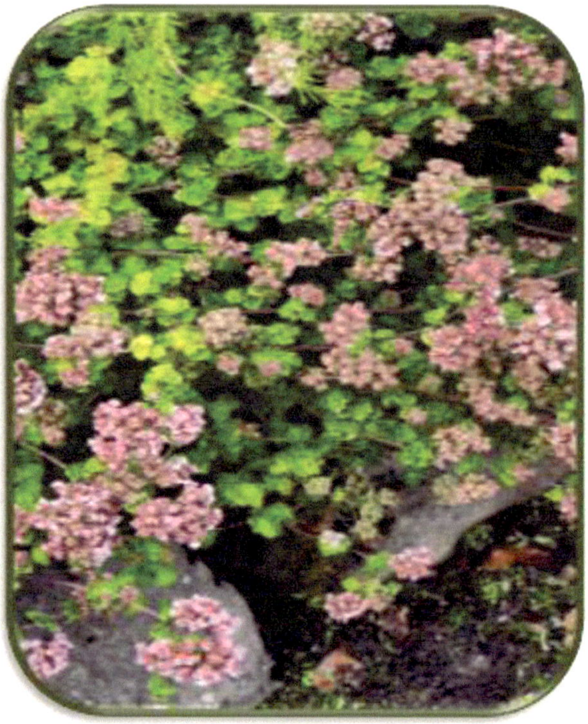

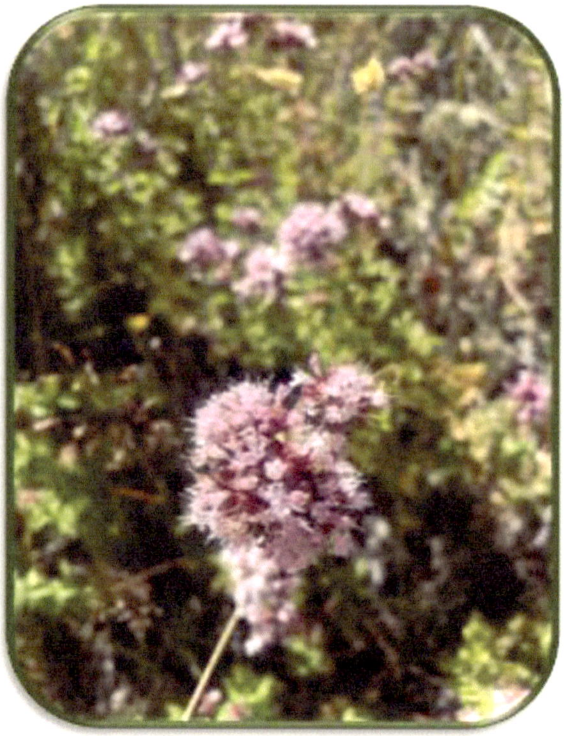

Occurrences :357,668 occurrences

Distribution in the world

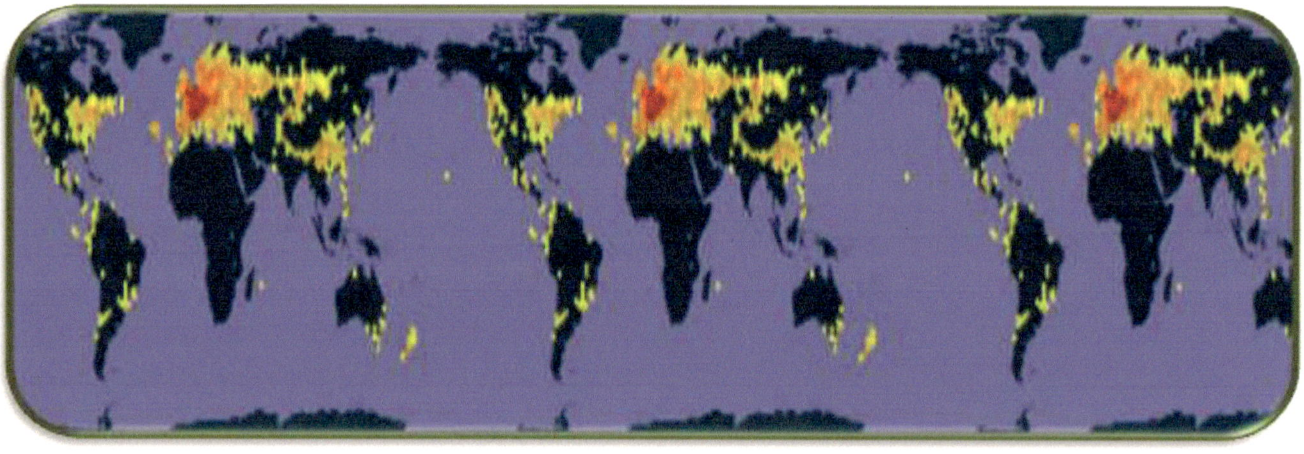

Botanical description:

A species similar to thyme, it is widespread in some Mediterranean countries (France, Italy, Spain). The plant contains a volatile oil rich in phenolic compounds: carvacrol 64%, thymol 4%, tannins, rosmarinic acid, resinous substances, and flavonoids.

Part used: Flowering plant, oil extracted from it.

Properties and medical uses: Similar to those of Syrian marjoram.

Origanum floribundum L.

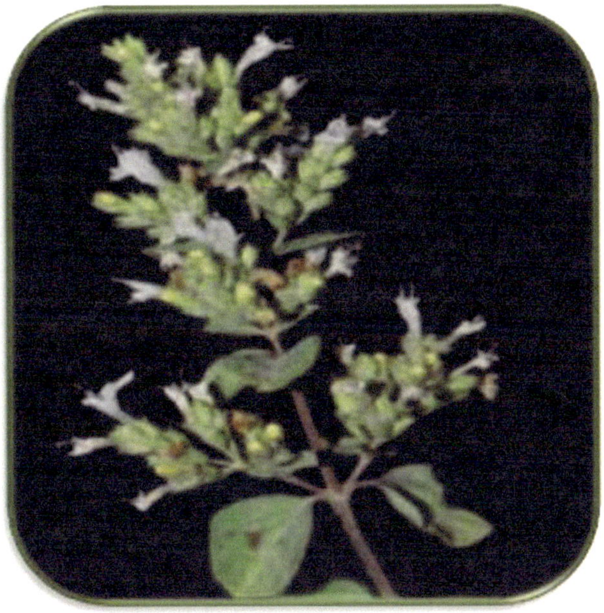
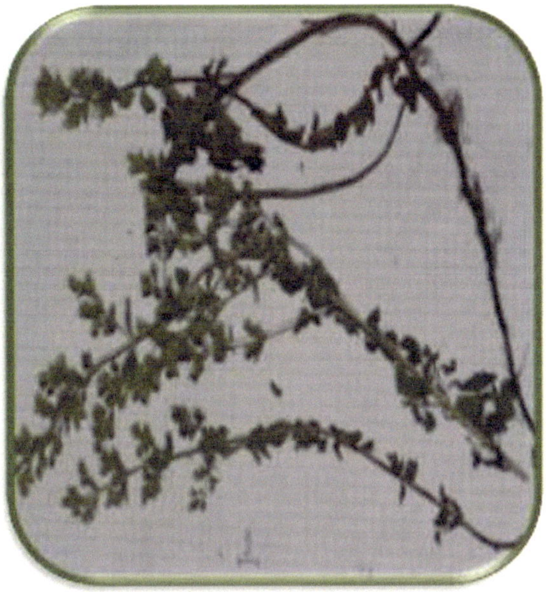

Occurrences : 124 occurrences

Distribution in the world

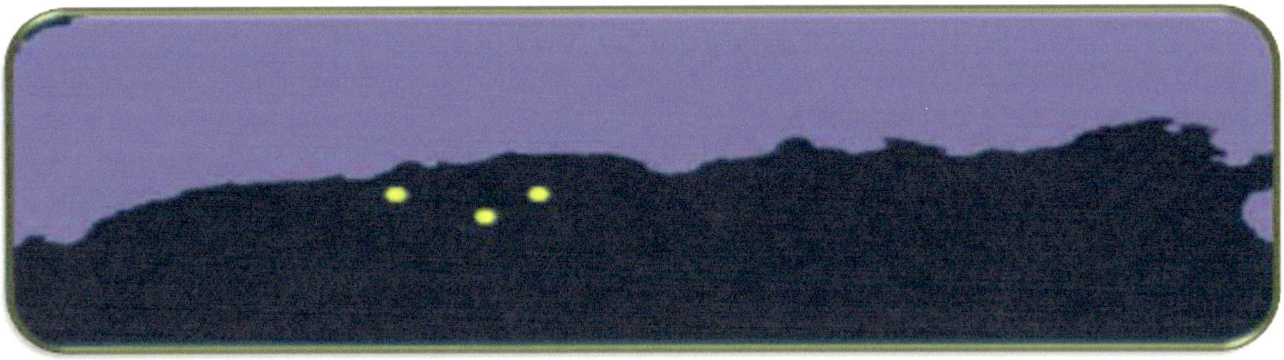

Botanical description:

Widespread in the Maghreb countries, especially in Algeria, the flowering plant contains a volatile oil rich in phenolic compounds (thymol). It is used for its appetite stimulating, antibacterial, stomach and intestinal disinfectant, digestive, antispasmodic, especially cough, and respiratory disinfectant properties.

Phlomis syriaca Boiss.

Occurrences : 71 occurrences

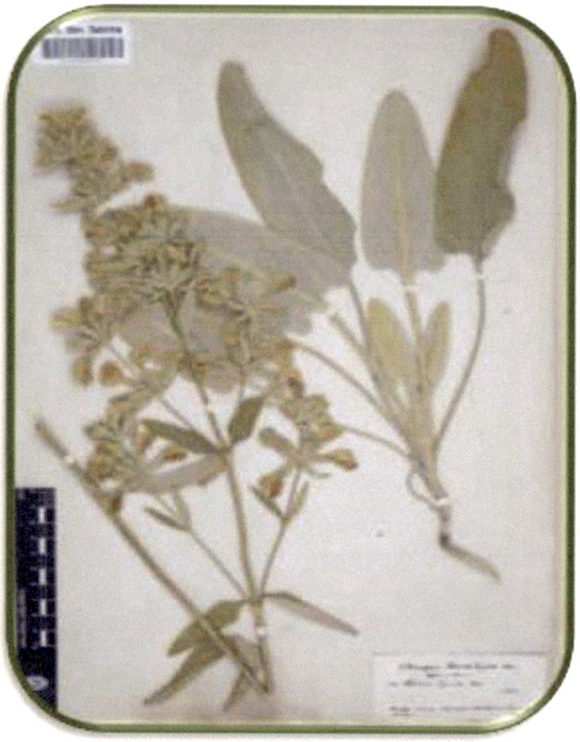

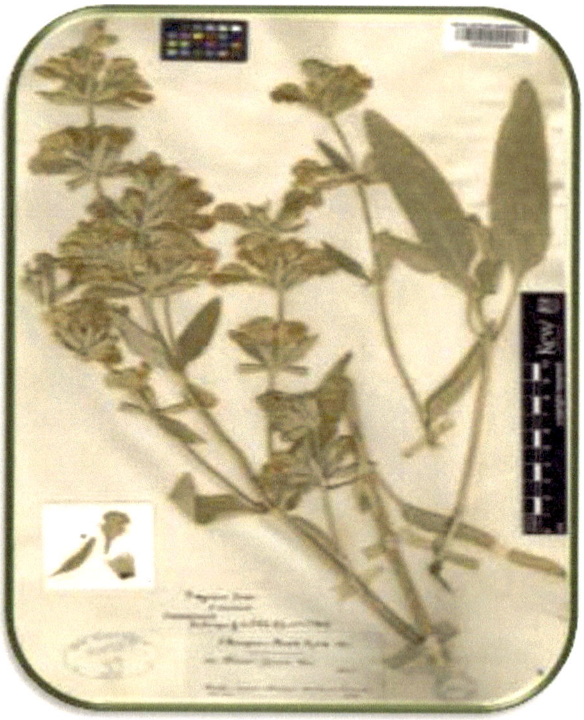

Family: Lamiaceae

Common names: Syrian flame, Nissoli flame

Foreign names: Phlomis Fr. Lampwick, Eng.

Distribution in the world

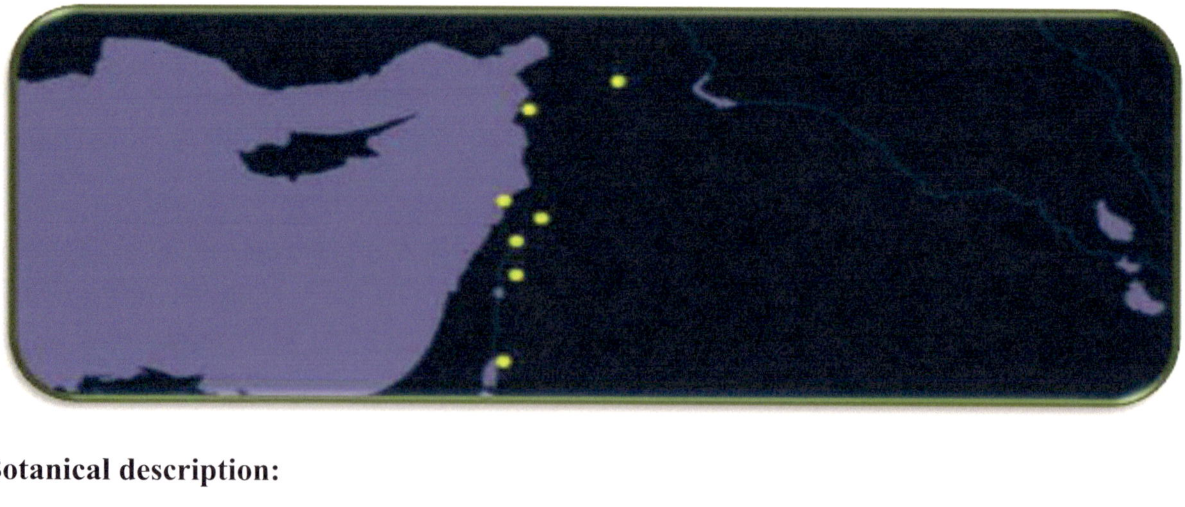

Botanical description:

A small shrub, 50-70 cm tall, yellowish in colour, covered with short felt hairs and star hairs, later becoming semi-growth. Stems erect, slender, simple or branched in the upper part in a pyramidal shape. Leaves are oblong, undivided, thick, stem oblong to lanceolate, base truncated, 1.5-4 x 2.5-10 cm, margin somewhat crinoline, floral leaves as long as whorls or longer. Flowers are gathered in few and widely spaced whorls, each containing 4-6 flowers of the raceme or semi-raceme. Bracts are few, conical, shorter than the calyx, 4-6 mm long. Calyx 5 sepals, 12-15 mm long, tubular with prominent ribs, teeth ovate, sharp-pointed, often ending in short barbs, lower teeth slightly longer than upper teeth. Corolla 5 petals, yellow, twice as long as calyx, tube included in calyx, upper lip shorter than lower, semicircular, downy above. Male dioecious, filaments without appendages. The female is bicarpal, bicameral, divided by a false septum into four chambers, each containing a single ovule. The fruit is ovate, ovate to triangular, smooth or almost smooth.

Flowering: May to June. Habitat and geographical distribution: Iranian-Turanian and Eastern Mediterranean (Amanus Mountains, Syria and Lebanon).

History and heritage:

The scientific name of the genus is derived from the Greek word phlox, meaning "flame" or "torch", referring to the fact that the leaves were used in the past as a wick for lamps. The descriptive name of the species syriaca refers to its distribution in Syria.

Part used: Aerial parts.

Chemical components:

The aerial parts contain several flavonoid glycosides, including: naringen- lamiide, acetoside, luteolin samioside, .in, The most important compounds are iridoids, phenylethanoid glycosides and volatile oils. 21 iridoids, 35 phenylethanoid glycosides and simple phenolic glycosides were identified, including two tetragly- lunarifolioside, physocalycoside, cosidic Quinic acid, Monomeric phenylpropanoids, neolignans and Lignans on the plant. It contains flavonoids, including glycosides chrysoeriol, luteolin, naringenin, methoxyflavonols, kaempferol, megastigmane triterpenoids, glycoside octenol, and acetophenone glycosides

Properties and medical uses:

Research indicates the antioxidant, antitumor, antiseptic and antipyretic properties of acetoside, as well as the antibacterial properties of samioside, and the antiulcer properties of naringenin. Anti-malaria. Syrian flame flowers are included in the composition of some herbal mixtures sold by herbalists in the herbal markets in Syria in the form of natural tea.

Environment:

It grows in semi-arid areas on sunny and stony plateaus and mountain slopes up to an altitude of 1500 m, and also grows in fields and pastures.

Cultivation and productivity:

It is propagated by seeds and division. The plant is generally not cultivated.

Prunella vulgaris L.

Prunella vulgaris subsp. *parviflora* Ehrh.

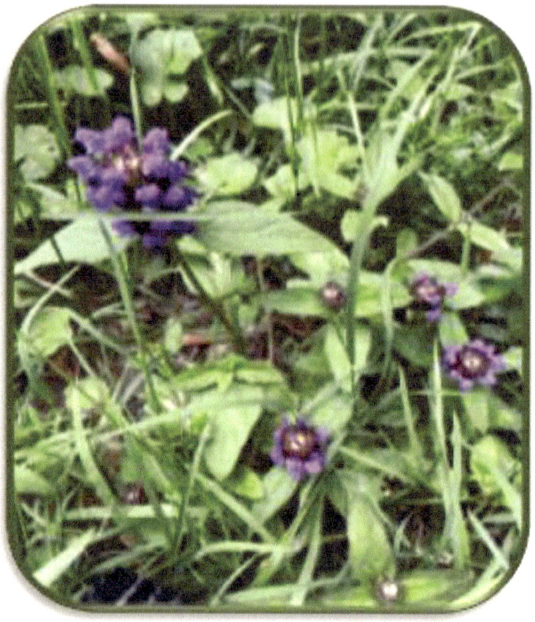

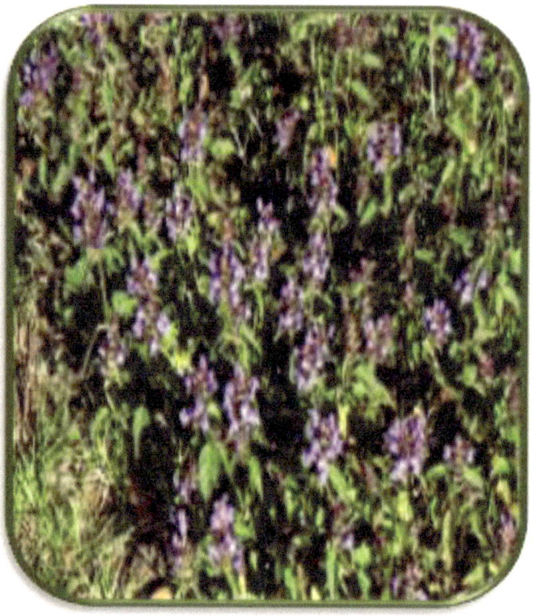

Family: Lamiaceae

Common names: Surgeon's weed, Surgeon's healer, Purple Surgeon's weed, Painkiller

Foreign names: Commune Brunelle Fr. Self-Heal, Eng.

Occurrences :882,490 occurrences

Distribution in the world

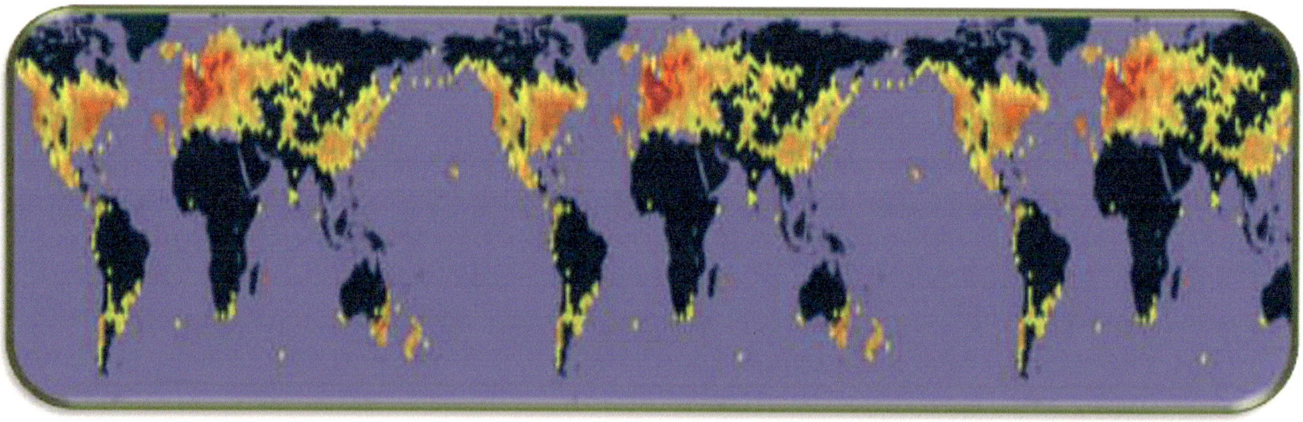

Botanical description:

Perennial herb, bare. Stems ascending, low height (rarely exceeding 15-20 cm),branched from the base, purple to red in color. Leaves are sessile (spikes length 7-25 mm), lanceolate to ovate, entire or slightly serrated, blunt at the apex, truncated or pedicelate at the base, blade dimensions 0.6-2.5×1.5-6 cm, glabrous to sparsely hairy, stem leaves are widely spaced. Inflorescence is spikelet, dense, ovate or oblong, 2-4 cm long, bracts broad, membranous, fringed, rounded, apex suddenly pointed. Calyx about 1 cm, bilipped, compressed and closed during fruit formation, upper lip teeth 3, very short, truncated, pedunculated, lower lip teeth 2, lanceolate. Corolla bilipped, violet, 10-15 mm long, tube slightly prominent, upper lip helmet-shaped, lower lip pendulous. Stamens 4, bipinnate, parallel, filaments ending in straight stigmas. Style bilobed. Fruit: 4 seeds, oblong, smooth, 1-2 mm long.

Flowering: June to August.

Habitat and geographical distribution: Semi-global, spread in Europe and temperate regions.

History and Heritage:

The plant has been known as a medicinal and edible herb for a long time. In Europe, it was said that "this herb is sacred, sent by God to heal all the organs of man and animal." It was also planted in home gardens because they believed that this "expels the devil." It was famous in the past for its properties in healing wounds and stopping bleeding. Its spike flowers were often used to treat mouth and throat infections because it was believed that plants heal the organs they resemble.

Part used: Flowering plant (leaves taste bitter and astringent.)

Chemical components:

bitter principles, flavonoids: hyperoside .rutin, tannins. triterpene saponins. triterpenic acids: ursolic acid, a. oleanolic acid, a. rosmarinic acid. sterol glucosides, volatile oil, candies. Vitamins K (C, B, A), and mineral salts Mg Cu, Ca, K, .

Properties and medical uses:

The plant has antibacterial and antiviral properties. A study has shown that the plant tincture is useful for inhibiting the action of the AIDS virus, and treating other types of viral infections, such as genital herpes virus. The plant has an astringent effect that reduces bleeding, and also reduces diarrhea. The plant is used topically for its astringent properties, as an antiseptic and a hemostatic. Its extracts are used in the form of gargles, creams and compresses to treat chronic ulcers, mouth, gum and throat wounds, burns, boils, bed sores, hemorrhoids and viral skin infections. The plant has great medical importance in treating throat diseases, colds and headaches, as the plant is boiled, the steam is inhaled, and a bath is made for women after childbirth, and in treating herpetic keratitis. It is used as an antibiotic, a blood pressure reducer, a fever reducer, a diuretic, an anti-rheumatic, anti-bacterial, antioxidant, and a worm repellent. It is also used in treating wounds and ulcers. The aqueous extract contains an active substance against HIV, which is the compound Pronlin, which is a polysaccharide and has an anti-herpes simplex virus effect. The aqueous extract of this herb prevents anaphylactic shock and allergic reactions. The plant protects the red blood cells of mice from hemolysis, protects the kidneys, and protects the brain against peroxide lipids. It contains a high percentage of rosmarinic acid, which makes the plant more suitable for use in its therapeutic applications. The plant has been widely used recently for its good taste and nutritional value, as it contains a good percentage of carbohydrates, proteins and fats. Analyses also confirm the high values of carbohydrates, fats and proteins. The plant contains good amounts of antibacterial phenols.

The plant is effective in treating typhoid fever and other bacterial infections, especially those caused by bacteria Escherichia coli, Bacillus typhi, and Mycobacterium tuberculli. Traditional healers in

Kashmir prescribe inhaling the steam of this herb to remove phlegm from the chest cavity and brain, thus reducing chest infections and headaches. It is common in Kashmir to use it as a decoction for bathing a month after childbirth. Traditional healers consider it a brain tonic that can give the head the ability to endure, and it works as a disinfectant and removes the general weakness of the mother's body. The herb also contains saponins, which are used to stop bleeding and treat wounds and ulcers, as they help in the clotting of red blood cells. It has also been used by nursing mothers to treat cracked nipples. Other secondary metabolites are alkaloids with analgesic, antispasmodic and antibacterial effects.

Other uses:

The leaves of the plant are eaten fresh or cooked, as part of salad or soup, and a refreshing tea is made from its dried or fresh leaves, which is a tonic for the body, a digestive that stimulates the liver and purifies it from toxins.

Environment:

The plant grows in neglected lands, meadows and on the edges of forests. It prefers alkaline and moderate soils. It is planted in moist soils in sunny or partially shaded places.

Cultivation and productivity:

Propagated by seeds. Seeds are scattered in the spring in the nursery or in greenhouse conditions, and when the seedlings reach a suitable size, they are transferred to bags or pots at a rate of one seedling per pot, and transferred to the permanent soil at the beginning of summer. Seeds may be scattered directly in the permanent soil if a sufficient quantity of them is available. The plant is propagated by division in the spring or autumn. Divided plants are planted directly in the permanent ground if they are large enough, or left in the nursery for some time if they are small. The plant blooms at different times depending on the climate and other conditions, mostly in the summer. The plant can sometimes become a weed that is difficult to get rid of.

Salvia rosmarinus Spenn.

Rosmarinus oficinalis L., *Rosmarinus angustifolius* Mill., *Rosmarinus latifolius* Mill., *Rosmarinus communis* Noronha, *Rosmarinus oficinalis* var. *angustifolius*) Mill.(DC., *Rosmarinus laxiflorus* de Noé.

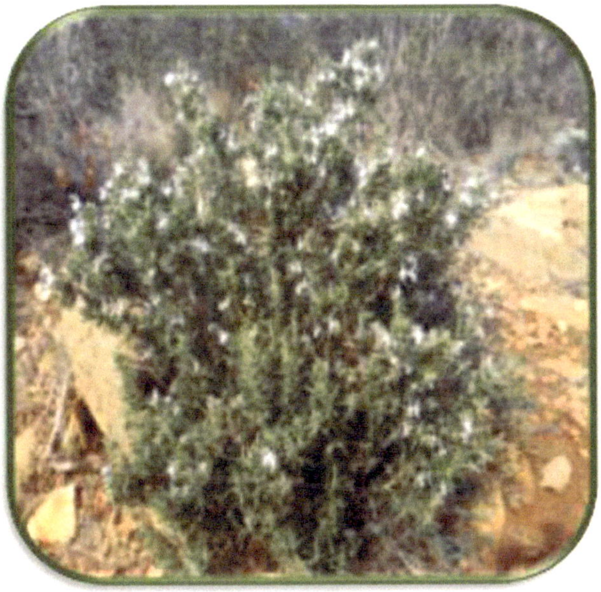 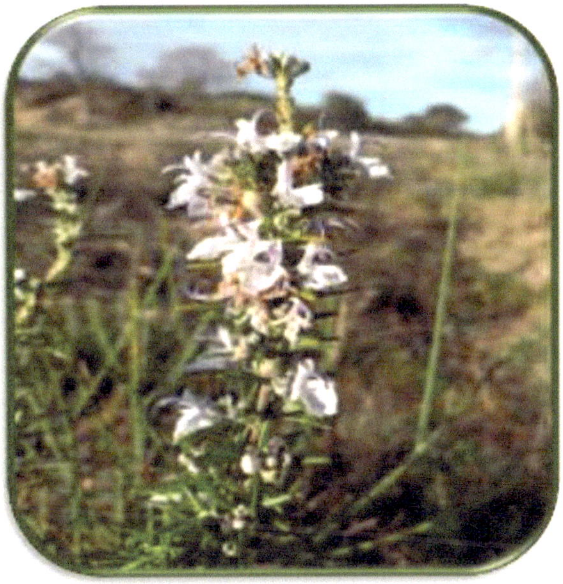

Family: Lamiaceae.

Common names: Rosemary, Rosemary, Rosemary.

Foreign names: Rosmarin Fr. Rosemary, Eng.

Occurrences : 413,879 occurrences

Distribution in the world

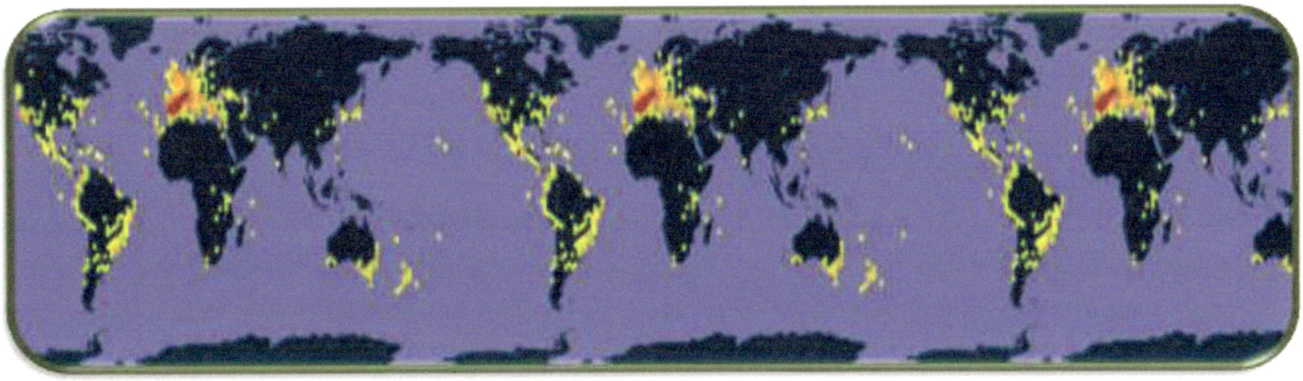

Botanical description:

A perennial, evergreen, woody, vigorous shrub. Many branches, 50-150 cm long. Leaves are aromatic, linear, The leaflets are entire, their margins are completely curled downwards. The main nerve is prominent on the lower surface and sunken on the upper surface, The upper surface is hairy, while the old ones are bare. Flowers semi- 2-3 cm long, 3-4 mm wide. Young leaves Pedunculate, blue or violet, rarely white, gathered in short racemes, calyx 5 sepals united, Villiform. Corolla bilipped, lower lip relatively large, deeply divided into two parts. Male Bilipped, of two stamens protruding from the corolla, the other two reduced to bracts. Fruit tetraechinoid, brown.

Flowering: February to September.

The species shows great variation, and many chemically distinct cultivars and genotypes have been identified. The plant is used to treat blood pressure problems, loss of appetite, and digestive disorders (in case of spasm, it helps relax the smooth muscles lining the digestive tract.) It helps in treating Alzheimer's disease. The decoction of the plant or its volatile oil is used topically to stimulate blood circulation and treat rheumatism, and in the form of compresses to cleanse and treat wounds, repair skin tissues and eczema, relieve muscle pain, nervous exhaustion and sciatica. The plant is currently considered one of the most promising herbal medicines due to its antioxidant, anti-inflammatory and antimicrobial pharmaceutical properties, and to treat inflammatory and infectious skin diseases, wound healing and anti-skin cancer. It has been used medicinally to treat claw edema in rats or mice, acute liver injury, and asthma. The aqueous extract was given by gavage, intraperitoneal, and orally. The most evaluated biomarkers were tumor necrosis factor, interleukin, myeloperoxidase, catalase, glutathione, glutathione peroxidase, malondialdehyde, and superoxide dismutase. The plant has great medical importance due to the presence of A diverse group of interesting specialized metabolites, particularly mono-, di-, hemi-, tri-, and tetraterpenes (mono-, di-, sester-, and tri-sesquiterpenes), as well as phenylpropanoids, phenolic acid derivatives, flavonoids, alkaloids, C23-terpenoids, C25-sesterterpenoids, and C30-triterpenoids (dammarane and uncommon triterpenoids) C20 + C10

Food and cosmetic uses:

Rosemary is used as an appetite stimulant and flavoring. The volatile oil is used in many food products (beverages and meats) to give them taste and smell and preserve them for a long time without spoiling or rotting. The volatile oil is used in cosmetics, inexpensive perfumes, shampoos and hair-strengthening soaps.

Precautions for use:

Rosemary is considered a safe herb for use by adults, except for pregnant or breastfeeding women. Rosemary is considered safe if used in the exact recommended doses.

Environment:

The plant grows wild on highlands and near forests in semi-humid and humid climates found in temperate and warm regions. It tolerates low temperatures at night down to zero, but its growth is greatly weakened or stops in this case. The species loves light and sun. It is grown in agricultural or forestry mountainous soils or on hills with light, well-drained, calcareous and yellow soil. It tolerates high salinity, so it is seen on sea coasts, and tolerates winds.

Cultivation and productivity:

The plant is propagated by seeds that are planted directly in the ground, or germinated in special beds from late winter until early summer, and when they become the appropriate length, they are transferred to permanent land. It is preferable to propagate it by root cuttings or by division at the beginning of spring. The cuttings are taken from one-year-old branches, 10-15 cm long, and contain at least 3 buds. They are then rooted in special beds for a week, and then transferred to the permanent ground. They are planted in the upper third of the line with a distance of 60-70 cm between each plant and are watered well. Fertilizers improve production. The plant blooms in spring, and again in autumn. The plants are harvested during the period from April to September starting from the second year at a height of 25-30 cm, then dried. The hectare yields 2.5-6 tons of dry grass and up to 60-70 kg of aromatic oil.

Salvia officinalis L.

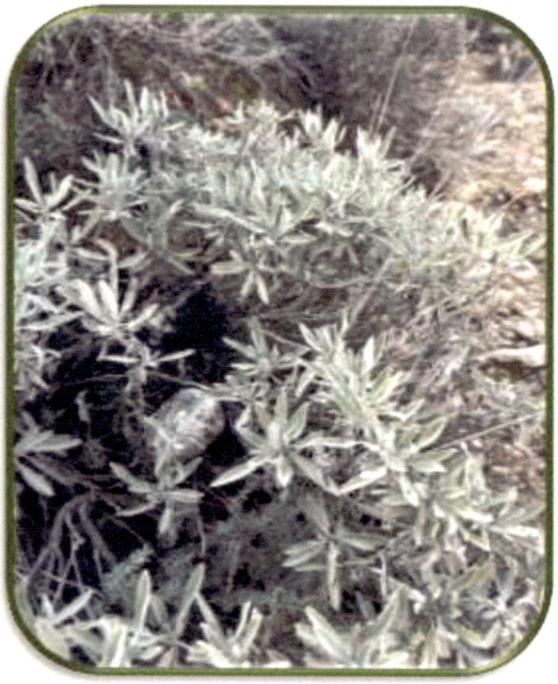

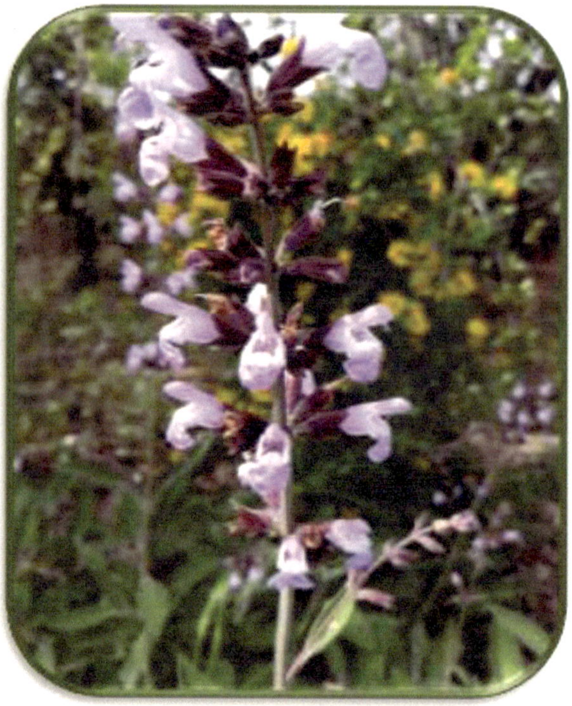

Family: Lamiaceae

Common names: Sage, Salvia officinalis, Salvia officinalis, Soft-skinned

Foreign names: Sauge Fr. Sage, Eng.

Occurrences : 31,490 occurrences

Distribution in the world

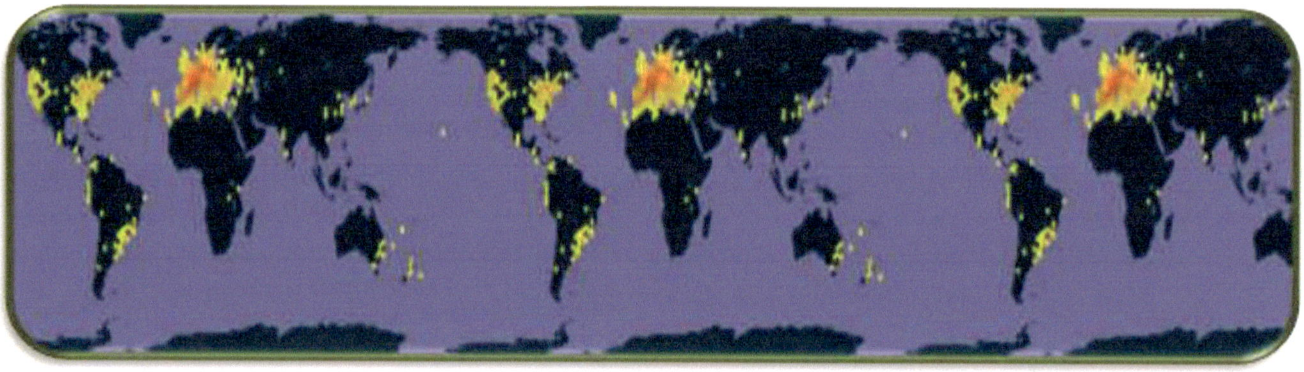

Botanical description:

A perennial shrub with strong growth, the stems are herbaceous but their bases are woody, erect, highly branched, velvety hairs, square section, its height reaches about a meter, and these branches dry up every year. The leaves are thick, distinctively aromatic, opposite, pendulous in the lower part of the stem, and petiolate in the upper part, oblong, elliptic or oval in shape, grayish green in color, due to the abundance of cotton hairs on their lower surface, the length of the blade is 8-1 cm, and its width is 35-8 mm, its base is rounded or semi-cut, the edge is crest-like. Flowers about 2 cm long, violet or blue, gathered in whorls, each containing 1-18 flowers, forming a spike-like inflorescence. Their length is 4-18 cm. The upper flower bracts are oval, pointed at the apex. The flower stalk is about 3 mm. The calyx is about 1 cm, becoming 1.5 cm in the fruit, two-lipped, hairy. The corolla is two-lipped. Male bi-stamens, the junction between the two anthers is about 3 mm long, the arms are equal. Fruit 4-spherical, brown, about 2.5 mm in diameter.

Flowering: April to June.

Homeland and geographical distribution: North Africa, Central and Southern Europe, widely cultivated in many countries.

Chemical components:

The leaves contain 0.08% volatile oil, which may reach 3.3%, which contains a high percentage of thujon, in addition to cineole, camphor, and borneol. Hydroxycinnamic acid derivatives, rosmarinic acid, and chlorigenic acid. Diterpenes, including carnosolic acid and rosmanol. Flavonoids, including Glucosides Apigenin and luteolin. Diterpene compounds of the abietan type, including salvin, lactone carnosol (Pikrosalvin) found particularly in dried or preserved plants. Triterpene compounds such as ursolic acid, ole-anolic acid, in addition to traces of mineral elements such as iron, magnesium and zinc.

Properties and medical uses:

Most of the plant's properties are due to its volatile oil content, which has antibacterial, antifungal, antiviral, antiperspirant, antihypertensive, stimulates bile secretion, and is a smooth muscle spasmolytic. It has a central stimulant effect, antidiabetic activity, and anti-edema activity. The oil is used topically as a gargle to treat inflammation of the mucous membranes of the mouth, throat, and gums (swollen or bleeding gums), and internally it is used in cases of loss of appetite, indigestion, excessive sweating, and hyperventilation. The plant is popularly used to treat diarrhea, gastritis (inflammation of the stomach lining), excessive or irregular milk flow from the breast, menstrual pain, and muscle spasms.

It is used to treat microbial infections, diabetes, cancer, and as an antioxidant, antimicrobial, and antibacterial. The essential oil distilled in the flowering stage showed inhibitory effects on amylase, glucosidase, lipase, lipoxygenase enzymes, and antibacterial. The essential oil has shown bactericidal effect on Listeria monocytogenes, Staphylococcus aureus, Salmonella typhimurium, Escherichia coli, Proteus mirabilis, Bacillus subtilis.

Pharmaceutical forms:

Sage is available in the form of dried and fresh leaves, fresh flower parts, and oils extracted from flowers and stems.

Other uses: It is used as a food flavoring and fragrance in soaps and perfumes.

Side effects, interactions and precautions for use:

Possible side effects of sage include stomatitis, epileptic seizures and skin irritation. Sage should be avoided with blood sugar-lowering medications, insulin, anti-narcotics (antabuse), and medications that affect epileptic seizures. Pregnant or breastfeeding women should also avoid using the plant.

Environment:

The plant prefers sunny areas and moist, well-drained soils, and is affected by heavy and acidic soils. It tolerates relative drought, but is affected by frost.

Cultivation and productivity:

The plant is easily propagated by seeds, when the temperature is 15-21° C. It can be propagated by cuttings.

Salvia fruticosa Mill.

Salvia triloba L. fil, *S. libanotica* Boiss. Et Gaill.

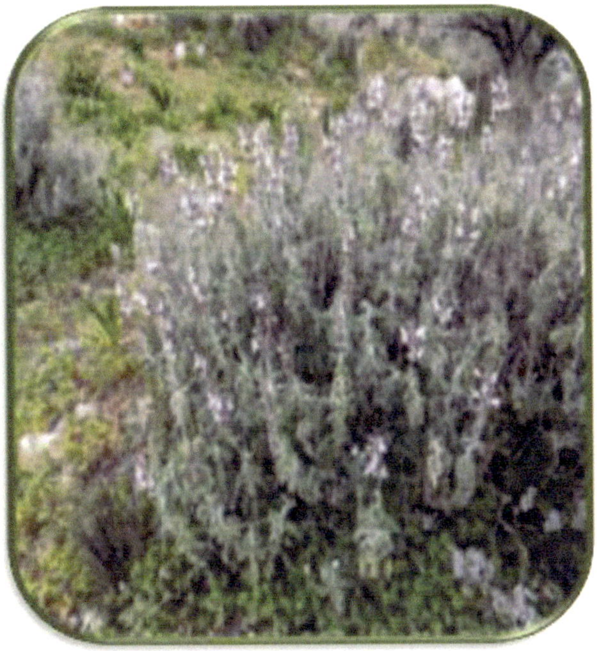

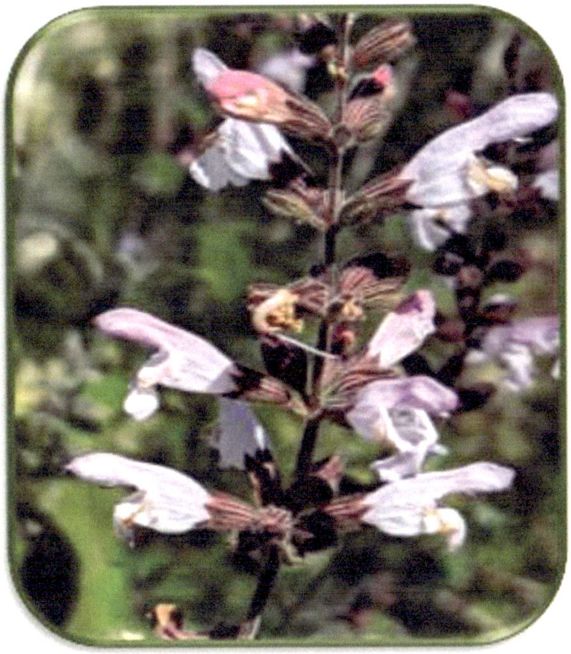

Family: Lamiaceae

Common names: Sage, Trilobite sage.

Foreign names: Sauge Fr. Sage, Greek Eng.

Occurrences : 3,078 occurrences

Distribution in the world

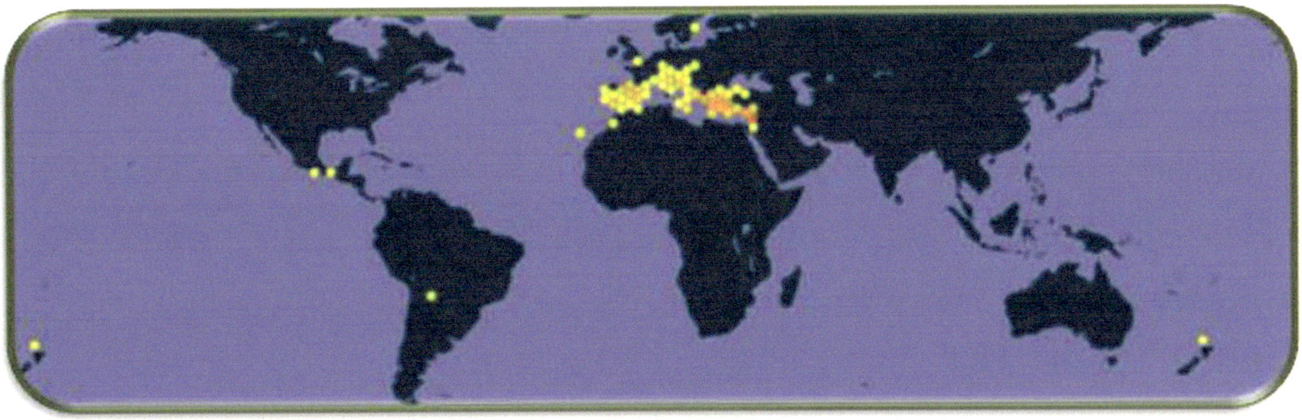

Botanical description:

A small shrub, densely covered with a woolly or pubescent hair. Stems are thick, square in section. Leaves are simple, petiolate, crest-shaped, the upper surface is more hairy than the lower surface, the base is heart-shaped or truncated, ovate-oblong to lanceolate, and in most parts of the plant are three-lobed as a result of the presence of two widely spaced lobes at the base. The floral leaves are short, pointed. The flowers are gathered in cymose inflorescences, located in whorls on the branches of the stem, and their group forms a cluster or panicle inflorescence, sticky and compact. Flower bracts short, membranous, pendulous. Calyx hairy, glabrous, semi-bilipped, triangular in teeth. Corolla pale violet, 21-81 mm long. Male stamens two. Ovary bicarpelic, tetracameral. Fruit 4 seeds. Some individuals lack lateral lobes at leaf base.

Flowering: February to July.

Homeland and geographical distribution: Folded in Greece, Albania, Cyprus, Turkey and Syria. Mediterranean

History and heritage:

The scientific name of the genus is derived from the Greek word salvare, meaning "healed", referring to the healing qualities attributed to some species of the genus. The descriptive name of the species triloba means "three-lobed leaves." Part used: Leaves (the leaves of wild plants are collected once a year, while the leaves of cultivated plants in the fields are collected three times a year), flowers, and the volatile oil extracted from them.

Chemical components: Volatile oil, the most important of which is cineol.

Medical properties and uses:

The cineol compound has antimicrobial properties. The plant has properties that lower blood pressure, resolve spasms, and lower blood sugar. It is an analgesic and sedative. Its extract is used as a gargle and mouthwash. The decoction of the plant is popularly used to treat diabetes, heart and lung diseases. It is used externally to treat skin infections. Plant extracts play a role in reducing nerve inflammation characteristic of Alzheimer's disease. Treatment of mice with plant extracts led to a significant improvement in biochemical parameters, as well as methanolic extracts, which have anti-neuro-inflammatory activities that characterize Alzheimer's disease.

Environment:

It is found in the maqui and agaric (similar to maqui but less high and dense) areas within Mediterranean forests, preferring sunny locations and sandy soils. Nitrogen-rich soils encourage abundant vegetative growth at the expense of flowering.

Cultivation and productivity:

The plant is propagated by seeds that are scattered in bags or pots in the nursery at the beginning of spring. Germination takes place within two weeks. After the seedlings reach a suitable size, they are transferred to the permanent soil at the beginning of summer. The plant can also be propagated by semi-woody cuttings during the growing season.

Teucrium polium L.

Chamaedrys polium (L.) Raf.

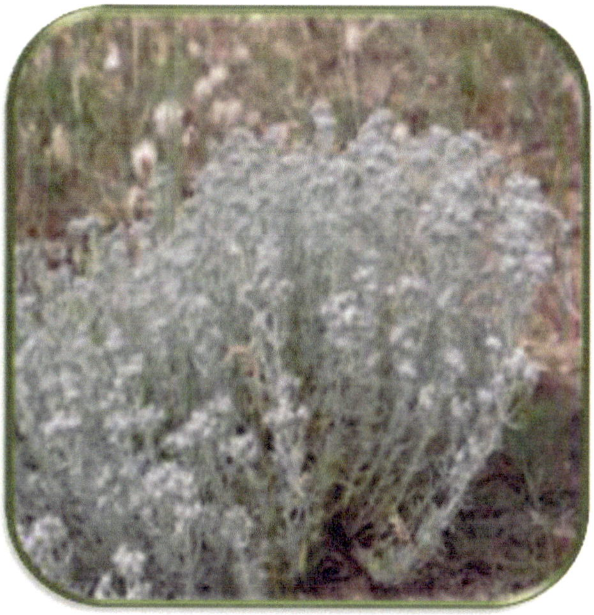

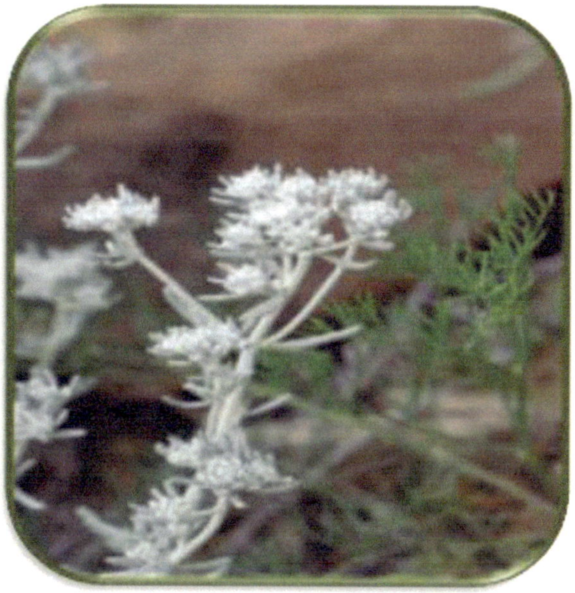

Family: Lamiaceae (Labiatae)

Common names: Grey curly, ryegrass

Foreign names: Germand golden, Germandrée tomenteuse

Occurrences : 40,0038 occurrences

Distribution in the world

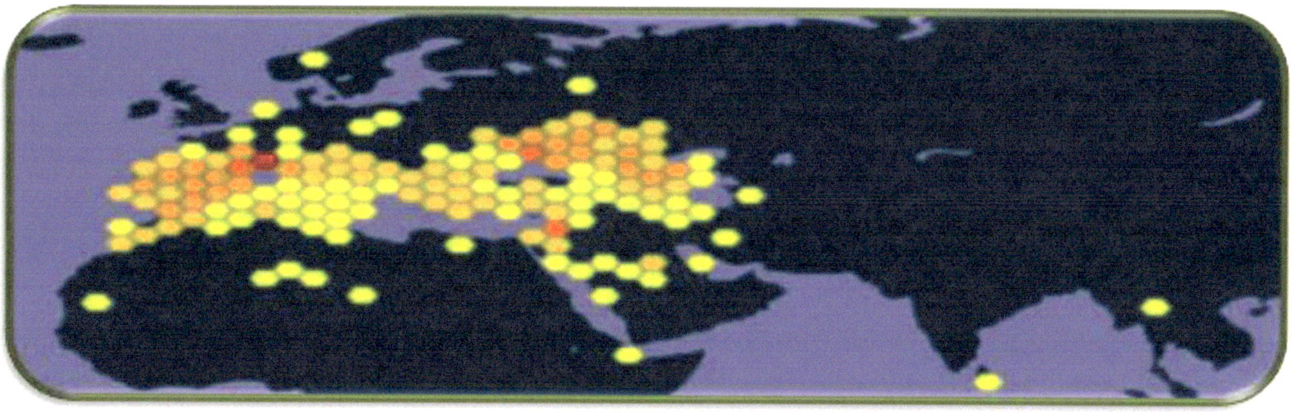

Botanical description:

A small shrub, 20-40 cm tall, covered with dense grey down, or white woolly hair, branching from the base. The branches are cylindrical, tapering at both ends, ascending to erect, 10-35 cm long, each ending in a comb or panicle inflorescence. Leaves are simple, oblong, oblong to linear, blunt at the apex, crenulate, strongly curled downwards, rarely flat, 1-3 cm long. Floral leaves are linear-oblong, also strongly curled, shorter than flowers. Flowers are hermaphrodite, bisymmetrical, gathered in dense whorls to form spherical to ovate heads, short panicles. Flowers are semi-oblong. Calyx densely hairy or woolly, about 4 mm long, bell-shaped, five-toothed, hidden in hairs. Corolla white to cream-coloured, apparently single-lipped, rapidly falling, consisting of a tube remaining embedded in the calyx, and a prominent, broad, flattened, five-lobed blade. Male bisexual, stamens projecting slightly from corolla. The female is bicarpal, bicameral, divided by a false septum into four chambers, each containing a single ovule. The fruit is tetracarpal, the ovule is inverted oval in shape.

Flowering: April to August.

Habitat and geographical distribution: Mediterranean and western Iran-Turanian.

History and heritage:

The scientific name of the genus is the Greek and Latin name for these plants and literally means "Trojan herb." The descriptive name of the species polium From the Greek polios meaning: "shiny gray-white."

Part used: Flowering plant

Chemical components:

Volatile oil 0.1 (-1)% rich in terpene and alcohol compounds (pinene), ß α, cedrenol, linalool, α-cadinol, α-hu- mulene, ß-caryophyllene, oxide caryophyllene terpine-4-ol, germacrene D D, etc.)..

Diterpenes compounds vary according to the source, including: picropolin, picropolinol, picropolinon, teucrin, montanines, tubulins, gnaphalidin.

Flavonoids: apigenin, luteolin, acacetine, cirsiliol, eupatorin, cirsimaritin, .salvigenin iridoid glycosides, including: harpagide, teucardoside, ß-sitosterol, stigmasterol, campesterol, brassicasterol, including sterols, sugars (glucose, fructose) tannins.

Medical properties and uses:

Research has proven the effectiveness of the aqueous extract of the aerial parts, which contain flavonoids, in reducing blood sugar levels, although this has not been proven clinically in a definitive manner. Animal experiments have shown positive indications of a reduction in ulcers after using the drug. The aqueous extract of the leaves and stems (flavonoids) has antioxidant properties (preventing the oxidation of beta-carotene, for example). Research has also shown the effectiveness of the leaf extract in reducing blood pressure. Research indicates the properties of the plant extract in reducing cholesterol (by approximately 40%) and triglycerides in mice. The volatile oil of the flowering plant has antispasmodic properties that help relieve digestive disorders accompanied by fever and diarrhea. The drug has antibacterial and antifungal properties (volatile oil, flavonoids, sterols). The plant extract is used topically as an antiseptic, in the treatment of skin infections, wounds and gingivitis. Boiled sage is popularly used as a diuretic, diaphoretic, antipyretic, and blood sugar lowering agent, and in the treatment of intestinal inflammation and ulcers.

The plant has been used since ancient times as an insecticide and to combat malaria. Traditionally, Palestinians have used hot water extracts of the plant's leaves for centuries to treat intestinal and heart disorders. The infusion of the leaves is drunk after each meal because of its antispasmodic and antidiarrheal effects. Also known in traditional Palestinian veterinary medicine as "Sibyan", it is used orally on sheep, cows and goats to treat diarrhea, colic, scabies and flatulence. The powder of the leaves is applied to the skin as a poultice to treat scabies. A standard decoction of 50 g of the plant leaves is prepared and taken orally, in an amount of 100 ml, three times/day to treat kidney and liver diseases, diabetes, stomach and intestinal pain, and inflammation. The aerial parts of the plant or the infusion of the young leaves are used by the Bedouins to treat fever, stomach and intestinal disorders, and as a worm repellent. The plant is also used in steam baths to treat colds and fever. It has been used in Saudi Arabia and Jordan to treat several diseases such as inflammation, pain, diabetes, kidney stones, cancer, fever, and rheumatism. It was found that there is a direct relationship between the antioxidant activity of the plant and its content of β-caryophyllene.

The effect of the plant on cancer cells was linked to the presence of a mixture of compounds α-bisabolol and (+) epi-bicy- closesquiphellandrene from the oil extracted from the plant or to compounds α-humulene-(caryophyllene, δ-cadinene, caryophyllene oxide, α-cadinol) in the leaves.

Precautions for use:

Long-term use of the drug in large quantities may cause hepatitis that appears in the form of jaundice and other symptoms. It has prevented Its use in France, for example, is due to these symptoms.

Environment: The plant grows on sandy steppe lands and dry stony slopes. It prefers sunny locations and neutral and alkaline lands. It is one of the species that indicate the deterioration of the vegetation cover and overgrazing. It grows in diverse habitats from coastal sandy areas to mountains and inland plateaus.

Cultivation and productivity:

The plant is propagated by seeds that are scattered in the spring in the nursery, and covered with a thin layer of soil. They are transferred to small pots after germination, then transferred to the permanent land after a year. The plant can be propagated by semi-woody cuttings or by division. In the latter case, the divided plants are planted directly in the permanent land if they are large, or left in the nursery until the following year if they are small, which is better.

Thymus syriacus Boiss.

Origanum syriacum)Boiss.(Kuntze.

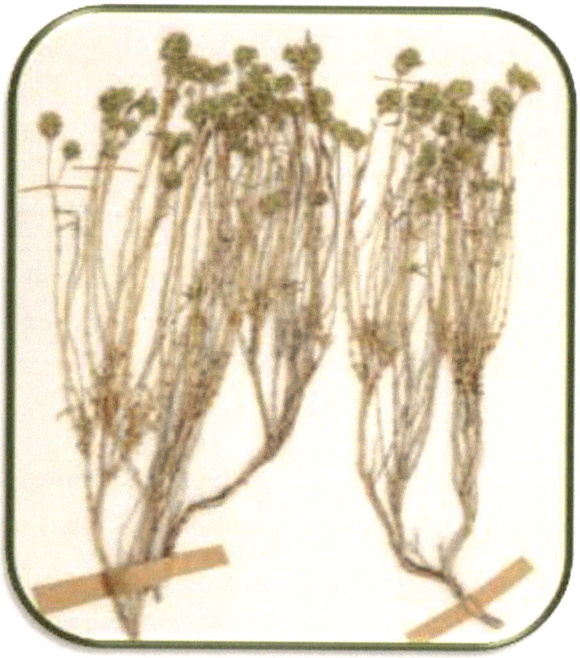

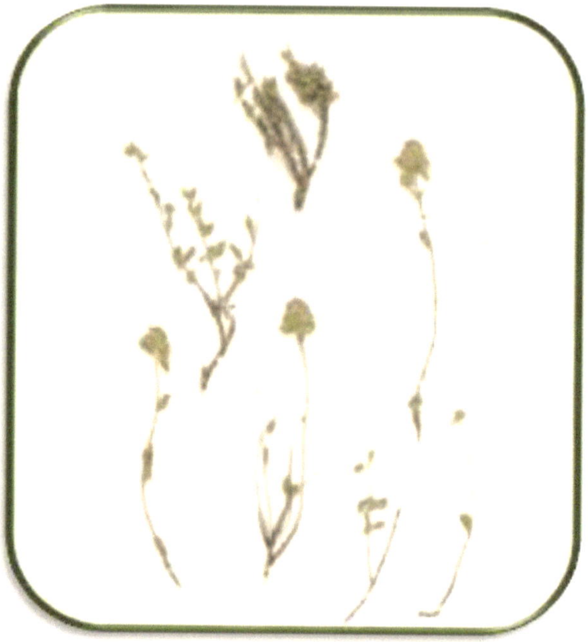

Family: Lamiaceae

Common names: Syrian thyme

Foreign names: Syrie de Thyme Fr. Thyme Eng.

Occurrences : 64 occurrences

Distribution in the world

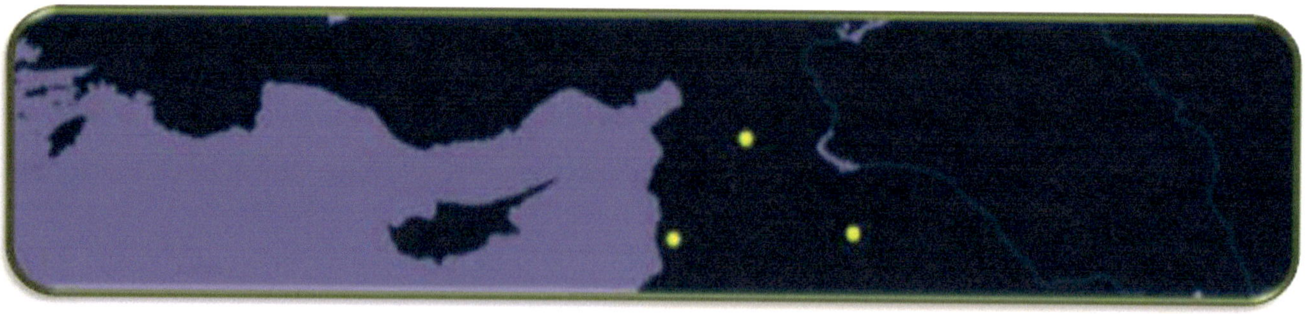

Botanical description:

A small shrub, varying in size, 30-50 cm long. The branches are erect, woody to varying degrees, hard, leafy, white and downy. The leaves are flat, hard, erect to flat, linear to lanceolate, sharp at the tip, abundantly covered with glands secreting volatile oils, 1-3 cm in size, distinctive. The flowers are gathered in dense terminal inflorescences, oval to semi-cylindrical in shape, 1-3 cm in size. The bracts are ovate-oblong, slightly pubescent. The corolla is white, composed of 5-7 nerves, equal in length to the calyx. The calyx is 6-7 mm, bilipped, a tube projecting slightly beyond the calyx, and splitting into two lips, the upper lip oblong, broad, and three-toothed, the lower lip two-toothed. Stamens 4. The fruit is an ovate or oblong-oblong acorn, short.

Flowering: June to October.

Habitat and geographical distribution:

Eastern Mediterranean regions, mainly distributed in Syria, Lebanon and Jordan.

History and heritage:

The scientific name of the genus is the ancient Greek and Latin name for a number of small plants from the Lamiaceae family, and is descended from the ancient Egyptian language tham, which is the poison of a plant that was used in the mummification process. The descriptive name of the species syriacus means "Syrian." Types of thyme have been known and used since ancient times, and Dioscorides described it in his treatments. Thyme was used as an antidote to snake venom and marine life venom, and the Romans used to burn it to treat headaches. It was introduced because they believed that its smoke repels scorpions. Pliny described wild thyme decoction in 77 AD. Types of thyme have been used in the pharmaceutical industry since the sixteenth century.

Part used: Flowering plant

Chemical components:

The flowering aerial parts contain volatile oil (1.3–1.7%) rich in phenolic compounds that may reach 70% carvacrol (thymol), paracymene (13%), terpinene, caryophyllene, dihydrocarvone, linalool, flavonoids and tannins.

Properties and medical uses:

The flowering plant has antioxidant, antiseptic and antibacterial properties, especially against Gram-negative bacteria and fungi. Experiments have proven its cleansing effect on the intestines from parasites, worms and colon bacteria. A decoction of the leaves and flowers is used popularly as a laxative and expectorant that is useful in treating dry cough, bronchitis, asthma, digestive disorders (antispasmodic, carminative, and for treating gastritis and peptic ulcers), urinary tract and bladder infections. The decoction of the plant is used topically in the form of gargles to treat inflamed gums, inflammation of the membranes lining the mouth and throat, and the volatile oil is used as a massage to reduce rheumatic pain, gout, arthritis, and to disinfect wounds.

Food uses:

Syrian thyme is used as an appetizing spice, and is often used in Syrian, Jordanian, and Lebanese cuisine, where it is added to many foods and pastries to give them a distinctive flavor. Young tender shoots are added to pickled olives, and a mixture of green shoots is prepared after drying and grinding them with the addition of sesame, sumac, etc. and eaten with olive oil as part of the breakfast meal in the Syrian kitchen.

Environment: It grows on sunny, stony, and limestone highlands in dry, semi-dry, and semi-humid areas.

Cultivation and productivity:

Thyme is propagated by seeds. Then the seedlings are planted in lines, 45-60 cm apart. It can be propagated by root cuttings. It needs irrigation if it is planted as an economic crop. The plant responds to mineral fertilization with essential elements. The vegetative mass is harvested once during the flowering stage and again after two months, dried in the shade for a week, then packed. If the goal is nutritional, the vegetative mass is harvested while tender and soft before flowering.

Thymus vulgaris L.

Origanum thymus Kuntze, *Thymus collinus* Salisb.

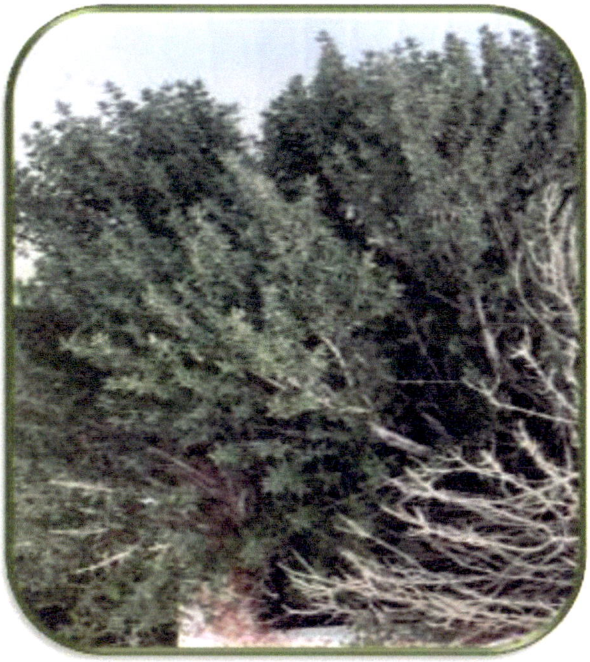

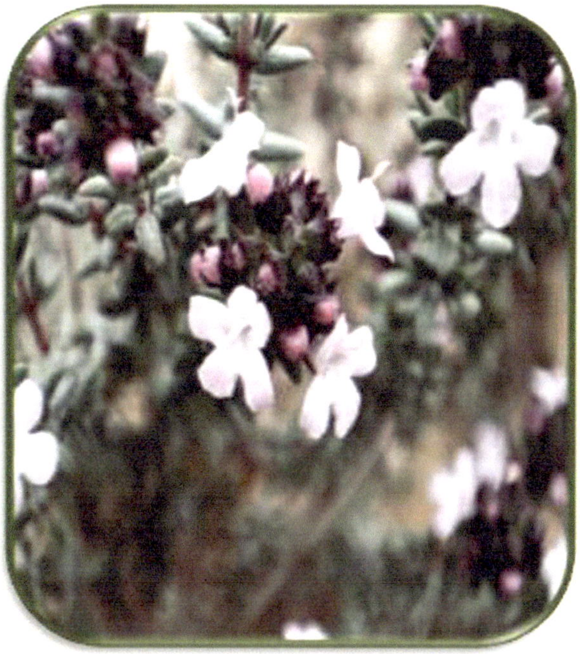

Family: Lamiaceae

Common names: Common thyme

Foreign names: Thym Fr. thyme, Common Eng.

Occurrences : 119,155 occurrences

Distribution in the world

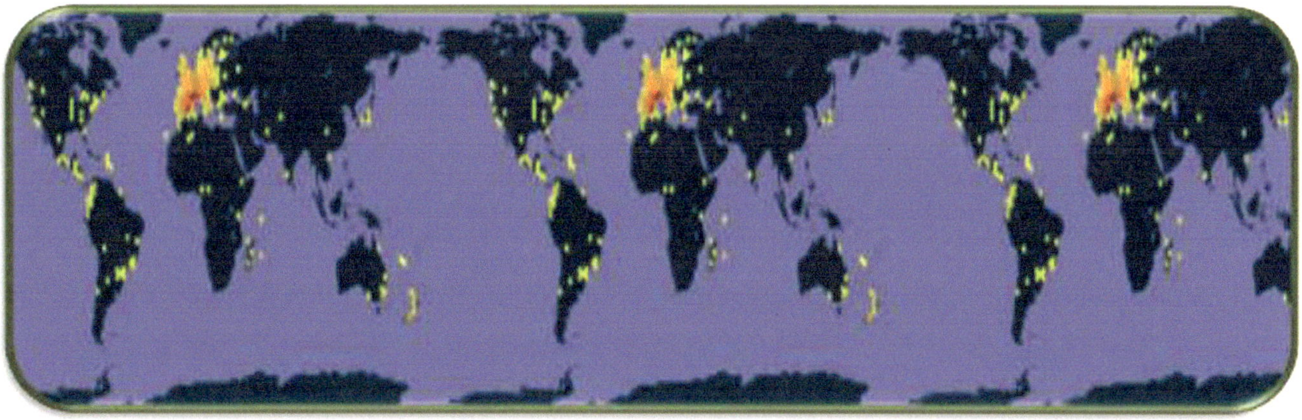

Botanical description:

A perennial herb, 20-40 cm tall, highly branched, its stem is erect, woody,A thicket, its color is reddish-gray. The leaves and inflorescences bear abundantly the thymus glands. The leaves are aromatic, small, linear or elliptical, entire, short-spinaled or petiolate, gray-green in color, 4-12 mm long, and about 3 mm wide. Their upper surface is green in color and the lower surface is covered with gray hairs, and bears some secreted hairs. The blade is leathery in texture, and its edges curl inward at the base of the blade. Flowers are violet or blue, gathered in clusters around the stem, forming in turn spikes or terminal heads, few Flowers, bracts are small. Calyx tubular, hairy, bilipped, bearing 10 nerves. Corolla slightly bilipped. Male 4 stamens. Female 2 carpels, ovary superior, quadri-chambered. Fruit 4 seeds.

Flowering: May to September.

Habitat and geographical distribution: Southern Europe and North Africa.

History and Heritage:

The scientific name of the genus is mentioned in the previous species, the descriptive name of the species vulgaris means "common." Thyme oil has been used as a therapeutic agent since ancient times.

Part used: Flowering plant.

Chemical components:

It should be noted that there are many chemically diverse strains of this species (about 7 strains). The percentage and type of compounds present in the volatile oil differ according to the strain studied. The most important strains are those dominated by phenolic compounds (carvacrol and thymol) and alcoholic (linalool). Volatile oil -2 2.5%, its most important compounds are thymol, carvacrol 60%, paracymene p-cymene, borneol, linalool, and others. Derivatives of caffeic acid, the most important of which is rosmarinic acid 0.15 1.35% and flavonoids including: luteolin, apigenin, naringenin, and thymusine. Triterpenes, the most important of which are ursolic acid 2%, and oleanolic acid 0.6%.

Properties and medical uses:

Common thyme has antioxidant, antispasmodic, expectorant, antibacterial, antiviral, antifungal, and antiparasitic properties. It is used to treat cough and bronchitis.

The decoction of the plant is used as a folk remedy, as a respiratory tract disinfectant, and to treat whooping cough and asthma. It is also used as an intestinal disinfectant, an intestinal antispasmodic, a gas expeller, a liver stimulant, and in the treatment of urinary tract and bladder infections, and as an expeller of worms and infectious parasites.

The essential oil shows antimicrobial activity against Staphylococcus aureus, Streptococcus pyogenes, Candida albicans, Salmonella thyphimurium, Escherichia coli, Pseudomonas aeruginosa without affecting the intestinal flora.

It is used to reduce colon and intestinal spasms as it helps relax the smooth intestinal muscles. The decoction of the aerial parts is used topically as a gargle to treat gum inflammation. Its oil is used as a massage to treat back pain, sciatica, rheumatic pain, to disinfect and treat wounds, acne, and eczema. It is an antioxidant and antimicrobial used in the food industry to increase the shelf life of food products.

Environment:

Many species of thyme grow wild in abandoned and stoned lands, meadows, the edges of forested sites, and on sunny slopes in mountainous highlands. It is suitable for semi-humid and semi-arid warm environments, and tolerates low temperatures and frost in winter, but environmental conditions with moderate and high temperatures and humidity of 70-75% are best for economic production. Thyme is a light-loving species, so it is planted on southern slopes with long sunlight. It can be grown successfully in all types of agricultural soils, the best of which is well-drained, aerated and rich in organic matter. It also grows in calcareous soils.

Cultivation and productivity:

Recent seeds that have not been stored for more than 3 years are planted at the end of summer in special nurseries.

The seedlings appear 15 days after planting, and are transferred to the permanent land the following spring, where they are planted in lines, with a distance of 45-60 cm between them. It can also be propagated by stem cuttings. Thyme can resist thirst, but it needs irrigation if it is planted as an economic crop. The plant responds to mineral fertilization with essential elements. The plant blooms in early summer until early autumn. The green mass is harvested once during the flowering stage, and again after two months, and dried in the shade for a week, then packed. The economic productive life of thyme is 5 years, after which it is recommended to renew the plant. One hectare of common thyme yields 0.5-2.5 tons of green grass and about 0.5-0.1 tons of dry grass.

Vitex agnus - castus L.

Agnus-castus alba Carrière, *Agnus-castus macrostachya* Carrière, *Agnus-castus robusta*) Lebas(Carrière, *Agnus-castus vulgaris* Carrière.

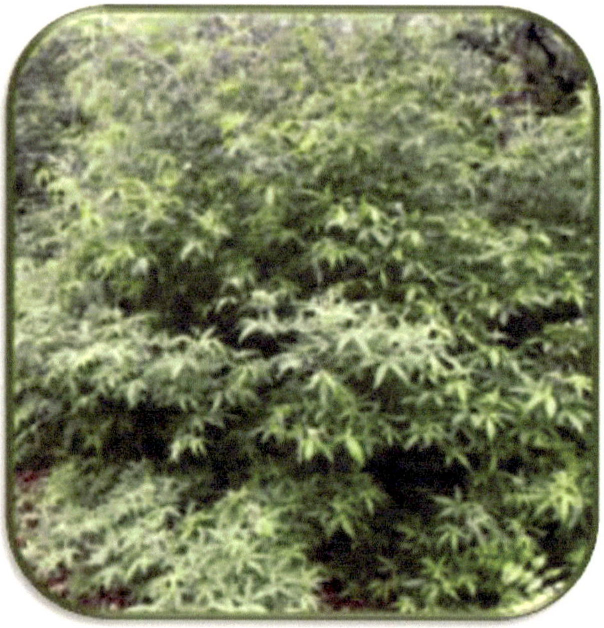

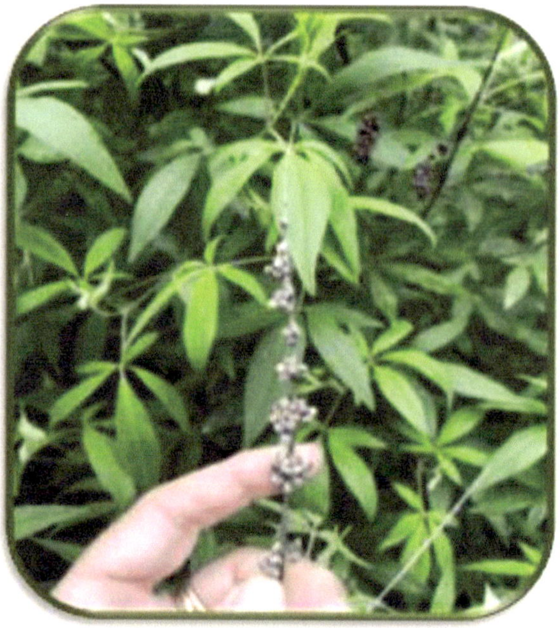

Family: Lamiaceae (formerly placed in the Verbenaceae family) Chaste tree, Abraham's tree, chaste tree.

Common names: Mary's palm, chaste, laurel

Foreign names: gattilier le Fr. tree, Chaste Eng.

Occurrences : 29,370 occurrences

Distribution in the world

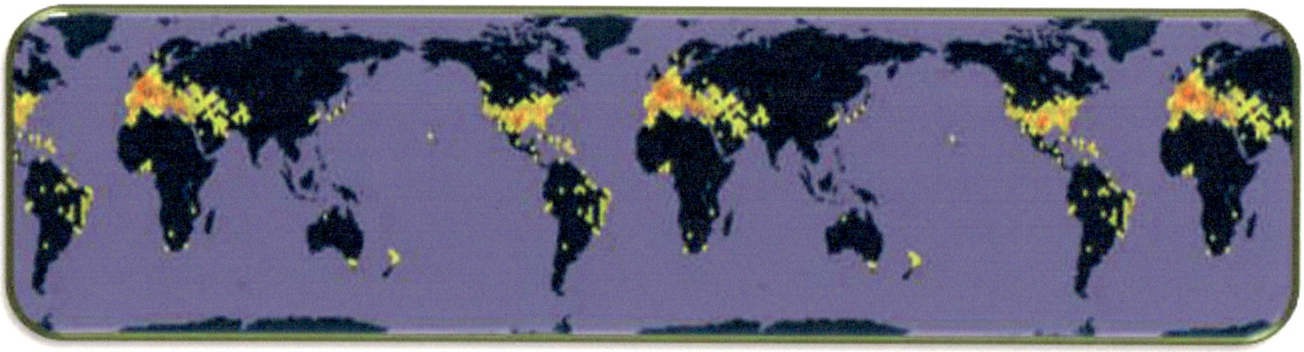

Botanical description:

Shrubs or shrubs, 1 to 6 m tall, young branches quadrangular, gray, hairy. Leaves are compound palmate, composed of 5 to 7 leaflets, opposite, falling, long-spikelet. Leaves are lanceolate, pointed at the apex, gradually tapering at the base, complete The margin, short-spooned, may reach 10 cm in length, its upper surface is green and the lower G. The flowers are pale violet (sometimes carnation or white), gathered in branched terminal inflorescences Grey-wine Semi-spike, 8 to 10 cm long. The calyx is 3 mm, densely hairy, its sepals are united in a tube ending in five short teeth. The corolla is composed of 5 petals united in the form of a semi-bilipped tube, exceeding Its length is about three times the length of the calyx. The male has 4 stamens of two different lengths. The ovary is quadripartite, each containing one ovule. The fruit is nuclear, spherical to oblong in shape, 3 to 4 mm in diameter, reddish-black in color when ripe, surrounded up to two-thirds by the calyx, which takes a cup-like shape. The outer fruiting shell bears short-stalked glandular hairs.

Flowering: From June to September. Fruiting in autumn.

Homeland and geographical distribution:

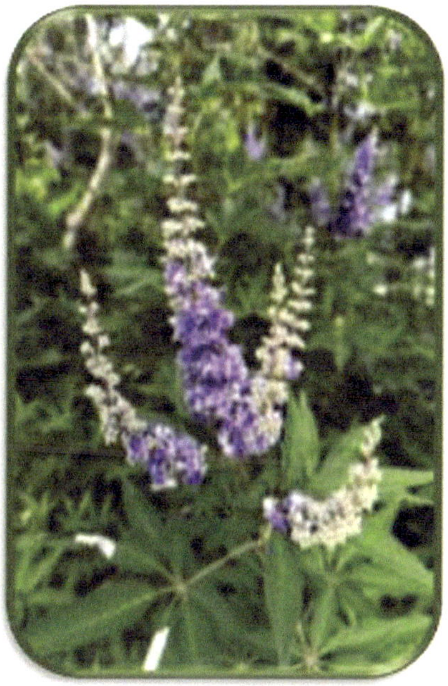

Mediterranean countries, extending to the Iranian-Turanian region. It is cultivated for ornamental purposes in many countries.

History and heritage:

The scientific name of the genus is the ancient Latin and Greek name of this shrub and is derived from the Latin word vieo, Salal. Agnus is from Greek and means "chaste", and castus is from Latin and has the same meaning, referring to the use of this type in ancient rituals of chastity among monks. This is due to the effect of its fruits that curb sexual desire. The fruits have been used since ancient times to reduce sexual desire.

Part used: Dried ripe fruits and dried leaves.

Chemical components:

The fruits contain iridoid glycosides, including: aucuboside, agnuside, cetosteroids, and eurostoside The leaves contain volatile oil -1.6%, rich in cineol, alpha and beta pinene α-ß, bornyl acetate, and flavonoids, including: luteoline7-glucoside, luteoline, chrysosplenol, casticine, homoorientine.The plant contains iridoids, diterpenes, steroids, flavonoids, and phenols. Nine iridoids were derived. Isolation of the antioxidant ethyl acetate extract. 6β diterpene Labdane, 14-diene, 7β-diacetoxy-13-hydroxy-labda-8 were also extracted from the hexane extract of the fruits, which have a strong affinity with the dopamine-D2 receptors. A new substance was isolated from the diterpene labdane containing nitrogen and was named vitexlactam A. Two other diterpene labdane alkaloids were isolated, called vitexlactam B and C.

Properties and medical uses:

The plant does not contain any hormone, but it exerts an anti-oestrogene and anti-androgen effect, through the activity of Chemically acting on the hypothalamic-pituitary axis, it restores the hormonal balance of estrogen/progesterone to its normal state by increasing the production of progesterone, and also limits the increase in prolactin and returns it to its normal rate. The plant is mainly used to treat premenstrual disorders resulting from a decrease in the level of progesterone hormone in the period preceding the menstrual cycle, menstrual disorders and pain (absence of menstruation, headache, fatigue, breast swelling and sensitivity, anxiety, irritability, sensitivity and irritability), treating menopausal disorders, and regulating milk production in mothers who suffer from hormonal problems.

It is popularly used to increase the pregnancy rate in women who suffer from infertility resulting from high levels of the hormone prolactin and low levels of the hormone progesterone. It is also used to treat acne resulting from hormonal disorders, treat prostatitis and testicular tumors, in addition to its famous ability to reduce and control excessive sexual desires in men.

Side effects and warnings:

There are some side effects of taking the drug if the drug is used for more than three months, and the side effects may include stomach upset, fatigue, and difficulty sleeping. The drug is likely to be unsafe for pregnant women and may increase the difficulty of pregnancy and harm the fetus. It may affect estrogen levels. The drug is not used in case of sensitivity to hormones. The drug contains chemicals that affect the brain in a manner similar to some medications used for Parkinson's disease, and may affect the treatment procedures for Parkinson's disease. It also affects a chemical in the brain called dopamine, which leads to a reduction in the effects of metoclopramide. Environment: The plant is widespread in humid environments and on the sides of coastal or inland waterways, however it tolerates fluctuating climate conditions and resists drought and thirst to a large extent. Its cultivation is successful in all bioclimatic levels with moderate, warm and sometimes fresh variables, as it tolerates a decrease in temperature in winter to -15°C provided that this decrease does not last for a long time, and in this case it may behave like deciduous plants. It tolerates high sunlight and exceptionally high temperatures in summer up to 48°C, provided that sufficient amounts of irrigation water are provided, which the plant needs in such conditions. It does not tolerate shade, even light shade, which results in a severe slowdown in its growth rate. The plant thrives in all types of soils, including clayey soils with temporary seasonal flooding, and tolerates salinity up to 4000 ppm. It has recently been used in primary afforestation of saline soils in Central Asia.

Cultivation and productivity:

It is propagated by seeds soaked in plain water for 24 hours, and it also responds to vegetative propagation by semi-woody cuttings without the need for rooting hormone.

***Ziziphora tenuior* L.**

Faldermannia tenuior)L.(Ter-Chatsch.

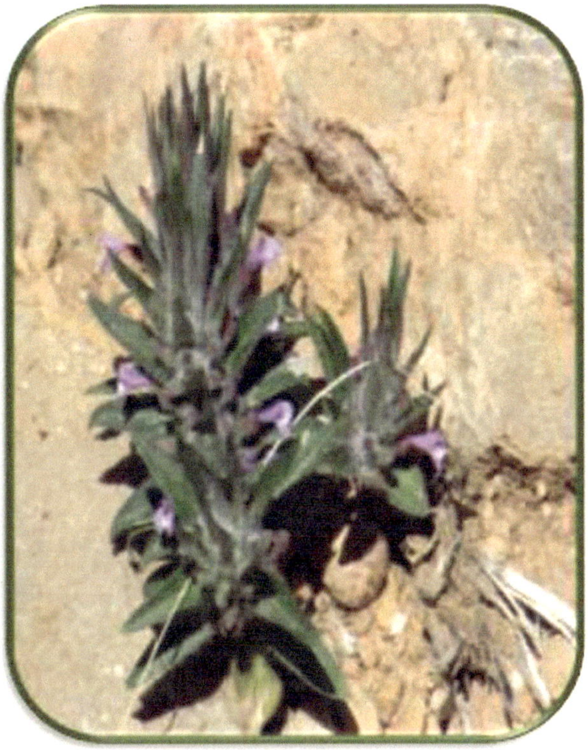

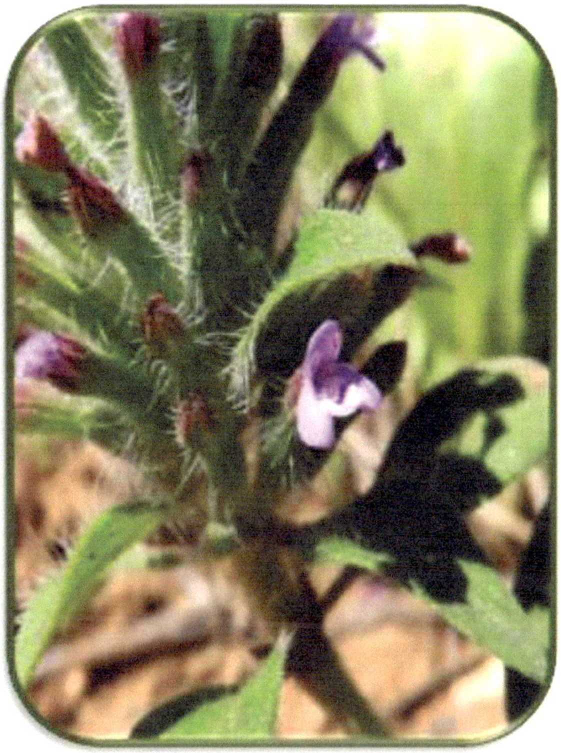

Occurrences : 791 occurrences

Distribution in the world

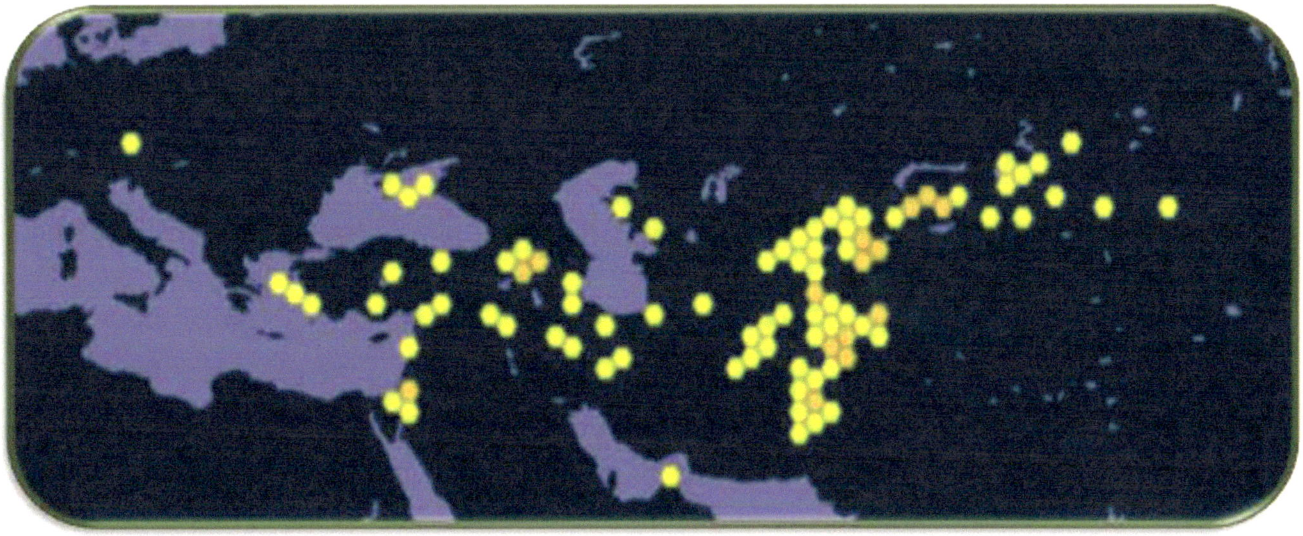

Botanical description:

An annual herb, 5-15 cm tall, covered with gray hair. The stem is slender, simple or branched from the base, and the branches are erect or ascending. The leaves are simple, entire, rough, 20-4x7-1 mm in size, few in number and spaced apart in the lower (sterile) part of the stem, elliptic to oval in shape, gradually tapering at the base. The floral leaves are more numerous and compact, lanceolate to linear in shape, sharp at the apex, fringed at the edge, prominently nerved, and longer than the flowers, erect to varying degrees, bearing glands that are not clearly visible. The flowers are hermaphrodite, bisymmetrical, small (10-12 mm), semi-sub-squamous, gathered in whorls of few flowers (2-5), supported by some leaves, and their group forms an elongated semi-spike inflorescence. Calyx narrow tubular, pentagonal, 2-1×9-6 mm, notched, covered with flat hairs and glands, teeth short, ovate to triangular. Corolla pentagonal, pink (rarely white), bilipped, tube only slightly protruding, upper lip erect, lower flat, trilobed, middle lobe slightly larger than lateral lobes. The male is composed of two fertile stamens contained in the corolla, bearing the true anthers resembling a ball. The female is bicarpal, bicameral, divided by a false septum into four chambers, each containing a single ovule. The fruit is an oval-shaped, smooth nut.

Flowering: March to May. In the Eastern Mediterranean countries there are other species Z. canescens (perennial) and Z. capitata (annual) similar in their popular uses to Z. tenuior.

Habitat and geographical distribution: Iranian-Turanian

History and heritage:

The plant has been known since ancient times as a spice, and was popularly used in some countries of Western Asia as a soothing drink.

Part used: Flowering plant (the plant has a strong aromatic smell)

Chemical components:

All parts of the plant contain 2% volatile oil rich in terpene compounds Pulegone (85%), thymol, isomyrcene, pinene, p-menth-3-en-8-ol, limonene, menthone .Only three and a half monoterpene compounds were identified in the oil (oxygenated sesquiterpenes) as secondary components: Caryophyllene oxide, Spatholinol, Viridiflorol, and Mannol diterpene (diterpene). The plant contains traces of tannins and flavones.

Properties and medical uses:

The flowering plant is used to treat diarrhea and digestive disorders (digestive and carminative properties). The oil has beneficial properties in treating cases of neurasthenia (anti-stress) in addition to its diaphoretic, expectorant, antibacterial and antioxidant properties. It is useful in cases of colds and coughs.

It is used in folk medicine to treat some heart diseases because it improves blood circulation.

A medicinal plant, it is included in many antimicrobial, antiseptic, expectorant and wound-healing preparations. It is used to treat fever, cough, stomach pain, dysentery and kidney stones. Bladder, fever, endometritis, enteritis, and painful menstruation. The plant has an antifungal effect, which justifies and enhances the use of this plant in traditional medicine and opens new ways in the development of health care products. In folk medicine in the Qalamoun Mountains region in Syria, it is used against coughs, stomach pains, and dysentery, and in ethnopharmacology, essential oils are used to treat edema, insomnia, lung abscesses, bronchitis, hemorrhoids, and high blood pressure. The methanolic extract showed significant antimicrobial activity against Morganella morganii and Candida al-bicans. The essential oil showed antibacterial activity. The essential oil is a good candidate for the treatment of candidiasis. The concentrations used were shown to be non-toxic to several mammalian cell types and to have anti-inflammatory activity, so the oil is suggested as a treatment for colorectal cancer. The results showed the presence of anti-cancer compounds that cause programmed cell death in HT-29 cells.

Other uses:

The volatile plant oil repels insects and is included in some insect repellent preparations. The essential oil is used in some types of food industries to give flavor.

Use warnings: The plant shows low toxicity characteristics and can cause some disorders if used internally in large doses.

Environment:

The plant is widespread in dry and semi-dry areas, and grows in steppes, on slopes, and on the slopes of hills and plateaus with sandy loam soils. Its spread indicates overgrazing.

Cultivation and productivity: It can be propagated by seeds.

Laurus nobilis L.

Laurus angusta Raf., *Laurus nobilis* var. *angustifolia* Nees, *Laurus papillosa* Demoly, *Laurus salicifolia* Nees, *Laurus tenuifolia* Mill., *Laurus undulata* Mill.

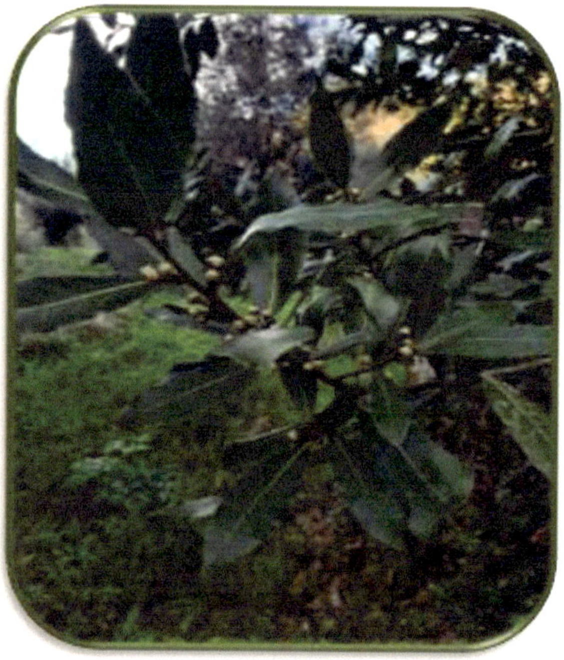

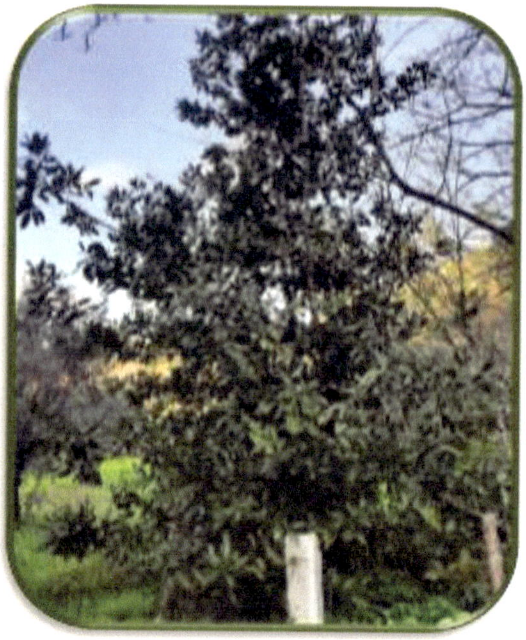

Family: Laurels Lauraceae

Common names: Noble laurel, Myrtle

Foreign names: laurier-sauce Fr. Laurel, Eng.

Occurrences : 65,679 occurrences

Distribution in the world

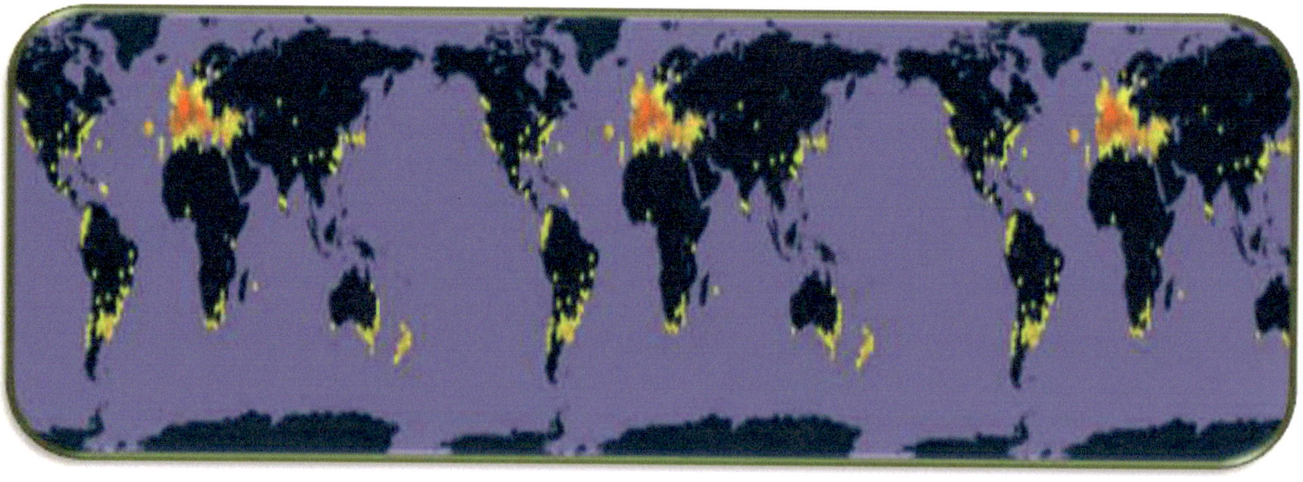

Botanical description:

An evergreen tree, 3-10 m high, all parts of which are Grave except for the flower spikes which are slightly hairy. The stem is straight, grey in the lower part, Green in the upper part. Leaves are simple, alternate, entire, short-spooned, leathery, oblong to lanceolate, wavy-edged, pointed at the apex, and pedunculated at the base, 8-12 cm long. Flowers are unisexual, and the plant is dioecious. The flowers are gathered in racemes composed of several small umbels, each containing 4-5 flowers, surrounded before opening by several bracts that fall quickly. The inflorescences are umbels and the flower spikes are short and downy.

The bracts are simple, pale yellow, composed of four bare segments, and do not last long. The stamens in the male flowers are numerous, located in more than one whorl, short filaments, and their anthers open by means of two valves that rise in an arch after maturity. The female flowers are few in number, the bracts are also four-segmented, and include 4 sterile stamens, the ovary is single-chambered, and the ovule is single-celled. The fruit is a black grape, located on the permanent flower seat, and resembles in shape and size a small olive.

Flowering: From March to April. The fruits ripen when they turn black in late summer and early autumn.

Homeland and geographical distribution: Mediterranean countries.

History and Heritage:

The scientific name of the genus is the old Latin name of this tree. The species name nobilis means "noble", referring to its use in wreaths to crown victors in wars among the Romans. Greek mythology mentions that the beautiful nymph Daphne could not attract and seduce Apollon (the god of art and the sun), who asked the gods to transform her into a laurel tree. Since then, victorious heroes, poets and scholars have worn laurel crowns as a symbol of nobility, victory and honor. It was also a symbol of protection from lightning during storms for the ancient Romans, and Emperor Tiberius used to cover his head with a laurel branch to protect him from lightning. This belief remained until the Middle Ages, for example, it is said that "lightning does not strike where there is laurel." The properties of laurel have been known since ancient times, and it was mentioned by Ibn al-Baytar, al-Antaki, and al-Ghasani. Ibn Sina also mentioned that laurel oil is useful in treating nerve pain.

Part used: Fruits, leaves, and the volatile oil extracted from the leaves.

Chemical components:

The leaves contain: volatile oil -1-3%, the most important compounds of which are cineol 1,8-cineol (-40)-50%, linalol 10%, eugenol, geraniol. Lactones: sesquiterpene, dehydrocostuslactone, coslaurenbiolide, furthermore, eremanthin, tunolide.

Isoquinoline alkaloids, including the alkaloid reticulin, tannins. The fruits contain: 1-4% volatile oil (its percentage varies depending on the method of harvesting and storage), its most important compounds are cineol citral, methylcinnamat, α, ß pinene, 1-8 palmitic a, lauric a, and linoleic acid. Its most important components: 25-55% laurel butter (laurel paste). The fatty oil is extracted by passing the fruits over water vapor until they soften, then they are cold pressed, and a green oily substance called laurel paste flows out.

Properties and medical uses:

It is grown as an aromatic plant Widely used in many parts of the world. The plant is important in the food and pharmaceutical industries. The commercial value of this type is derived from the essential oil, which may be applied to various industries. The leaf oil is used topically in the form of a poultice or ointments to treat rheumatism, joint diseases and relieve nerve pain. Its antiseptic and antimicrobial properties (bacteria, fungi, viruses) make its oil effective in treating gum and ear infections, wounds and bruises. And various skin diseases and inflammations (oily skin, psoriasis, acne.) A mixture of fatty and volatile oils is used to treat boils and pimples. The effect of essential oil in treating cancer has been proven.

Other uses:

Aromatic bay leaves are classified within the group of spices that stimulate digestion and are used to improve the taste of meat and fish. Bay butter is used in veterinary medicine to repel insects and treat parasites that infect animal skins. Laurel butter is one of the ingredients in the manufacture of laurel soap, which some Syrian cities are famous for, and which has gained a global reputation, due to its ability to maintain the softness and health of the skin. The plant resists diseases and insects, and protects surrounding plants from diseases.

Precautions for use:

It is not recommended for pregnant women to use volatile oil, due to the sensitivity it may cause due to the monoterpene lactones contained in the leaves.

Environment:

It is widespread in forest environments, and is considered one of the environmentally flexible species. It tolerates cold, but is affected by frost, which causes great damage to the leaf system. It is suitable for sunny, fertile, moist, well-drained soils, and well exposed to light.

Cultivation and productivity:

Laurel is propagated by seeds or dry or fresh fruits that are not dehulled, and treated by cold stratification, noting that laurel seeds lose their vitality quickly. It responds to vegetative propagation by layering and by woody cuttings treated with one of the hormones. Seedlings are planted at the age of 2-3 years, and need fertile soil in sunny or semi-shaded locations, and need abundant irrigation and constant moisture in the soil in the summer.

Linum catharticum.

Cathartolinum catharticum)L.(Small, *Cathartolinum pratense* Rchb., *Nezera cathartica*) L.(Nieuwl.,.*Cartholinum partense* Rchb., *Linum versifolium* Gilib.

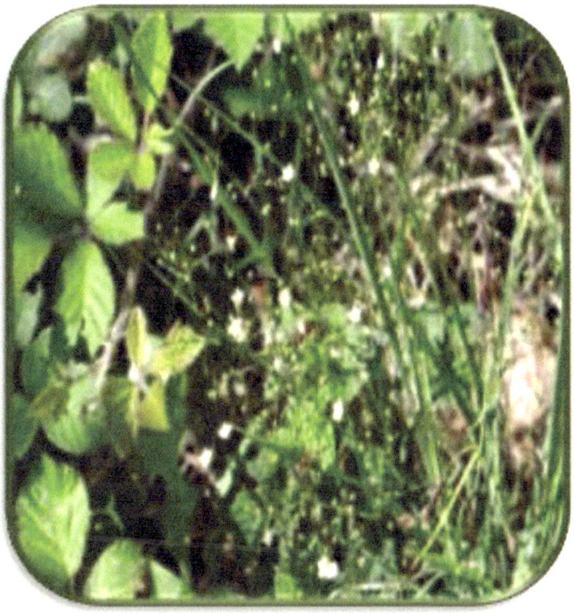

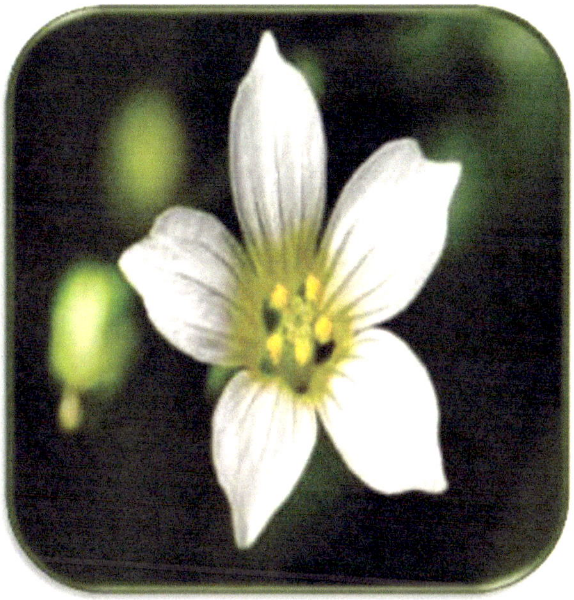

Family: Linaceae

Common names: Flax

Foreign names: flax, mountain flax, Fairy Eng. Fr. Lin sauvage purgative

Occurrences : 277,653 occurrences

Distribution in the world

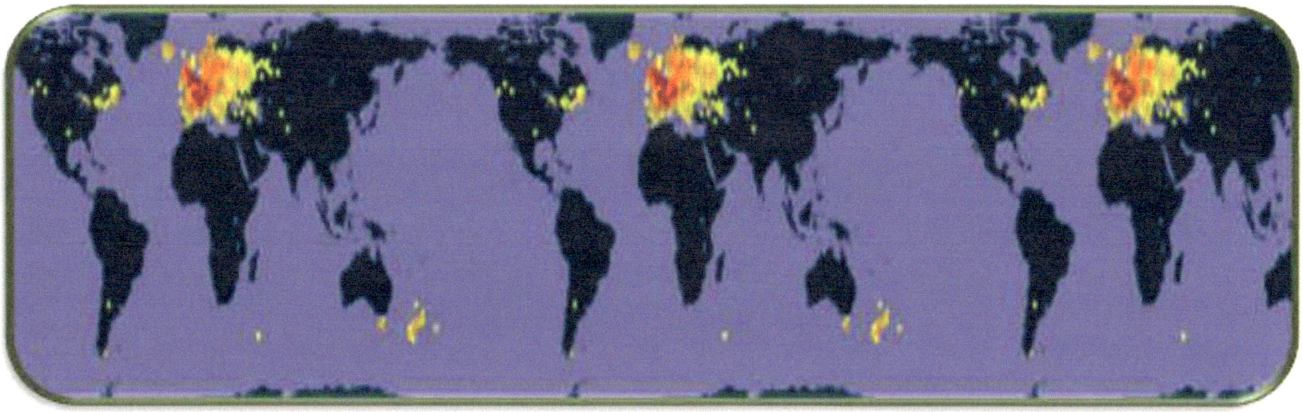

Botanical description:

An annual to biennial herbaceous plant, which may live for several years, with a height of up to 30 cm. The roots are long, thin, and whitish in color. The stem is erect or upright, or simple or branched at the base, thin and bare, with few leaves. The leaves are opposite, entire. The flowers are white to yellow in color. The fruits are spherical in shape and up to 3 mm long. The seeds are 1-1.5 mm, smooth, bare and pale brown in color. Flax is an important oil crop that is grown as a source of vegetable fibers or as fodder for livestock. Flax is the most economically important species.

Homeland and geographical distribution: Europe, the Mediterranean basin, and North Africa.

History and heritage: The scientific name of the genus is from the Greek linon, which is the Latin name for these plants, while the species name catharticum means "facilitator."

Part used: Herbaceous plant.

Chemical components:

0.5% lignans, including achromatin (bitter substance), tannins 2%, resin, 2%, and a little volatile oil 0.15%. The results showed the presence of 18 polyphenolic compounds. These results support the daily consumption of flax seeds for diabetics, and indicate that flax seed polyphenols are nutritional supplements or new herbal medicines for the treatment of diabetes and its complications, and have anti-diabetic and anti-inflammatory activities.

Properties and medical uses:

Flax seeds are oil seeds (45-50% oil based on dry weight). Its oil has shown many health benefits and industrial applications. The plant is anti-diabetic and anti-inflammatory. The plant has laxative and laxative properties, and if taken in large doses, it becomes emetic. The plant is popularly used to treat constipation, cases of urinary insufficiency, colds and rheumatic diseases, and cases of worm infestation.

Warnings for use: Causes gastritis and vomiting

Other uses: Many studies have shown that flax is highly accumulative, capable of absorbing large amounts of heavy metals such as cadmium and petroleum hydrocarbons from contaminated soil.

Environment:

Flax thrives in well-drained soils with a medium composition such as yellow clay or loamy soils, and is not suitable for light soils.

Cultivation and productivity:

It is propagated by seeds. The soil is prepared for cultivation by conducting deep autumn plowing and several shallow plowings, and fertilizers are added. Flax is a crop with relatively low nutritional requirements, and mineral fertilization is not recommended if the soil is fertile. The basic service operations after planting are weeding, weed, disease and insect control, as well as irrigation when needed.

***Linum usitatissimum* L.**

Linum angustifolium subsp. *usitatissimum*)L.(Rouy.

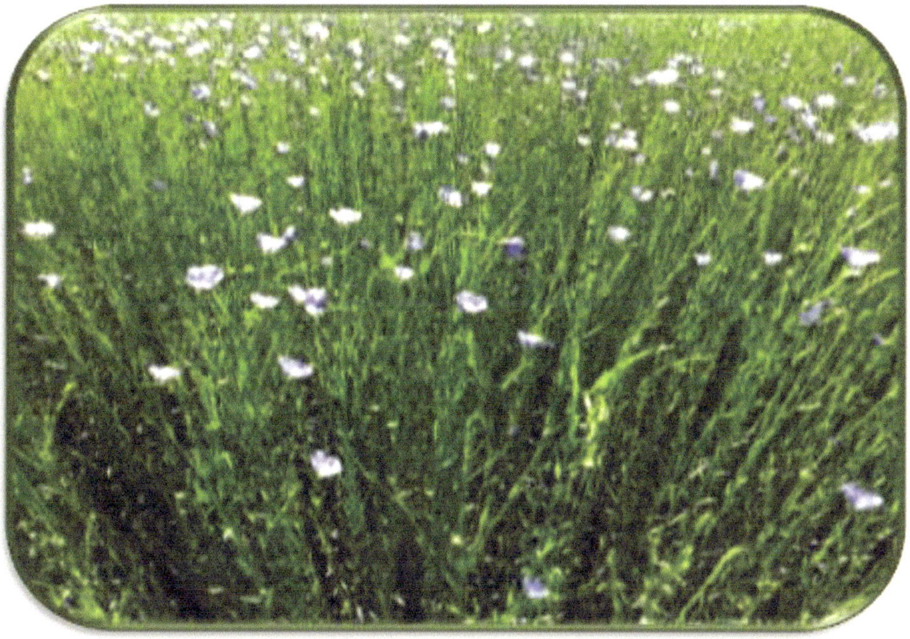

Family: Linaceae

Common names: Common Flax

Foreign names: Lin Fr. Flax, Eng.

Occurrences : 63,399 occurrences

Distribution in the world

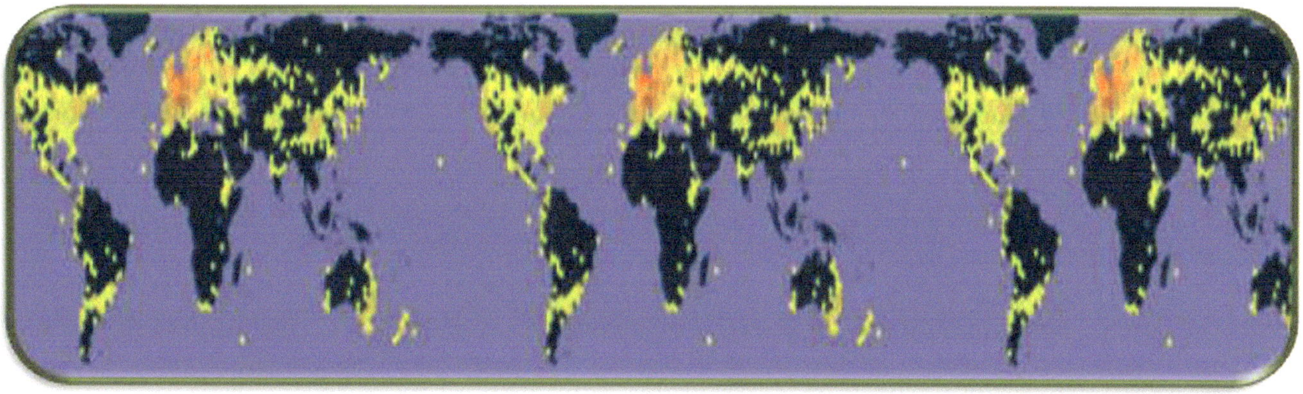

Botanical description:

An annual and sometimes perennial herb, its stem is erect, slender, rising to about a meter. The leaves are simple, petiolate, lanceolate, sometimes narrow and linear, glabrous, entire-edged, three-veined, 2-4 cm long, and about 3 mm wide. The flowers are hermaphrodite, radially symmetrical, gathered in cymose, axillary or terminal inflorescences, 15-25 mm in diameter. Calyx 5 sepals, perennial.

Corolla 5 petals, sky blue, opens only in the sun and falls easily. Male 5 stamens, broad filament bases, alternating with 5 stamens. Ovary pentagonal, containing two ovules in each chamber, styes 5 free. Fruit obovate, spherical, 7-9 mm, light brown, containing about ten seeds. Seeds are reddish-brown, shiny, oval or oblong, flattened, 4-6 mm long, 2-3 mm wide, 0.75-1.5 mm thick. One end is rounded and the other is pointed and hooked. The upper surface of the seed contains minute, irregular holes. The husk is easily barked off, covering a thin layer of endosperm and a straight embryo, both of which are salivary. Soaking the seeds in water leads to the formation of a salivary coat. The embryo pods are large, flat and rich in oil.

Home and geographical distribution:

Eastern Mediterranean and the Fertile Crescent, and is currently cultivated all over the world for its fibers, seeds and oil.

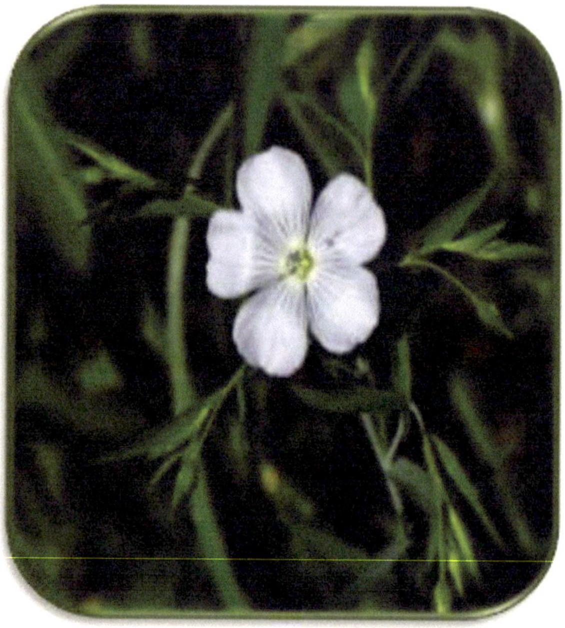

History and heritage:

The scientific name of the genus is derived from the Greek linon, which is the Latin name for these plants. As for the species name usitatissimum, it means "familiar." Flax has been known for more than five thousand years. The ancient Egyptians and Indians knew it and cultivated it to obtain its fibers. They used its seeds medicinally. The ancient Greeks also knew the medicinal properties of its seeds. Hippocrates recommended it to treat inflammation of the mucous membranes. In the 18th century, Charlemagne of France issued laws requiring the consumption of the seeds to preserve the health of his subjects, and Mahatma Gandhi said, "Where flax seeds are a common food item among the people, health is better." Part used: Flax seeds, flax oil produced by pressing the seeds. Constitutional flax oil is obtained by cold pressing of ripe fruits, its color is light yellow tending to brown or green, clear in appearance, and the smell is specific. Low viscosity, quickly solidifies, difficult to dissolve in ethanol, but mixes with ether, chloroform and benzene.

Chemical components:

The roots contain chlorogenic acid and cyanogenic glycosides.The leaves and stems contain flavonoids.Its seeds contain 30 (45-)% fatty oil composed of unsaturated fatty acids (linoleic acid 24% of the weight of flaxseed oil components, alpha linolenic acid (ALA) 40%, unsaponifiable saturated fatty acids (cholesterin, stigmasterine). The seeds also contain salivary substances and lignans 25%, phenylpropane derivatives, including li-nusitamarine in addition to a small amount of a cyanogenic glycoside compound: linamarin. Linamarin (cyanogenic glycoside) has a calming effect on the respiratory system.

Properties and medical uses:

Flaxseed oil has anti-inflammatory, anti-tumor, cardioprotective, defecation-regulating, cytokinase-inhibiting, lipid-lowering, antibacterial, and anti-carcinogenic properties, in addition to being rich in omega-3 fatty acids. It is used internally in cases of constipation, and is used topically in cases of skin inflammation. Diluted flaxseed oil is used popularly in cases of irritable colon, intestinal inflammation and hemorrhoids. It is also used topically in cases of burns, anal inflammation and chronic prostatitis. The decoction of the seeds is used popularly, as a laxative and treatment for cases of constipation, lowering blood sugar, and as an antispasmodic and anti-colitis. Compresses to treat respiratory problems and inflammations The paste made from ground seeds is used in the form of skin. The cooked seeds are popularly used to treat bladder infections, whooping cough, and gastrointestinal spasms.

Other uses:

Cooking oil, soap for grease, used in the composition of varnish and oil paints, and in the paper industry. It is also used as an excipient for skin pharmaceutical preparations.

Pharmaceutical forms:

The plant is available in the form of powder, soft gelatinous preserves, and oil. It is sold under names such as: Flaxseed Barlean`s Flax Oil, Barlen`s Vita-Flax

Side effects, interactions and warnings for use:

Symptoms of overdose are shortness of breath, rapid breathing, weakness, and poor muscle coordination that develops into paralysis and seizures. It is not given in cases of intestinal obstruction or severe constipation, acute inflammation of the digestive system and prostate cancer.

Flaxseed should be avoided with colon laxatives. Pregnant or breastfeeding women should avoid using the plant, because it may harm the fetus or cause miscarriage. Unripe flax seeds should not be consumed. When using flax, a large amount of fluids should be consumed to reduce intestinal gases.

Environment:

Flax is a long-day plant. The seeds begin to germinate at a temperature of 3-5 °C, and the seedlings can tolerate Decreasing temperatures to 4 °C. The appropriate temperature for its growth is 15-18°C, and its increase leads to increased branching of plants. and accelerating the formation of flowers and increasing seed production, while the quality of fibers deteriorates in this case. Flax needs moisture in all stages of its growth except the maturity stage. Flax grows well in well-drained soils with an average composition, such as yellow clay or loam soils. Light soils are not suitable for flax cultivation, especially in areas with little rainfall or irrigation water. Suitable pH: 5.9-6.5. Cultivation and productivity: The plant is propagated by seeds. Flax is planted in the fall in temperate regions, and in the spring in cold regions. The soil is prepared for planting by deep autumn plowing and several shallow plowings, and fertilizers are added. Flax is a relatively nutrient-intensive crop, and mineral fertilization is not recommended if the soil is fertile. The basic service operations after planting are hoeing, weed, disease and insect control, as well as irrigation when needed. The hectare yields 600-700 kg of seeds under normal conditions.

Lawsonia inermis L.

Lawsonia alba Lam., *Lawsonia spinosa* L.

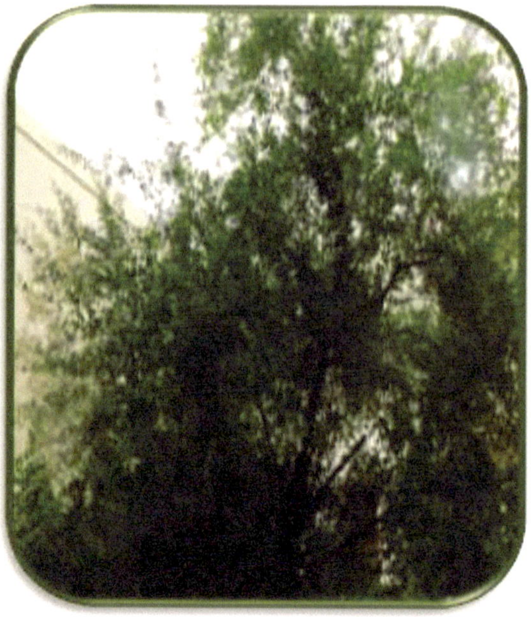

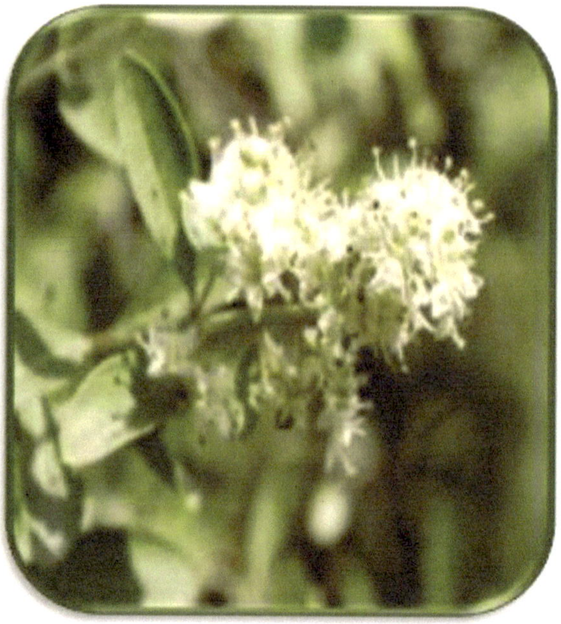

Family: Lythraceae

Common names: Henna

Foreign names: Eng. Henna, Egyptian priven, Fr. jalousie

Occurrences : 170,122 occurrences

Distribution in the world

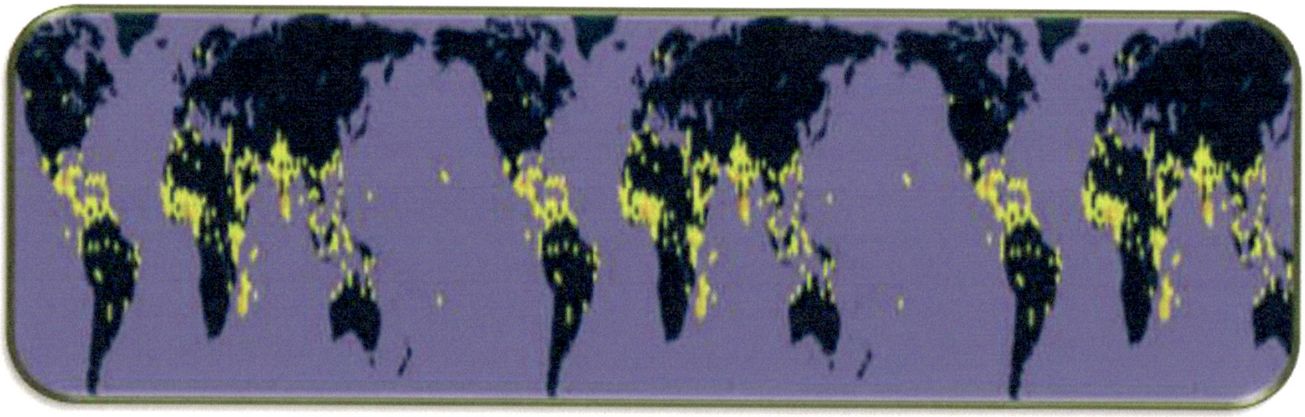

Botanical description:

A fragrant shrub, bare, up to 2.5 m high, its old branches become thorny. Leaves Simple, opposite, entire-edged, semi-lobed, elliptic, ovate or inverted-ovate, acute or blunt apex, 44-8 mm long, 20-2 mm wide. Inflorescence is paniculate, terminal, 22-3 cm long. Flowers hermaphrodite, radiate symmetrical, quadripartite, inflorescence 2-3.5 mm long. Sepals ovate, perennial with fruit. Petals wrinkled, inverted ovate, white to yellowish, 3-4 mm long, 4-5 mm wide. Male 8 stamens in pairs, filaments about 4 mm long. Ovary sub-spherical, quadripartite. Fruit capsule, 3-9 mm in diameter, wall with nerve network, irregularly opening. Seeds: Numerous, pyramidal.

Flowering:

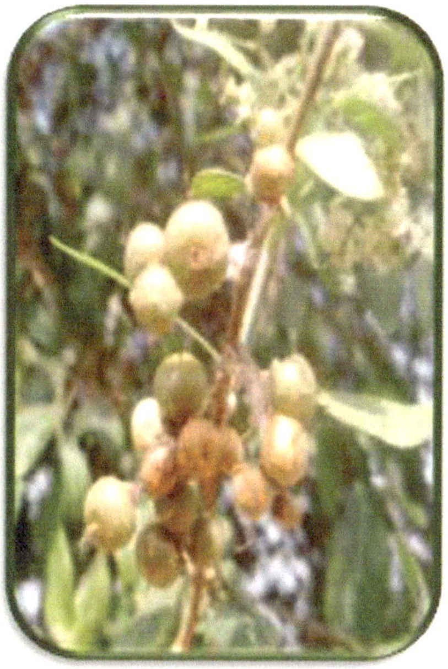

October to November. There are two varieties of henna shrub that differ in flower color: Alba has white flowers, and miniata has purple flowers.

Homeland and geographical distribution:

The original homeland of the henna plant is not known. It grows in hot tropical regions in southwest Asia, especially in the south of the Arabian Peninsula. From there, its cultivation spread to many countries in the world. The most important countries currently producing it are Egypt, Sudan, India and China.

History and Heritage:

The origin of the word Henna is taken from the Arabic "henna." The word inermis means thornless. The genus Lawsonia was named in memory of Dr. Isaac Lawson (died 1747) who financed the book "The System of Nature" written by Naeus. The species name inermis means "thornless." The plant has been cultivated since ancient times in the countries of the Eastern Mediterranean, Egypt, the Arabian Peninsula, Iraq, Iran, and India. Parts of it were found on an Egyptian mummy. The Arabs called it henna and used it a lot on the henna night for the bride to paint her hair and limbs before the wedding night. Ancient Islamic sources mentioned the use of henna to treat many diseases, and it was believed that the extracts taken from this plant were effective in protecting the person who dyed it from the effects of evil spirits. The ancients used henna flowers and placed them between the folds of their clothes to perfume them and protect them from being infested by clothes insects known as moths.

Part used:

Aromatic flowers, fruits, bark, powdered leaves and young branches.

Chemical components:

Henna leaves and young stems contain: 5-10% tannin compounds, known as "Henne tannins." Various glycosides (hennosides) that are enzymatically hydrolyzed into sugars and genin. The sugar radical (genin) is soon self-oxidized, giving a crystalline, reddish-orange compound soluble in water called Lawsone (-2-hydroxy 1-,4-naphthoquinone.) Coumarin compounds, flavones, gallic acid, sterols (sitosterol.) Sugary and resinous materials, the percentage of which is about 1 % It is noted that the amount of substances, especially the ozone compound, increases in henna leaves as the plant ages. The flowers contain a volatile oil, the most important components of which are alpha and beta ionone (ß, α).

Properties and medical uses:

Henna preparations relieve the pain of burns, help stop bleeding and heal wounds, especially chronic ulcers and eczema, and treat warts and ulcers that affect the feet, especially in diabetics.

Henna has an antibacterial, antiviral and antiparasitic effect. Henna purifies the scalp from microbes and parasites, reduces sweat secretion and excess oily secretions, and is beneficial in Treats dandruff and scalp infections. Nourishes the hair and gives it vitality and strength. The astringents in henna prevent cracking of the skin and provide it with vitality. Studies have proven the effectiveness of the two compounds Lawsone and isoplumbagin in eliminating cancer.

Henna is popularly used to treat duodenal ulcer bleeding, and is also used as an enema to treat ulcerative colitis. The infusion of the leaves is used as a topical poultice to treat headaches, skin diseases, and burns, and is used as an astringent and antiseptic gargle to treat mouth, gum, and tongue ulcers. Industrial uses: Henna is used in dyeing woolen, cotton and silk fabrics to give them color, clean them from greasy materials and stains, and in tanning leather, in addition to extracting a fragrant aromatic oil from its flowers, which is used in the perfume industry, including the famous perfume (Al-Tamrahna).

Beauty benefits of henna:

Henna is used in the manufacture of hair dyes, and to decorate hands and feet with different engravings and drawings according to taste and desire. Preparation of the dye: An orange and red dye is obtained by crushing the young leaves and buds into a green powder, which soon turns orange-red when exposed to air.

Precautions for use:

Sneezing, allergy to its components, henna is an abortive plant, and should not be used internally by pregnant women.

Environment:

Henna is widely grown in gardens, parks, the edges of green lawns and ponds, in warm areas. It can be successfully grown in all bioclimatic levels in both moderate and warm climates, and rarely in the sweet climate where frost is feared. Henna is a plant that requires light, and rarely tolerates shade. The plant grows well in humus clay soils and sandy soils, but tolerates clay and silty clay soils. It rarely tolerates salinity of more than 2500 parts per million in irrigation water. It tolerates drought relatively.

Cultivation and productivity:

Henna is cultivated for its fragrant flowers, and for the purpose of obtaining dye from its leaves. The plant is easily propagated

by seeds, and it also responds to vegetative propagation by woody cuttings with or without hormonal treatment. The leaves and growing tops are harvested, then exposed to the sun until they dry and stored until used.

Althaea officinalis L.

Malva althaea E.H.L.Krause, *Malva oficinalis*)L.(K.F.Schimp. & Spenn.

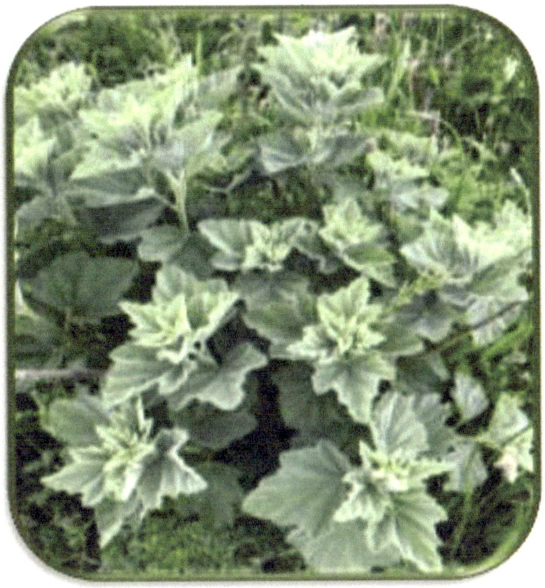

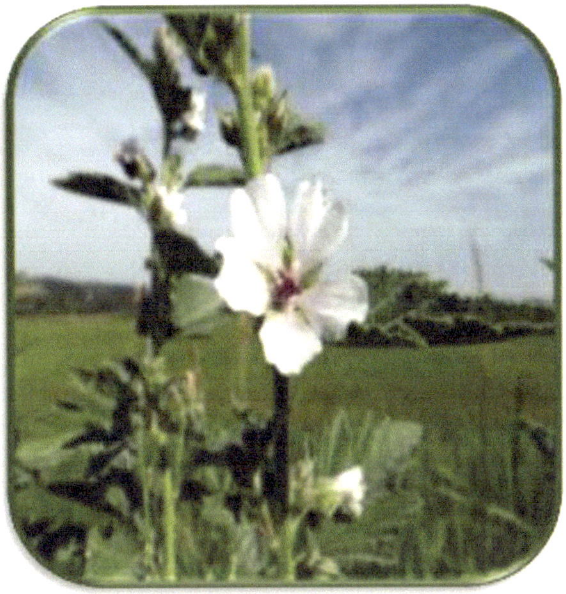

Family: Malvaceae

Common names: Marshmallow, Malvaceae officinalis, Marshmallow, Marshmallow, Sweet herb, Healing herb

Foreign names: Guimauve Fr. Marshmallow, Eng.

Occurrences : 56,206 occurrences

Distribution in the world

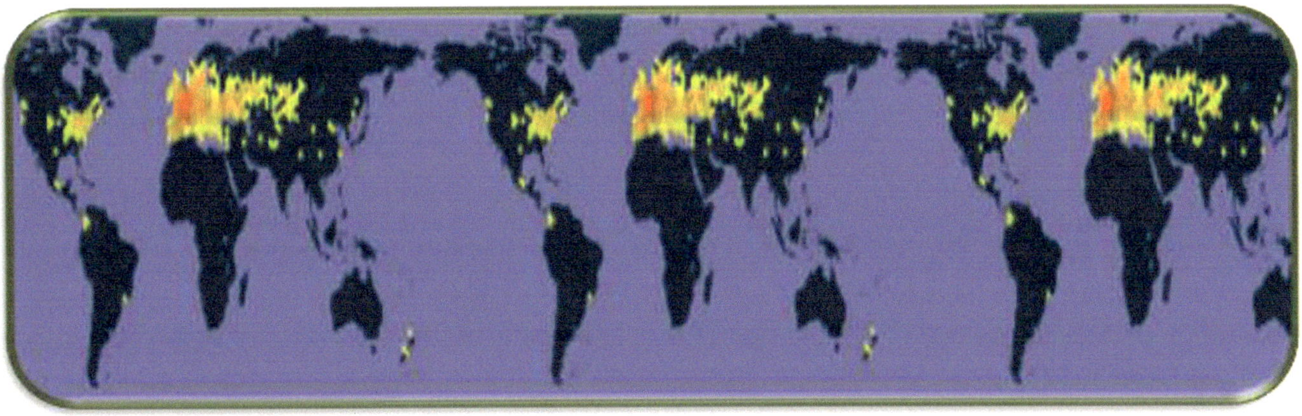

Botanical description:

A perennial herb, hairy, with a solid stem, woody at the base, few branches, 50-100 cm high. The roots are thick, fibrous, white in color. Leaves alternate, usually shorter than the blade, ears 3-5 mm, falling, blade serrated-crested, thick, hairy, whitish, palmately innervated, 2-7 x 4-10 cm, lower leaves ovate, cordate at base, almost entire to shallowly lobed to 3-5, upper leaves triangular in general shape, lobed to varying degrees, base truncated or pedicel. Flowers in axillary clusters of 1-3 flowers, the bract thick, shorter than the flowers, later elongating. The calyx 8-10 mm, pentagonal, hairy, supported by a calyx of 6-12 segments fused at their bases and twice shorter than the sepals, oblong to lanceolate in shape. The corolla is about 2 cm in diameter, composed of five white to pink petals, inverted ovate, notched at the apex, twice as long as the calyx. The stamen filaments fuse together to form a stamen tube surrounding the style, from which many branches branch out.

The ovary. The carpels are numerous, free, arranged in a ring around a shorter axis, and the ovary chambers are not divided by a septum. The fruit is disc-shaped, 7-9 mm in diameter, and consists of unicellular fruiting sections, hairy on the outside, and with radial veins. The seeds are black, brown, glabrous, kidney-shaped and slightly compressed.

Flowering: June to November.

Habitat and geographical distribution:

European-Siberian, Mediterranean, Iranian-Turanian. The plant is widespread in Syria, Lebanon, Palestine, Jordan, and most parts of Europe except the northern regions. It is also found in North Africa, Iran, and Afghanistan. History and heritage: The scientific name of the genus is derived from the Latin and Greek Althianô, meaning "healed", due to the use of some species of the genus Althaea in medicine. As for oficinalis, it is from the Latin and means "constitutional." The ancient Egyptians knew the medicinal properties of the plant and used it to treat many diseases since the ninth century BC. The Greek thinker Hesiod wrote about the plant: "It was famous among the ancient Greeks, who called it Herba omniborbium (i.e. herb for all diseases), and considered it a friend of the poor." It was mentioned by Theophratus and Dioscorides. Its use has been widespread since the times of ancient Egypt. Ibn Sina praised it and described it as a laxative and a solvent for phlegm and many symptoms of muscular and nervous diseases, as mentioned by Ibn al-Baytar and al-Antaki.

Part used: Roots (collected during October and November), leaves (collected after flowering), flowers (collected at the beginning of flowering).

Chemical components:

Hallmark roots contain mucilage 5-35%, (carbohydrate compounds), starch 35%, pectin 11%, asparagine 2%, betaine 4%, lecithin, tannins, flavonoids, scopoletol, phenolic acids, enzymes. The leaves contain 10% salivary substances, 10% starch and traces of volatile oil. The flowers contain: salivary substances 5-8%, starch, pentose and hexose sugars, pectin substances, tannins, traces of volatile essential oil, in addition to flavonoids. The amount of salivary substances in the leaves, flowers and roots increases with the age of the plant, and reaches its maximum when the flowers begin to form.

Properties and medical uses:

The medicinal value of the plant is due to the salivary substances it contains, which have protective properties against irritation of the mucous membranes. The root preparations are used internally as a soothing and laxative substance, in addition to adjusting stomach acidity and being useful in treating inflammation of the mucous membranes lining the digestive system (inflammation of the lining membranes, gastric and duodenal ulcers), and inflammation of the respiratory system (inflammation of the larynx, pharyngitis and bronchitis) by forming a gelatinous layer that covers the irritated part, and helps to relieve pain, renew cells and speed up their healing. The salivary substances found in the leaves and flowers are used in the preparation of expectorants, cough medicines, bronchitis and asthma, and are used in the form of enemas in the case of chronic constipation. The salivary substances are used in the preparation of mouthwashes (antiseptic mouth and gum gargles), ointments and pastes prepared to treat wounds and skin ulcers. The salivary substances are used in the manufacture of pharmaceutical tablets. The method of obtaining the salivary substance varies according to the purpose of use. If the use is internal, the salivary substance is obtained by soaking it in cold water to prevent the starch from spoiling. However, in the case of external use, the salivary substances can be extracted with the use of. Environment: Marshmallow is a light-loving species. It is successfully grown in warm, dry, semi-dry and semi-humid environments where there is a moderate temperature (15-35°C) and air humidity (75-85%). High temperature and low humidity cause poor vegetative growth and reduced fruit set. Khatmiah grows on different types of soils, but it thrives in fertile soils rich in organic matter, and in deep, moist yellow soils. It is well tolerant of soil salinity, and the appropriate acidity (pH) ranges between 5 and 8.8.

Cultivation and productivity:

The plant is propagated by seeds, which are planted in the spring in the nursery in basins or lines 50 cm apart, and are transferred to the permanent soil when they have four leaves. Seeds can also be planted directly in the permanent soil in Warm areas. The plant can also be propagated by division, by dividing the lower part of the large plants into several sections, each containing a small root system, which develops to give a complete plant after 7-8 months. The plants are cut at the beginning of the flowering stage from about 5 cm above the soil surface during the summer, then dried in a shaded place. The hectare gives 6-7 tons of green grass. The roots are collected when the plant is 2-3 years old and the productivity of the air-dry roots reaches 2-3 tons per hectare.

***Hibiscus sabdariffa* L.**

Sabdariffa rubra Kostel.

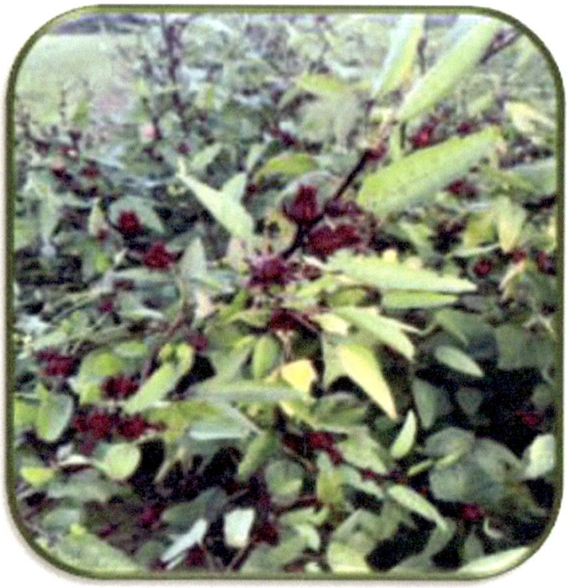

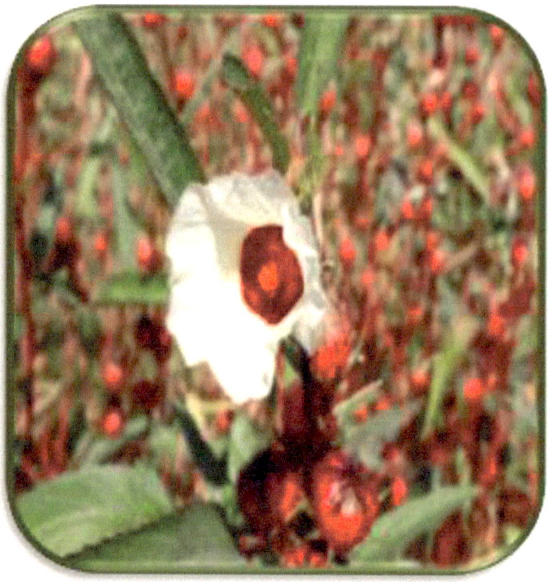

Family: Malvaceae

Common names: Hibiscus, Karkade

Foreign names: Karkade Fr. Roselle, Eng.

Occurrences : 3,728 occurrences

Distribution in the world

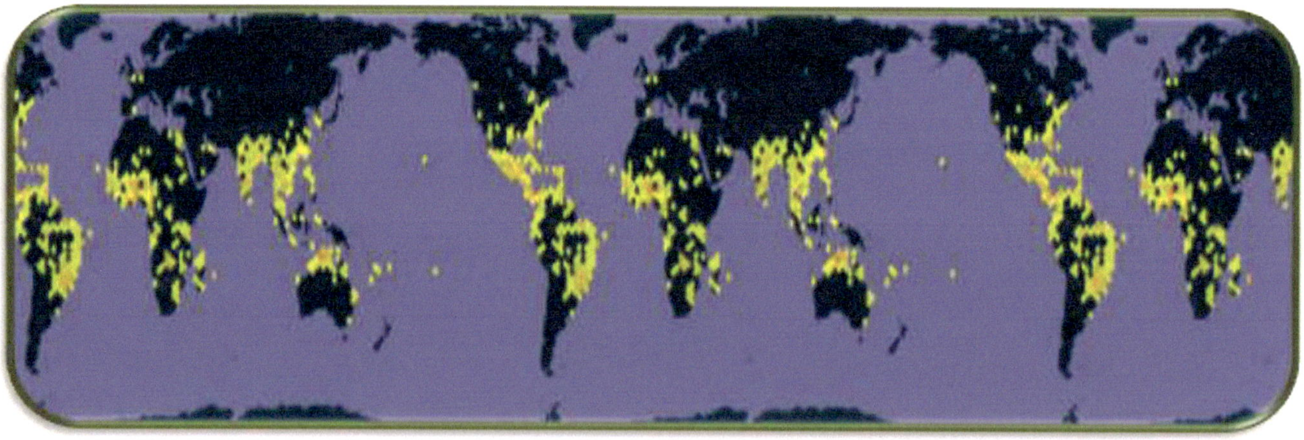

Botanical description:

Annual or perennial herb, can reach a height of up to 2 m. Stem simple or branched, solid, glabrous. Leaves simple, large, long-spiked (4-15 cm), bicolored, the lower ovate and unlobed, the upper lobed palmately, both glabrous. Ears 6-8 mm, filiform. Flowers relatively large, axillary, solitary, semi-spiked.The calyx is supported by a calyx composed of 8-12 segments, linear, 6-10 mm long, which becomes fleshy, reddish after flowering, and persists with the fruit. The calyx has 5 sepals, purple, fused at the base, 1-3 cm long, fleshy, woolly-haired and thorny, bearing at its base a linear gland on the median nerve. The corolla is yellow with a crimson spot in the center, the petals are 3-5 cm long, and fall off during drying. The stamen filaments are united to form a stamen tube. The fruit is a capsule about 2 cm long, containing many spherical seeds.

Flowering: Summer - Autumn.

Homeland and geographical distribution:

West Indies, Central Africa, currently cultivated in tropical and hot regions of the world. It is cultivated in Upper Egypt and Sudan. History and heritage: It is believed that the origin of the name of the genus goes back to the Greek from the word hibiskos, which is of the origin of ibis in relation to the bird "ibis" that eats from the plant, and the Indians used its leaves in ancient times for food.

Part used: The calyx and the red-colored sepals.

Chemical components:

The sepals contain organic acids (fruit acids) 15-30%, the most important of which are hibiscus acid, tartaric acid, citric acid, malic acid, and vitamin C. Anthocyanins pigments (red color): cyanidin-3-xyloglucoside, delphinidin-3-xylogluco- side, delphinidin-3-glucoside. Flavonoid compounds including: gossypetin, hibiscin. Quantities of calcium oxalate. Salivary (gelatinous) substances, including: arabinans, arabinogalactans, rhamnogalacturonans.

Properties and medical uses:

Hibiscus drink has a soothing, moisturizing, acidic taste that reduces the sensation of heat. It contains antiseptic and antibacterial compounds that infect many people when temperatures rise in the summer.The drink also has refreshing properties, stimulates digestion and secretion of digestive juices, is a mild laxative, dissolves phlegm, reduces the feeling of thirst, because it contains organic acids, especially hibiscus acid. It is a heart tonic, lowers blood pressure, and relaxes the muscles of the uterus. The aqueous extract of hibiscus has a stimulating effect.Studies have shown that hibiscus drink helps relieve the pain of gout and rheumatism. Research has shown the effect of hibiscus flower extract in eliminating tuberculosis bacteria, many other bacterial strains, and some parasites. It has also shown the soothing properties of the flowers and leaves for uterine, stomach, and intestinal contractions. Hibiscus tea is popularly used as a rich source of organic acids and vitamin C, a diuretic, a digestive system cleanser, a sedative for uterine and intestinal cramps, a nerve relaxant, and increases blood circulation. It also helps strengthen the heartbeat. It is often used in winter to treat colds and flu because it contains a high percentage of vitamin C. It has been used in folk medicine for thousands of years. Thanks to its many active compounds, polyphenols, And polysaccharides, organic acids, or pectins, which show hypoglycemic, antioxidant, hypotensive, anti-lipidic and many indirect effects associated with them. Hibiscus is a promising product that can be used either alone or added to conventional treatment regimens to prevent or treat diabetes and its associated diseases. Hibiscus and its extracts show an effect on blood sugar. It leads to an increase in insulin levels in the blood (by renewing Langerhans islets) and reducing HOMA-IR values. Hibiscus has antioxidant and disease-protective properties. The antioxidant properties of this plant improve the condition of low blood fats (dyslipidemia). Studies have shown that hibiscus has a protective effect on many organs, such as the pancreas, liver and kidneys, through different mechanisms. Hibiscus can help The extracts prepared from it also improve heart and blood vessel weakness. It also protects the testicles and sperm from damage resulting from diabetes. It improves cognitive dysfunction in the context of diabetes. In addition, antibacterial activity has been proven and its potential use as an antiseptic in diabetic foot. It has kidney-protective, anti-anemia, antioxidant, anti-inflammatory, and anti-dehydration effects.

Other uses:

Hibiscus drink is prepared from flower spikes by soaking them in water Cold or boiled for a short period and filtered. Hibiscus drink is served cold or hot and sweetened as desired. Sepals are used in the manufacture of jelly, jams, ice cream and sweets to add a healthy natural color and a pleasant flavor. Pharmaceutical and healthy soap factories use natural coloring materials extracted from the sepals of the hibiscus flower in their products. Sepals are used in the cosmetics industry as a natural colorant (lipstick, face powders). Hibiscus can be used as a safe drink for diabetics.The calyx leaves are widely used in cosmetics, foods, and in many medical applications.The drug has been used as an extract, in the form of enemas, decoctions, tea, drinks, in the form of capsules, pills, and in folk medicine to treat many diseases. Hibiscus plant is a major natural source for the production of plant fibers needed for the manufacture of ropes, paper and pure cellulose. Warnings for use: The saplings contain a high percentage of calcium oxalate, so it is not recommended for patients with kidney and urinary system problems in general, and it is also warned against its use by people with low blood pressure.

Environment:

Hibiscus grows in hot, dry areas with long days where the temperature is high and the humidity is low. Under these conditions, it gives a high flower yield in quantity and quality. The plant prefers light, fertile soil. The formation of anthocyanin pigments is affected by genetics and environment. The presence of a high concentration of sugar in the cells facilitates the formation of anthocyanin pigments. Lighting and low temperatures help increase the concentration of sugar and increase the pigments.

Cultivation and productivity:

The plant is propagated by seeds that are planted in the spring. Delaying their planting leads to a reduction in lateral branching and the formation of few and small flowers. Planting is done in lines 75 cm wide, leaving 60 cm between holes on the line and placing 4-5 seeds in the hole. The hectare needs 12-25 kg of seeds. The plant requires the necessary service operations of patching, thinning, fertilization and moderate irrigation of the plants. The process of collecting the flower cups attached to the fruits begins when they are spread out and open outwards, where they become easily broken, and this is done in early autumn until early winter at a rate of once every 3-4 days. After picking, the cups are transferred to the drying place, and placed on saws with a thickness not exceeding 10 cm, with daily turning to prevent rotting and fermentation and to speed up the drying process. The production of dry flower cups per hectare reaches 1.5 tons.

Malva sylvestris L.

Malva ambigua var. *microphylla* Rouy.

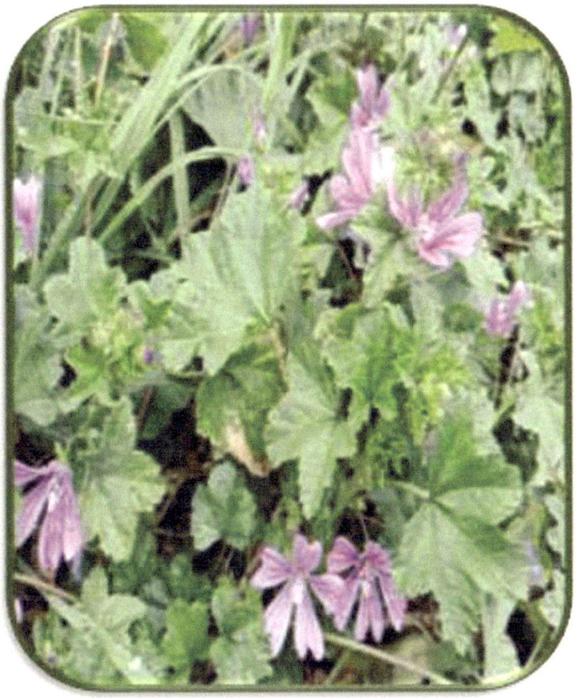

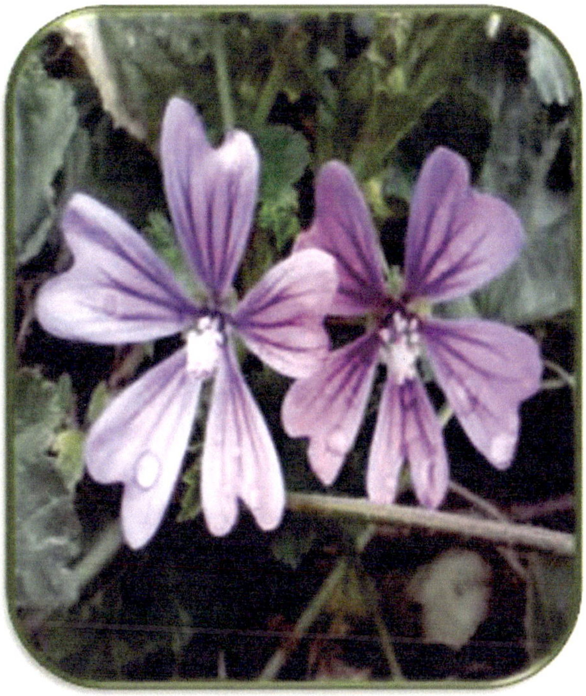

Family: Malvaceae

Common names: Forest mallow, Mallow, Muffin,

Foreign names: Eng. Common mallow, Fr. Mauve sylvestre

Occurrences : 234,065 occurrences

Distribution in the world

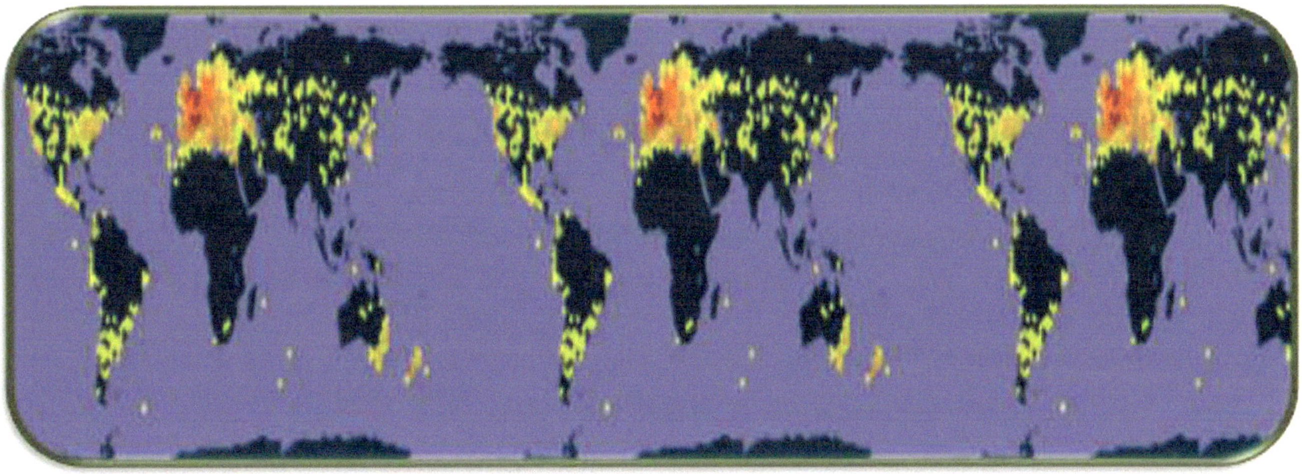

Botanical description:

An annual or biennial herb, hairy, 20-70 cm tall. Stem erect to ascending, sometimes lying, branched. Leaves simple, long-spined, rounded, 3-7-lobed, serrated at the margin, cordate at the base, hairy, palmately venated, and variable in size. Ears ovate to oblong, pinnate. Flowers axillary, in clusters of 2-3 or more. Inflorescences erect. The calyx is supported by a 3-segmented, free, oblong to lanceolate calyx, two-thirds the length of the calyx. The calyx has 5 sepals, 6-10 mm long, its lobes are convergent, ovate to triangular, bearing star-shaped hairs. The petals have 5, free, pink with purple veins, their length exceeds 3-4 times the length of the calyx, inverted ovate to oblong, truncated at the apex, and sphenoid and hairy at the base. The male has 5 stamens, their filaments are fused together to form a stromal tube that branches into many anthers. The female has many carpels. The fruit is a lobe, about 1 cm in diameter, consisting of a number of fruiting meristems equal to the number of carpels.

Flowering: February to April.

Habitat and geographical distribution: Mediterranean and European-Siberian extending to the Iranian-Turanian region. Introduced to South and North America and Australia.

History and heritage:

The scientific name of the genus is derived from the Greek word malakos meaning "soft", alluding to the softness of its leaves and its laxative properties. Malva was used as a popular food and medicinal herb, mentioned by Al-Ghasani and Al-Antaki.

Part used: Dried leaves and fresh flowering plant.

Chemical components:

The leaves contain flavonoids, including: hypolaetin-3-glucoside, gossypetin-3-glucoside salivary substances, (polysaccharides) 17%, including arabinogalactans and galacturonorhamane, The flowers contain anthocyanidin compounds, including malvin, and salivary substances 10% similar to those found in the leaves. The leaves and flowers contain many biologically active compounds such as flavonoids, gum, terpenoids, phenolic derivatives, coumarins, sterols, tannins, saponins, and alkaloids.

Properties and medical uses:

The plant has salivary substances that protect against irritation of the mucous membranes. Anti-haemolytic agents. The flowers and leaves are used in cases of dry cough, bronchitis and chest colds, mouth and throat infections, and digestive system infections. The flowers and leaves are popularly used to treat coughs, asthma, bronchitis and tonsillitis, throat and mouth irritation, and digestive system irritation. A decoction of the flowers or leaves is used topically to treat wounds and skin abrasions, swelling and irritation of highly sensitive skin, toothache, and insect bites. Extracts of the raw leaves and extracts of the flowers and leaves are anti-inflammatory. The plant has toxic effects on cells of various types of cancer cells. Work is currently underway to develop copper oxide nanoparticles using mallow leaf extract for potential use in food and medicine. Mallow is available in dry form and as a liquid extract. It is sold under names such as Malvedrin and Malveol.

Precautions for use:

The plant should be avoided by pregnant or breastfeeding women. It is also not recommended for long-term use.

Environment:

Mallow is a wild spring-summer plant that grows in diverse environments from dry and semi-dry to semi-humid temperate and warm. It is planted in various types of soil, and prefers moist red soil. It gives a high yield in medium-fertile soil, and responds well to irrigation.

Cultivation and productivity:

Mallow is grown as a winter crop in warm areas, and its vegetative and floral growth continues in spring, summer and until late autumn when suitable moisture is available, while it is planted in spring in cold areas. Cultivation is done in lines, with dimensions of 60X25 or 30X25 cm and sometimes with higher density within 3X4 m basins or basins. It is recommended to bury the seeds at a depth of 3 cm. Appropriate service operations such as weeding and pest and weed control are carried out.

Picking of leaves and flowers begins two months after planting, and continues during the summer. Flowers are collected on hot, dry, sunny days at midday, and dried in the shade at 40°C to preserve their color. Leaves are also collected and dried in the same way.

History and Heritage:

The genus name Ficus comes from the Greek Sykê or sykos, which is derived from the ancient Phoenician language. The descriptive name for the species Carica comes from Carra or Carie, an ancient country in the Near East (Turkey). Fig cultivation dates back more than 5,000 years, and was known to the Greeks and Romans. It is also said that figs were Cleopatra's favorite fruit, and that the snake that killed her was hidden in a basket of figs. The Phoenicians used it on their travels. Marine and land for food and treatment of skin diseases, pimples and gum infections. Many wars were fought throughout history with the aim of occupying lands where this species is widespread.

The fruits have been used since ancient times as a traditional treatment against constipation, and in the treatment of digestive disorders.

Part used: Fresh or dried ripe fruits, Latex sap (skin irritant.)

Chemical components:

The fruits contain simple sugars, especially dextrose at a rate of 50%, organic acids, especially citric acid, malic acid. Mucilage and minerals such as iron, copper, calcium, potassium, manganese and bromine and vitamins such as A, B1, B2 and C, pectins and flavonoids. The milky juice contains the enzyme ficin (a milk-coagulating enzyme), and salivary gums. Furanocoumarins, including: psoralen, and bergaptene. The total content of phenolics is 12.29 mg/100 g dry sample and of flavonoids 40.729 mg/g.

Properties and medical uses:

Figs are easily absorbed, rich in energy, and are given to children, during recovery periods, athletes, and thin people. Diabetics and obese people are warned against eating them. The fruits have laxative properties that are useful in cases of constipation in general, and in the elderly in particular, digestive (dissolving intestinal laziness), and for treating whooping cough, chest infections, and urinary tract infections.

The fruit extract is popularly used to treat throat ulcers, swollen gums, and is used as a poultice to treat tumors. A decoction of the leaves is used to treat diabetes and gingivitis. The milky juice secreted by the leaf stalks and young branches is popularly used to treat skin diseases (warts, boils and skin ulcers), and is also used as a laxative and anthelmintic. The methanolic extract of the plant has shown antioxidant activity.

The extract reduced ischemia-induced lesions, possibly due to the antioxidant activity, flavonoids and phenolic compounds in the extract. The methanolic extract of fig leaves has a protective effect against myocardial infarction. Studies have confirmed that latex plays a role in the early programmed death of cancer cells. A single dose of 2 g/kg of latex did not cause any death. Phytochemical analyses confirmed the presence of lupeol acetate and lupeol palmitate in the chloroform extract of the plant. Latex is used against skin warts caused by the human papillomavirus. It also has a role in inhibiting the cancerous cell lines of the cervix, CaSki and HeLa, as it reduces rapid growth. The results indicate that plant latex can be used in developing methods for treating, curing and preventing cervical cancer associated with the human papillomavirus.

Environment:

Figs are a light-loving species, resistant to cold up to -5°C in winter, but need protection and care to resist cold. Tolerates winds. Relatively resistant to drought, and its growth in relatively hot summer conditions is necessary to produce good quality fruits. It prefers fertile, well-drained soils, despite its ability to live on different types of soils.

Cultivation and productivity:

It is propagated by seeds that are transmitted and spread by birds, as well as by cuttings and grafting. It is planted at a distance of 5-6 m in rainfed agriculture and 6-7 m in irrigated agriculture. It is recommended to cut (prune) the tree in winter at a height of 60-70 cm and sometimes more to encourage branching and crown formation. The tree is then pruned by removing intertwined branches) to maintain the shape of the crown and produce fruitful branches. The trees are fertilized with organic fertilizer in winter and watered when needed, taking into account good soil drainage. A species sensitive to scale insects and red spider. The tree can be planted in orchards, gardens and on green areas in different conditions. The fruits appear in summer and continue until autumn. Fruiting begins 3 years after planting, depending on the variety planted.

Ficus salicifolia Vahl.

Ficus cordata subsp. *salicifolia*)Vahl(C.C.Berg, *Urostigma salicifolium*)Vahl(Miq.

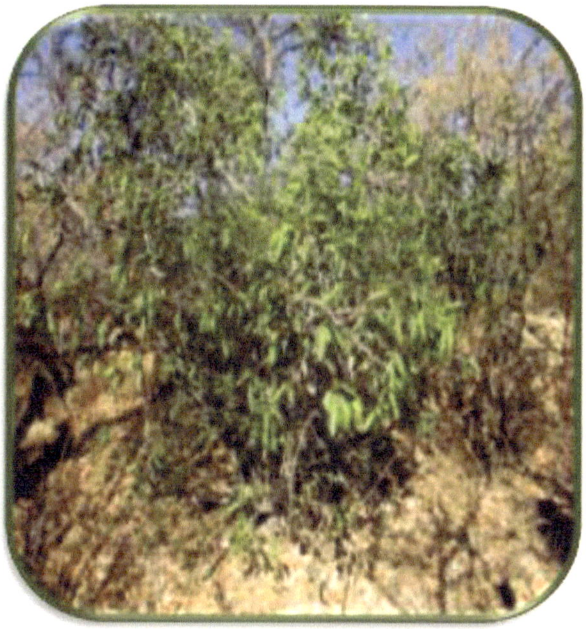

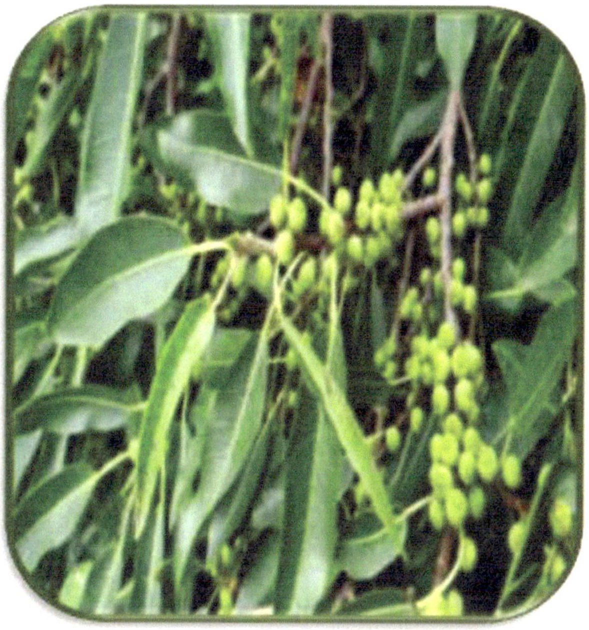

Family: Moraceae

Common names: Athb

Foreign names: Eng. Willow-leaved fig, Fr. Figuier sauvage

Occurrences : 1,588 occurrences

Distribution in the world

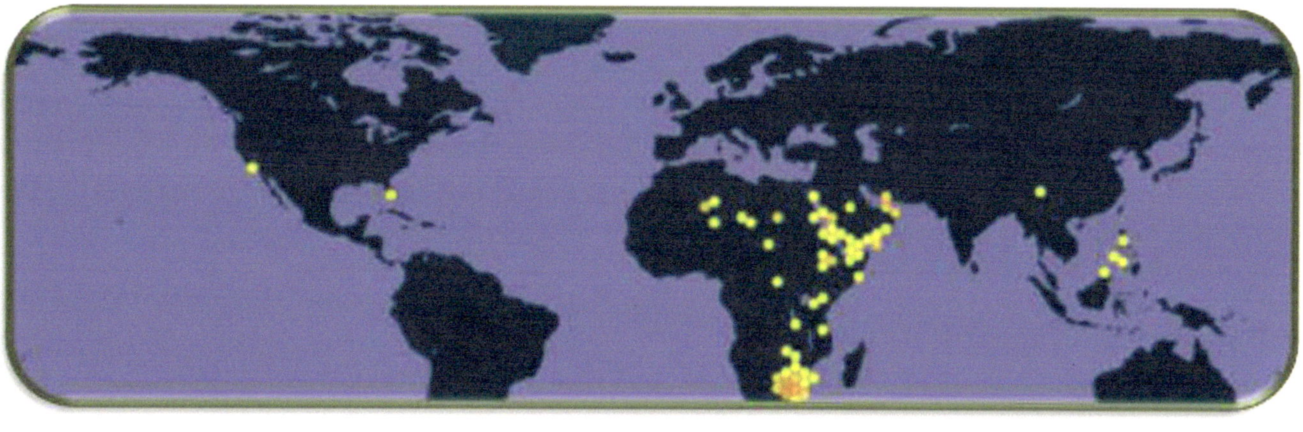

Botanical description:

An evergreen tree, reaching a height of about 8 meters, with a blue-green color, dense branches and leaves, bearing large lanceolate leaves that reach a length of 14 cm, and a width of 4 cm. The inflorescence is nut-sized, found in groups in the leaf axils. Flowers are unisexual, the female flower consists of two carpels and an ovary containing a single ovule, while the male flower contains a single stamen with a straight thread. The fruit is false, composed of both male and female flowers. Its fruits are formed as a result of the growth of the conical or spherical inflorescence, which contains inside it the fruits of the common fig, except that they are small, green before ripening and turning pink after ripening, and they are one of the edible fruits.

Homeland and geographical distribution:

India, and is widely spread in the cold regions of the Kingdom of Saudi Arabia, especially the Asir region. Its spread extends to South America.

History and heritage:

The descriptive name of the species salicifolia means "willow-leaf", due to the shape of its leaves that resemble the leaves of the willow. Salix It is said that consuming the fresh fruits may lead to attacks of tremors and hallucinations.

Part used: Aerial parts of the plant.

Chemical components: The fruits contain saliva and sugary substances. The leaves contain a milky juice rich in coumarin and tannin compounds. The aerial parts contain alkaloids, flavonoids, sterols and tannins.

Properties and medical uses:

Research has shown that the thuja contains a number of active substances, some of which are heart tonics, and some of which work to reduce blood pressure in the arteries and stimulate the central nervous system. Studies have also shown the properties of the leaves and bark of the tree, which are rich in astringent tannins that are useful in treating diarrhea, dysentery, and stopping internal or external bleeding. Studies have shown that the alcoholic extract of the latex kills bacteria, especially Staphylococcus aureus, Escherichia coli, and Candida albicans. Latex is rich in polyphenolic compounds, and is therefore an antioxidant and anti-proliferative. Studies have indicated that the latex substance has anti-proliferative and cytotoxic effects. The drug is used to treat wounds and prevent their expansion. Figs have been found to have genotoxic effects on cancer cells of the MDA-MB-23 type derived from breast cancer.The fruits, which are rich in saliva and sugars, are popularly used as a laxative in cases of constipation. The milky juice secreted by the plant is also used topically to treat some skin diseases such as warts and vitiligo. The juice is used as an eye wash and to treat hemorrhoids, joint pain and bruises.

Precautions for use:

Milky juice should not be used internally.

Environment:

It grows on steep slopes and is considered one of the most drought-resistant fig species.

Cultivation and productivity:

It is widespread in the wild and is rarely cultivated

Ficus sycomorus L.

Ficus chanas Forssk., *Ficus cocculifolia* Baker., *Sycomorus gnaphalocarpa* Miq., *Sycomorus rigida* Miq., *Sycomorus trachyphyllus* Fenzl ex Miq.

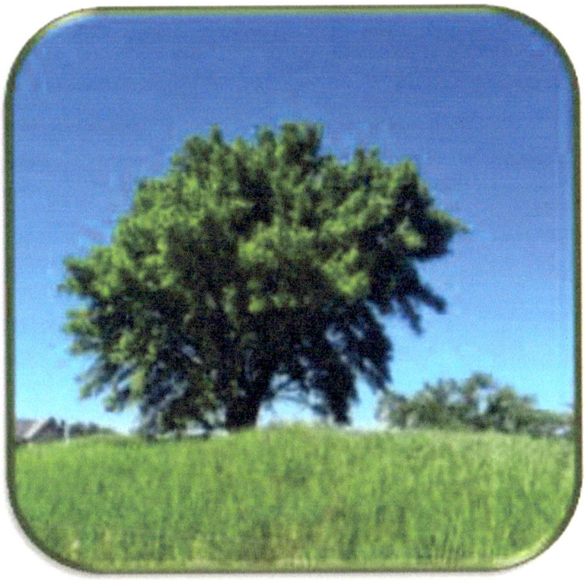

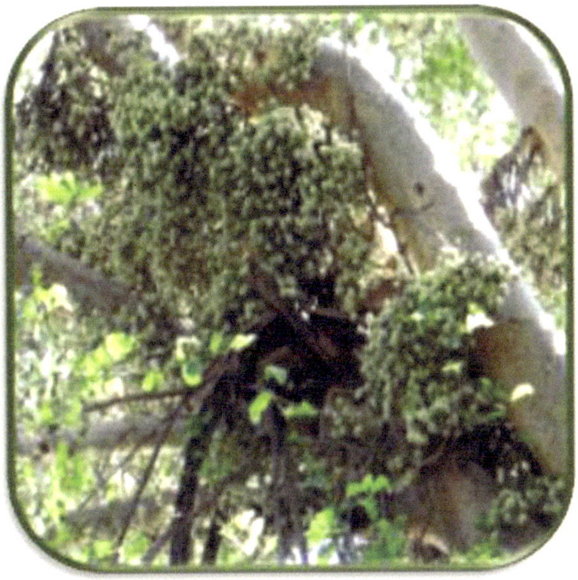

Family: Moraceae

Common names: Sycamore, Sycomore fig

Foreign names: Malberry fig, Sycomore fig, Sycomore, Fr. Figuier Sycomore

Occurrences : 4,532 occurrences

Distribution in the world

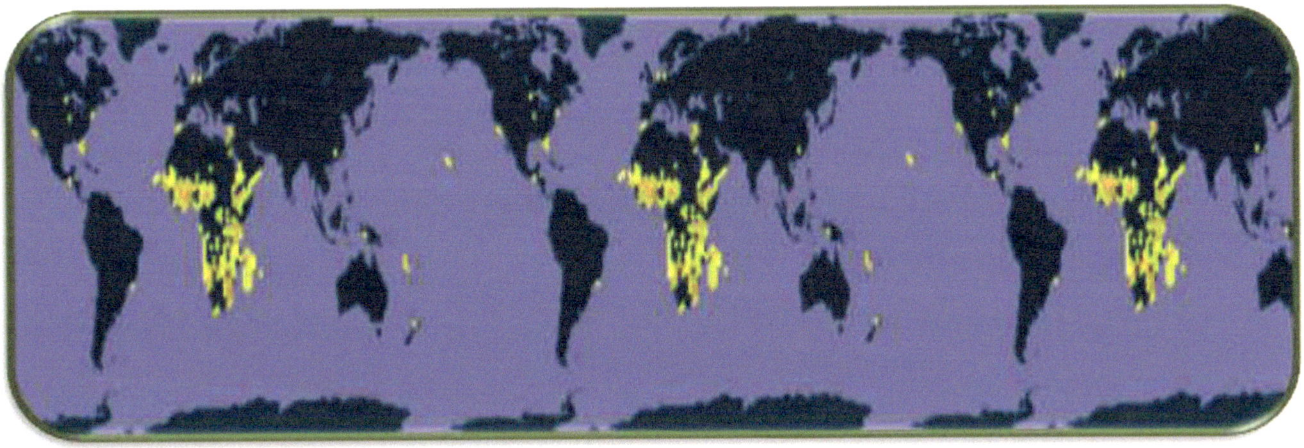

Botanical description:

An evergreen tree, its wood is characterized by its strength, especially when immersed in water. Its leaves are oval in shape, rough in texture, the fruits are somewhat similar to figs, but much thinner, there are no seeds in the fruit like figs, its taste is sweet, its color is yellow tending to red. The plant secretes abundant milky liquid when any part of it is cut. The tree begins to bear fruit about 5 years after planting.

Habitat and geographical distribution:

Southern Arabian Peninsula, Egypt, and Sudan. It was transferred long ago to the Levant, and spread in many countries, especially in temperate and hot environments.

History and Heritage:

The descriptive name of the species Sycomorus goes back to the Greek Sukomoros from Sukon meaning "fig" and moros meaning "berry." A tree known since ancient times to the Pharaohs, and was considered one of their holiest trees. They used the milky sap in therapeutic recipes for some skin diseases and in treating scorpion stings and snake bites. Sycamore was also included in Pharaonic recipes as a laxative and softener, and they used sycamore juice to treat liver diseases, intestinal infections and scurvy. It is said that the oldest tree of this type still exists in the Matariya area near Cairo, and is called the Virgin Mary Tree, and it is said that the Virgin Mary took shelter in its shade during her famous journey to Egypt.

Part used: Fruits, leaves and milky juice.

Chemical components:

Sycamore fruits contain plant milk, sugars, flavonoids and vitamins. The milky juice contains enzymes, salivary substances and furanocoumarin compounds, the most important of which are psoralen and bergaptene

Properties and medical uses:

Research has confirmed the antiseptic properties of milky juice, and it is used topically to treat wounds and some skin diseases such as ulcers and psoriasis. Fresh sycamore fruits are used as a laxative in cases of constipation, a stimulant for the stomach and intestines, a disinfectant for intestinal infections and a gas expeller. A decoction of the leaves is used in the form of gargles to treat gingivitis.

Environment:

A species sensitive to cold and friendly to light. It prefers fertile, well-drained soils. It can live in coastal areas or near them. It is planted on the banks of rivers and in gardens.

Cultivation and productivity:

A multi-purpose tree, mainly grown for its sugary fruits that resemble figs. Propagated mainly by cuttings in the spring, fruiting begins 5 years after planting, the fruit is a fig that does not ripen until a type of insect Sycophaga cressipes lays its eggs in the ovaries of the female flowers. Therefore, a slit must be made in the fruit to facilitate the insect's entry into it. The process is called circumcision, where the slit area darkens as the fruit ripens. The fruit is found on the tree almost all year round.

Morus nigra L.

Morus cretica Raf., *Morus laciniata* Mill., *Morus petiolaris* Raf., *Morus siciliana* Mill.

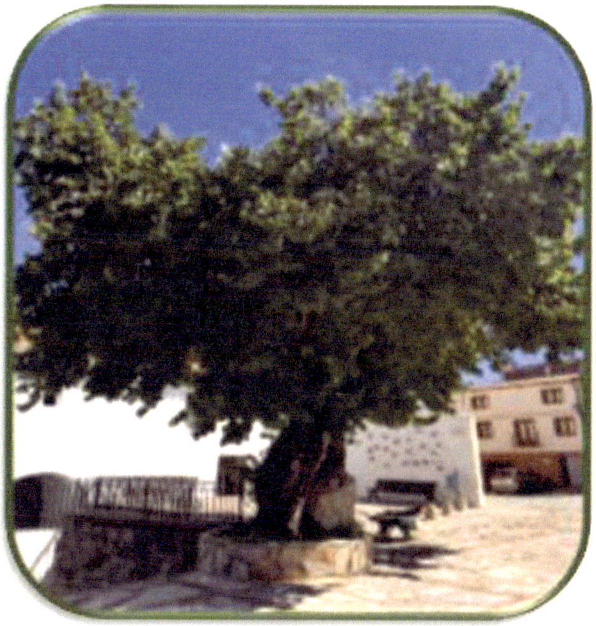

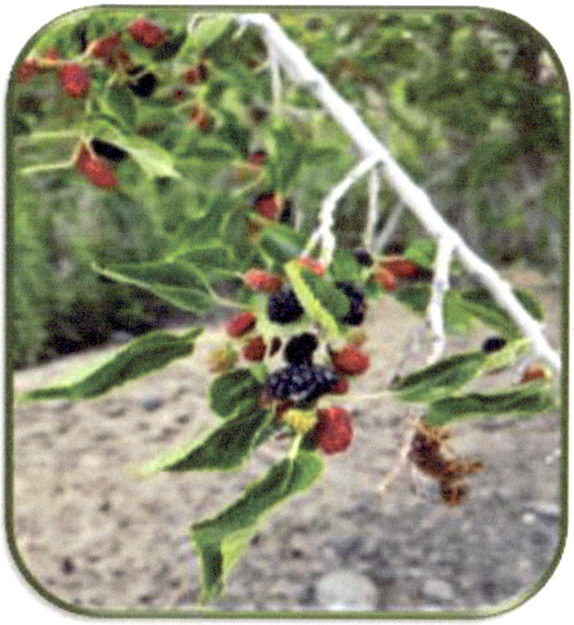

Family: Moraceae

Common names: Blackberry (Levantine).

Foreign names: noire Mûrier Fr. mulberry, Black Eng.

Occurrences : 4,975 occurrences

Distribution in the world

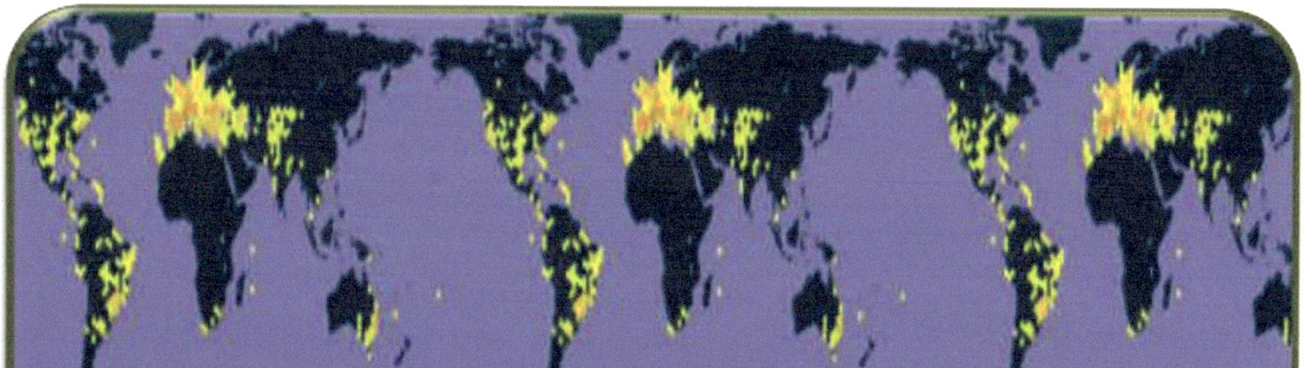

Botanical description:

A deciduous tree, up to 12 m high, dioecious or monoecious. The bark is brown-black. The leaves are simple,velvet, the leaf blade is broadly oval, not velvet. Spoons 1.5 - 2.5 cm, Alternate. The ears are lanceolate, membranous, lobed, its base is cordate, its tip is acute or slightly pointed. Its edge is serrated, its length is 10-20 cm longer than the length of the berry blade. White, thick, one surface of the leaf is pale green and downy, the other is dark green and rough. Male inflorescences Fluffy. Female inflorescences are elliptical, 2-2.5 cm long, the inflorescence is very short (shorter Cylindrical, 2-4 cm long, than in white mulberry.) The corolla is completely absent in mulberry, and the inflorescence is represented by four sepals, which take on a fleshy texture when the fruit is ripe. The male in male flowers is composed of 4 stamens. Female flowers have an unclear style, the stigma is two-branched. The fruit is clustered (flower product), without a stalk, black in color when ripe, its dimensions are 2 - 2.5 x 1.5 - 2.5 cm, its taste is very sour before full ripeness, then sour - sugary after ripening. The Middle East is interested in this type, and there are many agricultural varieties.

Flowering: Late spring and early summer, fruiting in summer.

Home and geographical distribution:

Northern Iran and Armenia, and its cultivation has spread to Syrian regions and many countries of the world.

History and heritage:

The name of the genus morus is derived from the Greek morea, which is the ancient name of the tree in Greece, while the descriptive name for the species nigra means "black" in reference to its black fruits.

Part used:

Ripped fruits and leaves (its leaves are not suitable for raising silkworms due to their hardness and thickness.)

Chemical components:

The fruits contain: Fruit acids 2%, the most important of which are: malic acid, citric acid, betulin-

ic acid and sucrose 10%, pectins, phenolic compounds, and flavonoids, the most important of which is rutin, Anthocyanin pigments (responsible for the black color of the fruits.)

Many vitamins: Vitamin C or ascorbic acid 0.17%, Vitamin B2 and B3.

Minerals: Potassium K, Calcium Ca, Magnesium Mg, Sodium Na, Iron Fe, Zinc Zn, Nickel .Ni

The leaves contain flavonoid compounds 2-6%, the most important of which is rutin. The bark of trees contains flavonoid compounds, including A - E albanin, M moracin, which have antioxidant properties.

The antioxidant capacity is attributed to the presence of phytochemical components such as polyphenols, flavonoids, and anthocyanins.

Properties and medical uses:

Blackberries, with their flavonoid compounds, phenols, and anthocyanins, have antioxidant and anti-inflammatory properties. The anthocyanins and acids contained in the fruit may help prevent colon cancer. Experiments on mice have shown that the leaf extract has anti-pain-reducing and anti-inflammatory properties for the mucous membranes of the respiratory system. Mulberry juice is used as a nutritious drink rich in sugars, minerals, acids and vitamins, and as a moisturizer. It relieves constipation, reduces blood sugar levels, and is useful in treating heat and thirst, stomach acidity, intestinal inflammation, anemia and liver weakness. Mulberry juice is used as a gargle to treat gingivitis, and the fruit puree is used to treat acne and cleanse the skin. Mulberry juice is also used to color and improve the taste of some types of medicines.

Environment:

A species that tolerates cold and high temperatures, and also tolerates thirst. It lives on different types of soil, although it prefers moist, well-drained soil. It tolerates salinity and alkaline gravel soils. It needs sunny places and is protected from the wind.

Morus alba L.

Morus sinensis G.Don., *Morus subalba* Steud., *Morus tatarica* L., *Morus tokwa* (Bureau) K.Koch, *Morus tortuosa* Audib. ex Moretti, *Morus venassainii* Steud., *Morus venosa* (Delile) Spach

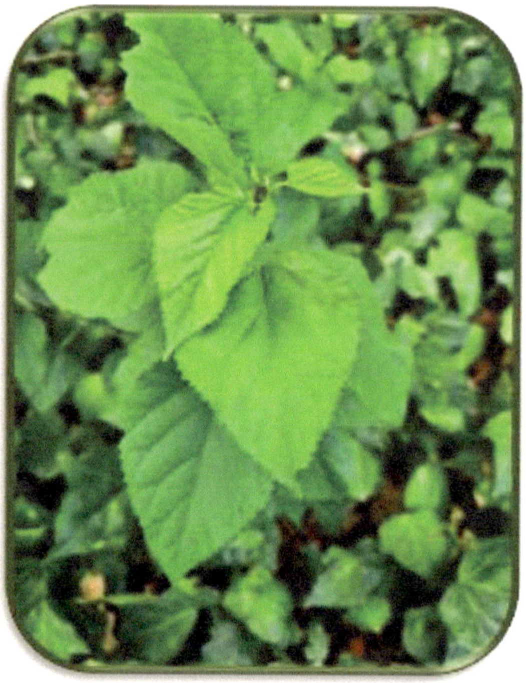

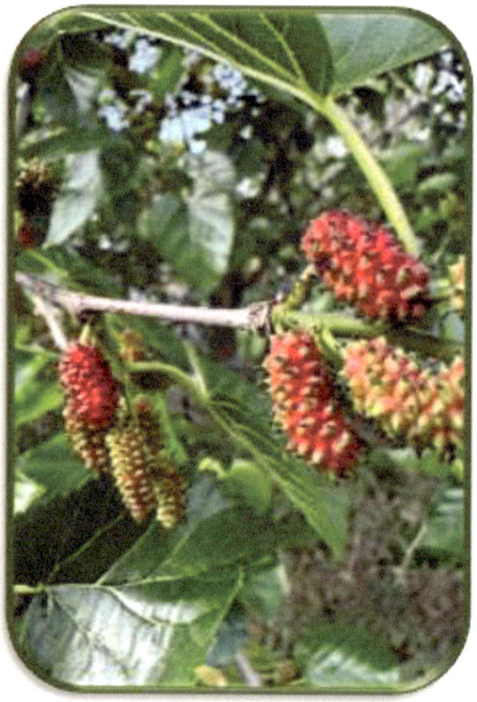

Family: Moraceae

Common names: White Mulberry

Foreign names: Blanc mûrier Fr., Mulberry White Eng.

Occurrences : 36,414 occurrences

Distribution in the world

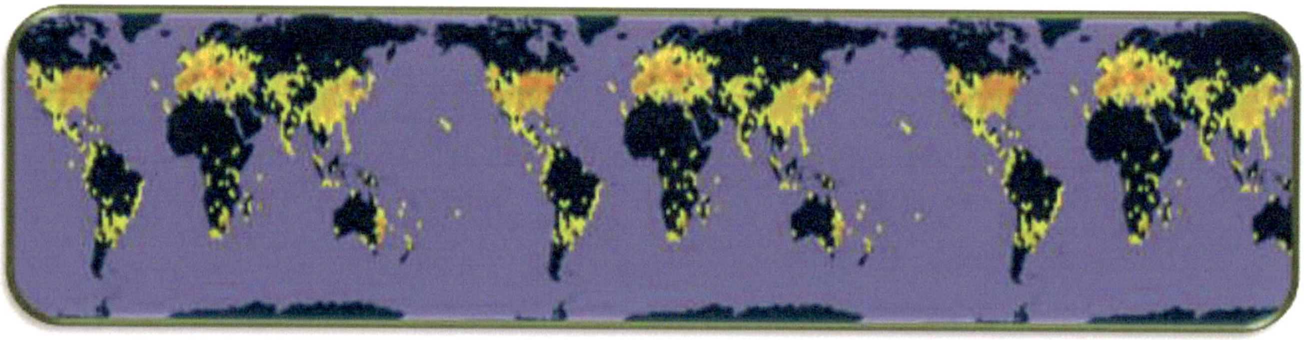

Botanical description:

A deciduous tree, 3-10 m high, produces vegetable milk. The bark of the stem is gray in color, its cracks are superficial, The branches are covered with soft hairs. The winter buds are reddish-brown in color, oval, and downy. The ears are lanceolate, downy. The leaf blade is oval, serrate to the cristae, round to hearty 2-3.5 mm. The obstructed 1.5-5.5 cm, base, apex pointed, 5-12 cm long, upper surface glabrous and hairy only, along the median rib on the lower side of the leaf. Flowers unisexual, without a corolla, and the plants are monoecious. Male inflorescences are cylindrical, drooping, cylindrical, 2-3 cm long, covered with dense white hair. Female inflorescences are semi-spherical cylindrical, 1-2 cm, panicle 5-10 mm. The calyx is quadripartite in male flowers, its lobes are broadly elliptical, and in female flowers its lobes are oval and bear hairs on their edges. The male has 4 stamens. The female has two carpels. The fruit is collected in a panicle, greenish-white in color when ripe, oval, elliptical or cylindrical in shape, 1-2.5 cm long. Its taste is slightly sweet before ripening and becomes very sweet after full ripening.

Flowering: April to May, fruiting from May to June.

Habitat and geographical distribution:

It is believed that its original habitat is Central Asia and northern China, from where it spread to many regions of the world, and it has been introduced to many countries for silkworm breeding.

History and heritage: The scientific name of the genus Morus is derived from the Greek Morea, which is the ancient name of the tree in Greece. The descriptive name of the species alba, meaning "white" in reference to its white fruits. The common Arabic name is berries, and it has been used since ancient times to name the genus.

Part used: Fruits and leaves

Chemical components:

A 100-gram berry fruit consists of 87 grams of water, 8.3 grams of monosaccharides, which may sometimes reach 20 grams, 1.5 grams of protein, 0.49 grams of fat, 1.4 grams of fiber, 0.9 grams of minerals, and a number of vitamins. The leaves contain aromatic amino acids gamma-aminobutyric acid.

Favones including: isoquercitrin, scopolin, astragalin Polyphenols including: bronthocanidin in addition to the compound deoxynojirimycin. The compound pentahydroxyflavone is one of the important compounds in many plants that belong to the Moraceae family. The compound Morin has antiviral, antibacterial and antioxidant activities. It inhibits Δ5-lipoxygenase, iodothyronine deiodinase, and aldose reductase enzymes and arachidonic acid secretion.

Properties and medical uses:

Berries have antioxidant properties. Research has shown the effect of the proanthocanidin compound in stopping the reproduction of the hepatitis C virus, which causes liver fibrosis or cancer. The gamma-aminobutyric acid compound helps reduce blood pressure, and the deoxynojirimycin compound helps reduce blood sugar levels. Eating the leaves led to a reduction in heart fibrosis and activation of mitogen-activated protein kinase (MAPK) and endothelin-1 and the catalytic factor. For the growth of the vascular lining (VEGF). This indicates that the leaves have great benefits for improving heart function and in cardiomyopathy resulting from myocarditis.

Other uses:

A multi-purpose tree, used as a fruit tree, and for raising silkworms. The wood is strong and suitable for carpentry, carving and making agricultural tools. It is planted in gardens and streets as a shade tree. The leaves have fodder value.

Environment: Tolerant of cold, high temperatures and salinity, and can be used in afforestation of saline lands.

Cultivation and productivity:

Propagation by seeds in spring In the fall, by cuttings or grafting at the end of winter, and by grafting with the eye in the summer.

Moringa oleifera Lam.

Gualandinia moringa L., *Hyperanthera moringa* (L.) Vahl, *M. edulis* Medic.، *M. erecta* Salisb., *Moringa parvifolia* Noronha, *M. polygona* DC., *M. pterygosperma* Gaertn., *M. zeylanica* Pers.

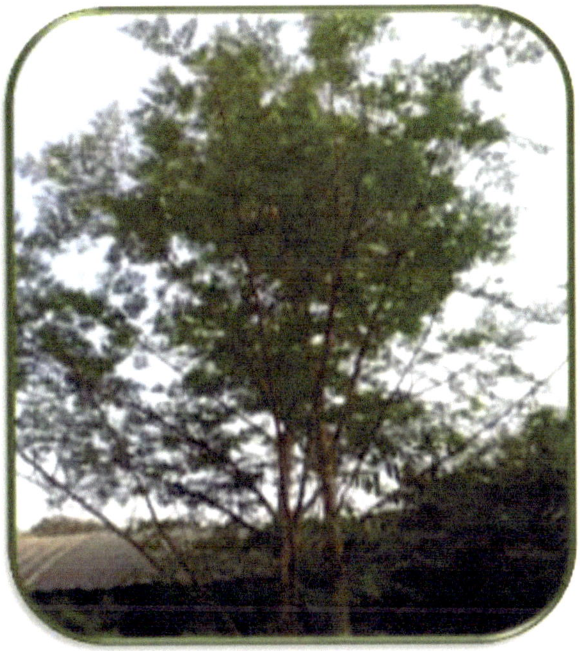

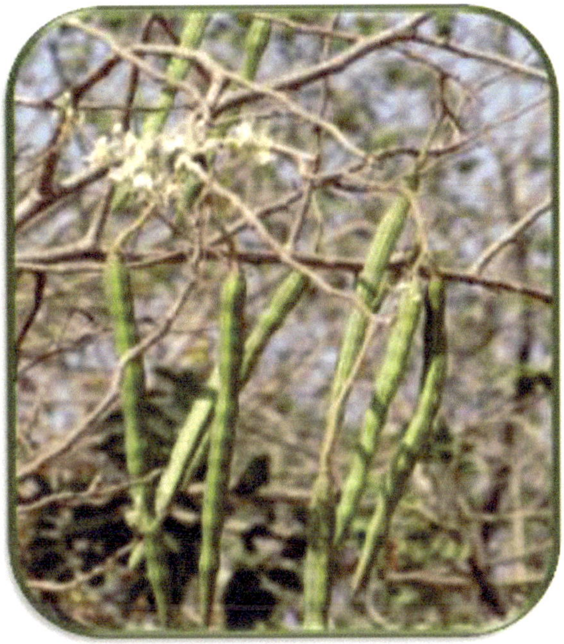

Family: Moringaceae

Common names: Moringa, horseradish tree, drumstick tree, shoa, bon tree

Foreign names: moringa Fr. tree, nut Ben Eng.

Occurrences : 11,328 occurrences

Distribution in the world

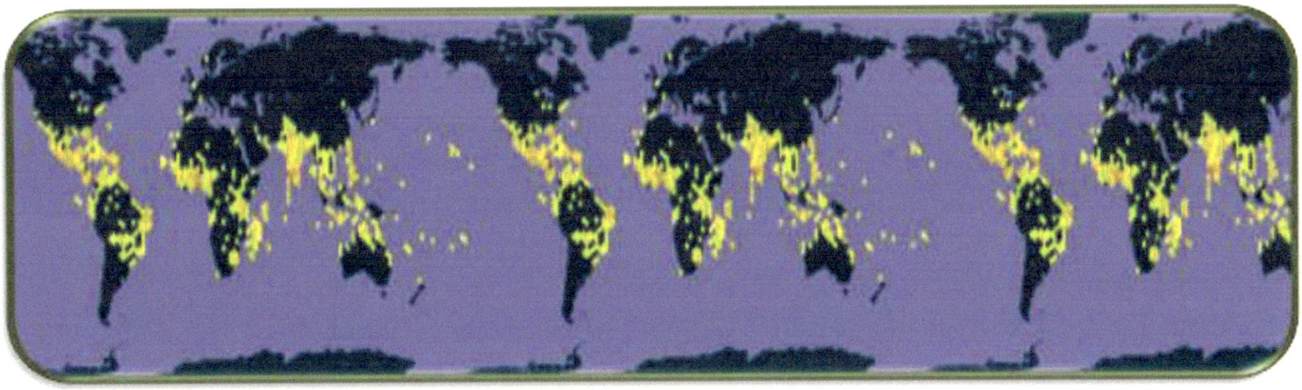

Botanical description:

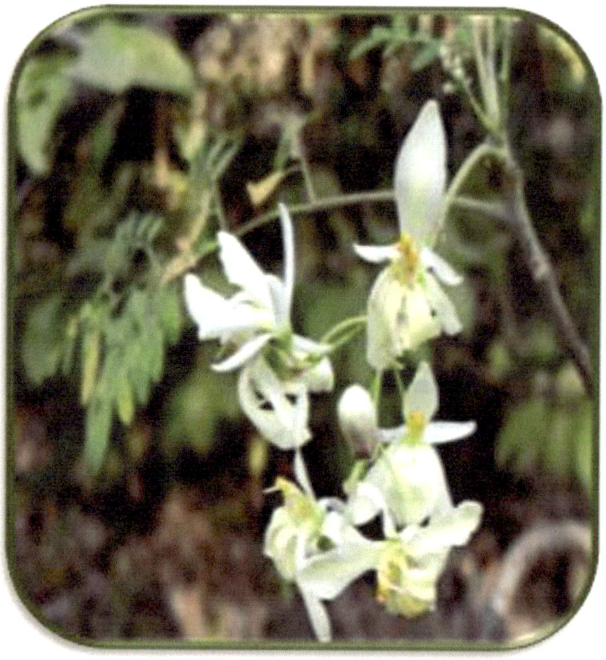

A large tree, with gummy bark, young branches Leaves alternate, deciduous, compound, triploid pinnate, can reach up to 60 cm in length (including the long leaf stalk of 4-15 cm). The main axis is slender, hairy, bearing 5-11 secondary axes 1-3 cm long, and the secondary axis bears 5-11 tertiary axes, which in turn bear 3-9 leaflets. The leaflet is 1-2 cm long, and 0.5-1.8 cm wide. The inflorescence is 8-30 cm long. The flowers are white, about 2.5 cm wide, and 1.3-2.1 cm long, with a honey-scented scent. The calyx is hairy, its lobes are unequal, petiolate, overlapping, linear to lanceolate, about 1.5 cm long, curved backwards, bearing yellow stripes in the center, complete, blunt at the apex. The petals are white, the front erect, the back curved backwar ds, spoon-shaped, bearing prominent nerves, about 1.5 cm long, and about 0.5 cm wide. The male has 5 stamens, its filaments are hairy from below. The ovary is oblong. The fruit is horny, pendulous, bearing 9 nerves, 30-40 cm long. The seeds are embedded in a hole within the ovary, triangular, winged, blackish, and spherical in general shape.

Flowering: January to April.

Habitat and geographical distribution: It is believed that its original habitat is in the Himalayan Mountains and tropical forests in India and the Arabian Peninsula, and it is cultivated in many tropical and subtropical countries.

History and heritage:

The name of the genus Moringa is derived from a local name in the state of Malabar in western India, while the name of the species is from ole meaning "oil", and ferre meaning "bearer", and the name is from the characteristic of the plant, as oil is extracted from its seeds. The plant is used as food and medicine. Al-Antaki mentioned that “all parts of the plant prevent tumors and catarrh, improve sweat, strengthen the body, and heal wounds.” Ibn Sina mentioned that “it is useful with vinegar and water for blockages in the viscera.” Al-Muzaffar mentioned that “the best of it is the large fragrant seed, which removes warts from the face and is useful for hard tumors if it is put in an ointment. It also removes liver and spleen infections if one drinks red vinegar from its seed.” It is called the miracle tree because it is used in the treatment of many chronic diseases.

Part used: fruits, seeds (the plant has a taste similar to that of hot radish), roots, and leaves.

Chemical components: The seeds contain 9% glucosinolates (in the seeds whose fatty substances have been removed) which include among other compounds benzyl glucosinolates, which produce benzyl isothiocyanates by the enzyme myrosinase.

Phenolic carboxylic acids. Fatty oil (50-20%), the main component of which is oleic acid (70-60%), palmitic acid (12-3%), stearic acid (12-3%), in addition to behenic acid, etc. The leaves contain a large amount of vitamin C, A and B complex, in addition to the minerals iron, calcium and selenium, and they also contain high concentrations of ten essential amino acids.

Properties and medical uses:

The seeds have antibacterial properties due to their mustard oil content.

Moringa extract is important in protecting the liver from carcinogenic factors and curing liver disorders. Experiments on rabbits have shown the effect of Moringa fruits in reducing the level of cholesterol, phospholipids and triglycerides in the blood. The level of lipids in the liver, heart and aorta also decreased, and an increase in the excretion of cholesterol through the stool was observed.

The root extract is used internally to treat gastrointestinal disorders, epilepsy, paralysis, heart disorders, blood pressure, fever, and colds. It is also used externally to treat gingivitis, abscesses, boils, rheumatism, and snake bites. The seed extract reduces the negative effects of chronic inflammation by inhibiting a series of pro-inflammatory factors. Isokercetin has antioxidant activity and shows an inhibitory effect on free radicals (ROS) by increasing antioxidant enzymes, such as superoxide dismutase (SOD), glutathione peroxidase (GPx), and catase. It also has immune-enhancing benefits.

Other uses:

Moringa leaves are an excellent nutritional supplement, and are rich in minerals and vitamins. The following are the estimated values found in 100 g of dry leaves compared to other types of food:

Nutrient Moringa dry leaves Other foods

Vitamin A mg 18 Carrots: 1.8 mg

Vitamin C mg 15 Oranges: 30 mg

Calcium mg 2000 Milk: 120 mg

Iron mg 28.2 Spinach: 1.14 mg

Potassium mg 1320 Bananas: 88 mg

Protein g 27.9 Yogurt: 3.1 g

Immature pods are The so-called "drumstick" is among the most valuable parts of the tree. It is eaten in India and is prepared similar to green beans. Its taste is mild and similar to that of asparagus. Moringa oil extracted from the seeds is considered a valuable oil like olive oil. It can be used in nutrition fresh or cooked (it spoils or goes rancid very slowly), and it can also be used in industry (paint, lubrication), or in the preparation of some cosmetics and perfumes. It is also suitable for use as lighting oil in oil lamps, as it gives a clear light that is almost smokeless.

Moringa leaf powder can maintain MDA (malondialdehyde) levels. The leaf extract helps regulate hyperthyroidism by inhibiting the synthesis of triiodothyronine. It is also used to treat atopic dermatitis (AD). The leaves are of great value as a supplement to the treatment of Alzheimer's disease. Moringa seeds can be used to purify contaminated water, eliminating 90-99% of bacteria. The seeds form a first-class coagulant, which can be used in treating river water containing solid suspensions (100 UTN units of turbidity). The seed powder can be replaced by the residues resulting from extracting oil from the seeds.

Precautions for use:

Large doses of the roots cause nausea, ringing in the ears and vomiting. Do not use in cases of pregnancy.

Environment:

A drought-tolerant plant, which grows in areas with an average of 250 mm of rainfall per year. Suitable temperature range: 25-40 C, tolerates high temperatures up to 48 C. It prefers neutral, acidic, well-drained loamy soils, and tolerates clayey soils, but does not tolerate flooding. Cultivation and productivity: It is propagated by seeds that are soaked a day before planting, watered after planting and germinate within 15 days. It can also be propagated by cuttings. Cuttings are taken with a length of 45 cm and a diameter of 10 mm, and planted in a mixture of sand and soil in a ratio of 3:1. The tree gives 300-400 horns per year at the age of 3 years, and large trees can give up to 1000 horns per year.

Eucalyptus camaldulensis Dehn.

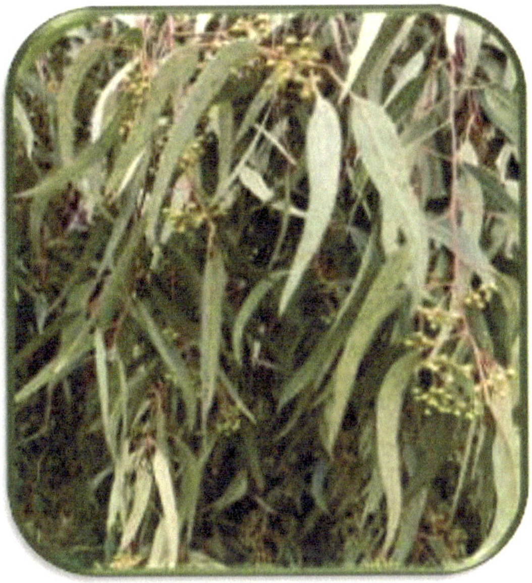

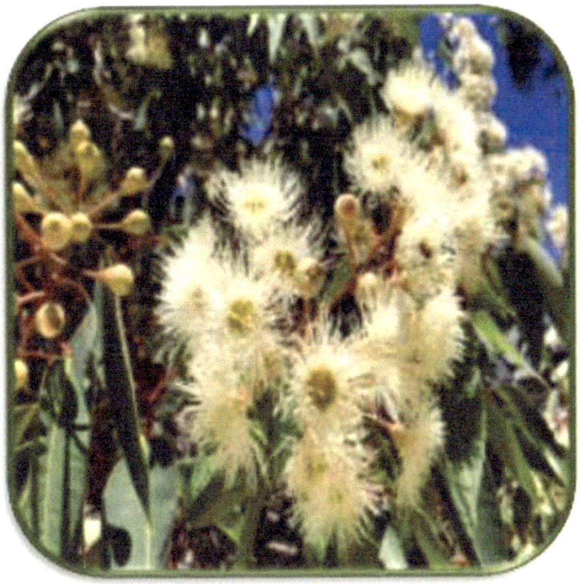

Family: Myrtaceae

Common names: Eucalyptus, Camphor (called Eucalyptus in Syria)

Foreign names: Eucalyptus Fr. Eucalyptus, Eng.

Occurrences : 42,230 occurrences

Distribution in the world

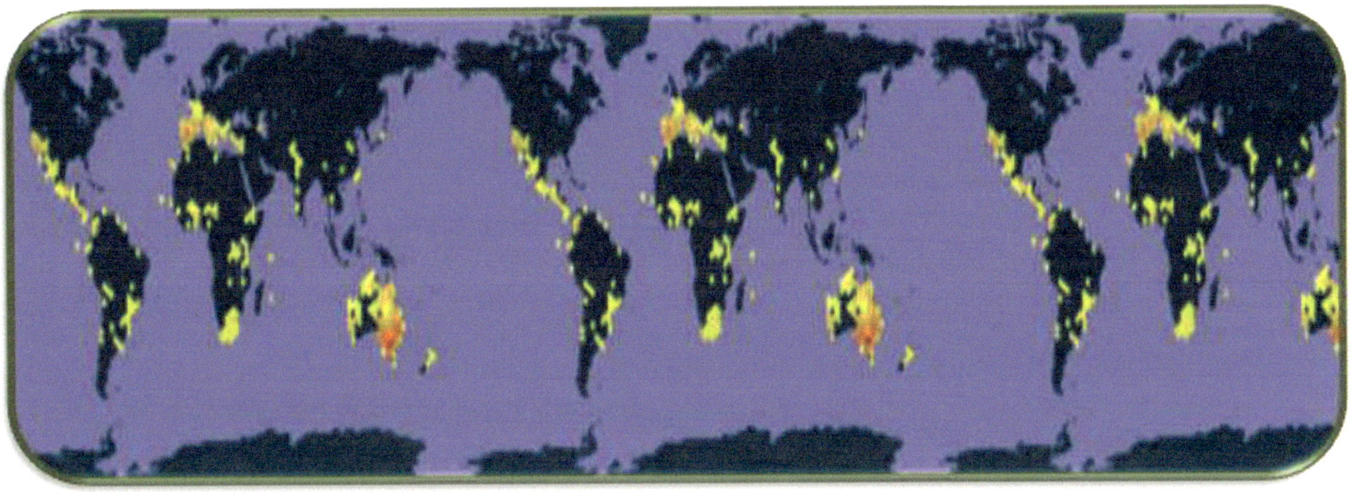

Botanical description:

A huge, evergreen, fast-growing tree, can reach a height of 50 m, and a diameter of 2 m. The trunk Smooth, bluish-gray in color, the bark separates in the middle section of the trunk every year in the form of elongated plates. The branches and leaves are drooping. The leaves are long, obtuse, and show a variety of shapes. They are oval-shaped and thin on young branches, and lanceolate to sword-shaped and thick on old branches. Their colour is grey to green, their edges are smooth and slightly thick. They can reach 25 cm in length and 1.5-0.7 cm in width. The flower has a distinctive shape, as the flower's calyx (the calyx and the corolla fused together) takes a conical shape that covers the male and female, gradually separates and falls, allowing the many stamens to appear. The fruit is a woody, semi-spherical capsule, topped by a prominent cylinder, 5-6 mm in diameter, containing the seeds, and opens with four valves. It flowers most of the year.

Habitat and geographical distribution:

Australia, widely distributed worldwide, especially in subtropical regions, and has adapted to the Mediterranean climate. The genus Eucalyptus includes about 400 species, the most important of which are: E. globules Labill, E. polybractea T. Baker, E. camaldulensis Dehn.

History and heritage:

The origin of the scientific name of the genus is derived from the Greek Kalyptos Eu- meaning "well-covered", in reference to the covering that covers the flower well, which resembles the rostrate beak of a bird, and from here came the name Eucalyptus beak. It is wrongly called Kena in Syria, and Kafour in Egypt, and both names indicate another species, as it is called Celtos in Tunisia. As for the name of the species camaldulensis, it is derived from the syllable camaldoli, which is the name of a region in Italy.

Part used: Young leaves, oil extracted from young leaves and tender branches.

Chemical components:

3% volatile oil, its most important compounds are Cineol (9%) 1,8-, paracymen ρ-cymen, alpha-pinen α, limonien, geraniol, and camphen. Acylphloroglucinol, euglobale. Flavonoids, including: quercetin, rutin, and eucalyptin. In addition to waxy compounds.

Properties and medical uses:

Volatile oil has antibacterial and antifungal activity, inhibits the biosynthesis of prostagandins, is a mild local irritant, expectorant, and causes an increase in Bronchial secretions, antitussive, improves lung function. Eucalyptus leaves have similar properties, they are expectorant, increase bronchial secretions, antispasmodic (volatile oil), antidiabetic, antibacterial, diuretic, and the compound Oglobal has anti-inflammatory and antioxidant activity. It is used internally in colds, and externally in the treatment of rheumatism.

The decoction of the leaves is popularly used to treat influenza, bronchitis, asthma, colds and congestion, indigestion (liver and gallbladder diseases), bladder and kidney diseases, and malaria fever. The decoction of the leaves is used topically as a wash to treat female infections, acne, stomatitis, and bleeding gums. Eucalyptus essential oil is effective against many gram-positive and gram-negative bacteria. Camphor essential oil and its extracts are among the most effective oils against bacteria compared to other species of the genus Eucalyptus.

Pharmaceutical forms:

Eucalyptus is available in the form of: oil and lotion, under names such as mint Eucalypta, Eucalyptus oil.

Side effects, interactions and warnings for use:

Overuse and overdose may cause blue-gray discoloration of the skin, a burning sensation in the stomach, muscle weakness, pupil constriction, delirium, dizziness, nausea and vomiting, and may cause constipation. Eucalyptus oil should not be taken while taking blood sugar-lowering medications. Pregnant and lactating women should avoid using it, and should not be given to those suffering from liver, intestinal and urinary tract diseases. The volatile oil should also be diluted before consuming it or applying it to the skin. Eucalyptus oil poisoning occurs in the elderly if the dose exceeds 3 ml, as blood pressure drops and suffocation occurs.

Note: Prostaglandins are hormone-like compounds that affect blood pressure and smooth muscle movement.

Environment:

A widely distributed species in Australia, where annual rainfall rates range from 250-600 mm/year. Through its use in afforestation outside its habitat, the species has shown flexibility in terms of climatic and soil conditions, as it lives on rainfall of up to 300 mm/year. The plant prefers sunny areas and moist, well-drained soils, and is flexible in terms of soil, adapting to dry and low-fertility soils, as well as to calcium and relative salinity. However, it fears extreme cold, and therefore it is not recommended to grow it economically in areas where the temperature drops sharply. This species contains multiple types and environmental patterns, characterized by special environmental and physiological characteristics, which must be taken into consideration in afforestation operations, especially the characteristic of resistance to lime, cold and wind.

Cultivation and productivity:

The plant is propagated by seeds that are planted in March in sunny and protected areas, noting that the collected seeds for 6-8 weeks. This type gives great growth from high areas that need to be stratified at a temperature of 2 in light and deep soils, and annual growth can reach 10-20 m/3 ha. This productivity is affected by insect infestations such as the piercing insect.

Myrtus communis L.

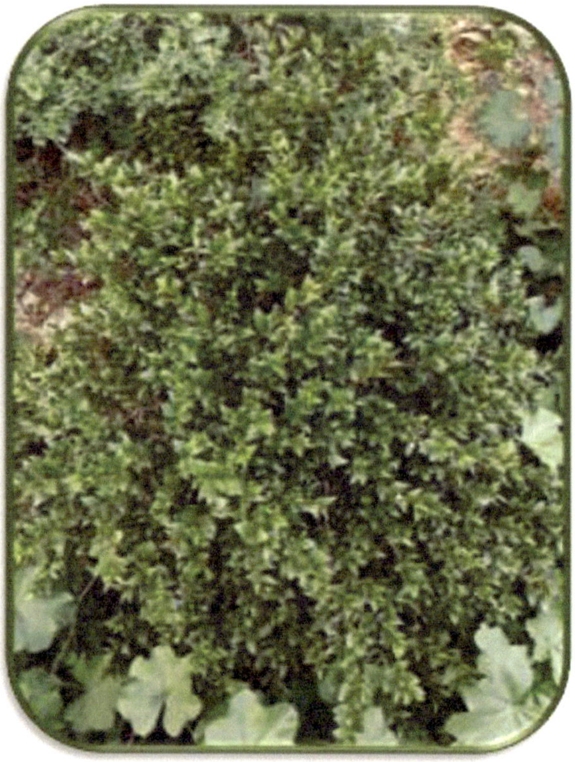

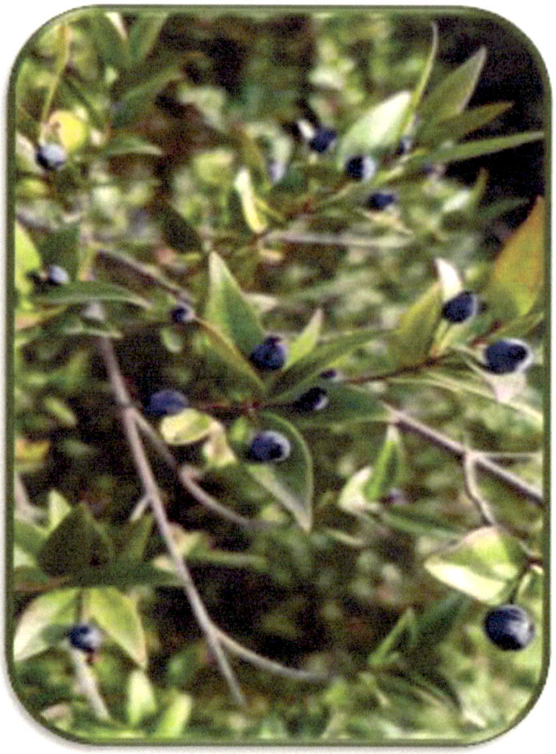

Family: Myrtaceae

Common names: Myrtle, Basil, Habbas, Hambas, Myrsine, Hades.

Foreign names: Myrtle, Common Eng.

Occurrences : 48,273 occurrences Distribution in the world

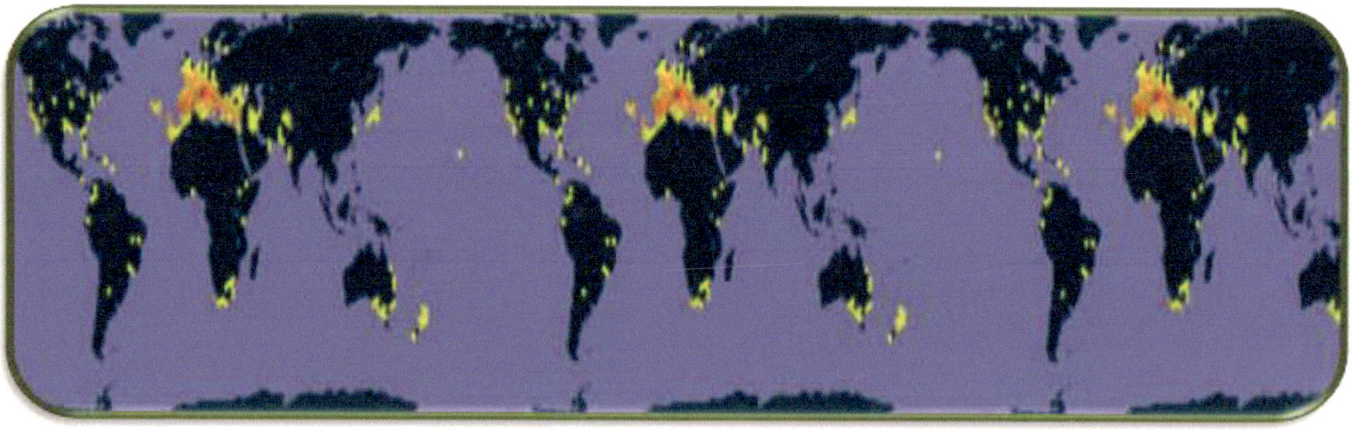

Botanical description:

An evergreen shrub, bare, 2-0.5 m tall and sometimes more. Stems numerous, branched, leaves 1-4 cm long, 7-20 mm wide, aromatic, especially when rubbed by hand, opposite or sessile, short-stalked, leathery, ovate to lanceolate to elliptic, pointed at the tip, shiny green, with transparent spots on the surface. Ears are deciduous. Flowers solitary, about 1.5 cm in diameter, sessile. Bracts 2, linear, deciduous. Calyx five-lobed, 2-3 mm long, ovate, acute. Corolla 5-lobed, white, inverted-ovate to rounded, about three times longer than the sepal. Stamens numerous and free. Ovary inferior, 2-3 chambered, each containing several ovules. The fruit is a fragrant grape, 8-10 mm long, broadly ellipsoidal to semi-spherical, white or blackish-blue in colour when ripe (depending on the variety), topped by a crown representing the lobes of the persistent calyx.

Flowering: From May to August, and the fruits ripen in November. The size of the flowers and fruits varies according to the species and variety.

Habitat and geographical distribution: The Mediterranean basin, extending to neighbouring areas. It grows abundantly in the coastal mountains in many Mediterranean Arab countries, as a companion to degraded forests.

History and Heritage:

The origin of the word myrtle is unknown, although there are similar words in Semitic languages, and the descriptive name for the species "communis" means "common." It has been known since ancient times, as scientists found branches of the plant in some Pharaonic tombs, and it was included in many ivory recipes in Pharaonic papyri to treat epilepsy, cystitis, and regulate urine. The Romans and Greeks knew it, and the Greeks used it to symbolize glory and victories. It was highly esteemed. Muslims have used and still use myrtle branches in some countries to decorate the graves of the dead during holidays. Ibn Sina and Ibn al-Baytar mentioned its various ivory properties.

Part used: dried leaves, young leafy and flowering branches, volatile oil extracted from the plant, The plant is collected during the months of May and June.

Chemical components:

The leaves contain volatile oil 0.1 - 0.5%, the most important compounds are: cineol - 1.8 at a rate of 15-45% (=)eucalyptole, alpha-pinene -15-38%, limonene 4-10%, alpha-terpineol 3-2%, geraniol 1.5%, myrtenol -1-5%, myrtol, geranylacetate 2%, myrtenylacetate 20-4% Tannins, α and β phloroglucinol derivatives, phloroglucinols β,α. The following compounds were detected in all parts of the plant: Quercitrin, myricitrin and myricetingalactopyranoside-β. The highest content of quercitrin was found in the flower buds, where it reached 18.5 ± 0.1 mg / g, while the highest content of myricetin was found in the leaves, where it reached 25 ± 0.4 mg / g.

Properties and medical uses:

The volatile oil and leaves have antiseptic, antibacterial, antifungal and antiviral properties. It is used to treat respiratory problems (bronchitis, sinusitis, whooping cough), intestinal and urinary tract infections (bladder, prostate). The leaves, with their volatile oil and tannins, are an antiseptic, astringent and hemostatic agent. It has been proven to prolong sleep and lower blood sugar. A decoction of the plant's leaves is popularly used to treat respiratory problems, prostatitis and diarrhea. The decoction of the leaves or the tincture prepared from the leaves or the volatile oil is used topically, as an antiseptic for superficial wounds, removing pimples, and in treating skin ulcers, psoriasis, and hemorrhoids. The paste of the leaves is used to strengthen the hair and reduce hair loss.

The fruits of myrtle are eaten fresh for their properties that stimulate the appetite and are useful in reducing diarrhea and intestinal gas. The water used in distilling the oil of the leaves and flowers is called , and is used as a nasal disinfectant.

Parts of the myrtle plant (Myrtus communis L.) are traditionally used to treat various disorders. The highest antioxidant activity was determined in the flower buds. In addition, luteolin, gallic acid, quercitrin, myricetin, myricetin and β-galactopyranoside-O-3 were found to contribute to the antioxidant activity of the extracts. The hydroalcoholic extract prepared from the leaves showed the highest anticancer activity using human colorectal cancer cell line. Test results showed that the leaves were most effective against the tested cell lines.

Other uses:

The essential oil is widely used in the perfume industry. Warnings for use: Myrtle oil should not be used internally in cases of inflammation of the digestive system and acute liver diseases, and the essential oil should not be used by pregnant women or children. Excessive doses of plant preparations sometimes cause headaches or nausea.

Environment:

It is widespread in semi-dry, semi-humid and humid bioclimatic floors. It lives on different types of soils, but prefers fertile and sunny soils. It is good for cultivation in warm areas that are not exposed to frost, and it succeeds in dry lands provided that they are protected from cold winds.

Cultivation and productivity:

It is propagated by seeds that are soaked in warm water for 24 hours, and planted in late winter. Service operations are provided to the seedlings, including irrigation, fertilization and weeding. The seedlings are transferred to the permanent land in late spring or early summer. Myrtle can also be propagated by stem cuttings, and the best time to collect them is at the end of autumn and the beginning of winter. The plant needs irrigation in the first year of planting it in permanent soil.

Nitraria retusa (Forssk.) Aschens.

Peganum retusum Forssk, *N. tridentata* Desf., *Nitraria senegalensis* Poir. *Nitraria sericea* Jaub. & Spach.

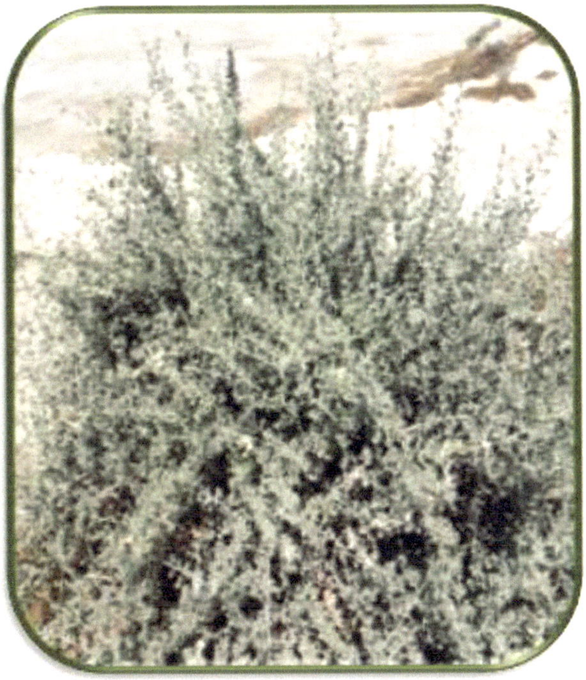

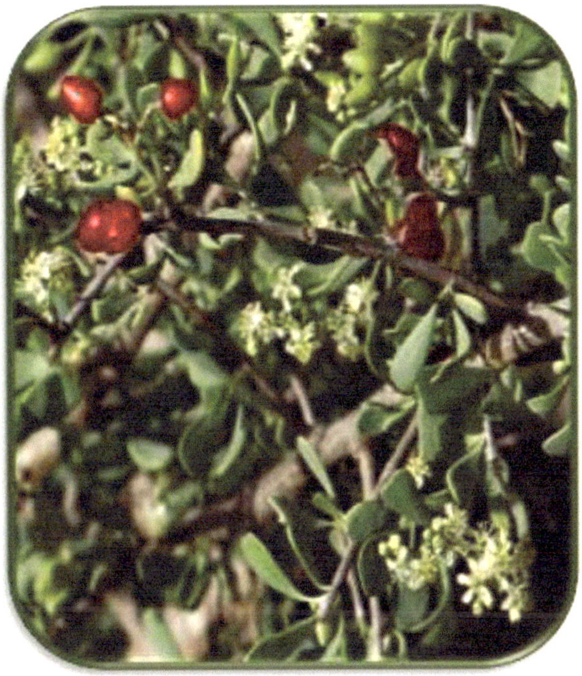

Family: Nitrariaceae

Common names: Gharqad, Ghardaq, Sakhnoon

Foreign names: Eng. Salt tree, Fr. Nitraire à feuilles rétuses

Occurrences : 1,569 occurrences

Distribution in the world

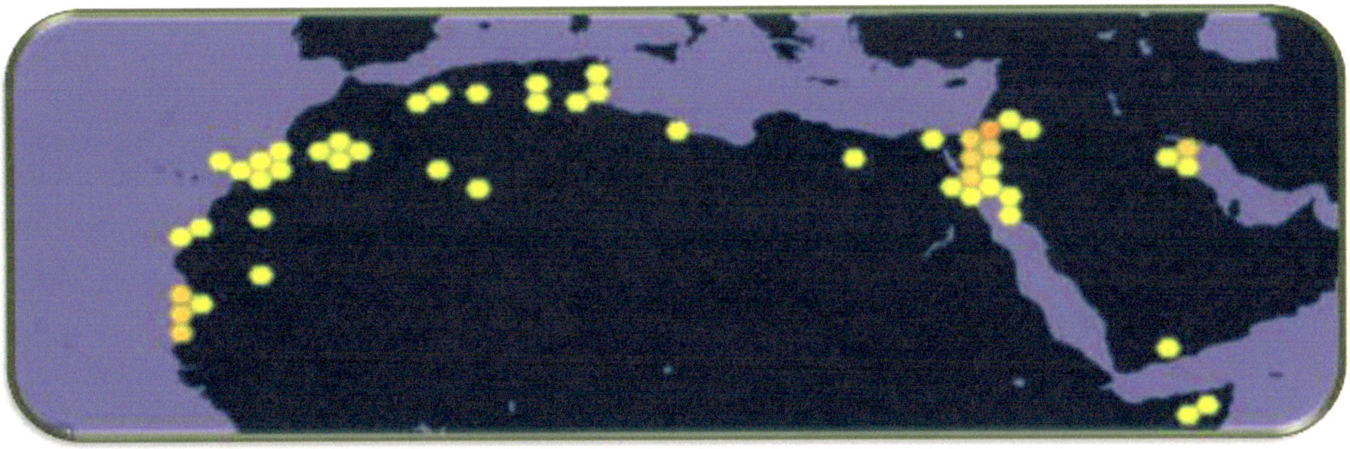

Botanical description:

A highly branched shrub, 1-2 m high, young branches covered with gray hair, their ends forming thorns. Stem numerous, erect, highly branched. Leaves simple, 1-2 cm long, obtuse, fleshy, fascicular or alternate, entire margin, inverted ovate to pedicel-shaped, their apex notched or bearing 3-5 teeth. Covered with hairs, or almost bare. Ears are minute, membranous, perennial. Flowers are hermaphrodite, long-stalked, 6-8 mm long, gathered in cymose, dichotomous inflorescences at the ends of young branches. Calyx 5 sepals partially fused to their bases, ovate, 2 mm long, bare or almost bare, perennial with fruit. Corolla 5 free petals, twice as long as calyx or more, greenish to white, hairy. Male 15 stamens arranged in three whorls, of equal length. Female tricarpal, ovary superior, tricameral, oblong to pyramidal, gradually tapering to a short stigma. Fruit nuclear, unicameral, monospermic, 10-6 mm long, ovate to triangular, apex pointed, purple to reddish, lengthwise crossed by stigmas. Seeds ovate.

Flowering: April to May.

Homeland and geographical distribution: Desert-Arab, spread in Palestine, Sinai, Egypt, Iraq, Kuwait, Saudi Arabia, Yemen and extends to the neighboring Sudanese region.

History and heritage:

It is the Faraj in the Arab Maghreb, and in Algeria it is Ghardaq, mentioned by Ibn al-Baytar and al-Antaki, but Ibn Sina did not address it. It was reported in the authentic hadith on the authority of the Prophet, may God bless him and grant him peace, that he said: "The Hour will not come until the Muslims fight the Jews, and the Muslims will kill them until the Jews hide behind rocks and trees, and the rock or tree will say, 'O Muslim, O servant of God, there is a Jew behind me, come and kill him,' except for the gharqad, for it is one of the trees of the Jews."

Part used: Leaves and young stems.

Chemical components:

The leaves and young stems contain polyphenols. Alkaloids: vasicinone. Favonoids: quercetin, isorhamnetin and its derivatives, 3-rutinoside isorhamnetin, isorhamnetin. 3-robinobioside, 3-glucoside

Properties and medical uses:

The plant has antioxidant and anti-cancer properties due to its phenolic and favonoid compounds. Anti-prolifrative The galactic property of the plant has shown a hypotensive effect. The leaves are used in folk medicine to treat flatulence and wounds.

Other uses:

The plant is used by locals in the soap industry, and a dye is extracted from its fruits for fabrics. Its fruits are eaten raw or cooked, due to their salty and pleasant flavor, and are also used in curdling milk. Its wood is used as fuel, due to its rapid ignition. Environment: The plant lives in a very dry, hot and moderate bioclimatic layer, and is concentrated in streams and valleys, and near water. It adapts to gypsum, clay or sandy soils that are relatively saline. The species indicates the presence of a shallow ground water layer. It resists burial with sand, and tolerates sea winds and sea spray. The plant contributes effectively to stabilizing sand dunes rich in marine salts.

Cultivation and productivity:

The plant is propagated by seeds, and can be propagated by cuttings. The seeds need to be treated by drying at a temperature of 50 ° C for 20 days, then treated with gibberellic acid 750 parts per million for 24 hours.

Peganum harmala L.

Harmala peganum Crantz, *Peganon harmalum* (L.) St.-Lag.

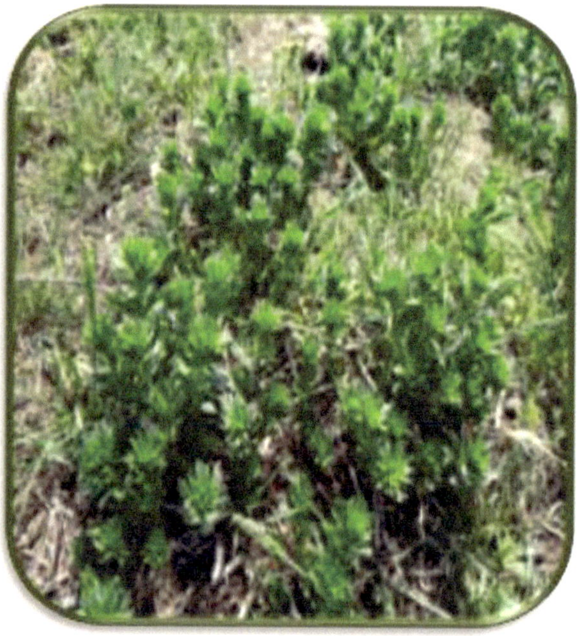

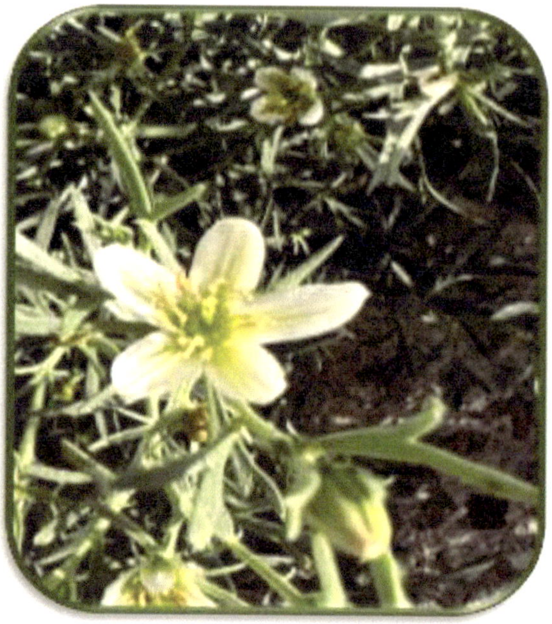

Family: Nitrariaceae (Zygophyllaceae)

Common names: Harmal, Wolf's hood, Desert harmal, Dog's lobes

Foreign names: Rue Fr.Syrian, hermala Engl.

Occurrences : 8,318 occurrences

Distribution in the world

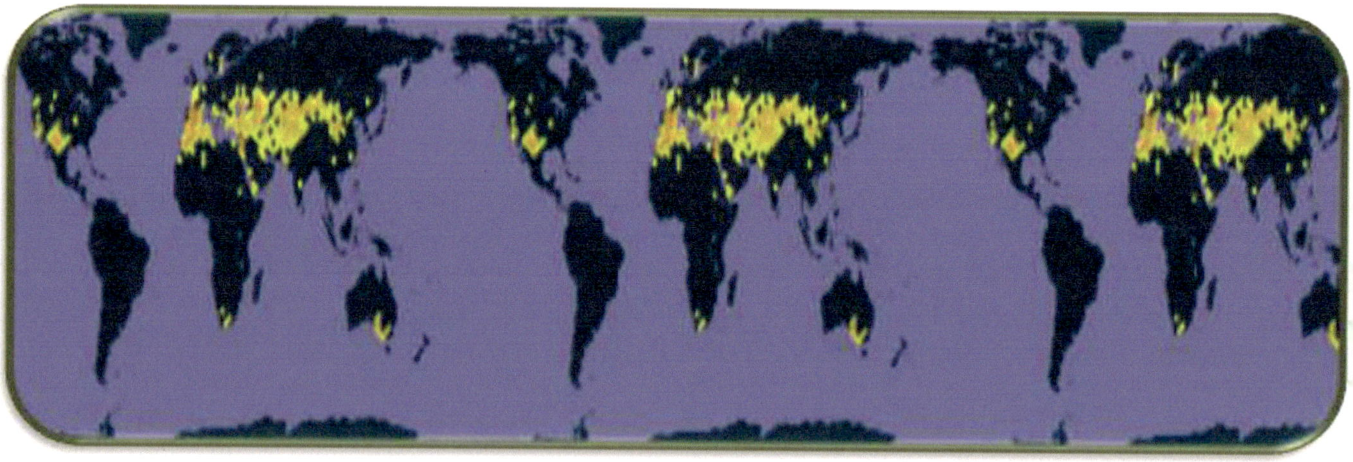

Botanical description:

A perennial plant, woody at the base, bare, ranging in height from 30 to 50 cm. The stem is highly branched, angular at the top. Erect or ascending. The leaves are alternate, 5-10 cm long, petiole, small ears (1.5-2.5 mm), conical, resembling hard hairs, the blade is deeply and irregularly divided to

Celestial erect, linear-lanceolate, entire, acute-apex, 2-4 cm long. Inflorescence terminally semi-ovate. Flowers hermaphrodite, large, long-stalked. Sepals five-lobed, perennial, 1.5-2 cm long, sometimes linear, three-lobed, with scales between the sepals (forming a cup-like shape). Sepals five-segmented, about 1.5 cm long and 0.5-0.7 cm wide, white or yellowish, oblong to Elliptical, numerous stamens (12-15) arranged in two rows on a cup-like disc. Ovary trichambered, spherical, ovules numerous. Fruit 1-0.8 cm (0.5-1.2 in), spherical, compact, trichambered, many-seeded, glabrous, pubescent, opening in three valves, style perennial. Seed about 2 mm, triangular, blackish to brown, tuberous.

Flowering: March to May.

Habitat and geographical distribution:

Iranian-Turanian, desert-Arabian, extending to the Mediterranean region in North Africa, the Middle East and the eastern Iranian region west of India, and grows spontaneously in semi-arid and pre-desert areas in southeastern Morocco.

History and heritage:

The genus name is derived from the Greek pêganon, and the species name harmala is derived from the Arabic name "harmal." Known for its toxicity, the ancient Greeks used the powdered seeds in ivory, and it was also used as a sexual tonic for men. Dioscorides mentioned that it "is beneficial for an open womb, so if it is crushed and made into an oil, it opens the mouths of the wombs." It was also mentioned by Galen, Masih al-Dimashqi, Isa ibn Masa, Ali ibn Razin, Habish, Ishaq ibn Imran, and Ibn Wafid. Part used: Seeds and the whole plant

Chemical components:

A poisonous plant in all its parts, due to its richness in many alkaloids of an indole-pyridine nature (harmaline, harmine, harman, and harmalol). The alkaloids are concentrated in the seeds in particular, where their percentage is 3-4% compared to the roots and stems where the percentage is 0.36% and in the leaves 0.52%. The alkaloid harmaline constitutes two-thirds of the total alkaloids in the seeds, and it is twice as toxic as Harmine.

Note : the high percentage of alkaloids during the summer season during the ripening period of the seeds and the subsequent pre-harvest stage.

It also contains amino acids (valine, proline, histidine) and vavones, coumarin compounds, tannins, citrullate and others. The outer shell of the seeds contains a red pigment known as "Turkish red."

Properties and medical uses:

Harmal has an inhibitory effect on monoamine oxidase (MAO), it is a stimulant for the central nervous system, especially the centers responsible for movement in the cerebral cortex, it accelerates breathing, reduces blood pressure, dilates peripheral blood vessels, and relaxes the muscles of various organs. It is used as a narcotic, hypnotic, antispasmodic, emetic, anthelmintic, and antiparasitic for malaria and dysentery. The seeds have anti-tumor and antioxidant properties. The seed extract is popularly used as a pain reliever, diaphoretic, anthelmintic, anti-colic and digestive disorders. It is used to treat hemorrhoids, and a decoction of the leaves is used to treat diabetics. The seed extract is used topically as an antiseptic, antibacterial and antifungal, helps heal wounds and burns, and treats some skin diseases (itching, allergies, boils, eczema). Studies have proven the effect of the seeds in aborting and causing infertility in women. Using the fragrant smoke resulting from burning dried seeds mixed with other ingredients is beneficial for people suffering from mental illnesses.

Warnings for use:

The seeds have a toxic effect. Large doses of it cause digestive disorders represented by vomiting accompanied by nausea and sweating, heart disorders (palpitations), and nervous disorders (visual hallucinations, tremors, convulsions, muscle tremors, numbness or paralysis of the limbs accompanied by dizziness and low temperature.) It is abortive in large doses. Long-term use may cause addiction. Some of the complications of harmala are due to the interaction between β-carbolines and MAO enzymes. Simultaneous use of products rich in tyramine can cause a sharp increase in blood pressure, known as the "cheese effect."

Other uses: The seed dye "Turkish red" is used in Turkey and Iran to obtain the colors used in the carpet industry.

Environment:

Harmal lives in arid and semi-arid temperate and cold regions, and tolerates drought thanks to the depth of its root system in the soil. It prefers sandy soils containing nitrogenous organic waste, and is found in cemeteries, roadsides and paths, where livestock dung is abundant. On the other hand, the plant can live under conditions of salt stress, and in highly alkaline soils.

Cultivation and productivity:

It reproduces by seeds, and can also be propagated by root cuttings. The fruits are collected after the seeds ripen.

Olea europaea L.

Olea pallida Salisb., *Olea sativa* Hoffmanns & Link.

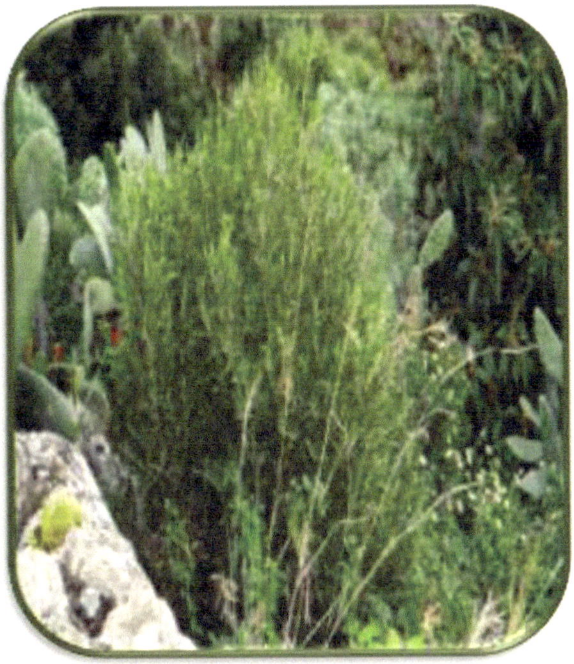 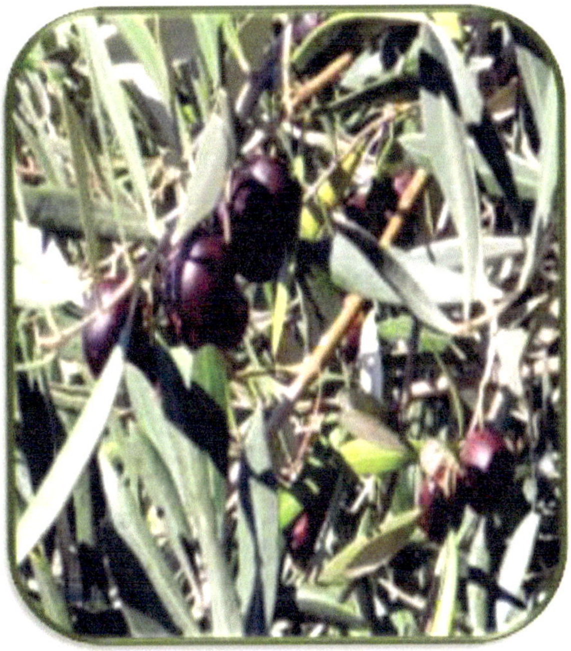

Family: Oleaceae

Common names: Olive

Foreign names: Olivier Fr. Olive. Eng.

Occurrences :388,678 occurrences

Distribution in the world

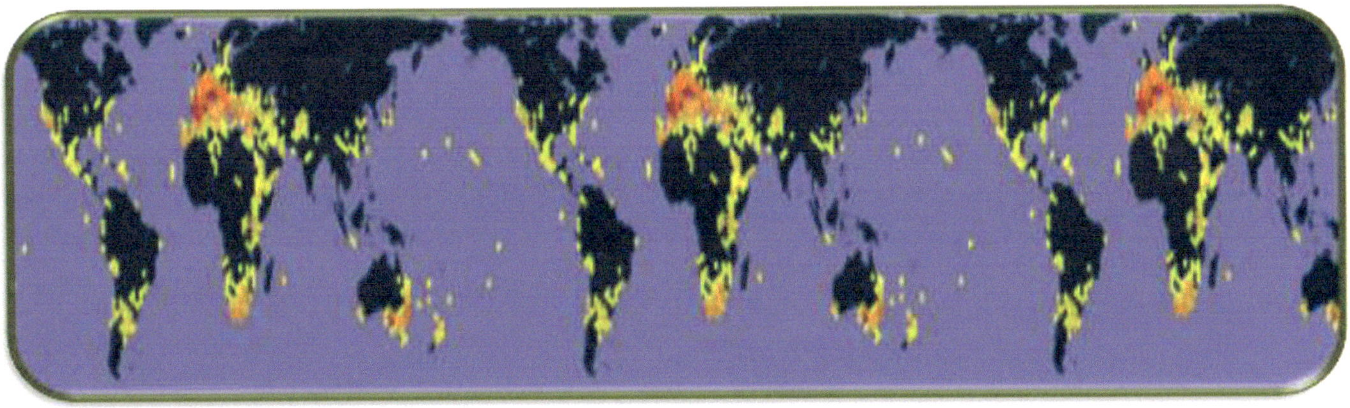

Botanical description:

A small, evergreen tree, reaching a height of 8 m. The stem is winding, abundantly branched, the bark is gray to brown in color, smooth on the young branches, cracking as the tree ages. The leaves are simple, opposite, entire, leathery, short-petiolate, oblong to lanceolate, shiny green on the upper surface, silvery covered with dense scales on the lower surface. Inflorescence axillary raceme.

Flowers small, hermaphrodite. Calyx 4 sepals fused. Corolla 4 petals fused, pinnate, white to cream-coloured. Male two stamens with short filaments and large anthers. Female carpels, unicellular ovary. Fruit nuclear, ellipsoid, truncated or tapering towards the ends, green in colour then blackening when ripe.

Flowering: April to May. The number of olive varieties grown worldwide is more than 200, and the amount of oil in them ranges between less than 10% and more than 30%.

Homeland and geographical distribution:

Mediterranean countries, most of which it was planted in, and from there it spread to many countries in the five continents, where similar climates are available.

History and heritage:

The origin of the genus name is from the Greek colloquial word elaï(f)a with the same meaning, and europaea means "European", in reference to the widespread distribution of this tree there. The olive is a fruitful, oil-bearing tree, wild and cultivated, known since ancient times in the Mediterranean basin and its fruits have been used as food and medicine since ancient times. It is mentioned that 3500 years ago, the Phoenicians, then the Greeks, Romans and ancient Egyptians developed the cultivation of this tree and spread it throughout the Mediterranean region. The olive tree had a high status among the Greeks and they mentioned it in their poems. Many numbers were discovered in the Kingdom of Eba that refer to olive oil, and that it was presented as a gift to kings and sports heroes. The olive tree was called the blessed tree, and it was mentioned in all heavenly books; The Holy Quran has referred to the importance of the olive tree and its oil in several verses, describing it as blessed, meaning abundant in giving and benefit, and the Prophet, may God bless him and grant him peace, ordered his companions and all Muslims to eat olive oil and anoint themselves with it. It was also mentioned in the Bible through the mention of the holy Mount of Olives near Jerusalem, where Jesus, peace be upon him, was. This tree remains distinctive to many civilizations as a symbol of peace, wisdom and strength.

Part used: Leaves, flowers and fatty oil extracted from the fruits.

Chemical components:

The leaves contain terpenoids including: oleuropein, triterpenic acids, and phenolic compounds, including flavonoids and alkaloids such as cinchonin and cinchonidin, in addition to choline. The fatty oil contains mono, di and triglyceride esters, and unsaturated fatty acids with a single double bond. In addition to polyunsaturated fatty acids with double bonds, the oil also contains triterpenoids, sterols, tocopherols, phospholipids, carotenoids, and vitamins. And bitter substances and secoiridoids, as it contains phenols, naphthalene, phenantrine, and sterols in addition to terpenoids, and vitamin E.

Properties and medical uses:

The leaves have properties that lower triglycerides and blood pressure, slow the heart, dissolve smooth muscle spasms, lower blood sugar, and are antifungal. The decoction of the leaves is popularly used to treat high blood pressure, hardening of the arteries, gout, rheumatism, diabetes, and fever, in addition to being used as a diuretic. The oil helps strengthen and stimulate the liver, helps treat fatty liver, protects against colon cancer, reduces the risk of breast cancer, has antioxidant activity, and protects against colon, uterine, ovarian, and melanoma cancer, in addition to its laxative effect in cases of constipation. Olive oil is used topically to soothe inflamed skin surfaces and soften skin flakes caused by eczema and psoriasis. Applying olive oil to the head for several hours helps get rid of lice. Olive oil is used as food and is also used in the manufacture of soap, especially that which is extracted from the second pressing of the thuja with special treatment.

Precautions for use: Olive oil is not recommended for people with gallstones.

Environment:

The olive tree is one of the trees that are resistant to difficult environmental conditions. The Mediterranean region is one of the best areas for growing olive trees, as it is characterized by cold, rainy winters and hot, dry summers. Exposing trees to high temperatures accompanied by dry winds and low humidity during the flowering, fruit setting and early fruit development period leads to dry flowers and incomplete pollination and fertilization processes, and consequently fruit drop to a large extent. Not depriving trees of water during this period limits these harmful effects. Olive trees can be grown in different types of soil provided that good drainage is available. Olive trees can also be grown successfully in calcareous soils, but their growth is negatively affected in heavy, poorly drained soils. The tree has the ability to tolerate drought and soil salinity.

Cultivation and productivity:

Olives are propagated vegetatively, and planting olive seeds does not produce plants identical to the variety. Therefore, vegetative propagation of the desired varieties is the best method for producing seedlings, whether by grafting onto seed or vegetative rootstocks, or by using cuttings of different types, or stems separated from trees growing on their roots. Care must be taken to ensure that they are free from disease or pests, and that they are taken from certified, highly productive mothers. Olive trees tolerate thirst and dry weather. The trees' need for irrigation varies depending on the soil, weather conditions, age of the trees, growth status, irrigation system used, and lack of water in the soil. Pruning is one of the most important service operations affecting production. It is usually done after harvesting the crop from December to January. In rain-fed agriculture, it is postponed until after the largest amount of rain falls, where pruning is light to moderate when there is plenty of rain, and excessive when there is little. Organic and chemical fertilizers should be added in the appropriate manner and at the appropriate time, which makes the trees stronger, more resistant to environmental factors and more productive. The tree begins to bear fruit in the second year, and in the sixth year the olive tree gives back the costs of planting it. The olive fruits are pressed to extract the oil, and olive oil soap is made from its oil. The wood of the olive tree is an excellent type of wood with a honey-brown color, rich in preservatives that prevent it from spoiling and being infested by insects.

Oxalis acetosella L.

Oxalis vulgaris Gray, *Oxys acetosella* (L.) Scop., *Oxys vulgaris* Rupr.

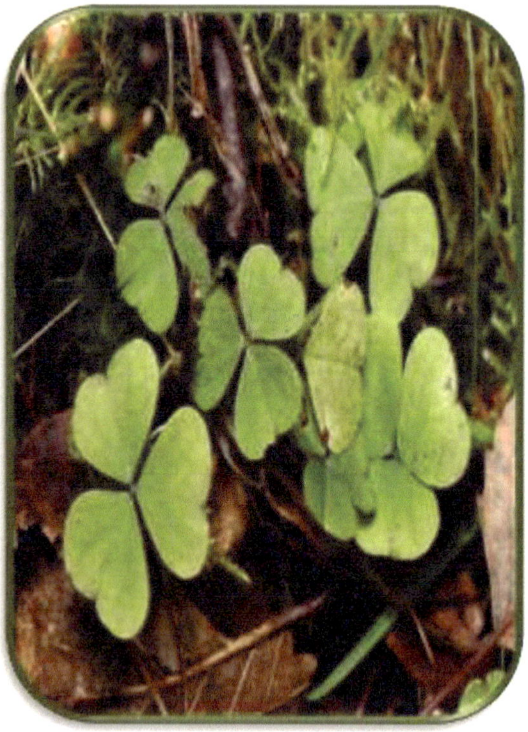

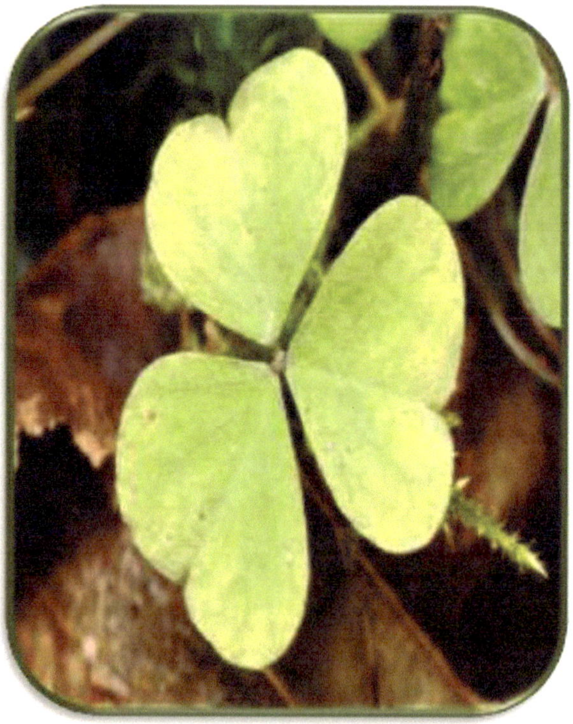

Family: Oxalidaceae

Common names: Sorrel, Purslane

Foreign names: Surelle Fr. sorrel, Common Eng.

Occurrences : 536,829 occurrences

Distribution in the world

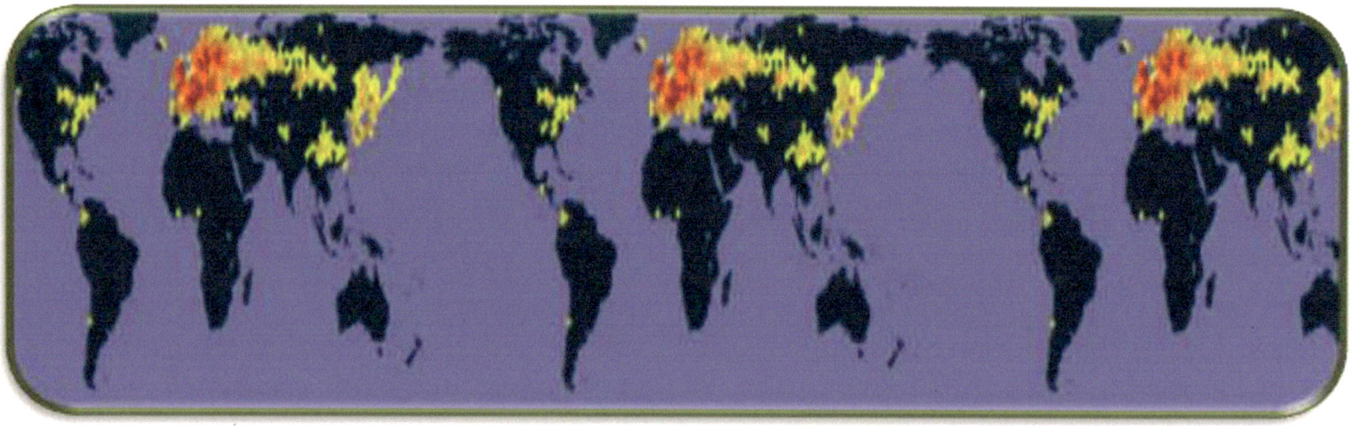

Botanical description:

A perennial herb with a rhizome. The stem is red to brown in color, highly branched, 20-50 cm high. The leaves are alternate, Trifoliate (similar to clover leaves), long-petiolate, the leaflet is heart-shaped, folded along the median nerve, The leaves and flowers contract at night and during rain. Flower diameter 3-4 cm, hermaphrodite, white or pink, with dark lines, solitary, insectivorous or self-pollinated. Calyx 5 free, overlapping sepals, about 1 cm long. Corolla 5 petals, free, about 2 cm long. Male: 10 stamens, Their filaments are slightly fused to their bases, located in two whorls (5+5), the stamens of the outer whorl have shorter filaments. Female: 5 fused carpels, the ovary is superior, five-chambered. The fruit is a capsule that opens spherically.

Flowering: From May to June.

Habitat and geographical distribution: The Mediterranean basin, and is spread in Europe, Africa and western Asia.

History and Heritage:

The scientific name of the genus is the ancient Greek name for a plant with a sour taste. The Arabs gave this name to this genus and to plants of the genus Rumex. The descriptive name for the species is acetosella, which means "grain cell" through acetum.

Part used: Green parts.

Chemical components: The plant contains 0.3 - 1.25% oxalic acid, represented in the form of potassium salt, especially vitamin C.

Medical properties and uses:

The green parts of the plant have diuretic activity. The fresh plant is a rich source of vitamin C. The plant is popularly used to treat digestive and liver disorders. A decoction of the green leaves was also used in the past to treat scurvy (vitamin C deficiency), wounds, and gum inflammation. The powdered leaves are used topically to treat gum inflammation, wounds, and boils (it has an astringent effect) and has an inhibitory effect on cutaneous leishmaniasis.

Other uses: The leaves are used in the kitchen, whether fresh by adding them to salads or cooked in soups or other, which gives the dish a delicious sour taste.

Use warnings: No health accidents or side effects have been known when the appropriate dose is given. With the possibility of oxalic acid poisoning only by eating large quantities of the leaves in a salad, for example. Note that cooking the plant reduces the percentage of oxalates. It is not recommended for use by people suffering from rheumatism, gout, and kidney stones.

Environment:

It grows on the banks of rivers and streams, in forests, and in humid and shady places. It likes humus-rich soils, and does not like very heavy and abundant soils. It tolerates low temperatures well.

Cultivation and productivity:

It is propagated by seeds that are planted immediately after they are ripe or in the spring in basins 25 cm apart, taking care to separate them after germination and water them regularly. The leaves begin to be harvested after 10 weeks in a light manner. It is also propagated by root cuttings taken from the roots of 3-year-old plants, after cutting their leaves above the soil surface at a height of 10 cm and burying them in the soil at a depth of 3 cm and a distance of 25 cm between them within a single line. The plant can scatter its seeds and spread automatically if the appropriate conditions are available. The seeds produced in early spring are less vital than those produced in summer.

Fumaria officinalis L.

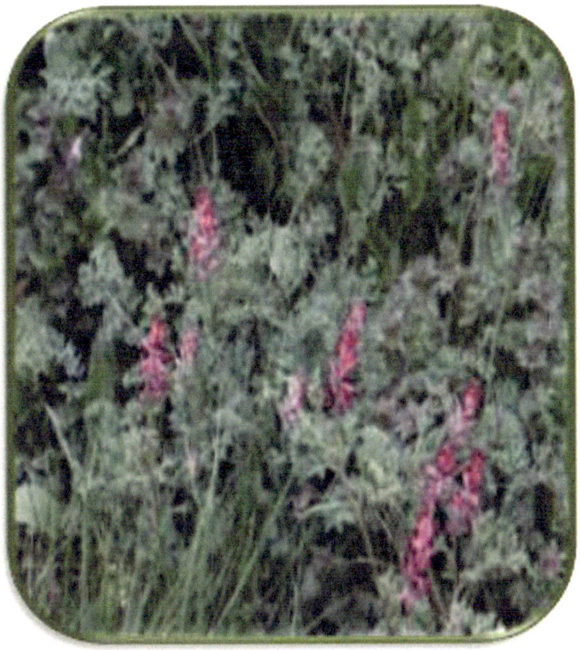

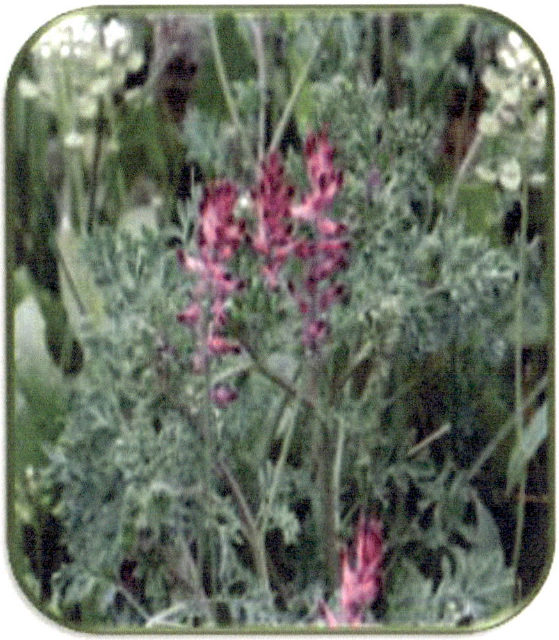

Family: Papaveraceae (formerly Fumariaceae).

Common names: Chatterj officinalis, purslane, earth smoke

Foreign names: Fumeterre Fr. Fumitory, Eng.

Occurrences :173,916 occurrences

Distribution in the world

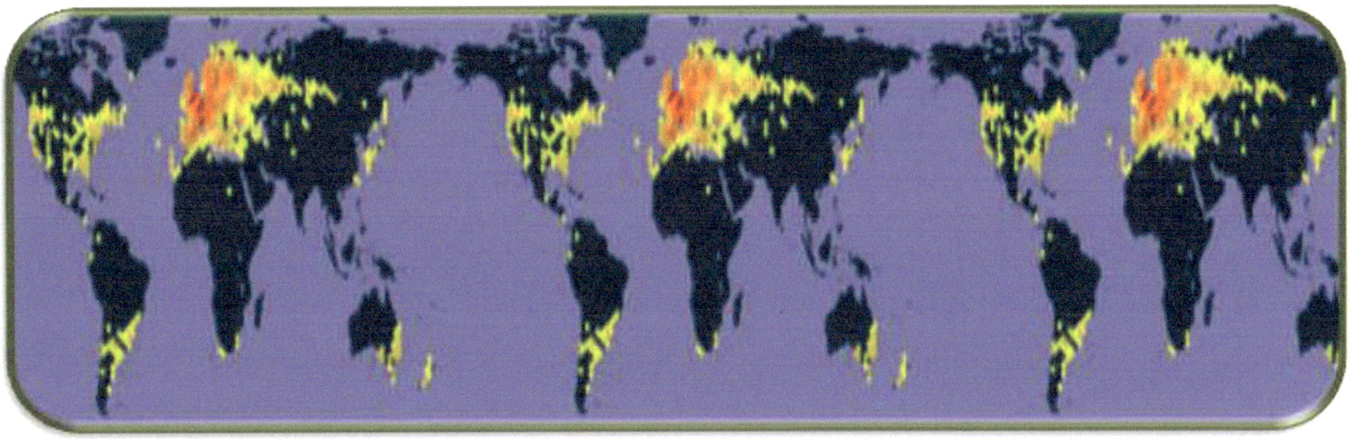

Botanical description:

Annual herb, 10-50 cm tall, slender stem, semi-lying on the soil, angular, branched, bare, gray-green in color. Leaves alternate, compound, pinnate, strongly divided, and their lobes are threadlike. The inflorescence is a terminal panicle. The flowers are tubular, 7-9 mm long, with a short, non-curved bract. The bracts are 10-15 cm long. Equal to the length of the stamen. The sepals 2, less wide than the petals. The corolla 4 petals, in two whorls, convergent, pink or violet, with red tips. The upper petal in the outer whorl is semi-cylindrical, winged at the top, its base elongated in the form of a spur. The lower petal in the outer whorl is narrow, takes the form of a canal, the petals in the two inner whorls are spoon-shaped. The male has two stamens. The ovary is monochambered, the ovule is monochambered. The fruit is a nut, indehiscent, spherical, 2.5-2 mm in diameter, notched at the top, containing one seed.

Flowering: February to June.

Habitat and geographical distribution:

Europe, the Mediterranean countries, and its natural distribution extends to Iran in the east.

History and Heritage:

The genus name is derived from the Latin fumus meaning "smoke", referring to the gray color of the leaves, which resembles smoke, or to their smoke-like smell, or to their tear-producing effect like smoke. The species name officinalis means "medicinal, constitutional." The plant has long been known for its ivory properties, especially in skin diseases. It was mentioned by Dioscorides, as well as by Ibn Sina, al-Antaki, and al-Ghassani.

Part used: Flowering aerial parts (odorless, bitter and salty taste.)

Chemical components:

Rutin flavonoid, 1.25% alkaloids, including: protoberberine derivatives such as scoulerine and protopine. Spirobenzyl isoquinoline alkaloids such as fumaricine and fumariline, indenobenzenzazepine alkaloids such as fumaritine and fumarofine. Hydroxycinnamic acid derivatives, including: acid. Caffeoylmalic Organic acids, including fumaric acid. Tannins, potassium, and vitamin C.

Properties and medical uses:

The drug has antispasmodic properties, especially in the upper part of the digestive system, and is used to treat disorders related to bile, bile ducts, and liver. The drug is popularly used to treat obstructive liver diseases, stimulate the digestive system and bowel movement, and treat cystitis. It is used topically to treat skin diseases, cleanse the skin, and eliminate pimples. In Italy, it is used to treat atherosclerosis, rheumatism and blood purification. In Bulgaria, after being freed from alkaloids, it is used to reduce blood pressure and sugar, as an anti-infective, tonic and anti-spasmodic. It is important in traditional medicine in many countries to treat some skin diseases such as cradle cap (cradle cap in newborns), eczema, scabies and others, or as a diuretic or laxative. Alcoholic plant extracts have a toxic effect on leukemia cells and multiple myeloma (MM) cells.

Pharmaceutical forms:

The plant is available in the form of dried herbal preparations, especially liquid, and tincture.

Side effects, interactions and precautions for use: Possible side effects include: Symptoms of low blood pressure such as dizziness, weakness, and slow pulse. In high doses, sage can cause seizures, and can increase pressure inside the eye, causing glaucoma (which leads to loss of vision). In particular, sage should not be taken with medications used to lower blood pressure, heart medications called beta blockers, such as Inderal, heart medications called calcium channel blockers, such as procardia Calan, Lanoxin, and other drugs that slow the heart rate. Pregnant or breastfeeding women should avoid using the plant, and those who suffer from glaucoma or a disease that makes them susceptible to seizures should avoid using it. The doctor should also be informed if they feel dizzy, weak, short of breath, or have a change in their pulse rate.

Environment: The plant grows wild in neglected lands, orchards, and on old walls. It is sometimes classified as a harmful weed that competes with agricultural crops for water and nutrients in the soil. Prefers light, well-drained soils and sunny places.

Cultivation and productivity: It is propagated by seeds that are scattered directly in the permanent soil at the beginning of spring in basins or beds isolated from agricultural fields.

Papaver rhoeas L.

Papaver rhoeas var. *vulgare* Roth.

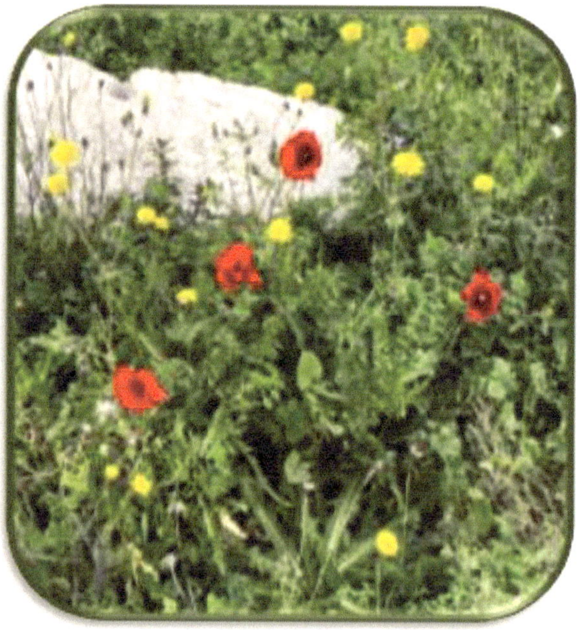

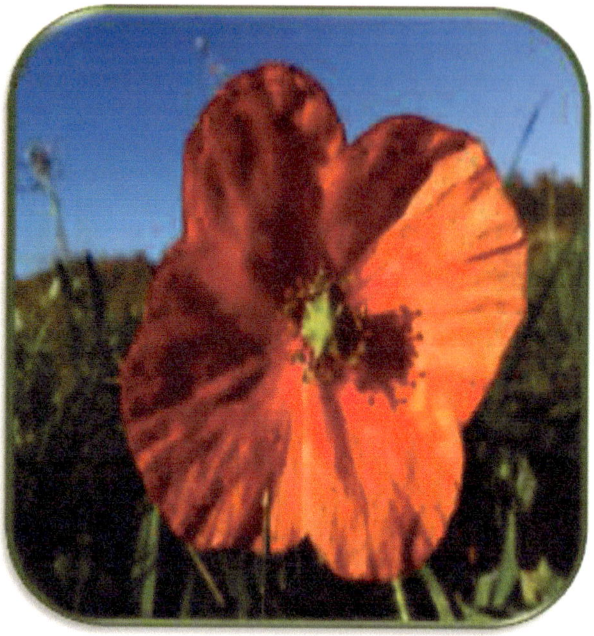

Family: Papaveraceae

Common names: Wall poppy, Scattered poppy, Anemone

Foreign names: Coquelicot Fr. poppy, Corn Eng.

Occurrences : 363,445 occurrences

Distribution in the world

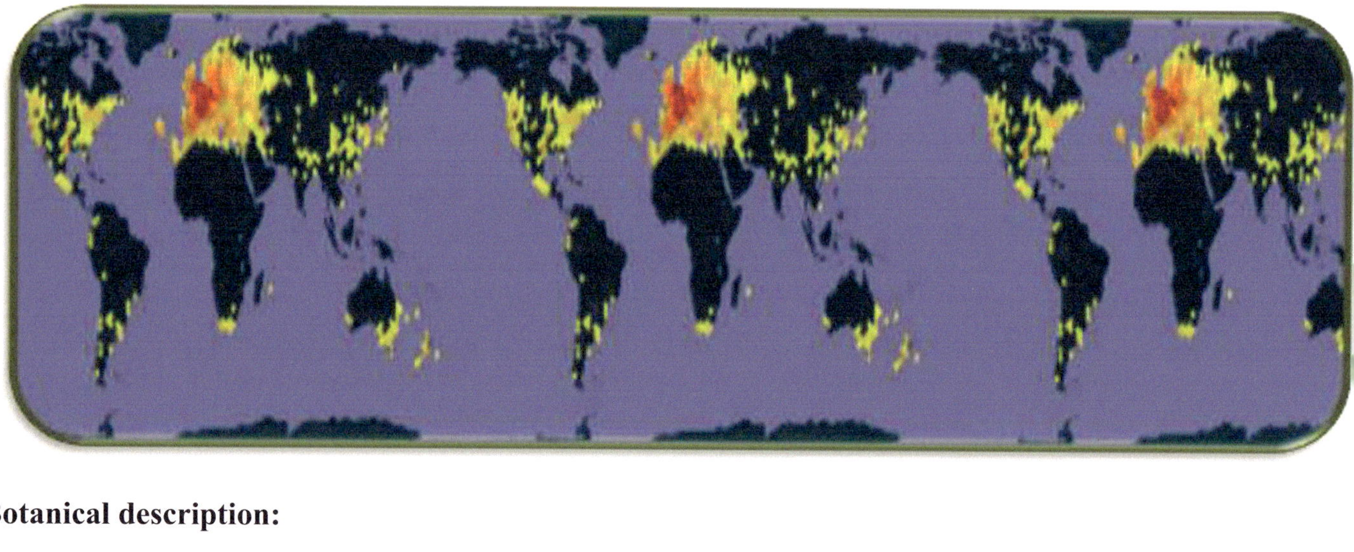

Botanical description:

An annual herb, covered with hairs, 20-90 cm high. Stem simple or branched, erect. Leaves have different shapes, they are usually medium or deeply lobed, rarely almost complete. Flowers are 5-8 cm in diameter, arranged singly at the end of long, erect, hairy panicles. Buds pendulous at first, then fully erect before opening, ovate to oblong, covered with hairs. Calyx sepals, Maubertine, rapidly falling. Corolla 4-petaled, 2-3 cm long, 2-4 cm wide, rounded to elliptic, red with a black spot at its base, male with many stamens. The female is composed of a number of carpels that form an ovary divided by incomplete septa, so it is considered unicellular, topped by radially arranged stigmas, forming a sessile disc (the stigmas are absent). The fruit is cap-shaped, bluish-green in color, semi-spherical or inverted oval to round to oblong in shape, its length is about 1 cm, the sessile disc is flat, exceeds the diameter of the capsule, its lobes are round, covering each other with their edges. The capsule opens Through small holes at the bottom of the disc. The seeds are small and numerous, and are dispersed outside the box by the wind.

Flowering: March to June.

Homeland and geographical distribution: Europe, the countries of the eastern Mediterranean and North Africa.

History and heritage: It is mentioned that the name of the genus Papaver is derived from the Latin "pappa", meaning "food" or "milk" in reference to the milky juice that comes out of the plant, while the name of the species rhoeas is derived from the Greek, meaning "red" in reference to the color of the petals.

Part used:

Flower petals (dry carefully, because they spoil quickly), and seeds.

Chemical components:

Flower petals contain: alkaloids of the isoquinoline group, the most important of which are: rhoeadine, isorhoeadine, rhoeagenine, coptisine, and isocorydine. Anthocyan pigments give the flowers their red color, including mecocyanin, cy-anin. Flavonoids, including the glycoside quercetol. Mucilages, muconic acid, and tannin.

Properties and medical uses:

The decoction of flower bits is used for its sedative and analgesic properties, and to help reduce hyperactivity, insomnia, and sleep disorders in children and adults (rhoeadine alkaloid). It is also used in the case of respiratory system disorders as an expectorant, and in treating cough and asthma (salivary substances). Flower bits are popularly used for their diaphoretic and antipyretic properties. Researchers from Ethiopia, Germany and India have discovered that anemone alkaloids help treat malaria, a common disease in tropical and subtropical countries.

Environment: Poppy is found scattered in fallow lands and agricultural fields. It can be grown from the equator to 56 degrees north latitude. Its seeds are sensitive and require a warm atmosphere to germinate. Poppy is a short-day plant. It needs a soil rich in humus, and it grows well in soil rich in calcium.

Cultivation and productivity:

Poppy is grown as a winter plant in warm areas or a summer plant in cold areas, by direct seeding or transplanting. Direct planting is done in scattering basins or in lines spaced 30-40 cm apart. When planting by transplanting, the land is marked into lines at a rate of 50 cm between the two lines, then the seedlings are transplanted at a distance of 40 cm between the two seedlings on the same line. The seedlings are transferred to the permanent field when 3-4 leaves appear.

About the Authors

Dr. Wathek Zair

Dr. Wathek Zair is a distinguished scientist, researcher, and industry leader, with expertise spanning pharmaceutical sciences, energy, environmental sustainability, agricultural science, and plant medicine. He holds a Ph.D. in Science from the University of Birmingham, a Master's in Sustainability from the University of Leicester, and a background in Agricultural and Plant Sciences, making him a leading expert in botanical medicine, natural product development, and environmental applications in pharmacology.

With over 100 published research papers, Dr. Zair has contributed significantly to scientific advancements in medicinal plants, pharmacognosy, and agrochemical innovations. His extensive research integrates traditional plant-based medicine with modern pharmacological applications, offering a scientific and evidence-based approach to herbal medicine.

Dr. Zair plays a vital role in manufacturing, regulatory compliance, and product stewardship. His deep knowledge of medicinal plants, agricultural sustainability, and pharmaceutical innovation ensures that this book serves as a comprehensive guide for researchers, clinicians, and plant enthusiasts alike.

Dr. Indre Howard

Dr. Indre Howard is a highly respected medical doctor with extensive clinical experience. She has dedicated her career to improving patient outcomes through a multidisciplinary approach.

A Collaboration of Science and Medicine

Together, Dr. Wathek Zair and Dr. Indre Howard have combined their scientific expertise, clinical experience, and research-driven approach to create an authoritative guide on medicinal plants. This book serves as a definitive reference for medical professionals, researchers, herbalists, and anyone interested in the therapeutic power of plants, offering a fusion of scientific precision and practical applications in plant-based medicine.

Made in the USA
Las Vegas, NV
03 November 2026

57424454R00305